HERBAL DRUGS

a modern approach to understand them better

HERBAL DRUGS

a modern approach to understand them better

Edited by

Dr Subhash C Mandal

MPharm, PhD (Pharmacy), Endeavour Fellow (Govt of Australia)
Distinguished Educator and Research Awardee 2009
[American Association of Indian Pharmaceutical Scientists (AAIPS)]
Associate Professor, Division of Pharmacognosy
Department of Pharmaceutical Technology
Jadavpur University, Kolkata 700 032, India

New Central Book Agency (P) Ltd

LONDON

HYDERABAD ERNAKULAM BHUBANESWAR

DELHI KOLKATA PUNE GUWAHATI

NCBA

REGD OFFICE

8/1 Chintamoni Das Lane, Kolkata 700 009, India
email: ncbapvtltd@eth.net

OVERSEAS

NCBA (UK) Ltd, 149 Park Avenue North, Northampton, NN3 2HY, UK
email: ncbauk@yahoo.com

EXPORT

NCBA Exports Pvt. Ltd, 212 Shahpur Jat, New Delhi 110 049
email: ncbaexp@ncbapvtltd.com

BRANCHES

212 Shahpur Jat
New Delhi 110 049
email: ncbadel@ncbapvtltd.com

Shop Nos. 3 & 4, Vinayak Towers
681/B Budhwar Peth, Appa Balwant Chowk
Pune 411 002
email: ncbapune@ncbapvtltd.com

Shop No. 15, Bharati Towers, Ground Floor
Forest Park, **Bhubaneswar** 751 001
email: ncbabub@ncbapvtltd.com

House No. 3-1-315, 1st Floor
Nimboliadda, Kachiguda, **Hyderabad** 500 027
email: ncbahydb@ncbapvtltd.com

GSS Shopping Complex, 1st Floor
Opposite College Post Office, Convent Road
Ernakulam 682 035
email: ncbaernk@ncbapvtltd.com

Radhamayee Complex (Second Floor)
Opp. SBI, Panbazar, Jaswanta Road
Guwahati 781 001
email: ncbaguwahati@ncbapvtltd.com

HERBAL DRUGS: A MODERN APPROACH TO UNDERSTAND THEM BETTER • Mandal

First Published: May 2011
Reprinted: March 2013

PUBLISHER AND TYPESETTER
New Central Book Agency (P) Ltd
8/1 Chintamoni Das Lane, Kolkata 700 009

PRINTER
New Central Book Agency (P) Ltd
Web-Offset Division, Dhulagarh, Sankrail, Howrah

COVER DESIGNER
Soumen Paul

COVER PRINTER
Liba Graphics, Kolkata

PROJECT TEAM
Suman Dutta, Kakoli Banerjee, and Prabhat Jas

ISBN: 978-81-7381-653-6

Price: ₹ 850.00

Dedicated to

elder brother
Late Dr. Manik Chandra Mandal
(1955-1995)

CONTENTS

FOREWORD

As a mentor of Dr Subhash C Mandal, it is indeed a pleasure for me to write a foreword for the upcoming book entitled *Herbal Drugs*, edited by him. There could not have been a better timing for bringing out a book of this nature, when there is emerging a great demand for all kinds of herbal drugs. The need to know more about such herbal drugs has become a necessity these days; consequent to the Thalidomide tragedy, people gradually began to realize that all is probably not well with the synthetic drug molecules. A great hunt for herbal options, therefore, began. And, it goes without saying, that India, with her diversified climatic zones, is a repository of medicinal plants. The chapters of this book have been authored by proven experts in their respective fields of specialization.

However, it should not be assumed that all herbal drugs are harmless. Pharmacological studies, involving short and long term toxicity are to be conducted on them. Freedom from adverse side-effects and drug interactions are to be investigated. Quality of herbal drugs is to be assured by proper statistically validated procedures. Freedom from pathogens is a must. Similarly, herbal drugs must be free from of aflatoxins and orchatoxins. Metallic impurity standard as prescribed by WHO must be strictly followed and pesticide residue should be meticulously determined for every batch of the herbal drug. Extensive research has already been done and many advanced research is on the anvil for finding lead moiety for every new drug discovery. This book will unfold some of these fascinating thrust areas of modern herbal research. Marker compound identification and reference standard isolation for quantification of herbal drug content is another important field of attraction. It is sincerely hoped that this book will be a useful reference for research scholars, students, teachers and the herbal drug industry.

I wish this book all success.

Professor B K Gupta
Formerly Professor and Head of the Department,
Pharmaceutical Technology,
Jadavpur University, Kolkata, India

PREFACE

Due to the rapidly expanding knowledge in the field of science and technology it becomes mandatory for an academician and a researcher to keep their knowledge always updated. However, in doing so, we need to understand that our roots should also go deep into the subject. In my fifteen long years of experience as an academician, I have experienced a tremendous growth in herbal drug research and its acceptability round the globe. The rapidly increasing volume of scientific output and literature makes one's job pretty difficult to collect and review the whole gamut of facts while planning any exciting project on herbal drug. Hence, this book was devised as a 'one-stop platform' where a perfect blend of comprehensive information pertaining to classical Pharmacognosy as well as the emerging trends can be put forward to the readers.

In preparing this book, various developments in drug discovery process through traditional medicine has been comprehensively weaved, which, I believe, will mesmerize the readers. Besides, chapters by specialist contributors give emphasis to a number of topics of current importance. Keeping in mind the era of interdisciplinary specialization within various fields which contribute to Pharmacognosy, an attempt has been made to produce a unified presentation and to provide pertinent references to the primary literature and review articles for the reader's convenience. The book will definitely be a treasurehouse for the young herbal drug researchers, planning different exciting projects, as they will find some invaluable pieces of text in a single volume.

I am much indebted to the contributors, who considered me capable enough to handle their expert opinion and rich experience which I have moulded in the form of this book. I am thankful to my editorial team for their technical support. I am indebted to all those difficulties as well, which came my way only to make my determination about this book even stronger.

I am greatful to my home university, Jadavpur University, for providing excellent research facilities which is the basic foundation behind this book. I am grateful to the publisher too for helpful assistance and understanding.

Subhash C Mandal
Department of Pharmaceutical Technology
Jadavpur University, Kolkata, India

chapter 1

Chemical Characters in Plant Taxonomy

Ambarish Mukherjee and Joydeep Acharya

INTRODUCTION

History of phytochemistry is quite long which incorporates innumerable chemical investigations concerning plants to explain biochemical mechanisms, physiological functions and medicinal principles. The possibilities for integration of chemistry with plant taxonomy remained unexplored for a long time. The first prophetic words came from Helen Abbot as early as 1886 that 'there has been comparatively little study of chemical principles of plants from a purely botanical view the external manifestations of a series of internal biochemical reactions'. Abbot's work (1886) on distribution of saponins in plants and general assertion about the value of chemical data in interpreting evolution is certainly one of the pioneering and most memorable endeavours in this direction. In spite of this, chemistry had to keep itself waiting till the mid 1950s for its recognition in the field of plant taxonomy when Hegnauer (1954, 1958) coined the term 'chemotaxonomy'. Simultaneous release of three books 'Chemotaxonomie der Pflanzen' (Hegnauer, 1962-86), 'Biochemical Systematics' (Alston and Turner, 1963) and 'Chemical Plant Taxonomy' (Swain, 1963) and subsequent publications of 'Comparative Phytochemistry' (Swain,1966) and 'Phytochemical Phylogeny' (Harborne, 1970) contributed enormously to chemotaxonomy and proved the efficacy of chemical characters in addressing taxonomic problems, improving traditional classifications and interpretation of phylogeny. Chemical information is fundamental and presence or absence of a chemical compound is *a posteriori* and consequently more important than those which are *a priori* since morphological characters are initiated at the level of genes. Chemical compounds, to which traditional taxonomists are usually indifferent, deserve special status, if not higher, at least close to morphological characters. This statement does not necessarily mean that a 'special purpose' system of classification can be expected from chemical compounds but it positively assures improvisation of the traditional systems of classification. In reality chemotaxonomy, also familiar as chemosystematics, biochemical systematics, taxonomic biochemistry etc., has become an integral part of taxonomy or systematic botany (Bate-Smith, 1962; Bisby et al. 1980; Gibbs, 1974; Hawkes, 1968; Harborne, 1984; Harborne and Turner, 1984; Heywood and Moore, 1984; Jensen and Fairbrother, 1983; Turner, 1969; Young and Seigler, 1981 and many others). The excellent review work of Giannasi and Crawford (1986) has contributed enormously to the visualization of the contemporary status of the subject and promotion of its further growth. The journey which chemotaxonomy started from the products of metabolism has progressed in course of time towards the information containing molecules. It has been working out various aspects of 'genetic-system vis-à-vis environment' interactions as well as plant relationships so as to resolve the micro-evolution.

COMPOUNDS USEFUL IN PLANT TAXONOMY

Although theoretically all chemical constituents are potentially valuable to taxonomists, in practice only the conservative organic substances find application in taxonomy. Such compounds are placed under three broad categories, viz. primary metabolites, secondary metabolites and semantides.

Primary Metabolites

The primary metabolites are the products of vital or life related metabolic pathways and hence indispensable and universal. Due to lack of variation in these substances even in respect of distant taxa, the primary metabolites have no systematic value. Only in certain cases the excess quantity of some characteristic primary metabolite, provides a basis for nomenclature. Excess quantities of aconitic acid, citric acid and oxalic acid have yielded the scientific names of the genera *Aconitum, Citrus* and *Oxalis* respectively. Similarly in *Sedum* the 7-carbon sugar sedoheptulose is present in quantities well above the amount which participates in the essential metabolism.

Secondary Metabolites

The secondary metabolites are the substances produced mostly as a consequence of nonvital processes or of nonuniversally vital processes in certain cases. Because of their characteristically restricted occurrence in plants these compounds are of great value in plant taxonomy. The most important compounds used in taxonomy include phenolics, terpenoids, tannins, glucosinolates, alkaloids, oils, waxes etc. The value of these substances in taxonomy is judged by their distribution in correlation with other characters.

Semantides

The semantides are information carrying molecules and can be classified into primary- (DNAs), secondary- (RNAs) and tertiary- (proteins) categories in the order of sequential transfer of genetic code. The sequence of nucleotides in the first two categories and the sequence of amino acids in case of proteins contain all the information regarding the characteristic forms and functions of all types of plants. The semantides offer a much better alternative to the use of secondary metabolites and cytological, anatomical, embryological features etc. in plant taxonomy since all these features are mere manifestations of the former. The protein taxonomy mainly involves amino acid sequencing and serology.

Molecular Interpretations

The chemical substances used in taxonomy are often interpreted in terms of micro- and macromolecules. The primary and secondary metabolites are regarded as micromolecules for having molecular weight less than 1 kDa. and the semantides together with larger polysaccharides are known as macromolecules for having molecular mass over 1 kDa.

Secondary Metabolites of Taxonomic Importance

The diversity of secondary metabolites is very wide for being the products of chemical behaviour of plants to the biotic and abiotic components of their environment for defense against prey, predators and pathogens, dehydration, success in cross pollination, tolerance, propagation, dispersal of fruits and seeds etc. For being highly conservative, importance of secondary metabolites is immense, some of which are introduced in the following.

Phenolics

The phenolic compounds have provided more taxonomic data than all other types of secondary metabolites.Taxonomic significance of phenolic constituents of plants has been appreciably revealed in the work of Bate-Smith (1958), Bate-Smith and Metcalfe (1962). These compounds are based upon phenol, C_6H_5OH, although each has its characteristic complication. Mostly these compounds are used strategically as defensive weapons against pathogens while others constitute the nonplastidial leaf, flower and fruit pigments rendering protection from sun, favouring pollination and dispersal of fruits and seeds.

Taxonomically the most important phenolics are the flavonoids mainly due to ease of their isolation, distinction, identification and stability as seen even in very old herbarium specimens. Further more variation is considerably wide showing taxon-specific pattern. Flavonoids are found in all plants except in most of the algae. These constitute a valuable source of comparative data especially at the lower level of taxonomic hierarchy and in documenting interspecific hybridization.

Flavones have relatively a common nucleus with a variation in types and patterns of side groups which characterize the individual compounds. These generally occur in a three ring system derived through cyclization of an intermediate from a cinnamic acid derivative and three malonyl CoA

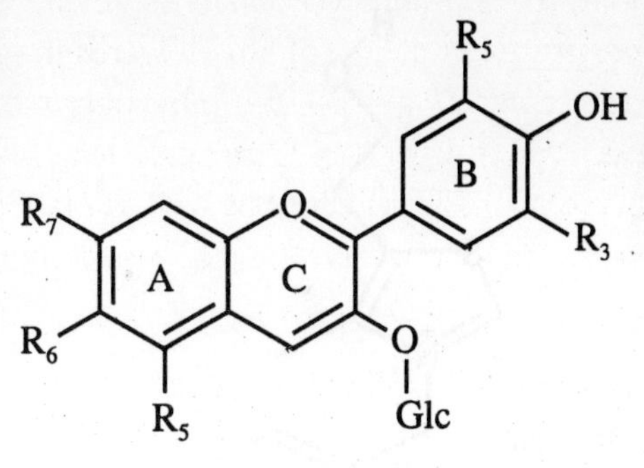

Anthocynidin

molecules. These compounds are mostly used in defense system of plants (Levin, 1971). One of the best examples of taxonomic value of flavonoids concerns flower pigments, particularly anthocyanidins. The hydroxyl groups at positions 3, 5, and 7 of malvidin is substituted by such sugars as glucose or rhamnose the resulting compounds is anthocyanin, which are widely distributed in flowering plants except in the members of Chenopodiineae of the Dicot order Caryophyllales.

Betalins

These are heterocyclic nitrogenous pigments found only in nine dicotyledonous families where anthocyanins are absent. Betalins could very well be regarded as alkaloids for their heterocyclic nitrogenous nature; but they are always given a sort of distinction for their colour and taxonomic value.

These are reddish (betacyanins) or yellowish (betaxanthins) pigments found in bracts, petals and other plant parts. Due to similarity in colours under ordinary light and identical UV reflection spectra these used to be called at one time nitrogenous anthocyanins. Inspite of the similarities, these pigments are quite distinct and never coexist in the same plant or taxon. The nine betalin containing families, viz., Aizoaceae (Ficodeae),

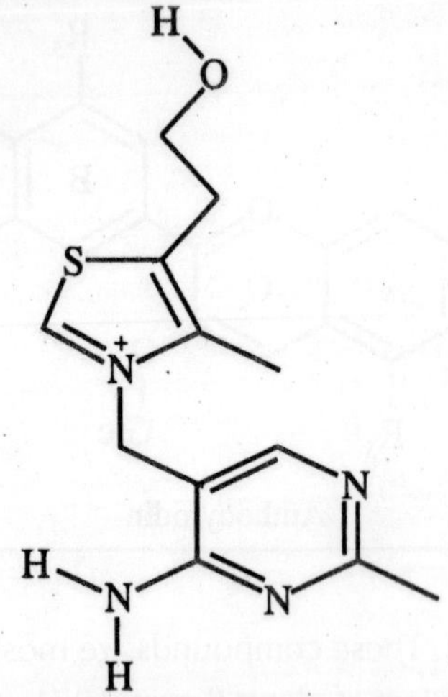

Betalin S (Thiamine chloride hydrochloride)

Portulacaceae, Cactaceae, Didiereaceae, Basellaceae, Phytolaccaceae, Amaranthaceae and Chenopodiaceae are aptly included in the suborder Chenopodiineae and two anthocyanins containing families Caryophyllaceae and Molluginaceae in the suborder Caryophyllineae of the same order Caryophyllales by Rodman *et al.* (1984).

Phenolic acids

Phenolic acids used in taxonomy include hydroxyl benzoic and the hydroxycinnamic acids. Angiosperm lignins are characterized by syringiç acid which is lacking in gymnosperms. Sinapic acid is predominant in non-woody species which undergoes β-oxidation to syringic acid in arborescent angiosperms. Relative proportions of these compounds enable to trace evolutionary relationship among various taxa.

Coumarins

These are C_6-C_3 compounds which are unsaturated lactones formed as a derivative of the amino acid phenylalanine. They occur in free form or as glycosides. Families like Fabaceae (Leguminosae), Poaceae (Gramineae), Apiaceae (Umbelliferae), Rutaceae, Solanaceae, Asteraceae (Compositae) etc. are rich in these compounds. Umbelliferones occur widely in Apiaceae while Scopoletins are more frequent in Solanaceae and Asteraceae. Diversity of coumarins enable distinction of genera, species and even infraspecific categories. viz. subspecies, varieties, forms (see Fig. next page).

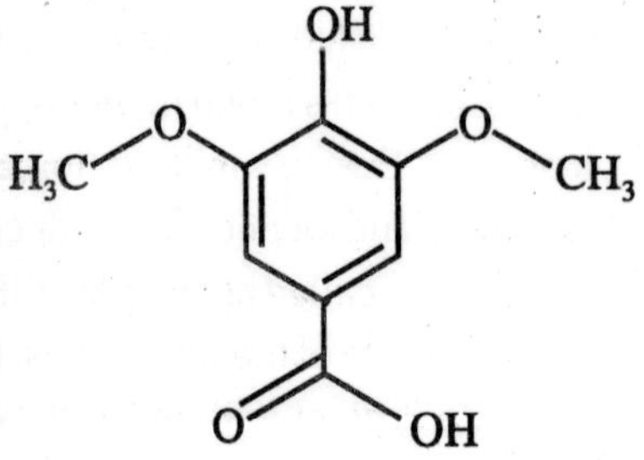

Syringic acid

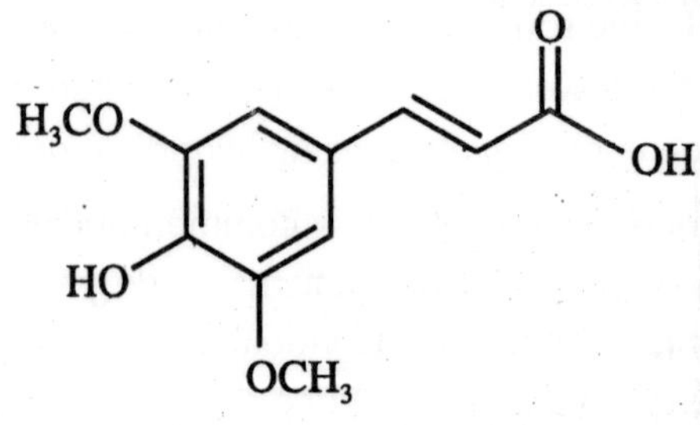

Sinapic acid

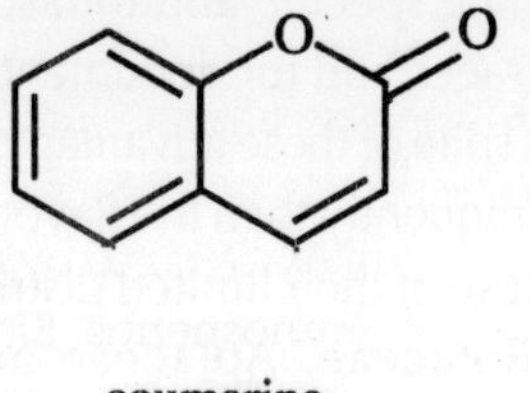

coumarine

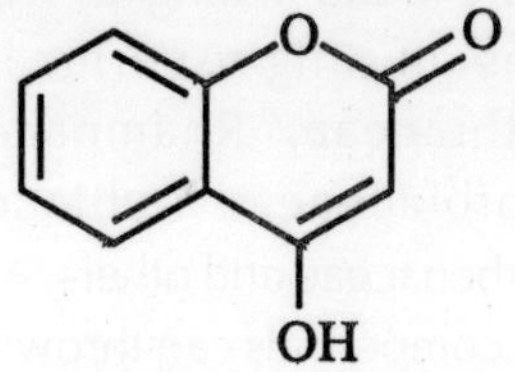

4-hydroxycoumarin

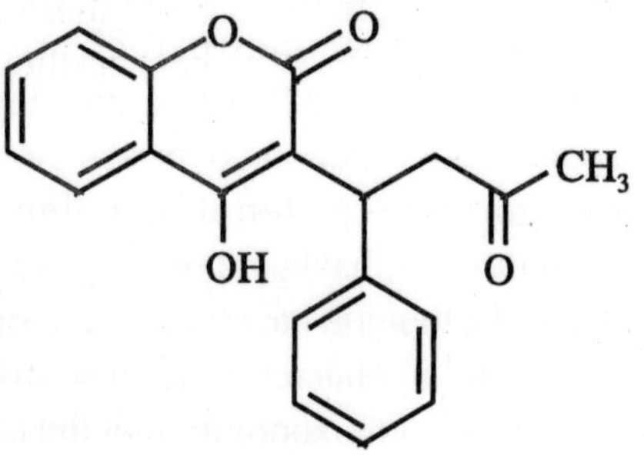

warfarin

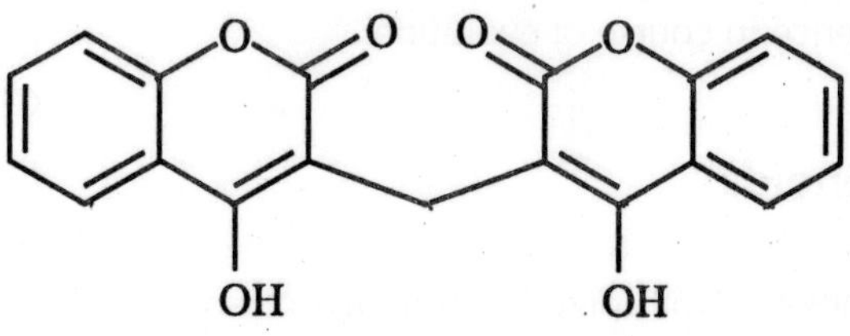

bishydroxycoumarine (dicoumarol)

Xanthones

Xanthones are C_6-C_1-C_6 compounds ($C_{13}H_8O_2$) having very restricted occurrence. They are yellow pigments and are often mistaken for flavonoids in routine chemotaxonomic surveys. But their characteristic spectra clearly differentiate them from flavones. The family Gentianaceae seems to be particularly abundant in such compounds and replacement of xanthones by flavonoids in the Menyanthaceae is a valid reason to support its separation from the Gentianaceae. The same argument holds good for elevation of the tribe Exacineae of Gentianaceae to the status of a distinct family Exacaceae.

Quinones

Quinones are α- β-unsaturated ketones of a rather special type being cyclic diketones of such a structure that they are converted by reduction to hydroquinones, the phenols with two –OH groups.

Benzoquinones are the common fungal pigments used as a criterion in their classification. Napthaquinones are satisfactorily frequent in higher plants although with a restricted occurrence. Plumbagin is one of such compounds which is found in Plumbaginaceae, Ebenaceae and Droseraceae and Juglone is characteristic for the family Juglandaceae.

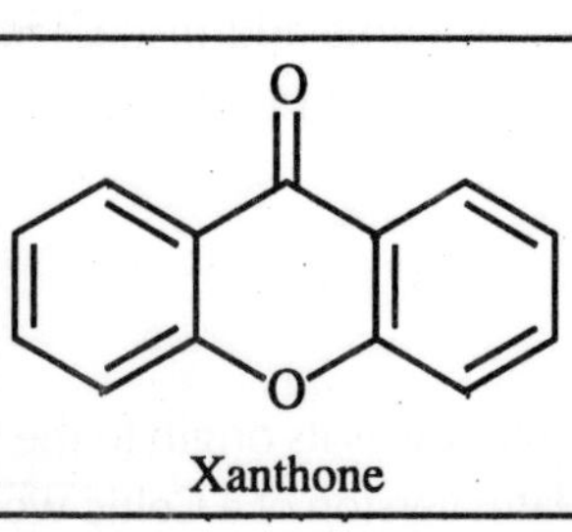

Xanthone

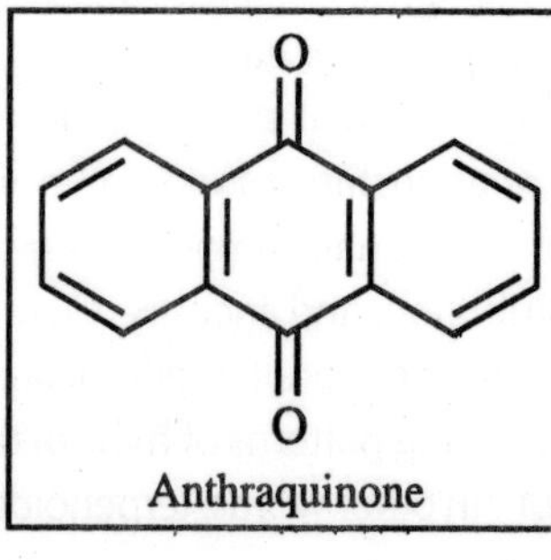

Anthraquinone

Anthraquinones are found in fungi as well as in diverse families of angiosperms like Polygonaceae, Lythraceae, Rhamnaceae, Ericaceae, Euphorbiaceae, Rubiaceae, Scrophulariaceae, Verbenaceae and others. A systematic study of these compounds can throw light on their taxonomic distinctiveness as well as relationship emerging from similar environmental experience in course of evolution.

Terpenoids

Terpenes are synthesized of multiples of isoprene units(2-methyl-1,3-butadiene) which are also extensively used in taxonomy. Terpenes containing 2 isoprene units are called monoterpenes (e.g. geraniol, limonene, menthol, pinene, camphor). Three isoprene units combine to handover sesquiterpenes (e.g. farnesol) and four such units give diterpenes (e.g. phytol).Triterpenes are formed by three isoprene units (e.g. squalene). Among higher terpenes carotenoids (tetraterpenes) and natural rubber (polyterpene) deserve mention.

Different types of terpenoids owe their origin to geranyl pyrophosphate pathway, including mono-, di- and tri-terpenes leading eventually to steroids. The most commonly used terpenoids in taxonomy include mon- and sesqui-terpenes.

Monoterpenoids are also known as essential oils for their fragrance. These are low molecular weight compounds and extremely volatile. The advantage of using this compound in taxonomy is that using gas chromatography these can be analyzed quantitatively by means of integration of areas under the peaks for each compound as also qualitatively giving great sensitivity to the determination of relationship. Monoterpenoids variation concerns individuals, ontogeny, seasons, geographical distribution, and ancestry. Owing to such kind of sensitivity the monoterpenoid data are very helpful for detecting patterns of hybridization and clinal variation. In other words, terpenoids are used for distinguishing specific and infraspecific taxa, geographical races and for documentation of hybridization. In spite of these advantages terpenoids are used less frequently than the flavonoids in systematics because of their limited distribution, e.g. Lamiaceae, Rutaceae, Apiaceae and gymnosperms.

Sesquiterpene lactones have been studied thoroughly in some families particularly the Compositae (Seaman, 1982). These compounds present appreciable variation - of both major and minor categories, e.g. tenulin, helenalin, vermcerin, parthenin, bakkenolide-A, glucolide-A, vernolepin, lactupicrin etc. These compounds are mainly helpful in characterization of categories at lower levels in taxonomic hierarchy and even at interpopulational levels (Miller *et al.*, 1968). The advantage of using sesquiterpene lactones over monoterpenoids is that the compounds are nonvolatile and plants getting dried up in field collections do not loose their sesquiterpenes. On the other hand since the monoterpenoids are volatile compounds the collected plant material necessitates immediate preservation at low temperature till the laboratory analysis is done.

Iridoid Compounds

Chemically these compounds are monoterpenoid cyclopentanoid lactones. Distribution of iridoid compounds is considered to be an evolutionary marker in plant taxonomy. Kubitzki (1969) attempted to link Rosalean and Guttiferalean complexes on the basis of iridoid compounds. Jensen *et al.* (1975) made an extensive survey of the iridoids in angiosperms and discussed their systematic implication and significance.

Tannins

The term 'tannin' owes its origin to the word 'tan' which is the latin version of a Celtic word for oak, a tree, the bark of which is a good source of tannin. Tannins include a group of chemical substances which are astringent, bitter chemical substances having a molecular weight between 500-3000 and contain number of phenolic hydroxyl groups (1-2 per mw) adequate enough to form effective link with proteins and penetrate between collagen fibrils of animal skin or hide so as to convert it into leather. Tannins are not compatible with alkalies, gelatins, heavy metals, iron, lime water, metallic salts, strong oxidizing agents and zinc sulphate.

Tannins are of two types, viz., hydrolysable- and condensed-tannins.

A hydrolysable tannin molecule contains a carbohydrate (usually D-glucose) at the centre. The hydroxyl groups of the carbohydrate are partially or fully esterified with phenolic groups such as gallic acid (in gallotannins) or ellagic acid (in ellagitannins). The carbohydrate and phenolic acids get released on hydrolysis with weak acids or weak bases. The gallic acid, esters of glucose in tannic acid ($C_{76}H_{52}O_{46}$), are found in the leaves and barks of many plant species.

Ellagic Acid

Extensive surveys of tannins in flowering plants have revealed that ellagitannins are exclusive to certain dicot taxa (subclasses Hamamelidae - Dilleniidae). Magnoliidae totally lacks ellagitannins so do all the monocotyledonous subclasses. This is an indication of a close relationship between Magnoliidae and the monocots and the latter taxa might have been derived from the former.

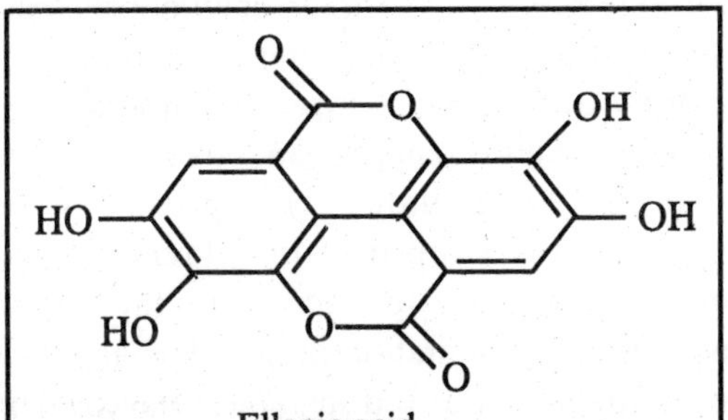

Ellagic acid

Condensed tannins are also known as proanthocyanidins. These are polymers of 2 to 50 or even more flavonoids units that are joined by carbon-carbon bonds which do not cleave on hydrolysis.

Glycosides

Glycosides are next to alkaloids in terms of toxic plant compounds. Chemically, the glycosides are acetals in which the hydroxyl of the sugar is condensed with a hydroxyl group of the non sugar component and the secondary hydroxyl is condensed with sugar molecule itself to give an oxide ring. These compounds yield one or more sugars among the products of hydrolysis. The non-sugar part is known as aglycone and the sugar part glycone. Only the beta forms of glycosides occur in plants. The most frequently occurring sugar is β-D-glucose although rhamnose, cymarose, digitoxose and others are not unlikely to be present. There are two main types of glycosides - cyanogenic and cardiac. The most frequently occurring cyanogenic glycosides belong to five groups, viz., prunasin, taxiphyllin, linamarin, gynocardin and cyano-lipid groups. These are highly conservative and hence capable of proving their worth in classification of plants even at higher systematic levels. Linamarin is characteristic to the tribe Calenduleae of Asteraceae and to Trifolieae and Phaseoleae of Fabaceae. Families like Rosaceae, Leguminosae, Compositae, and Gramineae are rich sources of these compounds. By themselves these compounds are relatively harmless. However when the plant organs containing them are damaged enzymes breakdown the glycoside to release the poisonous hydrocyanic acid or hydrogen cyanide as per the defense strategy of injured plant tissues against pathogens.

Cardiac glycosides, as the names imply, have highly specific and powerful action on cardiac or heart muscles. These are actually steroids occurring as glycosides. Sugars are attached at 3-position of the steroid nucleus. The steroid aglycones are of two types: cardenolide and bufadienolide. The more prevalent one in plants is cardenolide which are C_{23} steroids and the bufadienolides are C_{24} homologues of the cardenolides. The cardenolides are of more than 400 different types most of which are found in members of Liliaceae, Scrophulariaceae and Apocynaceae.

Alkaloids

Alkaloids are nitrogenous waste products of plants resulting possibly from decomposition of proteins. Chemically these are heterogeneous groups of compounds with carbon, hydrogen, oxygen and nitrogen. They occur in barks, leaves, wood and in storage organs like roots, modified stem (rhizomes, tubers, corms, bulbs etc.), seeds and other parts. Alkaloids are usually insoluble in water but soluble in alcohol. These bitter tasting compounds make up the largest group of poisonous substances in plants. More than 500 different types of alkaloids exist in plants and many of them enter into the composition of a large number of medicines.

From ethnobotanical, medicinal, poisonous, chemical and systematic view points alkaloids have elicited more intense interest and involvement than any other group of compounds. Relative to their value in plant taxonomy alkaloids are a rather difficult and very heterogeneous group of compounds. The great alkaloid diversity results from the number of nitrogen containing rings in the compound. For their physiological effects on human beings and animals these compounds have received much attention in medical science than for their systematic potential as seen in the overwhelming literature published on alkaloids.

Alkaloid distribution pattern has proved to be a very useful parameter in taxonomy. In *Veratrum* (Liliaceae) and relatives alkaloid data correlated well with morphology at generic level and gave insights into affinity (Kupichan *et al.*, 1961). Similar observations were also recorded for such genera as *Lycopodium*, *Lupinus* and taxa in the order Caryophyllales. Gibbs (1974) grouped Rubiaceae, Apocynaceae, Asclepiadaceae and Loganiaceae in the order Gentianales based on indole alkaloids. Papaveraceae and Fumariaceae accumulate isoquinolene where as berberin type is stored in these two families as well as Annonaceae, Ranunculaceae, Menispermaceae and Berberidaceae. Absence of alkaloids in *Buddleja* is one of the reasons for separating it from alkaloid-rich Loganiaceae and giving it the status of a distinct family Buddlejaceae. Interestingly isoquinoline alkaloids and related compounds, especially benzyl-isoquinoline and aporphine types, are confined to the subclass Magnoliidae.

Glucosinolates

These are sulphur containing compounds which on acidic or enzymatic hydrolysis with myrosinase yield glucose and isothiocynate. No less than 85 different structural types have been identified using gas and paper chromatography. Some of the typical glucosinolates are glucocapparin ($R{=}CH_3$), sinigrin ($R{=}CH_2{=}CH{-}CH_2$), glucoibervin [$R{=}MeS(CH_2)_3$], glucotropaeolin ($R{=}PhCH_2$), sinapine ($R{=}p{-}OH{-}C_6H_4$). These mustard oil glycosides are useful in classification of the order Capparales including Cruciferae (Brassicaceae) and Capparaceae. These are structurally most diverse in Cruciferae (Crawford and Giannasi, 1982). At one time Cruciferae, Capparaceae, Papaveraceae and Fumariaceae were included in the order Rhoeadales but presence of glucosinolates supports the placement of Cruciferae and Capparaceae in the order Capparales and separation of both Fumariaceae and Papaveraceae due to absence of glucosinolates. Bataceae and Gyrostemonaceae

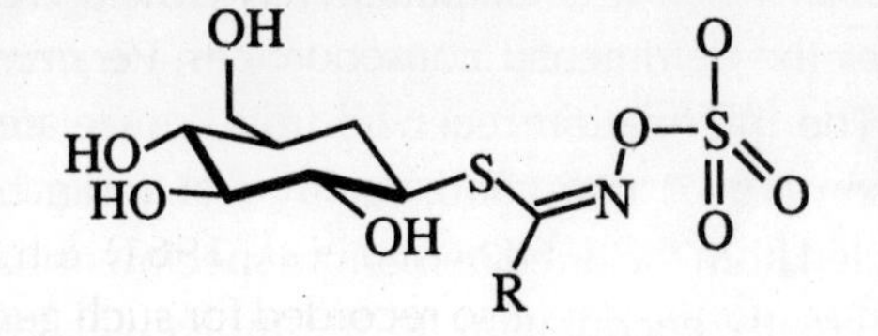

Glucosinolate structure; side group *R* varies

which were once in the order Caryophyllales are now included in Capparales for possessing glucosinolate compounds. Detailed studies undertaken by Rodman (1976) in the genus *Cakile* (Cruciferae) have shown that glucosinolates are very useful in infra-generic separation and the glucosinolate pattern may be used to document hybridization pattern. These data are mostly useful at the lower levels of the hierarchy. Rodman *et al.* (1981) found species specific profiles in *Caulanthus* and *Streptanthus* (Cruciferae) and even infra-specific variation in some species.

SEMANTIDES OF TAXONOMIC IMPORTANCE

Proteins

Proteins are molecules of one or a small number of polypeptide chains each of which is a polymer of amino acids linked through their amino and carboxyl groups by peptide bonds. The amino acid side chains can have a positive or negative charge, a short aliphatic chain or an aromatic residue. Since the 20 amino acids can be linked up in nearly all possible sequences, the potential diversity of structure and function is enormous. As tertiary semantides these serve as information carrying molecules, the language of their communication being scripted in their amino acid sequences. In view of this proteins have proved extremely useful in plant taxonomy. Moreover protein phylogeny is anticipated to be more conservative and a very trustful indicator of evolution. Electrophoresis of seed storage proteins, comparative protein and allozyme sequencing and systematic serology are the major areas integrating proteins with taxonomy.

Electrophoretic separation of proteins stored in seeds along an electrical gradient based on the polarities of their constituent amino acids hand over a series of bands. These electrophoretic patterns of proteins obtained from different taxa can be compared for ascertaining relationships. Moreover the data can very well be synthesized with character states obtained from other data sources for phenetic estimation of relationships. The work of Crawford and Julian (1976) on seed protein profile in the narrow-leaf species of *Chenopodium* occurring in Western United States deserves mention for having brought into light its taxonomic value and compared it with distribution of flavonoid compounds in the concerned species. The electrophoretic study undertaken by Mc Leod *et al.* (1979) has distinguished the species of *Capsicum* (Solanaceae).

Since the storage proteins are the outcome of additive inheritance from putative ancestors, studies concerning them are likely to explain with accuracy the cases of complex hybridization that might have taken place in nature in course of evolution. Levin and Schal (1970) were able to reveal through protein electrophoresis a reticulate pattern of evolution in the genus *Phlox*.

Amino acid sequences of specific proteins from different taxa can yield valuable taxonomic data. Cytochrome C has been sequenced for a number of animals and the findings used to construct dendrograms of evolutionary relationship comparable to those based on morphological data (Wilson *et al.*, 1977, Baba *et al.*, 1981). Moreover, any change in the amino acid sequence of the same protein or enzyme collected from two different populations of the same species occurring in two different ecological conditions is likely to give reliable information about the micro-evolution at infraspecific levels.

Allozymes [the same enzyme collected from two different plant sources (population/species) differing in amino acid sequences but performing the same function] have evoked much taxonomic interest since they provide clue to the genetic relationship of organisms (Soltis, 1982) since any change in the sequence of amino acids in an enzyme is a reflection of a change in the sequences of bases in DNA. Allozyme comparison, thus, provides an objective (quantitative) measure of genetic distance between populations, varieties and species under study (Nei, 1972) and a means to correlate genetic diversity and environmental association (Nevo *et al.*, 1982). Taxonomic comparison of amino acid sequences of ribulose-1,5-bisphosphate carboxylase and patterns of variability have adequate relevance to the study of phylogeny (Martin and Jennings, 1983).

Of the different proteins, comparative sequencing of Cytochrome C, plastocyanins, ferredoxin and ribulosebisphosphate carboxylase etc. are very reliable in taxonomic studies as can be evidenced from the work of Boulter (1972,1974, 1980); Boulter *et al.*, (1979); Martin and Stone, (1983); Martin and Dowd, (1986); Martin *et al.*, (1985).

Nucleic Acids

This is a general term for all such natural polymers in which nitrogenous bases (purines or pyrimidines) are attached to a sugar phosphate backbone. This can be single- or double-stranded. The nucleic acids (DNA and RNA) constitute the primary and secondary semantides (information carrying molecules). These compounds, especially DNA, have great potential for plant systematics and can offer significant insight into relatedness among plants (Bendich and Boulton, 1967; Bendich and Anderson, 1983). Nucleic acids have received preference to other molecules in taxonomic studies for their stability and the ease with which their preparations can be made. DNA can be prepared from a small amount of leaf tissue and even when it is taken from an endangered species the detrimental consequences are minimal. The information received from Doyle and Dickson (1987) that good quality DNA can be extracted from the dried herbarium specimens has been greatly encouraging to the molecular taxonomists. Moreover DNA analyses can access a nearly unlimited pool of genetic characters. Plant genomes range in size from 8.8×10^6 to more than 300×10^9 bp.

The venture in this direction started with DNA-DNA hybridization which is a direct method of assessing similarity between taxa at the molecular level of genetic material itself. Similarity is assessed by ascertaining the percentage reannealing of the DNA (single stranded) of one species with DNA (also single stranded) of another species. The rapidly reannealing fraction comprises the short, highly repetitive DNA generally thought to be concerned with gene regulation (Rose and Doolittle, 1983) whereas the slowly reannealing fraction represents structural genes.

Although the method is a refinement over analyses of chromosomal homologies technical difficulties reduced involvement of taxonomists. Especially confusing are the results when DNA strands are reannealed with those from the same species. This might be the fact hindering endeavours to enrich existing systems of classification and assess inter-taxa relationship based on nucleic acid hybridization.

Of the DNA-RNA hybridization programmes, certain efforts have set up very important mile stones in the development of chemotaxonomy. Chang and Mabry (1973) ascertained the relationships of the families of the Centrospermae. While preparing the DNA-RNA hybridization data for Centrospermous families Mabry (1976) concluded that the Caryophyllaceae (anthocyanin containing family) is quite close to the betalin containing families of Caryophyllales but not as close as the latter ones to each other.

Nucleotide sequencing has been quite popular for sometime in taxonomic assessment. Kossel *et al.*, (1983) investigated rRNA genes of some bacteria and chloroplasts from various plants ranging from unicellular algae to angiosperms and have shown that valuable phylogenetic inferences can be arrived at from such comparison.

The technical problems with DNA-RNA and DNA-DNA hybridizations and progress in techniques of genetic engineering have steered the taxonomic interest towards restriction endonuclease fragmentation of nuclear and chloroplast DNA (cp DNA) and mitochondrial DNA (mt DNA). Studies on mitochondrial DNA have been very much successful in animals and very rarely in plants. Plant mitochondrial DNAs are rather poorly studied compared to their counterpart in animals (Palmer *et al.*, 2000). Plant mitochondrial genome is unstable and inter- and intra-molecular recombinations occur frequently. Consequently, the gene sequence of mitochondrial DNA rearranges frequently.

The chloroplast DNA is more successfully used as a taxonomic tool in case of plants mainly for being relatively abundant component of total plant DNA to facilitate extraction and analysis.

The chloroplast DNA is a circular molecule ranging in size from 120-217 kb and in majority of angiosperms the size ranges within 135-160 kb. There are about 100 functional genes in the chloroplast genome and in most cases there are two duplicate regions in reverse orientation or inverted repeat (IR) ranging in size from 10 to 76 kb.

The circular cp DNA can be easily separated from its chloroplast and fragmented at numerous points by using different restriction enzymes that are specific for short (usually six) sequences of base pairs. These fragments can be separated by gel electrophoresis and a map of their sequence and size can be prepared. Compilation is eventually done in sequence and the circular map is developed for a taxon. These are then compared by synapomorphic cladistic technique to hand over a cladograms of the fragment data.

The chloroplast genome is free of deletions, insertions, transpositions and inversions and hence relatively conserved. Most of the genes of this genome conserve extensive molecular information about the concerned taxon. For this conservative nature a comparative study with data from different taxa can provide phylogenetic decisions at relatively higher levels of taxonomic hierarchy.

Chloroplast DNA is usually maternally inherited in angiosperms and paternally inherited in case of gymnosperms. As such cp DNA sequences together with nuclear data can ascertain maternal parental species in case of hybrids or allopolyploid species (Ackerfield and Wen, 2003).The rbcL gene in it which encodes ribulose-1,5-bisphosphate carboxylase has been widely sequenced for plants and has proved useful at higher taxonomic levels. It has contributed greatly to our understanding of angiosperm phylogeny alone or in combination with other markers (Martin and Stone, 1983; Martin and Jennings, 1983; Martin *et al.*, 1985; Xiang *et al.*, 1998; Ingrouille *et al.*, 2002). The *ndhF* gene which encodes subunit F of NADP dehydrogenase, a component of respiratory chain, has also been used at the family, genus and species levels (Wen *et al.*, 2003). Other chloroplast genes used for taxonomic purposes include the genes for α and β subunits of RNA polymerase II (*rpoA* and *rpoC2*, in the large single -copy region) and a maturase gene in the intron separating the coding region of *trnK* (*matK*, previously known as ORF, for open reading frame K), *AtpB*, the gene coding for β subunit of ATP synthetase etc.

Molecular plant taxonomy has also been emphasizing greatly the nuclear gene encoding ribosomal RNA (rRNA), commonly referred to as rDNA. This is arranged in tandem repeats in one or a few chromosomal loci. Each repeat has a transcribed region consisting of an external transcribed spacer (ETS) followed in sequence by the 18S gene, an internal transcribed spacer (ITS-1), the 5.8S gene, a second internal transcribed spacer (ITS-2) and ultimately 26S gene. Each repeat is separated from its adjacent ones by an intergenic spacer (IGS). In eukaryotes the ribosome consists of two subunits- a large subunit (LSU) and a small subunit (SSU) which is about half the size of the LSU. The 18S gene encodes the SSU and 26S and 5.8S encode LSU. The nuclear genes encoding rRNA are repeated thousands of times within the typical plant genome and can comprise no less than 10% of the total plant DNA.

The 18S region is a slowly evolving marker and is suitable for understanding phylogeny at higher taxonomic level (Soltis *et al.*, 1997) and for land plant phylogeny (Soltis *et al.*, 1999a, 1999b).

The nuclear ribosomal ITS region including the 5.8S gene has been most widely used molecular marker at the interspecific and intergeneric levels in plants (Starr *et al.*, 2004). ITS sequence variation is more amicable to sampling and comparisons within and among species of closely related genera (Martins and Hellwig, 2005).

The phylogenetic significance of the 26S sequence which is about 3.4 KB long with 12 expansion segments (ES), have not been widely explored. So far partial 26 sequences have been used among closely related families and within a family for assessment of phylogenetic position and relationship.

Concerted and coordinated efforts of a group of taxonomists in the mean time have started yielding modern systems of classification of angiosperms based principally on molecular data procured from nuclear and chloroplast genomes (e.g. APG System-III, 2009). These systems would further evolve to earn enormous appreciation and acceptance since molecular techniques provide powerful tools for studying natural relationship between taxa and their evolutionary perspectives. Moreover the ongoing improvisation of techniques has been adding much to their credibility.

CONCLUSION

The chemical data sources in terms of both micro- and macro-molecules and perpetuating technical advancement of phylogenetic analyses are certain to evolve to such heights so as to address all of sorts of problems related to taxonomic characterization, systematic position, affinity, classification and micro- and macro-evolution. However, no matter how powerful the chemical data be, morphological data will always remain critical and indispensable. A consistent correspondence and correlation of chemical characters with morphology and other structural and developmental data sources must always be maintained for accomplishment of taxonomy.

REFERENCES

Abott HC de S. Certain chemical constituents of plants considered in relation to their morphology and evolution. *Bot Gaz* 11, 270-272, (1886).

Ackerfield JR, Wen J. Evolution of *Hedera* (the Ivy genus, Araliaceae): insights from chloroplast DNA data. *Int J Pl Sc*, 164, 593-602, (2000).

Alston RE, Turner BL. Biochemical Systematics. Prentice Hall, New Jersey, (1963).

Angiosperm Phylogeny Group. An update of the Angiosperm Phylogeny Group classification for the orders and families of flowering plants: APG III. *Botanical Journal of the Linnean Society* 161(2): 105-121, (2009).

Baba ML, Darga LL, Goodman M, Czelusniak J. Evolution of cytochrome C investigated by the maximum parsimony method. *J mol Evol,* 17: 197-213, (1981).

Bate-Smith EC. Plant phenolics as taxonomic guides. *Proc Linn Soc (London)*, 169: 198-211, (1958).

Bate-Smith EC, Harborne JB. Differences in flavonoid content between fresh and herbarium leaf tissue in *Dillenia. Phytochemistry* 10: 1055-1058, (1971).

Bate-Smith EC, Metcalfe CR. The phenolic constituents of plants and their taxonomic significance. *J Linn Soc* (Bot.) 55: 669-705, (1962).

Bendich AJ, Bolton ET. Relatedness among plants as measured by the DNA-agar technique. *Pl Physiol* 42:959-967, (1967).

Bendich AJ, Anderson RS. Repeated DNA sequences and species relatedness in the genus *Equisetum. Pl Syst Evol* 143:47-52, (1983).

Bisby FA, Vaughn JG, Wright CA. (eds) Chemosystematics: Principles and Practices. Academic Press, London, (1980).

Boulter DE. The use of comparative amino acid sequence data in evolutionary studies of higher plants. In: Reinhold L, Liwschitz Y (eds) Progress in Phytochemistry, 3, 199-229. Interscience Publishers, London, (1972).

Boulter DE. Amino acid sequences of cytochrome C and plastocyanins in phylogenetic studies of higher plants. *Syst Zool* 22: 549-553, (1974).

Boulter DE. The evaluation of present results and future possibilities of the use of amino acid sequence data in phylogenetic studies with special reference to plant proteins. In: Bisby FA, Vaughan JG, Wright CA (eds) Chemosystematics: Principles and Practices. Pp. 235-240. Academic Press, London, (1980).

Boulter DE, Peacock D, Guise JT, Estabrook G. Relationships between the partial amino acid sequences of plastocyanin from members of ten families of flowering plants. *Phytochemistry,* 18: 603-608, (1979).

Chang CP, Mabry TJ. The constitution of the order Centrospermae: rRNA-DNA hybridization studies among betalin- and anthocyanin-producing families. *Biochem. Syst.* 1: 185-190, (1973).

Crawford DJ, Julian EA. Seed protein profiles in the narrow leaved species of *Chenopodium* of the western United States: Taxonomic value and comparison with distribution of flavonoid compounds. *Amer J Bot*, 63: 302-308, (1976).

Crawford DJ, DE Giannasi. Plant chemosystematics. *Bioscience* 32, 114-124, (1982).

Doyle JJ, Dickson EE. Preservation of plant samples for DNA restriction endonuclease analysis. *Taxon* 36: 715-722, (1987).

Doyle JJ, Soltis DE, Soltis PS. An intergeneric hybrid in the Saxifragaceae: Evidences from ribosomal RNA genes. *Amer. J. Bot.* 72: 1388-1391, (1985).

Giannasi DE, Crawford DJ. Biochemical Systematics II. A reprise. Evol. Biol.20: 25-248, (1986).

Gibbs RD. Chemotaxonomy of Flowering Plants: 4 vols. McGill Queens University Press, Montreal, (1974).

Harborne JB (ed) Phytochemical Phylogeny. Academic Press, London, New York, (1970).

Harborne JB. Chemical Data in Plant Chemosystematics. Academic Press, London, New York, (1984).

Harborne JB, Turner BL. Plant Chemosystematics. Academic Press, London, New York, (1984).

Hawkes JG (ed) Chemotaxonomy and Serotaxonomy. Academic Press, London, (1968).

Hegnauer R. Gedanken über die theoretische Bedeutung der chemisch- und chemisch-systematischen Betrachtung von Arzenei-Pflanzen. *Pharm Acta Helv*, 29, 203-220, (1954).

Hegnauer R. Chemotaxomische Betrachtungen.VI. Phytochemie und Systematik: Eine Ruckund • Vorausschau auf die Entwicklung einer Chemotaxonomie. *Pharm Acta Helv* 33, 287-305, (1958).

Hegnauer R. Chemotaxonomie der Pflanzen. Vols. 1-7. Birkhauser, Basel, (1962-1986).

Heywood VH, Moore DM (ed) Current Concepts in Plant Taxonomy. Academic Press, London and New York, (1984).

Ingrouille MJ, Chase MW, Fay MF, Bowman D, van der Bank M, Bruijn ADE. Systematics of Vitaceae from the view point of plastid rbcL sequence data. *Bot J Linn Soc* 138, 421-432, (2002).

Jensen U, Fairbrothers DE (ed) Proteins and Nucleic Acids in Plant Systematics. Springer-Verlag, Berlin, (1983).

Jensen SR, Nielsen BJ, Dahlgren R. Iridoid compounds, their occurrence and systematic importance in the Angiosperms. *Bot Not* (Lund) 128, 148-180, (1975).

Kössel H, Edwards K, Fritzsche E, Koch W, Schwarz Z. Phylogenetic significance of nucleotide sequence analysis. In: Proteins and Nucleic Acids in Plant Systematics (eds. U. Jensen, D.E., Fairbrothers) pp. 36-57. Springer-Verlag, Berlin, (1983).

Kubitzki K. Chemosystematische Betrachtungen zur Grosgliederung der Blutenflanzen. Taxon 18: 360-368, (1969).

Kupichan SM, Zimmerman JH, Afonso A. The alkaloids and taxonomy of Veratrum and related genera. Lloydia 24: 1-26, (1961).

Levin DA. Plant phenolics: An ecological perspective. *Amer. Naturalist* 105: 157-181, (1971).

Levin DA, Schal BA. Reticulate evolution in *Phlox* as seen through protein electrophoresis. *Amer. J. Bot.* 57: 977-987, (1970).

Mabry TJ. Pigment dichotomy and DNA-RNA hybridization data for Centrospermous families. *Pl. Syst. Evol.* 126: 79-94, (1976).

Martin PG, Boulter D, Penny D. Angiosperm phylogeny studied using sequences of five macromolecules. *Taxon* 34: 393-400, (1985).

Martin PG, Dowd JM. A phylogenetic tree for some monocotyledons and gymnosperms derived from protein sequences. *Taxon* 35: 469-475, (1986).

Martin PG, Jennings AC. The study of plant phylogeny using amino acid sequences of ribulose-1, 5-bisphosphate carboxylase I. Biochemical methods and patterns of variability. *Austral J Bot* 31: 395-409, (1983).

Martin PG, Stone SJL. The study of plant phylogeny using amino acid sequences of ribulose-1, 5-bisphosphate carboxylase II. The analysis of small subunit data to form phylogenetic trees. *Austral J Bot* 31: 411-418, (1983).

Martins L, Hellwig FH. Systematic position of the genera Serratula and Klasea of Centaureinae (Cardueae-Asteraceae) inferred from ETS and ITS sequence data and new combination in Klasea. *Taxon* 54(3): 632-638, (2005).

Mc Leod MJ, EshbaughWH and Guttman SI. An electrophoric study of *Capcicum* (Solanaceae): The purple flowered taxa. *Bull Torrey Bot Club* 106: 326-333, (1979).

Miller HE, Mabry TJ, Turner BL, Payne WW. Infraspecific variation of sesquiterpene lactones in Ambrosia psilostachya (Compositae). *Amer J Bot* 55: 316-324, (1968).

Nei M. Genetic distance between populations. *Amer. Nat.* 106: 283-292, (1972).

Nevo E, Golenberg E, Berles A, Brown AHD, Zohari D. 1982. Genetic diversity and environmental association of wild wheat, *Triticum dicoccoides* in Isreal. *Theor ApplGenet* 69: 241-254, (1982).

Palmer JD, Adams KL, Cho Y, Parkinson CL, Qiu YL and Song K. Dynamic evolution of plant mitochondrial genomes: mobile genes and introns and highly variable mutation rates. *ProcNat Acad Sci, USA* 97: 6960-6966, (2000).

Rodman JE. Differentiation and migration of *Cakile* (Cruciferae): Seed glucosinolates evidence. *Syst Bot* 1: 137-148, (1976).

Rodman JE, Kruckeberg AR and Al-Shehbaz IA. Chemotaxonomic diversity and complexity in seed glucosinolates of *Caulanthus* and *Streptanthus* (Cruciferae). Syst Bot 6: 197-222, (1981).

Rodman JE, Oliver ML, Nakamura RR, Bledsoe AH. A taxonomic analysis and revised classification of Centrospermae. *Syst Bot* 9: 297-323, (1984).

Rose MR, Dolittle WF. Molecular biological mechanisms of speciation. *Science* 220: 157-162, (1983).

Seaman FC. Sesquiterpene lactones as taxonomic characters in the Asteraceae. *Bot Rev* 48: 121-195, (1982).

Soltis DE. Allozyme variability in Sullivantia (Saxifragaceae) *Syst Bot* 7: 26-34, (1982).

Soltis DE, Soltis PS, Nickrent DL, Jhonson LA, Hahn WJ, Hoot SB, Sweere JA, Kuzoff RK, Kron KA, Chase MW, Swensen SM, Zimmer EA, Chaw SM, Gillespie LJ, Kress WJ, Sytsma KJ. Angiosperm phylogeny inferred from 18S ribosomal DNA sequences. *Ann Missouri Bot Gard* 84: 1-49, (1997).

Soltis PS, Soltis DE, Wolf PG, Nickrent DL, Chaw SM, Chapmany RL. The phylogeny of land plants inferred from 18S rDNA sequences: pushing the limits of rDNA signal? *Mol Biol Evol* 16: 1774-1784, (1999a).

Soltis PS, Soltis DE, Chase MW. Angiosperm phylogeny inferred from multiple genes as a tool for comparative biology. *Nature* 402: 402-404, (1999b).

Starr J, Stephen R, Harris A, Simpson D. A phylogeny of the unispicate taxa in Cyperaceae tribe Cariceae I: generic relationships and evolutionary scenarios. *Systematic Botany* 29(3): 528-544, (2004).

Swain T (ed) Chemical Plant Taxonomy. Academic Press, London and New York, (1963).

Swain T (ed) Comparative Phytochemistry. Academic Press, London and New York, (1966).

Turner BL. Chemosystematics: Recent Developments. *Taxon* 18: 134-151, (1969).

Wen J, Lee C, Lowryll PP, Hiep NT. Inclusion of the Vietnamese endemic *Grushvitzkya* and *Brassiopsis* (Araliaceae): Evidence from nuclear, ribosomal and chloroplast DNA. *Bot J Linn Soc* 142: 455-463, (2003).

Wilson AC, Carlson SS, White TJ. Biochemical evolution. *Ann Rev Biochem* 46: 573-639, (1977).

Young DA and Seigler DS (ed). Phytochemistry and Angiosperm phylogeny. Praeger, New York, (1981).

Xiang QY, Soltis DE, Soltis PS. Phylogenetic relationships of Cornaceae and close relatives inferred from matK and rbcL sequences. *Amer. J. Bot.* 85: 285-297, (1998).

chapter 2

BIODIVERSITY

Ranbir Sahu and Saikat Dewanjee

INTRODUCTION

Biodiversity demonstrates the variety and array of life on diversity is not only the spice of life, it is essential to life. The diversity of biological life (biodiversity) exists at three scales. These range from genes to species to ecosystems (Bodeker, 2003). A common measurement of biodiversity is the total number of species found in an area. Thus biodiversity can be defined as "The versatility of life on the Earth at all its levels, from genous to ecosystem, and the ecological and evolutionary processes that sustain it" (Epstein *et al.*, 2003).

TYPES OF BIODIVERSITY

Biodiversity can be broadly classified into three types.

1. *Species Diversity:* The extent of the world's species biodiversity is fewer than two million of an estimated 10-15 million species have been scientifically described. The depletion of the gene pool has serious implications as a considerable quantity (about 40 per cent) of the global economy is based on biological products and processes. Loss of species also has a direct impact at the local level – particularly on the 900 million people living in extreme poverty in rural areas who are highly reliant on the direct use of biodiversity for their food and livelihoods (Balmford, 2003).
2. *Habitat Diversity:* Habitat modification and destruction pose the greatest threat to biodiversity around the world (WEHAB, 2002). Growing human populations lead to rising resource demands namely food, fuel wood, shelter, land, etc. and pressure to convert habitat to other uses, such as agriculture and livestock-raising.
3. *Ecosystem Diversity:* Ecosystem diversity can be described as the number of ecosystems within a larger geographical unit, such as a country (William, 1992). Because human activities affect whole ecological communities, conservation efforts focused upon individual species alone will not adequately protect the various life-forms on this planet from extinction. It is useful to consider the various reasons to protect biological diversity in general and ecosystems in particular.

Some Important Points of Biodiversity

1. Biodiversity refers to the living pieces that shouldn't be discarded since we use the earth's resources to sustain us. Experience suggests to us that the first rule of intelligent tinkering is to keep all of the pieces. Because of the

interconnected nature of ecosystems, the loss or addition of one species has the potential to change an ecosystem.

2. High levels of biodiversity are associated with greater ecosystem stability. The more diverse a system is, the better able it is to cope with environmental stressors, such as floods or drought. Biodiversity gives us choices, options and flexibility to help us cope with variability, including long-term habitat changes.
3. When a system is simplified, such as having only one species of crop or type of grass, it increases the odds that environmental stressors will have a more pronounced impact or that a disease or pest will be able to spread rapidly. Animal and plant populations with low genetic diversity are much more susceptible to stress and vulnerable to extinction.
4. We all rely on the tremendous variety of species, genes and ecosystems in our world and the many benefits we receive from them - they deserve our respect and conservation (Ayensu *et al.*, 2000).

Factors Affecting Biodiversity

Site Selection

Medicinal plant materials derived from the same species can show significant differences in quality when cultivated at different sites, owing to the influence of soil, climate and other factors. These differences may relate to physical appearance or to variations in their constituents, the biosynthesis of which may be affected by extrinsic environmental conditions, including ecological and geographical variables, and should be taken into consideration.

Risks of contamination as a result of pollution of the soil, air or water by hazardous chemicals should be avoided. The impact of past land uses on the cultivation site, including the planting of previous crops and any applications of plant protection products, should be evaluated.

Ecological Environment and Social Impact

The cultivation of medicinal plants may affect the ecological balance and, in particular, the genetic diversity of the flora and fauna in surrounding habitats. The quality and growth of medicinal plants can also be affected by other plants, other living organisms and by human activities. The introduction of non-indigenous medicinal plant species into cultivation may have a detrimental impact on the biological and ecological balance of the region. The ecological impact of cultivation activities should be monitored over time, where practical.

The social impact of cultivation on local communities should be examined to ensure that negative impacts on local livelihood are avoided. In terms of local income-earning opportunities, small-scale cultivation is often preferable to large-scale production, in particular if small-scale farmers are organized to market their products jointly. If large scale medicinal plant cultivation is or has been established, care should be taken that local communities benefit directly from, for example, fair wages, equal employment opportunities and capital reinvestment.

Climate

Climatic conditions, for example, length of day, rainfall (water supply) and field temperature, significantly influence the physical, chemical and biological qualities of medicinal plants. The duration of sunlight, average rainfall, average temperature, including daytime and night-time temperature differences, also influence the physiological and biochemical activities of plants, and prior knowledge should be considered. WHO guidelines on good agricultural and collection practices (GACP) for medicinal plants (Aslam, 2006).

Soil

The soil should contain appropriate amounts of nutrients, organic matter and other elements to ensure optimal medicinal plant growth and quality. Optimal soil conditions, including soil type, drainage, moisture retention, fertility and pH, will be dictated by the selected medicinal plant species and/or target medicinal plant part (Aslam, 2006). The use of fertilizers is often indispensable in order to obtain large yields of medicinal plants. It is, however, necessary to ensure that correct types and quantities of fertilizers are used through agricultural research. In practice, organic and chemical fertilizers are used. Human excreta must not be used as a fertilizer owing to the potential presence of infectious microorganisms or parasites. Animal manure should be thoroughly composted to meet safe sanitary standards of acceptable microbial limits and destroyed by the germination capacity of weeds. Any applications of animal manure should be documented. Chemical fertilizers that have been approved by the countries of cultivation and consumption should be used. All fertilizing agents should be applied sparingly and in accordance with the needs of the particular medicinal plant species and supporting capacity of the soil. Fertilizers should be applied in such a manner as to minimize leaching. Growers should implement practices that contribute to soil conservation and minimize erosion, for example, through the creation of streamside buffer zones and the planting of cover crops and "green manure" (crops grown to be ploughed in), such as alfalfa (Catizzone, 1994).

Irrigation and Drainage

Irrigation and drainage should be controlled and carried out in accordance with the needs of the individual medicinal plant species during its various stages of growth (Hudson *et al.*, 1996). Water used for irrigation purposes should comply with local, regional and/or national quality standards. Care should be exercised to ensure that the plants under cultivation are neither over- nor under-watered. In the choice of irrigation, as a general rule, the health impact of the different types of irrigation (various forms of surface, sub-surface or overhead irrigation), particularly on the risks of increased vector-borne disease transmission, must be taken into account.

Plant Maintenance and Protection

The growth and development characteristics of individual medicinal plants, as well as the plant part destined for medicinal use, should guide field management practices. The timely application of measures such as topping, bud nipping, pruning and shading may be used to control the growth and development of the plant, thereby improving the quality and quantity of the medicinal plant material being produced. Good agricultural practices for medicinal plants any agrochemicals used to promote the growth of or to protect medicinal plants should be kept to a minimum, and applied only when no alternative measures are available. Integrated pest management should be followed where appropriate. When necessary, only approved pesticides and herbicides should be applied at the minimum effective level, in accordance with the labelling and/or package insert instructions of the individual product and the regulatory requirements that apply for the grower and the end-user countries. Only qualified staff using approved equipment should carry out pesticide and herbicide applications. All applications should be documented. The minimum interval between such treatments and harvest should be consistent with the labelling and/or package insert instructions of the plant protection product, and such treatments should be carried out in consultation and with the by agreement of the buyer of the medicinal plants or medicinal plant materials. Growers and producers should comply with maximum pesticide and herbicide residue limits, as stipulated by local, regional and/or national regulatory authorities of both the growers' and the end-users' countries and/or regions. International agreements such as the International Plant Protection Convention and Codex Alimentarius should also be consulted on pesticide use and residues (Aslam, 2006).

Significance of Biodiversity in Natural Medicine

There is a wide variety of naturally derived drugs which still serve as important therapies in medicine today. Many substances have been derived from traditional medicine, e.g. digitalis (from Foxglove), ergotamine (from contaminated rye), quinine (from Cinchona), etc. More recently, many antibiotic, antifungal and anticancer agents have been derived from bacteria, fungi, plant and animal sources.

The conservation of biodiversity throughout the world is of significance for the mankind and indeed to the constancy of the whole world. The vast genetic variety available in terrestrial plants, animals and micro-organisms offers a wealth of possibilities for the betterment of mankind in the production of foods and medicines (Young, 1999). Natural products offer a vast source of chemical diversity and yield unusual and unexpected lead structures. Although not always understood, secondary metabolites often have important biological function and are generally produced by plants, animals and micro-organisms for specific reasons. Biodiversity affects the metabolic pathways of species and modified phytoconstituents are produced thus there is an excellent chance to get newer molecules from corresponding species.

Discussion

Biodiversity is a vital component which acts as a highly sensitive system to provide the production of various types of medicinal plants and food according to their capacity. Total land area is only 2.4% of the total geographical area of the world, the country accounts for 8% of the total global biodiversity with an estimated 49,000 species of plants. The biodiversity of the Himalayas hills of north-eastern India, plane and plateau area of middle and south India contain nearly 90% of the country's higher plant species and are therefore of special importance to traditional medicine. Since centuries, many plant compounds have an outstanding role in medicine. Their pharmacological and consequently also their economical values have lost nothing of its importance until today. They are used either directly or after chemical modification. It should be mentioned that some plant products have psychopharmacological effects and morphine or mescaline are even counted among the 'hard' drugs.

List of the medicinal plant in various biodiversity (Aslam, 2006; Ghosh et al., 1985; Maikhuri et al., 2000)

Species	*Scientific names*	*Hill*	*Plane*	*Plateu*	*Annual growth rate (%) in India*	*State*
Amla	*Phyllanthus emblica* L.	–	+	+	22.5	Bihar, Chhattisgarh, Gujarat, Haryana, Orissa
Ashok	*Saraca asoca* DC. Wild	+	+	–	15.0	West Bengal, Orissa, Bihar, Himalayes
Ashwagandha	*Withania somnifer* Dunal	–	+	+	9.1	Chandigarh, Haryana, Delhi, Chhattisgarh
Atis	*Aconitum heterophyllum* Wall.	+	–	–	18.4	Uttaranchal, Jammu & Kashmir, Himachal Pradesh
Bael	*Aegle marmelos* L.	–	+	–	9.6	Bihar, Chhattisgarh, Madhya Pradesh, Jharkhand
Brahmi	*Centella aslatica* L.	+	+	–	20.1	Bihar, Delhi, Chhattisgarh, Chandigarh.
Chandan	*Santalum album* Linn.	–	+	–	19.1	Andhra Pradesh, Karnataka, Gujarat, Madhya Pradesh, Maharashtra, Tamilnadu, Bihar.
Chirata	*Swertia chirata*	+	–	–	10.1	Himalayas, Uttaranchal, Jammu & Kashmir, Himachal Pradesh
Giloe	*Tinospora cordifolia* Wild. Miers.	+	+	–	9.1	Chandigarh, North East India
Guggal	*Commiphora wightii* Bhandari.	–	+	–	19.2	Gujarat, Madhya Pradesh
Isabgol	*Plantago Ovata* Forsk.	–	+	–	–	Gujarat
Jatamansi	*Nardostachys jatamansi* De.	+	–	–	8.7	Sikkim, Uttaranchal
Kalmegh	*Andrographis paniculata* Nees	–	+	–	3.1	Himachal Pradesh to Assam, Mizoram, Gujarat, Bihar, South India
Kokum	*Garcinia indica* Linn.	–	+	–	–	West Bengal, Karnataka, Goa
Kuth	*Saussurea lappa* Clark	+	–	–	8.9	Uttaranchal, Jammu & Kashmir
Kutki	*Picrorhiza kurrooa* Royle. ex Benth.	+	–	–	12.9	Kashmir, Himalaya
Madhunashini	*Gymnema Sylvestre* R. Br.	–	+	–	–	Konkan, Tamilnadu, Karnataka, Uttar Pradesh
Safed Musali	*Chlorophytum borivillanum*	–	+	–	–	Southern Rajasthan, Western M.P, North Gujarat
Senna	*Cassia angustifolia* Vahl.	–	+	–	21.8	Tamilnadu, Maharashtra, Gujarat and Rajasthan.
Shatavari	*Asparagus racemosus* Willd.	+	+	+	15.1	Himachal Pradesh, Jammu & Kashmir, Madhya Pradesh, Uttar Pradesh, Uttaranchal
Tulsi	*Ocimum sanctum* L.	+	+	–	17.9	Chandigarh, Bihar, Uttar Pradesh

REFERENCES

Aslam M, Guidelines for Cultivation, collection conservation and propagation of medicinal herbs, Project On Introduction of Medicinal Herbs and Spices as Crop Ministry of Food, Agriculture and Livestock, Islamabad (2006).

Ayensu E, Claasen DV, Collins M, Dearing A, Fresco L, Gadgil M, Gitay H, Glaser G, Juma C, Krebs J, Lenton R, Lubchenco J, McNeely JA, Mooney HA, Pinstrup AP, Ramos M, Raven P, Reid WV, Samper C, Sarukhan J, Schei P, Tundisi JG, Watson RT, Xu GH, Zakri AH, Biosphere management: Some tools of the trade – Response. *Sci*, 287, 234-235, (2000).

Balmford A, Bruner A, Cooper P, Costanza R, Farber S, Green RE, Jenkins M, Jefferiss P, Jessamy V, Madden J, Munro K, Myers N, Naeem S, Paavola J, Rayment M, Rosendo S, Roughgarden J, Trumper K, Turner RK, Economic reasons for conserving wild nature. *Sci,* 297, 950-953, (2002).

Bodeker G, Traditional medical knowledge, intellectual property rights & benefit sharing. *Car J Int Com,* 11(2), 785-814, (2003).

Catizzone M, Soil Science Research in Developing countries: Towards a Holistic Approach. In: Soil Science and Sustainable Land Management in the Tropics, CAB International, Wallingford, U.K 268-274, (1994).

Epstein PR, Chivian E, Frith K, Emerging diseases threaten conservation. *Env H Pers,* 111(10), 506-507, (2003).

Ghosh SP. Horticulture in North Eastern India. *Ind J Hill Far*, 7, 11-21, (1985).

Hartmann HT, Kester DE, Davies FT and Geneve RL, Plant Propagation: Principles and practices. 6th edition. Prentices-Hall, Inc., Upper Saddle River, New Jersey, USA(1997).

Maikhuri RK, Semwal RL, Rao KS, Singh K, Saxena KG, Growth and ecological impacts of traditional agroforestry tree species in central Himalaya, India. *Agroforestry Systems,* 48, 257-272, (2000).

Oksman-Caldentey KM, Inze D, Plant cell factories in the post-genomic era: new ways to produce designer secondary metabolites. *Tr P Sci,* 9, 9, (2004).

WEHAB Working Group, A Framework for Action on Biodiversity and Ecosystem Management, Geneva (2002).

Young, R.N., Importance of biodiversity to the modern pharmaceutical industry. *Pure app Chem,* 71(9), 1655-1661, (1999).

chapter 3

Traditional Medicine versus Modern Phytomedicine

B. Parimala Devi and Subhash C Mandal

INTRODUCTION

The World Health Organization (WHO) estimates that about 80% of the population living in the developing countries relies on traditional medicine for their primary health care needs. In almost all the traditional systems of medicine, the medicinal plants play a major role and constitute their backbone. Indian Materia Medica includes about 2000 drugs of natural origin almost all of which are derived from different traditional systems and folklore practices (Narayana *et al.*, 1998)

The last three decades have shown a revival of interest in plant based drugs and aroma chemicals in the world. As people became conscious with the increased potency and the harmful side effects of newly isolated and synthetic compounds there is an increasing interest in the alternative systems of medicines and medicinal plants. It is very well-known that herbs do not have any side effects and some of the diseases can be cured by natural herbs. Modern herbal preparations involve identification, authentication, collection, testing, processing and marketing with necessary information.

In the broadest definition of medicinal plants, it includes all higher plants that have been alleged to have medicinal properties i.e. effects that relate to health or which have been proven to be useful as drugs by western standards or that which contain constituents that are used as drugs (Laird SA, Kate TK 2002).

1. Complicating the matter of identifying all such plants is that there are no readily available sources of information which are found scattered throughout the world in classical old literature & books on medical botany. In ethno –medico-botanical survey reports for specific geographic regions and or for different ethnic groups, in anthropological writings and as notes on voucher specimen in various herbaria, in variety of review articles and other sources.
2. Secrets locked in minds of indigenous peoples; traditional healers etc. are less likely to be discovered.

There are general and herb-specific concerns regarding herbal products and their ability to produce toxicity and adverse effects. A confusing nomenclature and issues of quality control and the accurate identification of plants are important concerns. There are no international conventions for naming plants, and there are many confusing synonyms. The common names of plants and herbal remedies can be archaic and variable depending on the geographic region. On global basis, it appears that only consolidated source of information on the monetary value of medicinal plant entering into global commerce is that provided by the international trade center (UNCTAD / GATT). The most recent compilation of data from this agency involving medicinal plants and their derivatives was published in 1982. However; this information must be considered as grossly complete. Major data on export / import of medicinal plants involve West Germany, Singapore and Hang Kong. However, these countries produce little medicinal plants.

TRADITIONAL INDIAN SYSTEMS OF MEDICINE

Herbs in the traditional Indian systems of medicine used for the variety of alleviations or sufferings of mankind from olden days (Nadkararni KM, Nadkarani AK 1976).

Although several hundred different genera are used medicinally most are used in herbal remedies and in indigenous system of medicine where either the whole plant or plant organs or its extracts are used. The species used for isolation of active ingredients may be indigenous species growing wild are taken into cultivation or hybrids or other cultivated varieties that have been bred for particular characteristic.

Traditional medicine covers health practices and approaches incorporating plant, animal and mineral based medicines, therapies, manual techniques and exercises employed for health care. However, this talk is biased towards the use of plant drugs because of the authors own background of drug research and also where the issues are more clearly definable and the problems easier to solve. But the same perspective can be extended to other areas of traditional medicine too.

The knowledge of traditional medicine and the medicinal plants used therein has been of great scientific value fir health care in many ways. Traditional medicine is still practiced widely in most of the developing countries. It is estimated that between 65-80% of the population in developing countries use traditional medicines for primary health care. Traditional medicine is attracting much attention in developed countries too; as an alternative to high cost modern drugs; for disease conditions with no or inadequate modern medicines; by and large being less toxic with fewer side effects.

TRADITIONAL AND MODERN MEDICINE

A pragmatic and realistic view has to be taken of the place and position of TMs for the healthcare of the community by drawing a proper balance between the use of traditional medicines vs the modern drugs in specific situations. What is important is the interest of the patient and not the promotion of a system of medicine. In life-threatening infectious diseases well proven modern drugs must be used while for life-style diseases, degenerative disorders or primary healthcare much grater use should be made of traditional medicine, with highly favorable pharmacoecomomics. It would be useful for each country to have a Standing Committee on Essential Drugs to draw guidelines for the use of Traditional Medicines vs. Modern Drugs. While many conventional drugs or their precursors are derived from plants, there is a fundamental difference between administering a pure chemical and the same chemical in a plant matrix. It is this issue of advantage of chemical complexity which is both rejected by orthodoxy as having no basis in fact and avoided by most researchers as introducing too many variables for comfortable research (Simon and Kerry, 2000).

The identification of crude herbs based on geographical origins is crucial in order to ensure authenticity, quality, safety and efficacy of the raw material before it is converted to the final product. Among all the quality control systems, fingerprint has gained more and more attention due to its ability to identify a particular herb and, moreover, to distinguish it from closely related species. Chromatographic fingerprints sometimes exhibit variations in peak height and retention time of a given sample running through identical columns under the same separation conditions. Because of this, appropriate consideration must be given to proper normalization of chromatographic fingerprints.

One of the major difficulties for undertaking medicinal plants cultivation in large scale i.e. the lack of scientific and appropriate agro technology for different climate zones. Experimental cultivation has been carried out nor in several places, but the recommended commercial practices have been neither worked out nor tested on industrial scale. Moreover, even if the cultivation is likely to yield economic returns, the dominant sector of cultivators in the country are conservative and are reluctant to abandon their time tested crops and turn to medicinal crops than modern drugs are preferred for promotive and preventive health care and for minor chronic ailments requiring long use. Traditional medicines have been of great value for modern drug research too by providing leads for the discovery of new single molecule medicines. Infact modern drug discovery started with the leads provided by traditional medicines and continues to this day. Many of the drugs thus discovered are still used in the modern system and many more carry the structural imprint of the parent molecular prototype which had led to their discovery. Herbals of course form the main stay of the material Medica of traditional medicine and are thus attracting much attention. In addition there are some societal concerns which add to the growing interest in plant drugs; their raw environment. There is thus now a global interest in the plant drugs.

- Quality control of herbal medicines is complicated and difficult, and high-technology could be of valuable support. However, when country capacity is limited, continued use of dependable basic technical methods and tests is recommended.
- Governments should provide adequate support for clinical studies, since there are few clinical studies and appropriate approaches for the assessment of efficacy. WHO should provide technical guidance of appropriate approaches for clinical studies and assessment of efficacy of herbal medicines.
- Traditional medicine plays an important role in primary health care in many developing countries and countries should consider categorizing herbal medicines based on available knowledge and the literature. Relevant appropriate requirements should be established for the assessment of safety and efficacy for different categorized herbal medicines to reduce cost and expenditure and meet demands of accessibility and affordability.
- A challenge for national health authorities is the lack of research information and data on herbal medicines. Sharing national information and experience, as well as setting up common accepted standards through bilateral recognition and through international.
- Regional regulatory cooperation for herbal medicines should be considered. WHO should continue to provide support to international and regional regulatory cooperative initiatives for herbal medicines.
- In order to ensure safe and effective use of traditional medicine, integration of traditional medicine into national health systems should be considered where appropriate.

Controlled clinical studies are needed to clarify and determine the clinical importance of drug herb interactions. Patients taking drugs with a narrow therapeutic index (cyclosporine, digoxin, hypoglycemic agents, lithium, phenytoin, procainamide, theophylline, tricyclic antidepressants, and warfarin) should be discouraged from using herbal products. (Kuhn, M., Winston D 2001). All drugs with a narrow therapeutic index may either have increased adverse effects or be less effective when used in conjunction with herbal products. More research is required to define the interactions. When adverse reactions are experienced with drug therapy, patients must always be queried as to their intake of herbal products: what they are taking in pills and tincture form, what they are drinking as teas, and what they are eating from their garden (Smith, M 2000, Kuhn M, 2001). The safety of herbal products may be related to the mixtures of active chemicals that they contain; their interactions with other herbs and drugs, contaminants, or adulterants; or their inherent toxicity. Plants have complex mixtures of terpenes, alkaloids, saponins, and other chemicals, increasing the risk of adverse reactions to any one of them or to the additive or synergistic effects of chemical interactions. For example, more than 100 chemicals have been identified in tea tree oil (Saxe, T.G, 1987, But, P.P 1994)

Active ingredients in herbs and dietary supplements can cause unexpected reactions when used with other herbs or medications. Effects on the distribution, metabolism, or excretion of drugs may be pronounced and may lead to drug toxicity. For example, sassafras reportedly inhibits microsomal enzymes and can increase the half-life of drugs metabolized by the liver. Contaminants and adulterants of herbal products can be pharmacologically active and responsible for unexpected toxicity (Moore and Adler, 2000) Ayurvedic medications have been known to cause lead poisoning in children because of their contamination with this heavy metal and others, such as arsenic and mercury. (Kew, et al., 1993). Many Chinese patent medicines contain drugs such as phenylbutazone and barbiturates, warfarin-like chemicals, and contaminants such as lead or arsenic (Abt, *et al.*, 1995).

Herbal products or folk remedies may be unsafe for example, aconite, a widely used Asian remedy, can produce life-threatening cardiac and neurologic toxicity (Fatovich. 1992) so stringent quality control measures are to be initiated to test such toxicity as per the recommendations of the pharmacopoeial standards. Modern phytomedicine emerging with the development of the latest techniques with sophisticated instruments to test the quality of the phytomedicines. eg. Gingerol and taxol in diabetes and cancer.

SUMMARY

The therapeutic use of Indian and Chinese herbal medicine has traditionally employed crude plants extracts while current medicinal practice favors the development of homogenous and purified pharmacologically active agents. In spite of that in the last two decades, one has witnessed a revival of interest in natural drugs and herbal products primarily due to the wide spread belief that natural medicines are healthier than synthetic drugs due to reduced side effects. Apart from that, medicinal plants continue to provide template for the development of other compounds that are capable of showing similar efficacy as that of western medicine.

Although isolating and identifying individual chemical constituents with relevant bioactivity provides the rational scientific basis for the medicinal use of a plant, synergistic bioactivity due to different constituents is common and a single plant may contain distinct chemical classes acting in different ways by mechanisms such as antioxidant & anti inflammatory activity, has to be justified on the basis for its specific use in herbal therapy is concerned.

The modern phytomedicine research reflects much about the molecular keys involved in therapeutic targets in disease prevention. Many of the bioactive constituents has been tested for its efficacy and it provides an avenue in the discovery of new compounds in the drug discovery from natural sources. Care to be taken to judge the safety and adverse effects of these molecules, so that the formulation will be successful to capture the pharmaceutical market and to meet with the demands of the public.

REFERENCES

Abt A, Oh JY, Huntington RA, Burkhart KK. Chinese herbal medicine induced acute renal failure. Arch Intern Med. 155:211-212, (1995).

But PP, Herbal poisoning caused by adulterants or erroneous substitutes. J Trop Med Hyg. 97:371-374. (1994).

Carson CF, Riley TV. Toxicity of the essential oil of *Melaleuca alternifolia* or tea tree oil. J Toxicol Clin Toxicol 33:193-194 (1995).

Fatovich DM, Aconite: a lethal Chinese herb. Ann Emerg Med. 21:309-311 (1992).

Kew J, Morris C, Aihie A, Fysh R, Jones S, Brooks D. Arsenic and mercury intoxication due to Indian ethnic remedies. BMJ. 306:506-507, (1993).

Kuhn M, Complementary Therapy-Gram. Vol 4, No.1. Hamburg, NY: Educational Services; April (2001).

Kuhn M, Winston D. Herbal Therapy and Supplements: A Scientific and Traditional Approach. Philadelphia, Pa: JBLippincott (2001).

Laird SA, Kate TK, Linking biodiversity prospecting and forest conservation. In: Pagiola, S., Bishop, J., Landell-Mills, N. (Eds.), Selling Forest Environmental Services. Earthscan, London, UK, pp. 151-172 (2002).

Moore C, Adler R. Herbal vitamins: lead toxicity and developmental delay. Pediatrics. 106:600-602 (2000).

Nadkararni KM, Nadkarani AK. Indian Materia Medica popular, vol 1. Bombay: Prakashan, (1976).

Narayana DBA, Katayar CK, Brindavanam, NB. Original system: search, research or re-search. IDMA Bulletin 29, 413-416 (1998).

Saxe TG, Toxicity of medicinal herbal preparations. Am Fam Physician); 35 :135-142 (1987).

Simon mills, Kerry bone Principles and practice of Phytotherapy: Churchill livingstone, p:22 (2000).

Smith M, Drug interactions with natural health products/dietary supplements: a survival guide. Paper presented at: Complementary and Alternative Medicine: Implications for Clinical Practice and State-of-the-Science Symposia; March 12, (2000); Boston.

chapter 4

Traditional Chinese System of Medicine

Saikat Dewanjee and Subhash C Mandal

INTRODUCTION

Traditional Chinese Medicine (TCM) is an inclusive coordination of medical contemplation, pathophysiological concepts and therapeutic interventions, that develops out of the matrix of Chinese civilization over a period spanning more than 4000 years. Chinese medicinal system has gotten its debut by taking references from Yellow Emperor's Classic of Internal Medicine (Huang De Nei Jing) based on the idea that all life is subjected to natural laws (Veith, 1949) and Yin-Yang theory (Gibert, 1998; Cheng, 2000). These two theories were developed separately and differ in terms of diagnosis and therapy. The primary modality of TCM is the use of an extensive Pharmacopoeia of over 6000 herbal and other natural products for the preventions and treatment of diseases and the promotion of health. TCM has been spread to Japan and Korea earlier during post-cultural revolution and gained its popularity as Kampoh system of medicine (Katsutoshi, 1993). Although it has developed its own characters giving due importance of the styles of corresponding countries their simplicity and spontaneity, still the basic ideas remain alike. Even in USA, TCM has gained its acceptability now a day (Patwardhan *et al.*, 2005).

COMPONENTS OF TCM

TCM has four main mechanisms: acupuncture, herbal medicine, tui na and qi gong. Herbal medicines are generally delivered in compound formulae specially formulated for a clinical syndrome or collection of symptoms. Tui na is the ancient Chinese massage used for lymphatic drainage and muscle rejuvenation. Qi gong is the practice of energy movement in the body through physical movement (Kapuchuk, 2000). The general theory of acupuncture is based on the principle that there are patterns of energy flow (Qi) through the body that are essential for health. Aberration of this flow is believed to be responsible for disease condition. Acupuncture is used to correct imbalances if Qi flow at particular anatomical locations just below the skin, the acupuncture points, by the stimulation of a variety of techniques. The studied mechanism of stimulation of acupuncture points employees penetration of the skin by thin, solid, specially tipped, metallic needles, which are manipulated manually or by electrical current (Birch, 2001).

MAJOR CLINICAL APPLICATIONS

TCM has found its utility to alleviate the ailments like hypertension and other cardiovascular diseases, allergic condition, respiratory illness like asthma, gastrointestinal complaint such as gastric and irritable bowel syndrome, muscular skeletal conditions such as low back and neck pain, inflammatory conditions such as osteoarthritis, autoimmune disorders like rheumatoid arthritis, menstrual complaints such as premenstrual syndrome, endocrine disorders like hypothyroidism and type II diabetes, and dermatological conditions like eczema. In addition to a positive clinical-therapeutic outcome, reported benefits to patients comprise evasion of toxic side effects of drugs, accelerated healing process, enhanced immunity, reduction of stress, neuro-endocrine balancing lead to greater sense of well being (Yuan and Lin, 2000).

ROLE OF INDIGENOUS MEDICINAL PLANTS IN TCM

Chinese herbal medicine is a major part of Chinese therapeutics both in nutrition and as a form of drug therapy (Bensky and Barolet, 1990; Bensky and Gamble, 1986). The vast majority of traditional Chinese drugs are of botanical origin with less than 10% being of animal and mineral origin. Some drugs are consumed as foods and are also used for health promotion or treatment of diseases depending on the dose. TCM practioners employ single herbs and formulations with multiple herbs to treat the ailments.

List of some important medicinal plants are used in Chinese medicine (Huang, 1999; Tang et al., 1995; Ye et al., 2003; Mamedov et al., 2005; Attele et al., 2002; Bensky and Gamble, 1986)

Plant name	*Functions and clinical uses*
Acanthopanax gracilistylus	Anti-inflammatory, analgesic, strengthen the sinews and bones, used for rheumatoid arthritis chronic wind damp painful obstruction with deficiency of the liver and the kidney.
	Cardiotonic, anti-inflammatory, anti-shock analgesic, tranquilizing effects. It also increases blood pressure.
Alisma orientale	Diuretic, antidiabetic, hypotensive and stimulant agent. Used for difficult urination, edema, diarrhoea, dizziness caused by congested phlegm.
Allium macrostemon	Used for cough, weezing, chest pain caused by stagnation, dysentery like disorder.
Andrographis paniculata	Antibiotic, antiviral effects, dried dampness, uses for pulmonary abscesses, pharyngitis, dysentery, snake bite, carbuncles.
Angelica pubescens	Tranquilizing, hypnotic, analgesic, antihypertensive. Used for wind cold dampful obstruction.
Areca catechu	Antiparasitic, antifungal, antiviral effect.
Aristolochia manshuriensis	Diuretic effect. Drains the heart and promotes lactation. Used for painful scanty urine, mouth ulcers, and irritability.
Artemisia apiacea	Antibiotic, antimalarial, summer heat syndrome, deficiency fever.
Asarum heterotropoides	Antipyretic, analgesic antibiotic effects. Used for headache, toothache, mouth ulcer.
Astragalus membranaceus	Immunostimulant, diuretic, increase the contraction of heart, hypotensive, antiaging effect.
Atractylodis lancea	Strengthens the spleen and dried dampness, used in night blindness and keratomalacia.
Belamcanda chinensis	Antiviral antifungal, increase secretion of saliva, expels phlegm, benefits throats, used for tonsillitis, pharyngitis and bronchitis.

Bletilla striata	Shorten the thrombin time, inhibits fibrinolysin, and increases platelets counts. Antibiotic effect. Used for bleeding from lung and stomach, bleeding caused by traumatic injuries, bleeding ulcers, chapped skin, pulmonary abscess.
Buthus martensi	Anticonvulsive, tranquilizing effects, hypotensive. Relaxation effect on skeletal muscles. Used for acute or chronic infantile convulsion, facial paralysis, tetanus, carbuncle, migraine, headache.
Cannabis sativa	Nourishes and moistens the intestine. Used for constipation from deficient blood or deficiency of body fluid and chronic constipation.
Catharanthus tintorius	Stimulates the contraction of the uterus. Lower cholesterol levels. Used for dysmenorrhoea, amenorrhoea, postpartum abdominal pain and angina pectoris.
Chaenomeles lagenaria	Anti-inflammatory effect. Comforts the sinews and activates the channels. Used for wind damp painful obstruction, abdominal pain, vomiting, spasm, and diarrhoea.
Cinnamomum cassia	Antibiotic, antipyretic, diuretic effects. Warms the channels, disperses cold, strengthen heart. Used for edema and dysmenorrhoea.
Citrus aurantium	Anti-shock, diuretic effect, hypertensive, increases the intensity and frequencies of peristalsis, excites uterus. Used for food stagnation, constipation, gastopsis.
Citrus sarcodactylis	Antispasmodic effect on duodenal spasm, used for chronic cough with diffused phlegm.
Croton tiglium	Laxative, expels phlegm, epilepsy.
Curcuma zedoaria	Antineoplastic, cardiovascular effects. Inhibit early pregnancy.
Dryobalanops aromatica	Antianginal, antibiotic effects. Clears heart and alleviates pain. Used for fainting, convulsion, boils, sore throat, muscle ulcer.
Eudia rutaecarpa	Antibiotic, analgesic, hypotensive, used for cold epigastris and abdominal pain, chronic diarrhoea.
Euphorbia kansui	Laxative expels water and reduce swelling, used for edema ascitis, pleurisy, intestinal obstruction and epilepsy.
Forsythia suspense	Antimicrobial, antiemetic, diuretic, cardiotonic effects. Used for carbuncles and tonsillitis.
Gardenia jesminoides	Antibiotic effect, used for fibril disease, jaundice, epistaxsis, haematuria, trauma.
Gentiana macrophylla	Anti-inflammatory, sedative, analgesic, antibiotic effects. Used for rheumatic arthritis.
Hedyotis diffusa	Antineoplastic, analgesic effect. Clear heat poisons, reduces abscesses, carbuncles, and snake bite.
Hordeum vulgare	Dissolve food stagnation, strengthen the stomach, restrains lactation.
Imperata cylindrica	Haemostatic, antibiotic, cools blood, used for nephritis, jaundice.
Isatis tinctoria	Antimicrobial, antiviral effects. Used for influenza, mumps, sore throat.
Leonurus heterophyllus	Stimulates the contraction of uterus. Antianginal, sedative effects. Promotes urination, used for irregular menstruation, postpartum abdominal pain, traumatic injuries, edema.
Lindera strychnifolia	Increases peristalsis, relieve flatulence, antibody effects.

Lonicera japonica	Antibiotic, antiviral, anti-inflammatory, antipyretic. Used for wind heat exterior syndrome.
Lysimachia christinae	Diuretic, increase the secretion of bile, used for acute hepatitis, jaundice, painful scanty urine, biliary and urinary stones, snake bite.
Magnolia officinalis	Antimicrobial, antiviral, purgative.
Melia toosendam	Antimicrobial effects, antispasmodic.
Mentha haplocalyx	Antibiotic, antipyretic, diaphoretic effects. Used for measles.
Morus alba	Endocrine, hypoglycemic effects. Promotes the healing of sores. Clears the liver and eyes used for cough, acute conjunctivitis.
Panax notoginseng	Shorten bleeding time and thrombin time. Lower blood pressure, antibiotic and antidiabetic effect.
Patrinia scabiosaefolia	Antibiotic, antiviral, expels pus. Used for acute appendicitis, pulmonary abscesses and carbuncles.
Perilla frutescens	Antipyretic, antibiotic, used for restless fetus or morning sickness.
Phragmites communis	Antidiabetic effect. Clears heat and generate fluid. Stops vomiting, used for high fever, pulmonary abscesses.
Pinellia ternate	Antitussive, antiemetic effects. Dissipates lumps and reduces distension. Used for cough with profuse phlegm, nausea, vomiting, morning sickness, stuffiness in the chest, scrofula.
Plantago asiatica	Diuretic, expectorant, antitussive, hypotensive. Used for vertigo, cataract.
Pogostemon cavlin	Antibiotic effect, promotes the secretion of gastric juice, antiemetic.
Polygonum cuspidatum	Antibiotic, antiviral, expectorant and antitussive effects. Used for amenorrhoea, rheumatic arthritis, traumatic injuries, damp heat jaundice, burns, boils, carbuncles, sores, lung heat cough, constipation.
Poria cocos	Diuretic, tranquilizer, hypoglycemic. Used for difficult urination, congested fluid, deficient spleen syndrome, and insomnia.
Prunella vulgaris	Antibiotic effect, decreases blood pressure, used for acute conjunctivitis, goiter.
Prunus humilis	Moistens and moves stools, promotes urination.
Pueraria lobata	Antispasmodic, antipyretic, antidiabetic effects. Decreases blood pressure, nourishes the fluids used for fever, damp heat diarrhoea.
Raphanus sativa	Antimicrobial antifungal, used for GI disorder.
Rheum palmatum	Purgative, antimicrobial, cholagogic and haemostatic effects. Jaundice, amenorrhoea, appendicitis.
Rubia cordifolia	Shorten thrombin time, antitussive, expectorant and antibiotic effect. Used for various types of bleeding, dysmenorrhoea, traumatic injury.
Salvia miltiorrhiza	Cardiovascular, hypoglycemic, sedative effects. Decreases serum cholesterol levels. Used for amenorrhoea, postpartum abdominal, abdominal masses, boils, carbuncles, high fever, delirium palpitation, insomnia, angina pectoris.

Sargasum pallidum	Antifungal and hypotensive effects. Soften hard masses, promotes urination. Used for thyroid disorders, scrofula, edema.
Schizonepata tenufolia	Diaphoratic, haemostatic effects, releases exterior and expel wind. Used for wind cold exterior syndrome. Measles, epistaxis, menorrhoea.
Smilax glabra	Detoxifies fire poison, used for syphilis, painful scanty urine and carbuncles.
Sophora japonica	Haemostatic, antihypertensive, anti-inflammatory effect. Relieve intestinal spasms, cools the blood, used for bloody stool.
Traxacum mongolicum	Antimicrobial antibiotic, diuretic, cholagogic effect. Used for breast and intestinal abscesses, jaundice, carbuncles and sores.
Trichosanthes kirilowii	Abortive effect. Promote decharge of pus. Used for high fever with thrust, cough, sores, carbuncles.
Tussilago farfara	Expectorant, antitussive, antiasthmatic effects. Used for various types of cough.
Uncaria rhynchophylla	Antihypertensive, sedative, antispasmodic effects. Used for epilepsy, tremors, seizures from liver wind.
Viola yedoensis	Antimicrobial effect, clear heat and detoxifies fire poisons, used for breast and intestinal abscesses, carbuncles, mumps and snake bite.
Viscum coloratum	Diuretic, antiviral, hypotensive. Used for arthritis, lower back pain, threatened abortion.
Zingiber officinale	Diaphoretic, antibiotic. Increase the secretion of gastric juice. Alleviates coughing. Stop vomiting, reduces poisonous effect of other herbs.
Zizipus jujube	Sedative, hypnotic, antispasmodic, analgesic effects. Used for insomnia, palpitation caused by deficient blood of liver and heart. Also used for spontaneous sweating and night sweating.

STATUS OF TCM IN CHINA AND ITS ROLE ON ECONOMY

There are more than 2800 TCM hospitals in China provide one third of total outpatient medical care of country. In addition there is a well established training system for TCM professionals with 27 colleges and 44 departments in universities and medical colleges, teaching 6,00,000 students. There are also about 100 research based institutes for TCM, hosting more than 11,000 scholars to provide more acceptable out come. TCM industry is well developed in China in term of providing infrastructure, manpower, innovative ability and market. Infrastructure includes TCM medical network, training and research systems. Innovative capacity in TCM is reflected by the augment in number of molecular development of newer drugs. Data showed between 2003 and 2004, about 203 new and licensed drug molecules were discovered. For quality control they are using modern stylish analytical techniques like HPLC and HPTLC fingerprints for standardization of products.

As per national economy of China TCM is most rapidly expanding field. In the year of 2004, industrial output was 95.8 billion RMB (50 times higher than it was in 1978), 2003-2004, out put was considered 19-23% of total pharmaceutical output whereas percentage of sales was 25-30%. About 11 TCM pharmaceutical companies have annual sales over 1 billion YMB. Among them two have annual sales over 5 billion YMB.

CHALLENGE FACED BY TCM

Although enormous progress has been made in expansion of TCM industry but industry is clearly facing problems related to sustainability and international competitiveness. Major problems associated with TCM are:

- Lack of break through in basic science of TCM.
- Lack of criteria for clinical diagnosis and evaluation.
- Problem associated with quality control of TCM formulations.
- Increase over exploitation of herbal resources.

In order to over come aforementioned challenges following measures were suggested to be taken for meeting solution (The State Administration of traditional Chinese medicine of the People's Republic of China, 1997).

- Development of innovative network for TCM. It includes TCM related research, clinical studies, development, production sales and management to demand best product.
- Development of modern methodologies technologies and standards.
- Maintenance of herbal resources. It is related to reproduction, cultivation, germ protection, dynamic monitoring as well as alerting herbal resources.
- Strengthening international collaboration. It may promote scientific collaborations, exchanges.

DISCUSSION

TCM has passed a long history of success not only confined in China but also in other countries like Japan, Korea and Vietnam. The prospect of TCM in term of modern development is peerless in term of adjusting integration of traditional literature with modern research, particularly in respect to the information and associated data based discovery. Accelerated modernization of TCM to meet the obligation of present era has given a new dimension of modern alternative therapy.

REFERENCES

Attele AS, Zhou YP, Xie JT, Wu JA, Zhang L, Dey L, Pugh W, Rue PA, Polonsky KS, Yuan CS. Antidiabetic effects of Panax ginseng berry extract and the identification of an effective component. *Diabetes*, 51(6), 1851-1858, (2002).

Bensky D, Barolet R. Chinese Herbal Medicine, Formulas & Strategies. Seattle: Eastland Press, (1990).

Bensky D, Gamble A. Chinese Herbal Medicine Materia Medica. Seattle: Eastland Press, (1986).

Birch S. An overview of acupuncture in the treatment of stroke, addiction, and other health problems. Springer, Berlin. pp 131-139, (2001).

Cheng JT. Review: drug therapy in Chinese traditional medicine. *J Clin Pharmacol* 40, 445-450, (2000).

Gibert TF. Reflections on traditional Chinese medicine and its pharmacopoeia. *Annales Pharma Franca,* 56, 282-285, (1998).

Huang TK. Handbook of Composition and Pharmacological Action of Commonly Used Traditional Chinese Medicine. Chinese Medical Science Publication Co. Shanghai. (1999).

Kaptchuk TJ. The Web That Has No Weaver: Understanding Chinese Medicine. McGraw-Hill, New York. (2000).

Katsutoshi T. Kampo: Japanese-Oriented Medicine. Translated by Bacowsky H, Gerz A. Tokyo, Japan: KK Standard McIntyre.pp. 32, (1993).

Mamedov N. Adaptogenic, geriatric, stimulant and antidepressant plants of Russian Far East. *J Cell & Molecul Bio,* 4, 71-75, (2005).

Patwardhan B, Warude D, Pushpangadan P, Bhatt N. Ayurveda and Traditional Chinese Medicine: A Comparative Overview. *eCAM*, 2(4), 465-473, (2005).

Shan BE, Yoshita Y, Sugiura T, Yamashita U. Suppressive effect of Chinese medicinal herb extract on human lymphocytes *in vitro. Clin & Exper Immu*, 118, 41-48, (1999).

Tang X, Ma Y, Li P. Seperation and identification of anti-inflammatory diterpene from the root cortices of *Acanthopanax gracilistylus. Chung Kuo Chung Yao Tsa Chih,* 20, 231-253, (1995).

The State Administration of traditional Chinese medicine of the People's Republic of China. Anthology of Policies, Laws and Regulations of the People's Republic of China on Traditional Chinese Medicine. Shangdong: Shangdong University. (1997).

Veith I. The Yellow Emperor's Classic of Internal Medicine. Berkeley, The University of California Press. (1949).

Ye YP, Sun CR, Li XY, Suncand HX, Panb YJ. Alisol B monoacetate from the rhizome of *Alisma orientale. Acta Crystallograp*, E59, 1858-1859, (2003).

Yuan R, Lin Y. Traditional Chinese medicine an approach to scientific proof and clinical validation. *Pharmacol & Therapeu,* 86(2), 191-198, (2000).

chapter 5

Phytopharmacological Research for the Treatment of Cancer

Brigitte Binneman and Namrita Lall

Cancer treatment via chemotherapy was introduced more than 50 years ago into the clinic. Toxic drugs are needed in most cases of chemotherapy treatment in patients which often result in unpleasant side effects, but the beneficial effects of these toxic drugs outweigh their adverse reactions. Plant materials (edible and nonedible) have phytochemicals present which may function as chemo preventative or chemotherapeutic agents. Modern medicine has benefited significantly from anecdotal results of their empirical methodology. Presently large numbers of illnesses are treated by choosing necessary candidates for a pharmacopeia that is inadequate. Natural products also had a major impact on cancer chemotherapy. It has been reported that more than 60% of the approved drugs for cancer treatment are natural products or derived from natural products. There are many plant-derived anticancer agents which are in clinically use these days. These include the vinca alkaloids/ natural alkaloids vinblastine and vincristine that were isolated in minute quantities from *Catharanthus roseus* G. Don. Another two semisynthetic derivatives are etoposide teniposide of the parent compound epipodophyllotoxin, a natural product, which is an isomer of podophyllotoxin. The medicinally used Podophyllum species (Podophyllaceae) from the Indian subcontinent, *Podophyllum peltatum* Linnaeus (commonly known as the American mandrake or Mayapple), and *Podophyllum emodii* Wallich, have been used extensively for the treatment of skin cancers and warts throughout history. The taxanes were more recently added to the armamentarium of plant-derived chemotherapeutic agents, Paclitaxel (taxol®)was isolated originally from the bark of *Taxus brevifolia* Nutt. Paclitaxel is used alone or in combination with other cancer drugs primarily for the treatment of ovarian, breast, and non-small cell lung cancer (NSCLC). Furthermore it showed efficacy against Kaposi sarcoma, potential treatment of multiple sclerosis, psoriasis and rheumatoid arthritis. 'Homoharringtonine' (HHT) was isolated from *Cephalotaxus harringtonia* var. drupacea (Sieb and Zucc.) (Cephalotaxaceae). In China, acute myelogenous leukaemia and chronic myelogenous leukaemia is treated effectively with the use of a harringtonine and HHT racemic mixture. Elliptinium, a derivative of ellipticine, was isolated from a Fijian medicinal plant *Bleekeria vitensis* A.C. Sm. (known for anticancer properties) and species of several genera of the Apocynaceae family, is marketed for treatment of breast cancer in France. Natural products for cancer chemotherapy are often very potent but have limitations in terms of solubility in aqueous solvents and they show narrow therapeutic indices, this caused the termination of a large number of pure natural products such as bruceantin and maytansin (isolated from *Maytenus serrata*).

Development of new derivatives from natural products with improved antiproliferative profiles and chemo preventive activities is essential, but it can only happen if their molecular mechanism of action, their effects on cellular signalling process is entirely understood as well as their structure-activity relationships. Revival is taking place in medicinal botanicals (including herbal remedies) as part of complementary medicine for disease prevention and therapy as conventional medications have high costs, side effects and therapeutic limitations. Therefore, there are great interests and enthusiasm in naturally occurring phytochemicals for cancer chemoprevention.

WHAT IS CANCER ?

Cancer is generally considered to comprise more than 100 different diseases, each characterized by uncontrolled growth and spread of abnormal cells, resulting from a chain of multiple genetic changes causing a loss of typical growth controls, leading to unregulated growth, lack of differentiation, apoptosis, genomic instability, and metastasis (Bishop, 2005). The genetic alterations are caused by both external factors (tobacco, chemicals, radiation, and infectious organisms) and internal factors (inherited mutations, hormones, immune conditions and mutations that occur from metabolism). To initiate or promote carcinogenesis these factors can work jointly or in sequence. Cancer knows no boundaries and is able to develop in any tissue within any organ at any age and the frequency of cancers intensifies exponentially with age. According to Bagchi and Preuss (2005), two in five persons will be diagnosed with cancer some time in their life, and finally three out of every four families will be affected. A long latent period of ten or more years was found to be one of the hallmarks of tumour development. No obvious clinical evidence of disease can be seen during this latent period. Studies suggested that for the full development of cancer it is required that three to seven rate-limiting mutations should take place (Bishop, 2005). Both animal carcinogenesis models and human clinical data support the stepwise sequence of cancer (Fig. 5.1).

Many genes that take part in normal cells processes and therefore, cancer cells can be damaged by any of these genes (Bagchi and Preuss, 2005). Multiple genetic modifications and biochemical defects underlie cancer development, they are crucial for converting normal cells into a cancerous cell mass with atypical growth. It is crucial for tumorigenesis that genetic modifications occur in the cells genes responsible for cell cycle progression and growth so that they can achieve the proliferative advantage. Proteins are encoded via growth-regulating genes. Mutations in these genes will then alter levels or function of these proteins, equipped to alter cell division successfully (Bishop, 2005). Oncogenes and tumour suppressors (loss of function) are two main types of genes mutated in cancer.

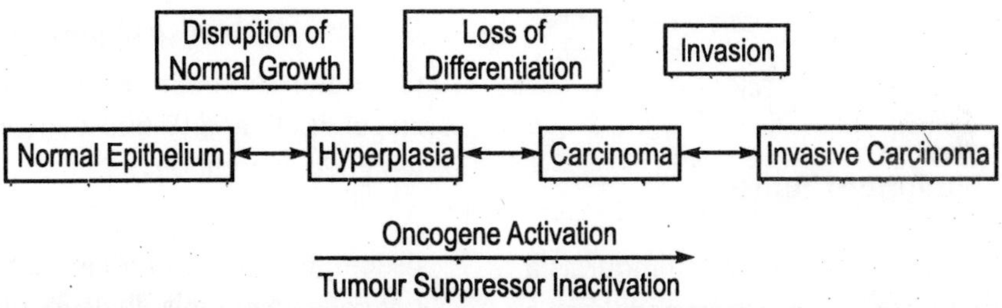

Fig. 5.1: The upper row represents disturbances in growth, differentiation, and tissue integrity that lead to the phenotypes that characterize the different stages of cancer, shown in the lower row (Bishop, 2005).

TYPES OF CANCER

There are many different types of cells in the body and all the different cells can grow into cancer. Cells from different body parts do behave differently, some may grow faster or slower, some produce different symptoms, others respond differently to the same treatment and some might be more or less likely to spread to a specific part of the body. Cancers are divided into four main groups according to the body tissue from which they arise (Table 5.1) (Bagchi and Preuss, 2005).

Table 5.1: Cancer terminology (Bagchi and Preuss, 2005)

Cancer	*Developed from*	*Examples*
Carcinoma	Epithelial cells, such as the cells that line the digestive tract and make up organs such as the liver, kidney and pancreas.	Glandular, e.g., prostate: adenocarcinoma Squamous, e.g., cervix: carcinoma
Sarcoma	Cells that form things such as muscle, nerves, or blood vessels.	Smooth muscle: leiomyosarcoma; benign hyperproliferation is called a leiomyoma (fibroid) Bone: osteosarcoma Fat cells: liposarcoma; benign hyperproliferation is called a lipoma
Lymphoma	Cells in a lymph gland	Solid tumour derived from B- or T-lymphocytes
Leukemias	Blood-forming tissue	Myeloid cells: myelocytic leukaemia Lymphocytes (white blood cells): lymphocytic leukaemia

Benign and Malignant Tumours

Bagchi and Preuss (2005) defined a tumour as a mass of abnormal cells which are formed when a cells starts to divide uncontrollably. The tissue surrounding the cancer is firstly invaded and thereafter spreads upto a blood or lymph vessel, then it is said that the cancer have metastasized. Benign tumours contain cells that are not able to spread to a different site in the body, therefore, they are most of the time not cancerous, and are contained within a covering of normal cells, they grow slowly and is most of the time harmless and therefore, no treatment is required, whereas malignant tumours contain cells that are capable of spreading beyond the original tumour to another part of the body, this is dangerous because as the cells invade surrounding tissue they can damage them and stop them from working properly, and these tumours are cancerous.

Cancer Stages

At the time of cancer diagnosis a staging is a process used to explain the degree or spread of the disease. Staging is vital for determining the selection of therapy and measuring the prognosis. The size and location of the primary tumour determines a cancer's stage and also whether or not it has spreads to the other areas of the body. Different staging systems are used for all the different cancer types in order to assist in describing the progress of that cancer (Bagchi and Preuss, 2005). The different types of staging used to classify tumours are:

1. TNM — this classification system measures tumours in three ways: extent of the primary tumour (T), regional lymph node involvement (N) absence or presence, and distant metastases (M) absence or presence.
2. Once the TNM is assigned stages of I (early stage), II, III, and IV (most advanced stage) is assigned in addition.
3. Another system is used for descriptive and statistical analysis of tumours: in situ — if cancer cells do not invade deeper into the tissue and are present only in the layer of cells where they developed; invasive – if cells have spread

to nearby tissue beyond the original layer; local – an invasive malignant cancer confined entirely to the organ of origin; regional – a malignant cancer that (1) has extended beyond the limits of the organ of origin directly into surrounding organs or tissues; (2) involves regional lymph nodes by way of lymphatic system; or (3) has both regional extension and involvement of regional lymph nodes; distant – a malignant cancer that has spread to parts of the body remote from the primary tumour either by direct extension or by discontinuous metastasis to distant organs, tissues, or via the lymphatic system to distant lymph nodes (Bagchi and Preuss, 2005).

Selection of the most suitable type of treatment for a specific type of cancer can only be done when the stage of the cancer is known since it is important to decide on the right treatment for that specific stage of cancer. After a biopsy, grading is done in the lab where cancer cells are graded according to how much they look like normal cells and also their aggressiveness. Many different types of grading systems exist and depend on the type of cancer. The Gleason system is the most commonly used grading system which is based on a number from 0 to 10, the lower the number the lower the grade. According to Bagchi and Preuss (2005), grades under 4 mean that the cancer cells look similar to normal cells and that the cancer is less likely to be aggressive, where grades 5 to 7 are the intermediates which means that these cancer cells do not look like normal cells and are more likely to be aggressive and more likely to grow faster and grades 8 to 10 means that the cancer is very aggressive in growth.

The staging system of the Gleason system according to Bagchi and Preuss (2005) is as follows:

Stage 0 (Carcinoma in situ):	Very early cancer. The abnormal cells are found only in the first layer of the primary site and do not invade deeper into the tissue.
Stage I:	Cancer involves the primary site but did not spread to nearby tissue.
Stage IA:	A very small amount of cancer was found to be visible under the microscope and is found deeper in the tissue.
Stage IB:	Here a larger amount of cancer cells were found in the tissue.
Stage II:	The cancer has spread to the nearby tissue but is still found inside the primary site.
Stage IIA:	Cancer has spread beyond the primary site.
Stage IIB:	Cancer has spread to other tissue around the primary site.
Stage III:	Cancer has spread throughout the nearby area.
Stage IV:	Cancer has spread to other parts of the body.
Stage IVA:	Cancer has spread to organs close to the pelvic area.
Stage IVB:	Cancer has spread to distant organs, such as the lungs.
Recurrent:	Cancer has recurred at the same location where the original tumour was or at a different location after it has been treated and supposedly eliminated.

CANCER GLOBALLY

Each year cancer is newly diagnosed in 10 million people worldwide and account for 7.1 million deaths (12.5% of the global total). It is second to cardiovascular disease as a cause of death in developing countries, which causes overall 10% of all deaths in the world. People usually regard it as a problem of the developing world, but more than half of all cancers are seen in the three-quarters of the world's population who live in the developed countries. According to the World Health Organization (WHO) global cancer rates could increase by 50% to 15 million by 2020. This sharp and alarming increase in cancer rates both in developed and developing is due to steadily aging populations in countries, present trends in smoking prevalence along with the growing adoption of unhealthy lifestyles (WHO, 2003).

Malignant tumours were responsible for 12% of the nearly 56 million deaths worldwide, it developed in 5.3 million men and 4.7 million women. Altogether 6.2 million died, in the year 2000. In developing countries cancer has appeared as a main public health problem. However, the likelihood of being diagnosed with cancer in developed countries is twice as high as in developing countries. The highest over all cancer rates for industrial nations are: United States of America (USA), Italy, Australia, Germany, The Netherlands, Canada and France, and the lowest cancer rates for developing countries were Northern Africa, Southern and Eastern Asia (WHO, 2003).

Lung cancer is the most common cancer worldwide, accounting for 1.2 million new cases annually, of which the main cause is smoking and other causes include domestic and industrial pollution. A clear linear dose-response relationship exists between magnitude of cancer and the period of smoking as well as the amount smoked. Cancer of the breast follow lung cancer by, just over 1 million cases; colorectal, 940 00; stomach, 870 000; liver, 560 000; cervical, 470 000; oesophageal, 410 000; head and neck, 390 000; bladder, 330 000; malignant non-Hodgkin lymphomas, 290 000; leukaemia, 250 000; prostate and testicular, 250 000; pancreatic, 216 000; ovarian, 190 000; kidney, 190 000; endometrial, 188 000; nervous system, 175 000; melanoma, 133 000; thyroid, 123 000; pharynx, 65 000; and Hodgkin disease, 62 000 cases. One should however note that the three leading killers differ from the three most common forms of cancer. Of all the cancer deaths in the world, according to the WHO (2003) the three leading killers are: lung cancer responsible for 17.8% fatal cases, then stomach cancer at 10.4% and liver cancer at 8.8%.

More than a quarter of deaths are attributed to cancer in many countries. As many as one third of cancers worldwide could be prevented by healthy lifestyles, and tobacco use the most preventable cause of cancer in the world. Although, childhood cancers (aged one to 14) are rare and largely curable if detected early through modern molecular and imaging technology e.g. PET scanning for lymphomas, the treatment options is limited. Cancer causes the second most deaths, in children world wide. Three in five children (80 116 or 92%) still die in developing countries because of cancer and 133 931 (83%) cases are newly diagnosed each year. In developed countries childhood cancers are newly diagnosed in 26 864 (17%) children and account for 6 863 deaths annually (Tynes *et al.*, 2003).

Unproven Methods or Medical Intervention for Cancer Treatment

Regardless of widespread positive research data from experimental and preclinical studies the existing importance and potential of botanical medicines used in cancer treatment remains largely untapped, but at the same time it is recognized with the rising of an integrative model. Multiple factors including, historical, political, and cultural factors in conjunction with confusion within the principles and practice of botanical medicine are invariably responsible for this.

All over the world cancer patients use various forms of treatments, drugs and other unproven or questionable methods such as homeopathy, folk medicines, vitamins, healing "psychological" treatments, herbs, different dietary patterns rich in fruit, vegetables and herbs. In German speaking countries a high frequency (52%-65%) of complementary or conventional methods are used as curative or alternative treatment. Some products or medicine are country specific (in the Netherlands the Moerman diet, Ayurvedic medicine in India, Chinese medicine) and others are however used world wide: mistletoe and vitamins. From countries in Asia, Africa and the entire Africa there is a lack of data although it is know that traditional/folk medicine are used there.

Complementary and/or alternative methods are ones that include diagnostic tests, methods of treatment or preventative treatments which are not scientifically tested or proven. Most of the time these methods or treatments for cancer are either unique or extra treatments (complementary to classical ones) that can be given either according to classical concepts of cancer treatment or according to a new concept of the world and life. It was found that women and the members of the upper socioeconomic class (in the Western countries) are more frequently using these unproven methods since they are sometimes expensive. Unproven methods or treatments, easily accessed world wide via the Internet, are mostly used by patients with a chronic or terminal disease.

Cancer Prevention

The WHO world cancer report (WHO, 2003) provides clear evidence that healthy lifestyles and public health action, governments and health practitioners could stem this trend, and prevent as many as one third of cancers world wide. If we all take action now today we can prevent one third of all cancers, cure another third and provide good palliative care to the remaining third. Cancer chemoprevention is defined as pharmacological intervention with synthetic or naturally occurring compounds that may prevent, inhibit, or reverse carcinogenesis, or prevent the development of invasive cancer.

Examples of where this immediate action can make differences are as follows:

- The reduction of tobacco (major preventable cause) and alcohol consumption. Complete prevention is possible for all cancers due to cigarette smoking and excess alcohol consumption (WHO, 2003).
- A healthy lifestyle and diet which consists of frequent high fruit and vegetable consumption (more than 400 g/day) and physical activity is the second preventable cause of cancer (WHO, 2003). An overall energy imbalance is the result of a Western lifestyle (highly caloric diet, rich in fat, refined carbohydrates and animal protein) together with low physical activity. In western countries, approximately 30% of cancers are caused by dietary factors and in developing countries about 20% (WHO, 2003). About 20% of all cancers could be prevented with a healthy diet. Daily consumption of fruit, vegetables and herbs such as broccoli, grapes, cabbage, sprouts, peanuts, ginko biloba, and garlic prove to reduce the incidence of cancer especially stomach cancer associated with *Helicobacter pylori*. It was also found that woman could reduce the risk of ovarian cancer by 60% with a dietary supplement derived from ginko biloba and a daily sulphide supplement can reduce DNA damage in breast epithelial cells treated with carcinogens produced when protein-rich foods are cooked at high temperatures (WHO, 2003).

Early detection through screening especially for breast, cervical, colon, rectum, cervix, prostate, oral cavity, and skin may cure cancer. Today more than 80 per cent of all cervical cancer deaths occur in developing countries because they do not have excellent public health infrastructure. Other good examples are that of breast cancer which is detected by mammography, it may reduce breast cancer mortality by 25 to 30 per cent and in nationwide screening programmes a reduction of 20 per cent appears feasible. Lower mortality rates for prostate cancer due to screening by assessment of serum prostate specific antigen (PSA) levels, but early lesion management is still extremely invasive. A colonoscopy for colon cancer is considered the gold standard although extensive medical resources are needed for use in population-based screening programmes (WHO, 2003).

- Curb infections which cause cancer, because up to 23% of malignancies in developing countries are caused by infectious agents. These agents include hepatitis B and C virus (liver cancer), *Helicobacter pylori* (stomach cancer) and human papilloma viruses (cervical and ano-genital cancers). Roughly eight per cent of all malignancies at some stage in cancers are caused by chronic infections in developed countries (WHO, 2003). The solution designed for preventing these cancers could be vaccinations. In high-incidence countries it was shown that liver cancer could be prevented by Hepatitis B virus (HBV) vaccination and in a few years time vaccination might be possible for human papilloma virus (HPV).

CANCER TREATMENT

Cancer is treated by:

Surgery

Surgery is the oldest and most frequently used cancer therapy utilized to eradicate cancer. However, a very drastic measurement, but is the most efficacious in the treatment of local disease in the region of the primary tumour and in regional lymphatics. Although surgery is no longer believed to be the sole therapy for several neoplasms it is still preferred in a high percentage of cases. In the management of the disease especially with multiple metastasis, once a neoplasm has spread from the primary site to a distant organ surgery should have little role since many types of cancer are currently managed by the use of chemotherapy and radiation therapy in combination with surgery (Fang, 2006). The extent of surgery procedure required has therefore, reduced considerably.

Radiation

Today, a wide range of malignancies are treated with radiation and it has become a standard treatment option. Radiation treatment is frequently included in primary oncological treatment as revealed by the data from the Epidemiology and End Results (SEER) program (US Surveillance). More than half of all cancer patients receive radiotherapy in their care if subsequent palliative interventions are included (Fang, 2006). Small to moderate amounts of radiation can enhance apoptosis in certain tissue without producing necrosis. Radiation therapy/radiotherapy act mainly by inducing apoptosis and the degree differ extremely from one tumour to another. Cancer cell resistance can occur as a result of defects in the apoptotic pathway. Cells that are mostly susceptible are differentiating spermatogonia, gut crypts, rapidly proliferating cells in the fetus and lymphocytes. The way in which radiation triggers the apoptotic cascade in normal and neoplastic cells seems to involve the p53 tumour suppressor gene (Kerr et al., 1994).

Chemotherapy

Cancer treatment via chemotherapy was introduced more than 50 years ago into the clinic (Johnstone *et al.*, 2002). Toxic drugs are needed in most cases of chemotherapy treatment in patients which often result in unpleasant side effects, but the beneficial effects of these toxic drugs outweigh their adverse reactions. Bagchi and Preuss (2005), therefore, defined chemo preventative agents as any or all natural or synthetic compounds that can suppress, inhibit or reverse the development and progression of cancer.

The focus during cancer therapy is on strategies to trigger the apoptotic program so that tumour growth can be suppressed in the cell. Ear-

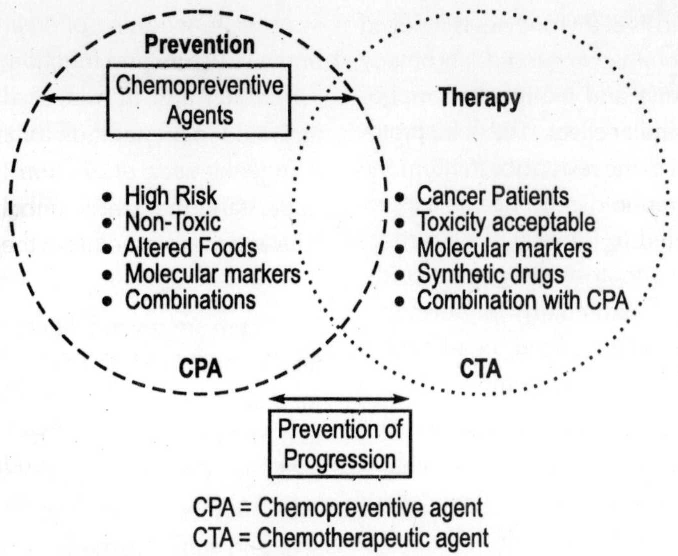

Fig. 5.2: Schematic diagrams showing the range of efficacy of chemopreventative agents (Bagchi and Preuss, 2005).

lier, various cancer chemotherapy agents were proofed to affect tumour cell killing by launching apoptosis (Lee *et al.*, 2003). Secondary metabolites from natural products such as plants and microbes contribute towards chemotherapy and play an important role in the amelioration of cancers. Plant materials (edible and nonedible) have phytochemicals present which may function as chemo preventative or chemotherapeutic agents (Bagchi and Preuss, 2005). Newman and his co-workers conducted a study on the analysis of the antineoplastic drugs that are available in western countries and Japan, out of the 140 compounds, 54% were found to be from natural products (14%), natural product derivatives (26%), or compounds made by total synthesis, but modelled on natural product leads (14%). Three major types of chemo preventive agents derived from their activities have been identified to be of plant origin i.e. inhibitors of carcinogen configuration (mainly by formation of nitrosoamines from secondary amines), blocking agents (to prevent carcinogens from reaching or reacting to target sites) and repressing agents or anti-progression agents (Mukherjee *et al.*, 2001).

With carcinogens there are a sequence in which things happen — initiation, promotion and progression. Chemotherapy begins where chemoprevention ends, at the stage of progression. The stage where promotion ends and progression begins (Fig. 5.2) is not very clear. Chemo preventative agents can conceptually reach a point in time where they can be effectively made use of for blocking cancer progression (Bagchi and Preuss, 2005).

Hormones

According to Kerr and his co-workers (1993), "apoptosis is involved in the atrophy of endocrine-dependent organs, such as prostate and adrenal cortex, that follows withdrawal of hormonal stimulation, and as might be expected, it also is enhanced in hormone-dependant tumours after successful ablation therapy". In contrast to this they also found that, apoptosis of thymocytes is induced by increased levels of glucocorticoid, and many lymphocytic leukaemia and malignant lymphomas demonstrated a similar effect. The bcl-2 proto-oncogene is involved in the resistance to hormone therapy. In some lymphoid cell lines its expression has been revealed to be related with resistance to induction of apoptosis via glucorticoids. No effective cure exists particularly for hormone-independent cancer and advanced breast cancer that is highly resistant to chemotherapy.

Cancer is a global problem since intrinsic and acquired drug resistance occurs due to the adaptability of tumour cells and therefore, the need for new anticancer agents is urgent. Most of the cell killing anticancer drugs used today also affect normal cells; therefore the challenge remains to find way to kill cancer cells specifically.

Cell Death

Lately, researchers from a range of various fields of biology and medicine (such as cell and molecular biology, oncology, immunology, embryology, endocrinology, haematology, and neurology) took interest in of cell death (irreversible loss of vital cellular structure and function) as focus topic (Darzynkiewicz *et al.*, 1997). Cell death, or "point-of-no-return" (Trump *et al.*, 1997), was also termed cell necrobiology since it is associated with a variety of life processes. Humans and animals depend permanently on cell death as part of their development and it continues into adulthood. Other functions of cell death include the elimination of lymphocytes that have reached their age, it also plays an important role where it helps control cell numbers by removing excess cells: neutrophils (a type of white blood cell), and during fatal development it carves out cavities or divide digits to sculpt the different parts of the body. A complex cascade of biological processes, also normally part of a cells life (pathways, enzyme systems, functioning of organelles, plasma membrane structure and function, modulation of transcriptional and translational activities etc.) was activated in preparation for and during cell death (Darzynkiewicz *et al.*, 1997). It is also vital to understand that every cell is programmed to die subsequent to a suitable stimulus (Trump *et al.*, 1997).

There are several different forms of cell death. Studies of dying cells have demonstrated the need for precise definitions of various forms of cell death that include apoptosis, oncosis, necrosis and autophagy. Cell death is generally divided into two different mechanisms which are mutually exclusive and stand in sharp contrast, apoptosis (programmed cell death) and necrosis (accidental cell death) which are the two fundamental types of cell death (Table 5.2) (Darzynkiewicz *et al.*, 1997). Apoptosis and necrosis differ in their mechanism of induction.

Different forms of cell death are: 'apoptosis', 'necrosis', 'oncosis' and 'autophagy'. The pre-lethal response (reaction to injury prior to cell death often reversible) to cell death can be divided into two major categories known as apoptosis and oncosis, the pattern linking between these two types obviously depend on both the cell type and the injury. The post-mortem autolytic and degradative cellular changes are termed necrosis; in fact there are anyhow two forms of necrosis: apoptotic necrosis and oncotic necrosis (Trump *et al.*, 1997). The necrotic step can either follow apoptosis or oncosis, these cells are termed late necrotic cells (Darzynkiewicz *et al.*, 1997). This makes cell death even more complex. According to (Darzynkiewicz *et al.*, 1997), studies of the proceedings that take place throughout both apoptosis and oncosis could be referring to the term cell necrobiology, whereas the post-mortem events of necrosis refer to cell necrology. The detailed description of all four forms of cell death is as follows:

Table 5.2: Apoptosis and Necrosis

Apoptosis	*Necrosis*
Trigger for cell death	
Intrinsic (pathway mitochondria-dependant)	Extrinsic (ligand receptor interaction)
Generated by signals within the cell	Triggered by death activators binding to receptors at the cell surface
Involves the participation of the mitochondria that release caspase-activating proteins.	Represented by tumour necrosis factor (TNF), family of receptors
Proteins of the Bc12 family proteins govern mitochondria-dependant apoptosis	TNF receptors utilize protein interaction modules known as death domains and death effector domains (DEDS) to assemble receptor-signalling complexes. Receptor-signalling complexes recruit and activate cell death proteases, namely pro-caspase 8 and 10.
Cell morphology	
Cell shrinks dramatically due to blebbing and produces apoptotic bodies	Cell swells and lose integrity of cell membrane due to influx of H_2O
Membranes and organelles remain intact	Outer membrane and organelle membranes rupture leading to non-specific release of damaging enzymes like DNAase and proteases
Nucleus condenses	Nucleus swells
Pyknosis and karyorrhexis (dense condensation of chromatin)	Karyolysis preceded by irregular chromatin clumping
Single cells affected	Groups of cells affected
DNA degradation	
Apoptosis exhibits internucleosomal DNA degradation	Necrosis exhibits random DNA degradation
Caused by activation of specific nucleases	Caused by intracellular enzymes released upon organelle membrane rupture or caused by random enzymes
Inflammatory response	
No inflammatory response because membranes remain intact	Extensive inflammatory response due to release of intracellular material from the necrotic cell
Synthesis of anti-inflammatory agents occurs that results from actual upregulation of certain apoptotic gene products	Inflammation can further damage normal tissue
Activation of proteases	
Activation of caspases (cysteine proteases) that specifically cleave substrates with aspartic acid residue	Lyposomal rupture leads to release of many non-specific destruction of cell proteins
Genetic regulation	
Under strict genetic control	Induction by harsh cellular environment

Apoptosis

Kerr *et al.*, (1993) was first to describe the distinct morphological features of programmed cell death, and coined the term apoptosis (Huppertz *et al.*, 1999). Apoptosis was derived from a Greek word which is put in plain words as "falling off" as used to describe the leaves falling from trees. Generally it is accepted that cells have the ability to undergo an internally controlled cell suicide process known as apoptosis, which happens in response to an environmental agent, or given stimulus (Schwartzman and Cidlowski, 1993). Directed destruction of a cell by apoptosis can only happen if sufficient time was given to arrange a sequence of intracellular events (Huppertz *et al.*, 1999). Dying by apoptosis is therefore, an energy-dependant (Halestrap, 2005), tidy regulated and controlled death (quickly and neatly) that expends energy in the ATP form (Edinger and Thompson, 2004). Programmed cell death is used synonymously with apoptosis (multifocal single-cell death) as a type of "natural" death. The functional term, programmed cell death, is used to explain a cell death that is typical of life for a multicellular organism, alternatively, apoptosis (descriptive term) is used to explain a type of cell death that display a unique set of several morphological features that does not come for free. However, the characteristic features of apoptosis together with the organization of multiple gene-directed energy-dependant biological processes that is crucial for apoptosis to take place need to be observed during programmed cell death to classify it together with apoptosis. Therefore, to avoid misunderstanding, it is suggested that apoptosis and programmed cell death have to be used with care (Martin *et al.*, 1994).

The apoptotic mechanism of cell death or programmed cell death plays a fundamental role in the normal development of tissues and organisms through monitoring tissue homeostasis by balancing cell proliferation (opposite role to mitosis) (pathological cell accumulation occur in cancer) (Kerr *et al.*, 1993; Van Engeland et al., 1998) and takes place in a variety of settings following a range of microbiological and chemical injuries in various different organ systems (Trump *et al.*, 1997). It also affects numerous pathological and physiological processes (Schwartzman and Cidlowski, 1993), such as death of tumour cells and viral hepatitis (acidophilic bodies), alternatively to, embryonic tissue modelling and adult tissue turnover and differentiation, respectively (Buja *et al.*, 1993). It is frequently marked with atrophy (for example in the prostate following castration) and regression in adult disease (Trump *et al.*, 1997). Apoptosis is similar to proliferation and differentiation and is frequently started by specific receptor-ligand interactions (Huppertz *et al.*, 1999). Via an asynchronous way, apoptosis affects small groups of cells or single cells. Apoptosis is characterized by a distinct set of morphological, specific structural alterations and biochemical features as a consequence of these complex mechanisms it lead to (or consist of the following characteristics): dehydration (loss of intracellular water and ions which leads to condensation of the cytoplasm), cell shrinkage, cytoplasm condense, formation of blebs in the cell surface or multiple cytoplasmic protrusions (typically containing organelles), nuclear/chromatin condensation/coalesce/clumping, proteolysis, nuclear fragmentation, internucleosomal deoxyribonucleic acid (DNA) cleavage, apoptotic body formation, on a background of resolute reliability of the plasma membrane (Huppertz *et al.*, 1999; Martin *et al.*, 1994).

During the process of apoptosis, DNA fragmentation (double-stranded DNA cleavage) involves activation of endonuclease, which characteristically breaks the DNA between the clumps of chromatin (DNA cleavage at inker regions between nucleosomes) that are referred to as nucleosomes (Buja *et al.*, 1993), the consequence of this is that the DNA breaks into fragments of rather precise sizes that are multiples of about 200 DNA base pairs (bp) (180 bp and multiplicity of 180 bp) in length (Fang, 2006). The products of DNA degradation are nucleosomal and oligonucleosomal DNA fragments (Kerr *et al.*, 1993), which create a distinctive "ladder" pattern during agarose gel electrophoresis. However, some cell types stop at the creation of 300 to 50 kilo-base pair (kb) sized DNA fragments (Darzynkiewicz, 1997). They do not continue with DNA fragmentation until nucleosomal sized fragments are formed. During the DNA cleavage process the nucleus starts to break into fragments, similarly the cell splits into pieces, this was referred to as karyorrhexis (Fang, 2006). Sealed package fragments / membrane-enclosed (plasma membrane) (apoptotic bodies) with well-preserved organelles (Kerr *et al.*, 1993), are formed as a result of apoptosis and by this avoid inflammation that is caused by the uncontrolled release of intracellular contents and therefore apoptosis can be regarded as an injury-limiting mode of cell disposal. However, some exceptions do exist even though the inflammatory response is rare (Trump et al., 1997). Thereafter, healthy neighbouring epithelial cells gradually digest or engulf these fragments by phagocytosis that forms a phagosome (Kerr *et al.*, 1993; Buja *et al.*, 1993). These apoptotic bodies are then degraded within the neighbouring epithelial cells by their lysosomes, which happen within hours.

There are numerous triggers well-known to be involved the activation of apoptosis such as the action of activators, effectors, and negative regulators for example removal of growth factors, DNA damage, Fas ligand (FasL) binding, use of chemotherapeutic agents, etc. (Van Engeland *et al.*, 1998). During the apoptotic cell death process a complex cascade-like sequence of biological of events can be observed (Huppertz *et al.*, 1999; Darzynkiewicz, 1997). These processes involves the activation of many diverse enzymes systems, regulatory pathways, maintenance and frequently modulation of transcriptional and translational activities, transformation of cell organelles activity, alteration of the cell plasma membrane structure. A relatively short launch of the alleged 'execution phase' of the apoptotic process is determined by the activation of the proteolytic cascade. Breakdown of cellular proteins (the nuclear matrix, cytoskeleton and the poly-adenosine diphosphate (ADP)-ribose polymerase) is a consequence of either the direct activation of the caspase family proteases or through lunching other cellular proteases (calpain or proteasomes) (Van Engeland *et al.*, 1998).

Among individual cell types differing in the steps of the apoptosis cascade may occur. This cascade of molecular events leads to the cells' total disintegration. There is a close link between apoptosis and the differentiation process that simultaneously create additional complexity in the difficulty of the apoptosis cascade. Both pathways (apoptosis and the differentiation process) was found to partly use the same machinery (1) association of caspases (termed executioners through the apoptosis cascade) in lens fibre differentiation; (2) Cleavage of lamins as well as TUNEL (TdT-mediated dUTP nick end labeling) reactivity (DNA cleavage) in the deadly differentiation of erythroid cells; (3) in syncytial fusion apoptosis-induced phosphatidylserine flip result in the formation of placental syncytiotrophoblast (Huppertz *et al.*, 1999).

Different patterns of apoptosis have been identified: early and delayed apoptosis, homo-phase, homo-cycle and post-mitotic apoptosis. On exposure (for a few hours) to a fairly high concentration of toxic agents, many cell types (especially "apoptosis primed cells") rapidly undergo apoptosis..Here, apoptosis occur in the same cell cycle, or the same phase when the injury is brought on the cell, it is an example of early apoptosis. Homo-phase apoptosis is the term used to define the apoptosis that happens in the same phase of the cell cycle wherein the cells are originally exposed to the apoptosis inducing agent. At a particular phase, during homo-phase apoptosis, the cells stay arrested (or traverse it slowly) and die without continuing into the next phase of the cell cycle. Homo-cycle apoptosis is used to define when apoptosis is taking place in the same cell cycle where the cells are exposed to the noxious agent (initially), excluding the specifying cell cycle phase, so the cells die before, or during the first mitosis following induction of the injury. The phrase post-mitotic apoptosis is used to describe the process of apoptosis happening in the cell cycle(s) after the one where the cells are originally exposed to the harmful agent, it is also indicative of a delayed apoptosis which frequently happen as the cells are pulse-exposed to a fairly low concentration of noxious agents and afterwards they are permitted to grow within drug free media (Darzynkiewicz *et al.*, 1997). During post-mitotic apoptosis, apoptosis occurs due to damage to the genes which are vital for survival.

In recent years, an explosion of studies on apoptosis has clarified that it represents the mode of death that is a complex process actively driven by the cell (Fang, 2006). Currently there is an avalanche of interest, excitement and revelation in understanding of how cells undergo the process of apoptosis or evolutionary conserved process programmed cell death and basic mechanism that triggers it. Solving the puzzle of apoptosis by knowing how, why and when cells are instructed to die will improve our understanding of many basic biological processes and may provide insights to the aging process, autoimmune syndromes, degenerative diseases and malignant transformations. It will point to the development of potentially new targets for therapeutic treatment of diseases that show an imbalance between cell proliferation and cell loss and can result in major therapeutic implications for anticancer drugs (Martin *et al.*, 1994; Van Engeland *et al.*, 1998; Kuan and Passaro, 1998). One of the major obstacles in the successful treatment of cancer with drugs is failure to activate apoptosis (Cummings *et al.*, 2004).

It is however, surprising to see that in cancer cells the death programme never give the impression that it is completely inactivated, since cancer cells get progressively more malignant as they improve their ability to survive and proliferate through the accumulation of mutations. Cancer cells have evolved with random selection and mutation a process and therefore, mutations that inactivate apoptosis have to be beneficial to cancer cells. Viability assays or colorimetric assays are commonly used when anticancer substances screenings are completed. This approach however has an inherent problem: all compounds which are toxic and growth inhibitory will give positive results, irrespective of the mechanism used to kill the cells (Hagg *et al.*, 2002). Therefore, a great need exist for an assay that is able to screen compounds that specifically induce apoptosis.

Necrosis

Necrosis, an ancient word, "accidental" cell death or degenerative cell death is induced by a wide variety of external and noxious stimuli such as lethal chemicals, biological or physical events, that include hyperthermia, complement attack, ischemia, metabolic poisons, hypoxia and direct cell trauma (Huppertz *et al.*, 1999; Schwartzman and Cidlowski, 1993). As a result, cells die by an uncontrolled, energy-independent process (Halestrap, 2005), and is the consequence of a passive (Kuan and Passaro, 1998), catabolic, degenerative process (Darzynkiewicz *et al.*, 1997), which is identified primarily by the loss of membrane integrity and their contents (Fang, 2006). Necrosis explains the alterations that cells and tissue endure following their death in a living organism (Trump *et al.*, 1997).

The alterations in the phase of necrosis are alike subsequent to either apoptosis or oncosis

(Trump *et al.*, 1997). Necrosis exhibits distinctive morphological and biochemical characteristics. Early changes include swelling of the cytoplasm and organelles (endoplasmic reticulum, lysosomes, and other vesicles), especially mitochondria (intracellular organelles that produce ATP), with only minor changes in the nucleus (Schwartzman and Cidlowski, 1993). Pathologic in that injury is produced and the insult causes lyses/rupture of cell membranes after which the cytosol leak into the surroundings or extracellular space (Kuan and Passaro, 1998). These morphological alterations are caused by failure in the control of the plasma membrane's selective permeability and is in reaction to the early loss of membrane ion-pumping activities that are either directly caused by injury to the membrane or secondary to cellular energy exhaustion. Tremendous cellular swelling occurs as the outcome of fluid shifts associated with cations that move across the membrane along concentration gradients. Prior to membrane-bound phospholipases activation, free cytosolic calcium (Ca^{2+}) increases. Widespread disruption of membranes arises based on the activation membrane-bound phospholipases that bring about disruption of membrane phospholipids (Schwartzman and Cidlowski, 1993). This then leads to an irritant effect on the nearby cells and therefore, causes exacerbated injury which leads to consequent inflammation. Kinins are released from cytosol, of organelles without strong membranes (easily injured) such as the mitochondria, into the surrounding tissue to incite inflammation, edema (capillary dilation) and macrophage aggregation ensue (Kuan and Passaro, 1998). Strong membrane organelles (e.g. nucleus) on the other hand remain intact. Thereafter, it can take hours or days for the inflammatory response to occur around the dying cell and eventually will subside and leaves traces of its presence by the formation of a scar. Three stages occur during the pathophysiology of membrane injury: (1) distinct change in ionic transport systems of membranes, (2) non-specific increase in membrane permeability, and (3) physical membrane disruption and violation (Buja *et al.*, 1993).

Cells start to die by necrosis, for example, after a heart attack or stroke, when the blood supply to an area of the heart or brain is disrupted by a clot (Halestrap, 2005). Significant ATP depletion (level incompatible with cell survival) allegedly are initiated primarily by cellular 'accidents' such as toxic insults or irreparable physical damage (Edinger and Thompson, 2004). If a cell is deprived from a supply of ATP or if violation of the plasma membrane occurs every cell is entirely programmed for death, and this is however, what is frequently overlooked (Trump *et al.*, 1997).

Oncosis

Oncosis is derived from the Greek word "swelling", originally used by von Recklinghausen in 1910, hence, pathologists use the term to explain cell death related with cell swelling. Early changes in oncosis include obvious alterations in the cell shape and volume. These marked adjustments occur with in seconds to minutes following application of injury (Trump *et al.*, 1997). During slow ischemia, for example in during bone formation the loss of osteocytes entombed in the bone, is when oncosis occur. In a variety of systems it has been found that the features of oncosis are identical to that observed in the early phase of accidental cell death (Darzynkiewicz *et al.*, 1997). Key features of oncosis viewed during in vivo (affects broad areas or zones) studies include displaying blebs (detaching later) along the luminal borders and vascular spaces and formation of casts in the lumens of the nephrons in the kidney. The common characteristics of oncosis are plasma membrane transport violation, dissolution of remnants of chromatin (karyolysis, autolytic processes etc. early and reversible protein denaturation. Formerly, in some situations oncosis was described to take part in programmed cell death (Trump *et al.*, 1997).

Autophagy

Non-apoptotic forms of programmed cell death have been described and classified as programmed necrosis or autophagic cell death (Edinger and Thompson, 2004). Cellular signal pathways are therefore used to set off necrosis in response to specific cues before accidental death occur. Autophagic cell death was formerly classified as separate type of non-apoptotic death although morphological similarities exist. It is different from necrosis and the term autophagy means to eat oneself. In times of famine (nutrient stress), autophagic plays a catabolic role, energy production is used for a survival mechanism, that is activated during the degradation of cellular constituents that arise when cells change to a catabolic metabolic program. In the cytosol a double membrane vesicle is formed to facilitate encapsulation of whole organelles and bulk cytoplasm, this is called an autophagosome, and thereafter, fuses with the lysosome where degradation and recycling of the contents take place. Autophagy also provides a return for injured organelles and long-lived proteins via a turnover mechanism (Edinger and Thompson, 2004). In the end direct contradiction exists on the role of autophagy, it seems as if autophagy is more of a survival strategy than a programmed mechanism of cell kill. But further testing of this theory will go on, particularly with the aim of identifying the genes involved in these processes, so that autophagy could be separated from necrosis.

THE ROLE OF NATURAL PRODUCTS IN WESTERN MEDICINE

Modern medicine has benefited significantly from anecdotal results of their empirical methodology. Presently large numbers of illnesses are treated by choosing necessary candidates for a pharmacopeia that is inadequate (Lewis *et al.* 1995). It is estimated that about 25% of all modern medicines are directly or indirectly derived from higher plants, and 11% of the drugs considered as basic and essential by the World Health Organization (WHO), are of plant origin. More than half of the world's 25 top selling pharmaceuticals, for 1991, owe their origin to a variety of natural source materials. Two of these top selling pharmaceuticals (cyclosporine and mevinolin) are natural products and 12 others are natural product derived (O'Neill, 1993).

The world market in 1997, for over the counter phytomedicinal products was (US) $ 10 billion, with an annual growth of 6.5%. The North American market for products of plant origin reached US$ 2 billion in 1997. Fifty per cent of the phytomedical products in Germany are sold on medical prescriptions. Well-established herbal medicine industries are found in China and India (Rates, 2001). About 60% of the medicines currently available on the market that are derived from natural products are mainly from higher plants as well as most of those are in the trial stages (Calixto, 2000). Higher plants therefore, contribute about one quarter of the prescriptions dispensed. Ethnomedicines represent an important class of natural therapeutics that are used and accepted worldwide. Numerous examples from medicine impressively demonstrate the innovative potential of natural compounds and their impact on drug discovery and development. Traditional healers today still use plants in their crude form of herbal remedies although Western technologies have transformed these plant products into more palatable forms. The search for new plant derived drugs and the recognition and validation of traditional medicine could lead to new strategies to control various diseases. Current literature suggests that traditional healers, operating within many rural communities where local products are more accepted, should become the subject of intense research to establish new ways to strengthen collaboration between the traditional healers and modern health care providers (Ndubani and Hojer, 1999). Natural products play a significant role as source of drug leads in the discovery and understanding of cellular pathways that are a vital component of innovation in the drug discovery process (Guallo *et al.*, 2006).

Development of naturally derived drugs (pharmaceuticals) to clinically active agents took 30 years until in the 1990s. New drugs originating from natural sources in the areas of cancer and infectious diseases are 60% and 75%, respectively (Guallo *et al.*, 2006), between 1981 and 2002. Twenty three new drugs (derived from natural products) between 2001 and 2005, were introduced for the treatment of disorders such as bacterial and fungal infections, cancer, diabetes, dyslipidemia, atopic dermatitis, Alzheimer's disease and genetic diseases such as tyrosineamia and Gaucher disease. Furthermore, a total of 136 natural–product-derived drugs have undergone various stages of clinical development that might be used to treat human diseases in all major therapeutic areas in the future (Lam, 2007). Natural products also had a major impact on cancer chemotherapy. It has been reported that more than 60% of the approved drugs for cancer treatment are natural products or derived from natural products. Currently more than 30% of compounds of microbial origin are undergoing various stages of clinical development for cancer treatment. Marine organisms led to the discovery of two novel anticancer agents which are in Phase I clinical studies (Lam, 2007).

There are several advantages to screen natural products for drug discovery that outweigh their limitations and some are more important, 'quantifiable' advantages: (i) Natural products offer unmatched chemical diversity together with their structural complexity as well as biological potency; (ii) A complementary region of chemical space is occupied by natural products as compared to that of synthetic compounds; (iii) In combinatorial chemistry natural products are used as templates which enables the creation of libraries of analogs, which might have enhanced drug-like properties (e.g. pharmacokinetics, solubility); they also might increase our understanding of the genetics and biosynthesis of natural products so that the guidelines of natural product biosynthesis can be optimized; (iv) Compounds from natural products could possibly lead to the discovery and better understanding of the disease process and pathways involved by using these targets, (v) Synthetic drugs are typical due to their structural modifications where natural products can go straight from 'hit' to a drug (Lam, 2007).

Cancer represents one of the most severe health problems worldwide and two fields that are of utmost importance in drug discovery and clinical therapy is the development of new anticancer drugs and more effective treatment strategies (Altmann and Gertsch, 2007). Today most research is focused on cancer-specific mechanism and its corresponding molecular targets. Also research is focussed on discovering improved cytotoxic agents in the functional inhibition of cellular microtubules for better treatment strategies.

PLANTS AS A SOURCE OF ANTI-CANCER AGENTS

Since the earliest times naturally occurring substances from plants, animals and minerals provided a source of medicine for man. For a long time man has exploited particularly the plant kingdom, which has proved to be very useful for treating most of our ailments. During the course of history, experimentation has succeeded in distinguishing those plants which have beneficial effects from those that are toxic or merely non-effective (Lall, 2000). Throughout the centuries, humans have found through trial and error ways to relieve their pain and sickness. Every cultural group has responded by developing a medicinal system and making use of natural products to cure various aliments because of the fear of disease and death. These traditions may seem strange and magical, others appear rational and sensible, but all of them attempt to overcome illness, suffering and enhance quality of life (Finimh, 2001).

Plants have adapted to the diverse habitats of the world through their physical and biomedical modifications. For thousands of years plants have been used traditionally as a source of treatment for various ailments throughout the world among all human races. Plants have always provided an important source of medicines, and were first used in folk medicine. In ancient times in various cultures worldwide people have always been using holistic means of healing. In contrast to the frequent assumptions, the medicines used by traditional healers are surprisingly effective.

Historically the development of many important classes of drugs relied on natural products that have served as templates (McChesney, 1993). Six major fields of study contribute to the studies on natural products. These include: ethno ecology, traditional agriculture, cognitive ethnobotany, material culture, traditional phytochemistry and paleoethnobotany. Ethnobotany is defined by Cotton (1996) as all the studies, which describe local people's interaction with the natural environment, as well as all the studies, which concern the mutual relationships between plants and traditional people. This definition is a very broad description of a large range of subjects such as ethnomedicine, ethnotaxonomy, ethnoecology etc. Ethnopharmacology on the other hand is known as the scientific evaluation of traditional medicine, which usually excludes spiritual and mythical aspects of plant use. The ability to correlate the ethnobotanical reports with corresponding scientific studies could lead to the improved selection of plants for study in the healthcare system (Lall, 2000). Ethnopharmacology provides an alternative approach for the discovery of medicinal compounds. The results obtained by researchers, ethnobotanists and scientists often justified the use of plants in folk medicine and is a serious basis for the improvement of the efficacy, safety and quality of the plant remedies used worldwide. Conventional western medicine accepts folk medicine only when their efficacy is confirmed (Philp, 2004).

Historically plants have been valuable sources used in the treatment of cancer and many other diseases (Hartwell, 1982). Hartwell published a long list of more than 3000 plants that are being used in the treatment of cancer. In many instances the cancer is undefined and is reported on symptoms that apply to the skin or other visible conditions that sometimes correspond to cancerous conditions. This is a problem because cancer is poorly defined in traditional medicine and folklore. Despite these observations, an essential role have been played by plants as a source of effective anti-cancer agents. Natural sources derived from plants, marine organisms and micro-organisms account for over 60% of currently used anticancer agents (Cragg and Newman, 2005). Nevertheless, a well reputable armamentarium of valuable chemotherapeutic agents have come from approximately five decades of systemic drug discovery and development, together with several significant achievements in the treatment and management of human cancer (Mann et al., 2002). In reality, chemotherapy effectiveness has endured different confounding factors that include systemic toxicity due to lack of specificity, rapid drug metabolism, and both intrinsic and acquired drug resistance. Furthermore the most unpredictable factor affecting chemotherapy is multidrug resistance since tumour cells are very adaptable (Johnstone *et al.*, 2002).

In the 1950s the search for anti-cancer agents from plants sources started to intensify. It was also during this time when the discovery and development of vinblastine and vincristine (vinca alkaloids), and the isolation of the cytotoxic podophyllotoxins took place. This led to the intensive plant collection from temperate regions in the 1960s plus the discovery of novel chemotypes such as the taxanes and camptothecins, which showed a range of cytotoxic activities. Revival of plants and other organisms took place when new screening technologies were developed in the 1986, now the focus was on the tropical and subtropical regions of the world. Even though several anticancer agents are now in the preclinical development no new clinical agents from plants have reached the stage of general use (Cragg and Newman, 2005).

There are many plant-derived anticancer agents which are in clinically use these days. These include the vinca alkaloids/ natural alkaloids vinblastine and vincristine that were isolated in minute quantities from *Catharanthus roseus* G. Don. (Apocynaceae) (Fig. 5.3a, b). Vincristine possesses a formyl group where as vinblastine has a methyl group and despite these small differences their toxicological properties and spectra of antitumour activities differ (Hill, 2001).

During the search for potential oral hypoglycaemic agents it was found that extracts of *C. roseus* reduced white blood cell counts and caused bone marrow depression in rats, and afterwards in mice studies these extracts were active against lymphocytic leukaemia (Cragg and Newman, 2005). Combinational chemotherapy regimes use vincristine as a key component for the treatment of acute lymphocytic leukaemia, a number of childrens solid tumours, acute childhood leukaemia, Hodgkin and non-Hodgkin lymphomas as well as multiple myeloma, breast and small-cell lung cancer in adults. Vinblastine, alternatively, is an essential component of curative chemotherapy regimes used for testes germ cell cancers and advanced Hodgkin disease and it is also frequently used to treat carcinoma of the bladder, breast and Kaposi's sarcoma through combinational therapy with other anti-cancer drugs (Hill, 2001). Vinblastine and vincristine remain in wide spread clinical usage even today. Analogs produced via synthetic modification could possibly have activity against other tumour types, less toxicity and side effects. Several semi-synthetic ana-

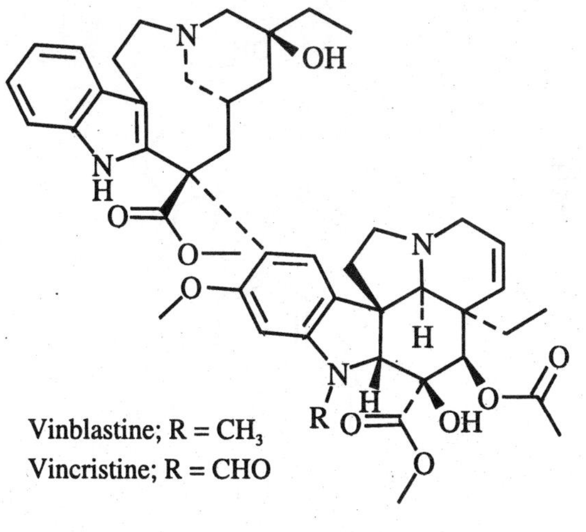

(a)

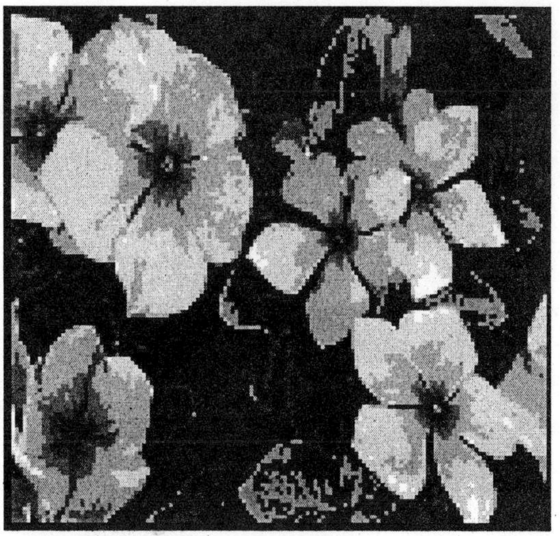

(b)

Fig. 5.3: (a) Natural alkaloids 'Vinblastine' and 'Vincristine' isolated from (b) *Catharanthus roseus* (Cragg and Newman, 2005)

logs were made and the most recent are vinorelbine and vindesine (the C-3 amidoanalog of 4-deacetyl vinblastine). Vindesine when compare with other natural vinca alkaloids has less neurotoxicity, but causes complete remission in acute lymphocytic childhood leukaemia and adult nonlymphocytic leukaemia (Lee, 2003). These semi-synthetic analogs are used in combination with other cancer chemotherapeutic drugs and used against a variety of cancers, breast, lung and highly developed testicular cancers as well as Kaposi's sarcoma (Cragg and Newman, 2005).

Another two semi-synthetic derivatives are etoposide (Fig. 5.4a) teniposide (Fig. 5.4b) of the parent compound epipodophyllotoxin (Fig. 5.4c) (natural product), which is an isomer of podophyllotoxin (Fig. 5.4d). Etoposide and teniposide are clinically used for the treatment of testicular, lymphomas, leukemias and bronchial cancers, but their use is limited due to problems such as drug resistance, poor bioavailability and myelosuppression therefore they need further structural modification. The medicinally used Podophyllum species (Podophyllaceae) from the

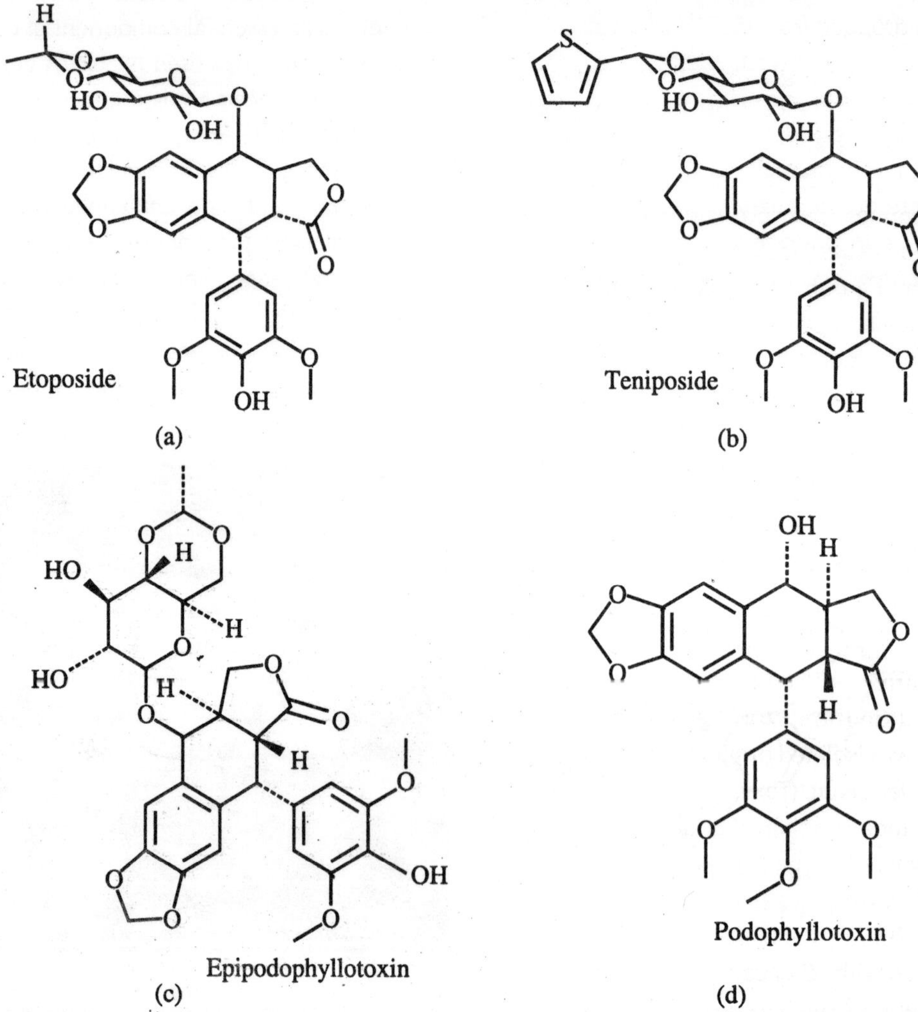

Fig. 5.4: Semi-synthetic derivatives of epipodophyllotoxin, an isomer of podophyllotoxin (a) etoposide and (b) teniposide which are clinically active (c) epipodophyllotoxin (d) podophyllotoxin (Cragg and Newman, 2005).

Indian subcontinent, *Podophyllum peltatum* Linnaeus (commonly known as the American mandrake or Mayapple), and *Podophyllum emodii* Wallich, have been used extensively for the treatment of skin cancers and warts throughout history (Cragg and Newman, 2005). In 1880 the major active constituent, 'podophyllotoxin' was first isolated and only in the 1950s its correct structure was reported. Podophyllotoxin functions as a mitotic inhibitor by binding reversibly to tubilin and it inhibits microtubule assembly (Lee, 2003). Many ligans directly related to podophyllotoxin (podophyllotoxin-like) were reported; several of them were dropped from the clinical trials, due to their unacceptable toxicity and lack of efficacy (Cragg and Newman, 2005). Etoposide and its thiophene analog teniposide are structurally related to podophyllotoxin, but at C-4 they have opposite stereochemistry (â in etoposide and teniposide, á in podophyllotoxin) and different substituents (glycosyl in etoposide and teniposide, OH in podophyllotoxin). The antitumour action of etoposide and its analogs is to inhibit DNA topo II (an essential enzyme) and, then increase DNA cleavage. Etoposides other actions include covalent protein binding by a bio-oxidized E-ring orthoquinone, and metal- and photo-induced cleavage of DNA caused by hydroxyl radicals formed from metal-etoposide complexes (Lee, 2003).

The taxanes were more recently added to the armamentarium of plant-derived chemotherapeutic agents (Kingston, 2005) Paclitaxel (taxol®) (Fig. 5.5a) was isolated originally from the bark of *Taxus brevifolia* Nutt. (Taxaceae) (Pacific Yew) (Fig. 5.5b), and today paclitaxel, together with several key precursors (the baccatins), are found in the leaves of various Taxus species (Cragg and Newman, 2005). Paclitaxel is used alone or in combination with other cancer drugs primarily for the treatment of ovarian, breast, and non-small cell lung cancer (NSCLC). Furthermore it showed efficacy against Kaposi sarcoma, potential treatment of multiple sclerosis, psoriasis and rheumatoid arthritis. It has a unique mode of action; it acts as a mitotic inhibitor by promoting the assembly of microtubules (Lee, 2003) and interacts with the polymerized form of $\alpha\beta$-tubulin (Altmann and Gertsch 2007). Taxol induces apoptosis in proliferating cells through cell cycle arrest at G2/M. From early on, supply was a major obstacle in the development of paclitaxel since it is present only in minute quantities. It led to the synthesis of 'Taxotere', a form of 10-deacetyl-baccatin III which is more readily available. This compound was isolated from the European yew tree (*Taxus baccata* L.). A major renewable natural source was made available to this important class of drugs through the semi-synthetic conversion of baccatins to paclitaxel, and biologically active paclitaxel related analogs, such as docetaxel (Taxotere®) (Cragg and Newman, 2005). Docetaxel is used in the treatment of breast cancer and NSCLC, and has microtubule-stabilizing properties (Altmann and Gertsch 2007). It has also shown efficacy in combination with other cancer drugs such as anthracyclins, prednisone and cisplatin, paclitaxel. Other Taxus species such as *Taxus canadensis* Marshall, *T. baccata* L. and other parts of *T. brevifolia* were used by the Native American tribes for non-cancerous conditions. Only one report for the use of cancer was found for T. baccata in the traditional Asiatic Indian (Ayurvedic) medicine system. Currently another 23 taxanes are in the preclinical stage, 9 are undergoing PhaseI/II clinical development for new and improved as anti-cancer agents, and several other second generation taxanes were selected for clinical development to improve their solubility and activity against drug resistant tumours (Cragg and Newman, 2005; Altmann and Gertsch 2007). Taxanes are popular antitumour agents but clinical resistance poses a treat to their successful treatment. Effective conventional chemotherapy treatment of cancer is difficult due to multidrug resistance (Lucci *et al.*, 1999).

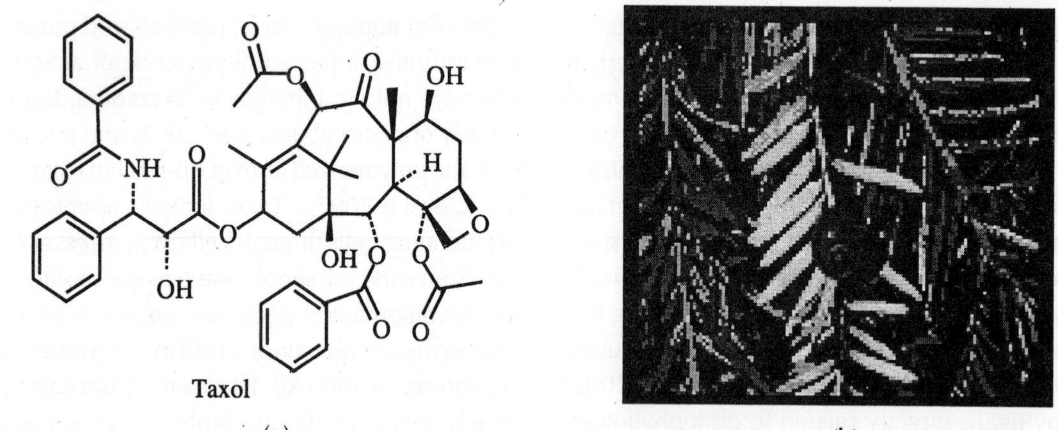

(a) (b)

Fig. 5.5: (a) Taxol isolated from (b) *Taxus brevifolia* (Cragg and Newman, 2005).

From *Camptotheca acuminate* Decne (Nyssaceae) 'camptothecin' (Fig. 5.6), a natural alkaloid, was isolated. Camptothecin is another important addition to the anti-cancer drug armamentarium of clinically active agents. The National Cancer Institute (NCI) (US), advanced camptothecin (as sodium salt) to clinical trials in the 1970s. It caused severe bladder toxicity and was consequently dropped. Topotecan (used for treatment of ovarian and small cell lung cancers) and irinotecan (used for treatment of colorectal cancers) (CPT-11; Camptosar) were developed throughout extensive research and structural modification as more effective derivatives of camptothecin (Cragg and Newman, 2005; Tazi *et al.*, 2005; Lee, 2003). These compounds together with camptothecin were potent antitumour and DNA topo I inhibitory agents (Lee, 1999). Both derivatives are amine-hydrochloride salts. Topotecan was made to be 100-fold more water soluble than the parent compound camptothecin, which is poorly water soluble. Irinotecan was metabolized to be more potent, about 200 to 1000 times more than camptothecin, and in vivo is a phenolic topo I inhibitor. Several second- and third-generation camptothecins e.g. exatecan and diflomotecan are currently undergoing clinical trials (Tazi *et al.*, 2005). Five less toxic, water soluble

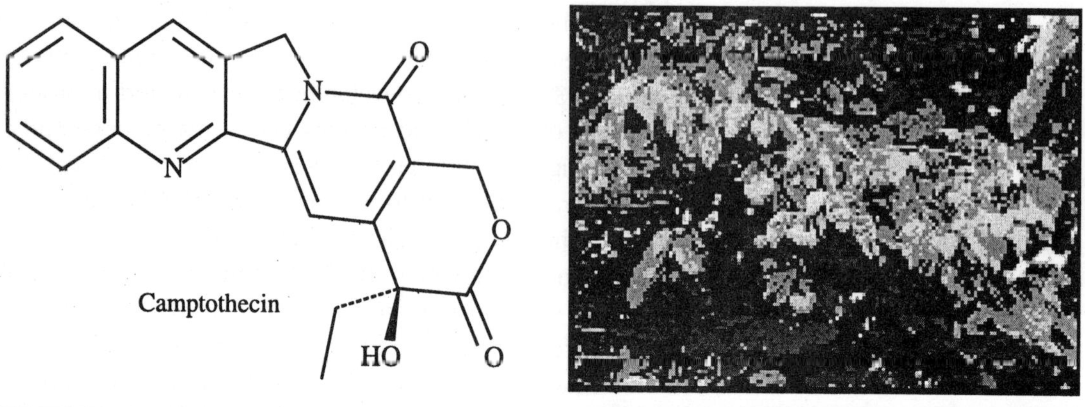

Fig. 5.6: A natural alkaloid 'camptothecin' from *Camptotheca acuminate* (Cragg and Newman, 2005).

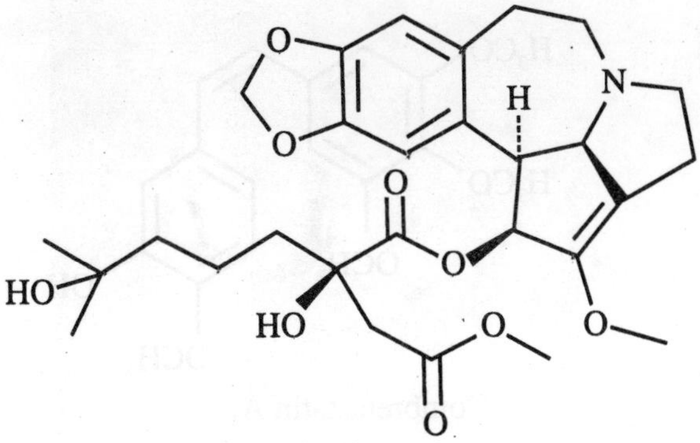

Homoharringtonine

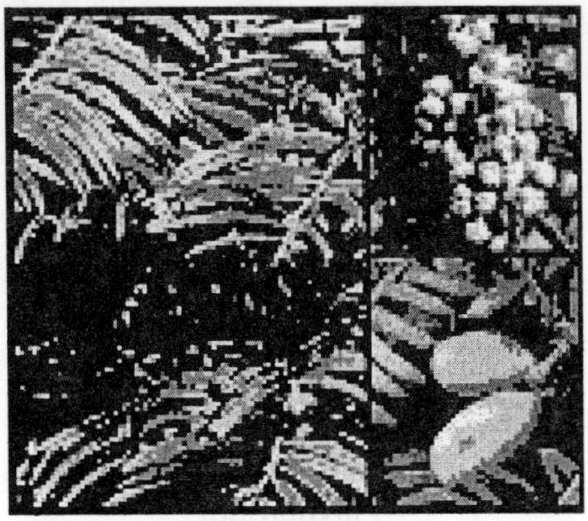

Fig. 5.7: (a) 'Homoharringtonine' isolated from the Chinese tree (b) Cephalotaxus harringtonia var. drupacea (Cragg and Newman, 2005).

synthetic 7-(acylhydrozono)-formyl camptothecins were found to be more potent than camptothecin in causing protein-linked DNA breaks and DNA topo I inhibition (Lee, 2003).

'Homoharringtonine' (HHT) (Fig. 5.7a) was isolated from *Cephalotaxus harringtonia* var. drupacea (Sieb and Zucc.) (Cephalotaxaceae) (Fig. 5.7b). In China, acute myelogenous leukaemia and chronic myelogenous leukaemia is treated effectively with the use of a harringtonine and HHT racemic mixture. In patients with chronic myelogenous leukaemia (CML) in the late chronic phase complete hematologic remission (CHR) has been reported by homoharringtonine and it is effective against various leukaemia. Elliptinium, a derivative of ellipticine, was isolated from a Fijian medicinal plant *Bleekeria vitensis* A.C. Sm. (known for anticancer properties) and species of several genera of the Apocynaceae family, is marketed for treatment of breast cancer in France (Cragg and Newman, 2005). These plant derived agents are also clinically in use.

By systematically screening plant extracts, clinically active agents with antitumour properties can be isolated, their metabolism can be explained as a result more active molecules might be synthesized (Hill, 2001).

PLANT DERIVED ANTICANCER AGENTS IN CLINICAL DEVELOPMENT

From *Dysoxylum binectariferum* Hook. f., Meliaceae family, rohitukine was isolated and this flavonoid structure formed the basis for a novel synthetic flavonoid structure, flavopiridol (Fig. 5.8a). During a structure activity study over 100 synthetic analogs were synthesized. These analogs were tested against a series of breast and lung carcinoma cell lines, in the course of these studies it was found that they have tyrosine kinase activity and potent growth inhibitory activity (Cragg and Newman, 2005). Flavopiridol showed the most potent activity. *In vivo* (in mice) broad spectrum activity was found against human tumour xenografts. The NCI then selected it for preclinical and clinical studies in collaboration with the Hoechst Company; currently it is in 18 Phase I and Phase II clinical trials. Flavopiridol is effectively used alone or in combination with other anticancer agents to treat a broad range of tumours, leukemia, lymphomas and solid tumours (Cragg and Newman, 2005).

In the 1970s the NCI and United States Department of Agriculture (USDA) were working together with the South Africa Botanical Research

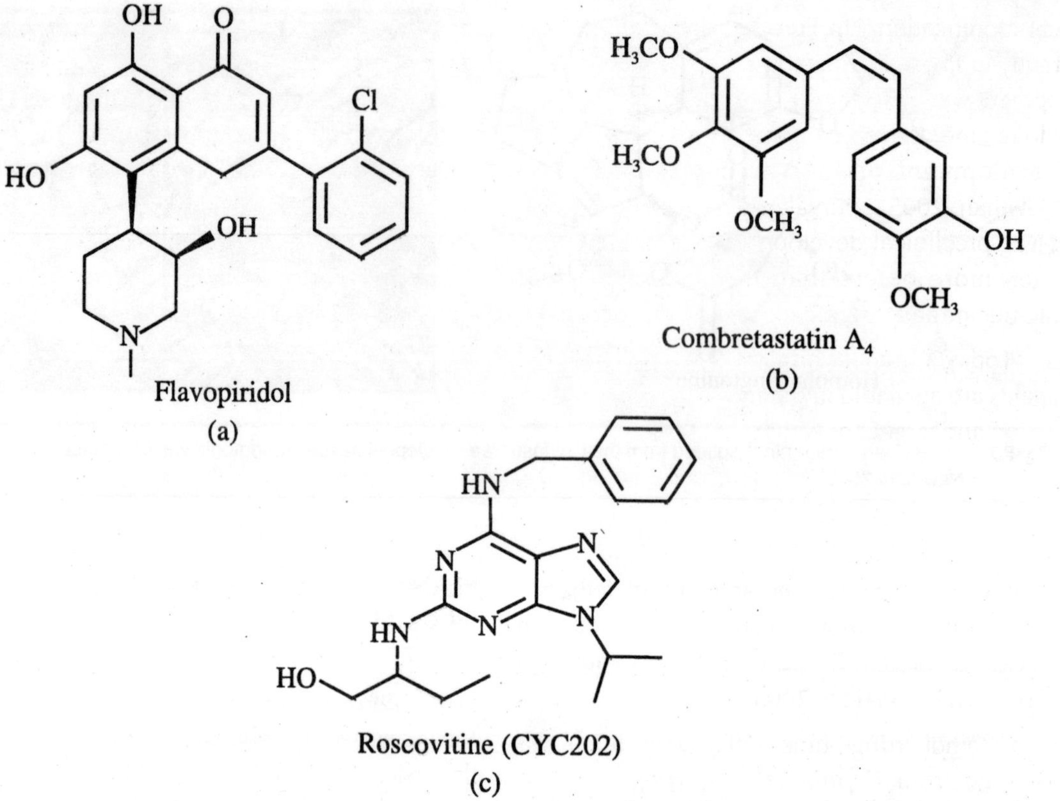

Flavopiridol (a) — Combretastatin A_4 (b) — Roscovitine (CYC202) (c)

Fig. 5.8: (a) A novel synthetic flavonoid 'flavopiridol' (b) One of the water-soluble analogs of the combretastatins, 'combretastatin' phosphate (CA4). (c) 'Roscovitine' derived from olomucine (Cragg and Newman, 2005).

Institute on a random collection program. Combretastatins, a family of stilbenes, were isolated from the South African *Combretum caffrum* (Eckl. & Zeyh.) Kuntze, which was collected as part of that random collection program. The genera Combretum and Terminalia both belong to the family Combretaceae that are used for malaria, hepatitis and a variety of other diseases in Indian and African traditional medicine. Reportedly, several of the Terminalia species have been used for cancer treatment. The combretastatins act as anti-angiogenic agents, they cause tumour necrosis through vascular shutdown in tumours (Cragg and Newman, 2005). One of the water-soluble analogs of the combretastatins, A4 phosphate (CA4) (Fig. 5.8b), has shown promising activity in early clinical trials, and now several mimics are being developed of which three is in clinical trials and another 11 in the preclinical development. By combining medicinal and combinational chemistry a multitude of analogs were synthesized from this chemical class that served as a model which had a relatively simple natural product structure. All of them containing the crucial trimethoxy aryl moiety linked to substituted aromatic moieties through a variety of two or three atom bridges together with heterocyclic rings and sulfonamides.

Olomucine was first isolated from the cotyledons of Raphanus sativus L. (Brassicaceae) (radish) (Meijer and Raymond, 2003). Olomucine inhibit cycline-dependent kinases (Ddk), proteins which play a major role in cell cycle progression. Roscovitine (derived from olomucine) (Fig. 5.8c) is a more potent inhibitor that resulted from chemical modification. In Europe, roscovitine is currently in Phase II clinical trials and further development was also taking place within this series of olomucine derived compounds which led to the development of 'purvalanols' (Cragg and Newman, 2005). Purvalanols is currently undergoing preclinical development because they are even more potent than the natural product olomucine and its synthetic derivative roscovitine.

Today a number of plant derived anticancer agents are available in the market. Their mode of action and target are well known (Table 5.3).

TARGETING NATURAL PRODUCTS

Drug discovery and clinical therapy are extremely important for the development of more effective new anticancer drugs as targeted therapeutics with tailored treatment strategies and regimes. Currently research is focused, due to progress in cancer biology, on cancer-specific mechanisms and molecular targets corresponding to that (Altmann and Gertsch, 2007). Natural products for cancer chemotherapy are often very potent but have limitations in terms of solubility in aqueous solvents and they show narrow therapeutic indices, this caused the termination of a large number of pure natural products such as bruceantin and maytansin (isolated from *Maytenus serrata*) (Cragg and Newman, 2005). Alternatively these agents should be investigated and developed as potential "warheads", by attaching these agents to monoclonal antibodies that are targeted specifically to epitomes on the tumours of interest (Sausville *et al.*, 1999). With the emergence of novel technolo-

Table 5.3: Summary of anticancer agents derived from natural products (Fang, 2006).

Compounds	*Drug name*	*Source*	*Cancer use*	*Mode of action*	*Arrested cell cycle*
Doxorubicin	Adriamycin® Rubexâ	*Streptomyces peucetius* var. caesius (Microbe)	Lymphoma, breast, ovary, lung and sarcomas	Topoisomerase II inhibition and DNA binding	G_2/M phase
Etoposide/Teniposide	Etopophos® VePesid®	*Podophyllum peltatum* (Plant)	Testicular and small cell lung cancer	Topoisomerase II inhibition	S and G_2/M phase
Mitomycin C	Mutamycin®	*Streptomyces lavendulae* (Microbe)	Gastric, colorectal, anal and lung cancer	DNA alkylation and cross linking	Non-specific
Paclitaxel/Docetaxel	Taxol®	*Taxus brevifolia* (Plant)	Ovary, breast, lung, bladder, and head and neck cancer	Promotion of microtubule stabilisation	G_2/M phase
Topotecan/Irinotecan	Hycamtin®	*Camptotheca acuminate* (Plant)	Ovarian, lung and paediatric cancer	Topoisomerase I inhibition	S and G_2/M phase
Vinblastine	Velban® Velbe®	*Catharanthus roseus* (Plant)	Bladder, kidney, lung, leukaemia, prostate and germ-cell ovarian cancer	Microtubule assembly inhibition	M phase
Vincristine	Oncovin® Vincrex®	Catharanthus roseus (Plant)	Leukaemia, lymphoma, neuroblastoma and rhabdomyosarcoma	Inhibition of tubilin polymerization	M phase

gies revived interest in "old" agents could make it possible for them to be developed into effective drugs. Dedicated research over a 20-30 years period for clinical agents such as topotecan, paclitaxel (taxol®), irinotecan and the camptothecin derivatives eventually led to the confirmation of their efficiency.

Revived interest was also found for 'bruceantin' isolated from *Brucea antidysenterica* J.F. Mill. (Simaroubaceae), since it showed substantial activity against panels of leukaemia, lymphoma and myeloma cell lines, as well as in animal models bearing early and advanced stages of the same cancers, (Cragg and Newman, 2005). Previously, bruceantin showed activity in animal models. However, during its clinical trials no objective response was found. Further development was therefore ended. Currently there is strong evidence supporting further development of bruceantin for the treatment of haematological malignancies. Its activity was linked with the down-regulation of (c-MYC), a key oncoprotein (Cragg and Newman, 2005).

Development of new derivatives from natural products with improved antiproliferative profiles and chemo preventive activities is essential, but it can only happen if their molecular mechanism of action, their effects on cellular signalling process is entirely understood as well as their structure-activity relationships. Another vital clinical problem that needs to be tackled is drug resistance (Johnstone *et al.*, 2002).

RATIONALE FOR STUDYING ANTICANCER BOTANICALS

Revival is taking place in medicinal botanicals (including herbal remedies) as part of complementary medicine for disease prevention and therapy as conventional medications have high costs, side effects and therapeutic limitations. Enthusiasm and exceptional growing public interest for botanicals are not only found in the United States where about 40% of the Americans are using alternative medicine, but also in other parts of the world. Reduced risk of cancer was suggested by high consumption of fruits and vegetables in epidemiologic studies. Therefore, the great interests and enthusiasm in naturally occurring phytochemicals for cancer chemoprevention.

Whole botanicals (extracts) are seen as effective and safe to the general public, but investigative and conceptual scientific evidence is difficult to obtain. Extracts, herbal preparations or botanical medicine contain many compounds and pose significantly more conceptually challenges during research than that of a single compound, because they contains unknown components with unknown properties, the different components may act together as a barrier to the toxic effects of a single compound (buffer) and number of different compounds in combination may have synergistic activities (Vickers, 2002). They are also not subjected to the same regulatory standards than the other conventional medicine. Furthermore, possible drug interactions, recommended dosage and schedule create a lot of concern.

There are several reasons why whole botanical extracts, containing many compounds, should be used or may benefit in anticancer treatment because there is the possibility is that whole botanical extracts can decrease the adverse effects as well as synergistic activity. Some have speculated that synergy result from the existence of "redundancy and back-up mechanisms found in the key regulatory and metabolic pathways of the cell". A number of different compounds in combination may have synergistic activity by targeting both primary and back-up mechanisms simultaneously (Darzynkiewicz *et al.*, 2000). The use of whole plant botanicals or extracts could also reduce toxicity because of buffering taking place between the different constituents.

REFERENCES

Altmann KH, Gertsch J. Anticancer drugs from nature-natural products as a uniquesource of new microtubule-stabilizing agents. *Nat Prod Rep*, 24, 327-357, (2007).

Bagchi D, Preuss HG. Phytopharmaceuticals in cancer chemoprevention. CRC Press LLC, pp 32-40 (2005).

Bishop JM, Enemies within: the genesis of retrovirus oncogenes. *Cell,* 23, 5-6, (1981).

Buja LM, Eigenbrodt ML, Eigenbrodt EH. Apoptosis and necrosis basic types and mechanisms of cell death. *Arch Pathol Lab Med*, 117(12), 1208-1214, (1993).

Calixto JB. Efficacy, safety, quality control, marketing and regulatory guidelines for herbal medicines (phytotherapeutic agents). *Braz J Med Biol Res*, 33, 170-189, (2000).

Cotton CM. Ethnobotany principles and applications. John Wiley and Sons, Chichester, pp 1-18, (1996).

Cragg GM, Newman DJ. Plants as a source of anticancer agents. *J Ethnopharmacol*, 100, 72-79, (2005).

Cummings J, Ward TJ, Ranson M, Dive C. Apoptosis pathway-targeted drugs- from the bench to the clinic. *Biochim Biophys Acta*, 1705, 53-66, (2004).

Darzynkiewicz Z, Juan G, Li X, Gorczyca W, Murakami T, Traganos F. Cytometry in cell necrobiology: analysis of apoptosis and accidental cell death (necrosis). *Cytometry*, 27, 1-20, (1997).

Darzynkiewicz Z, Traganos F, Wu JM, Chen S. Chinese herbal mixture PC SPES in treatment of prostate cancer. *Int J Oncol*, 17(4), 729-736, (2000).

Edinger AL, Thompson CB. Death by design: apoptosis, necrosis and autophagy. *Curr Opin Cell Biol*, 16, 339-663, (2004).

Fang R. Investigation of some traditional Chinese medicines used to treat cancer. Dessertation, University of London (2006).

Finimh AC. Encyclopaedia of medicinal plants. Doring Kindersley, London, pp 1-53, (2001).

Guallo VP, McAlpine J, Lam KS, Baker D, Petersen F. Drug discovery from natural products. *J. Ind. Microbiol Biotechnol*, 33, 523-531, (2006).

Hagg M, Biven K, Ueno T, Rydlander L, Bjorklund P, Wiman KG, Shoshan M, Linder S. A novel high-through-put assay for screening of pro-apoptotic drugs. *Invest New Drugs*, 20(3), 253-259, (2002).

Halestrap A. A pore way to die. Nature, 434, 578-579, (2005).

Hartwell JL. Plants used against cancer. Quarterman, Lawrence, MA, pp 75-79, (1982).

Hill BT. Vinflunine, a second generation novel vinca alkaloid with distinctive pharmacological profile, now in clinical development and prospects for future mitotic blockers. *Curr Pharm Design*, 7(13), 1199-1212, (2001).

Huppertz B, Frank HG, Kaufmann P. The apoptosis cascade-morphological and immunohistochemical methods for its visualization. *Anat Embriol.* 200, 1-18, (1999).

Johnstone RW, Ruefli AA, Lowe SW. Apoptosis: a link between cancer genetics and chemotherapy. *Cell*, 108, 153-164, (2002).

Kerr JFR, Winterford CM, Harmon BV. Apoptosis its significance in cancer and cancer therapy. *Cancer*, 73(8), 2013-2026, (1993).

Kingston DGI, Toxol and its analogs. In Cragg GM, Kingston DGI, Newman DJ (Eds.) Anticancer agents from natural products. Brunner-Routledge Psychology Press, Taylor & Francis Group, Boca Raton, FL, pp 89-122, (2005).

Kuan N, Passaro E. Apoptosis: programmed cell death. *Arch Surg*, 133, 773-775, (1998).

Lall N. Isolation and identification of Naphthoquinones from Euclea natalensis with activity against Mycobacterium tuberculosis, other pathogenic bacteria and herpes simplex virus. Dissertation, University of Pretoria, (2000).

Lam KS. New aspects of natural products in drug discovery. *Trends Microbiol*, 15(6), 279-289, (2007).

Lee K. Novel antitumour agents from higher plants. *Antitumour agents*, 197, 569-596, (2003).

Lewis WH, Lewis MPE. (1995) Medicinal plants as sources of new therapeutics. *Ann Mo Bot Gard*. 82:16-24.

Lucci A, Han T, Liu Y, Giuliano AE, Cabot MC. Multidrug resistance modulators and doxorubicin synergize to evaluate ceramide levels and elicit apoptosis in drug-resistant cancer cells. American cancer society. *Cancer*, 86(2), 300-311, (1999).

Martin SJ, Green DR, Cotter TG. Dicing with death: dissecting the components of the apoptosis machinery. *TIBS*, 19, 26-30, (1994).

Mann J. Natural products in cancer chemotherapy: past, present and future. *Nature Rev*., 143–148, (2002).

McChesney DJ. Biological and chemical diversity and the search for new pharmaceuticals and other bioactive natural products. In Kinghorn AD and Balandrin MF. Human medicinal agents in plants. American Chemical Society, Washington, pp 38-47, (1993).

Meijer L, Raymond E. Roscovitine and other purines as kinase inhibitors. From starfish oocytes to clinical trials. *Account Chem Res*, 36, 417-425, (2003).

Mukherjee AK, Basu S, Sarkar N, Ghosh AC. Advances in Cancer Therapy with Plant Based Natural Products. *Curr Med Chem*, 8, 1467-1486, (2001).

Ndubani P, Hojer B. Traditional healers and the treatment of sexually transmitted illnesses in rural Zambia. *J Ethnopharmacol*, 67, 15-25, (1999).

O'Niell MJ. The renaissance of plant research in pharmaceutical industry. In Kinghorn AD & Balandrin MF. Human medicinal agents in plants. American Chemical Society, Washington, pp 48-55, (1993).

Philp RB. Herbal remedies: the good, the bad, and the ugly. *J Compl Int Med*, 1, 1-11, (2004).

Rates SMK. Plants as source of drugs. *Toxicon,* 39, 603-631, (2001).

Sausville EA, Zaharevitz D, Gussio R, Meijer L, Louarn-Leost M, Kunick C, Schultz R, Lahusen T, Headlee D, Stinson S, Arbuck SG, Senderowicz A. Cyclin-dependent kinases: initial approaches to exploit a novel therapeutic target. *Pharmacology & Therapeut*, 82, 285-292, (1999).

Schwartzman RA, Cidlowski JA. Apoptosis: the biochemistry and molecular biology of programmed cell death. *Endocr Rev*, 14(2), 133-151, (1993).

Tazi J, Bakkour N, Soret J, Zekri L, Hazra B, laine W, Baldeyrou B, Lansiaux A, Bailly C. Selective inhibition of topoisomerase I and various steps of spliceosome assembly by diospyrin derivatives. *Mol Pharmacol*, 67(4), 1186-1194, (2005).

Trump BF, Berezesky IK, Chang SH, Phelps PC. The pathways of cell death: oncosis, apoptosis and necrosis. *Toxicol Pathol*, 25(1), 82-88, (1997).

Van Engeland M, Nieland LJW, Ramaekers FCS, Schutte B, Reutelingsperger CPM. Annexin V-Affinity Assay: A review on an apoptosis detection system based on phosphatidylserine exposure. *Cytometry*, 31, 1-9, (1998).

Vickers A. Botanical medicines for the treatment of cancer: Rationale, overview of current data, and methodological considerations for phase I and II trials. *Cancer Invest*, 20, 1069-1079, (2002).

Doe J (2003). Title of preprint. http://www.who.int/tb/publications/2003/en/index1.html Cited 25 Dec. 2003.

Tynes T, Klaeboe L, Haldorsen T. Residential and occupational exposure to 50 Hz magnetic fields and malignant melanoma: a population based study. *Occup Environ Med,* 2003;60(5):343-347.

chapter 6

THE ANTIQUITY AND HISTORY OF MEDICINAL PLANTS AND TUBERCULOSIS

Sannah Patience Nkami Mativandlela and Namrita Lall

INTRODUCTION

History of Herbal Medicine and Plant Derived Drugs

Herbal medicine, sometimes referred to as herbalism or botanical medicine is the use of plants for their therapeutic or medicinal value and has been used by all cultures throughout history. Plants produce and contain a variety of chemical substances that act upon the body. Herbalists use the leaves, flowers, stems, berries and roots of plants to prevent, relieve, and treat illnesses. About 25% of the prescription drugs dispensed in the United States contain, at least, one active ingredient derived from plant material, some are made from plant extracts and others are synthesized to mimic a natural plant compound (Balick, 1990). A number of herbal plants and their compounds have been used, and have served as models for modern medicine (Farnsworth, 1984). Many drugs listed as conventional medications were originally derived from plants. Salicylic acid, a precursor of aspirin, was originally derived from 'white willow bark' and the 'meadowsweet plant'. Well known examples of plant derived drugs include the antimalarial 'quinine', extracted from the bark of the 'Cinchona' species. 'Vincristine', which is being used to treat certain types of cancer, comes from the 'Madagascar periwinkle' (*Catharanthus roseus*). In 1819, the isolation of the analgesic morphine, codeine and paregoric laid down the foundation for the purification of pharmacologically active compounds for the treatment of diarrhoea. 'Laudanum', a tincture of the 'opium poppy', was the favoured tranquilliser in Victorian times. Even today, morphine, the most important alkaloid of the opium poppy, remains the standard against which new synthetic analgesic drugs are measured (Phillipson, 2001; De Smet, 1997).

Use of Medicinal Plants

The use of plants as the source of remedies for the treatment of many diseases dates back to prehistory and people of all continents have this old tradition. Plants continue to be a major source of medicines, as they have been throughout human history (van Wyk *et al.*, 1997). Up to 80% of the world population, South Africa population use medicinal plants as remedies for various ailments. Plant species serve as a rich source of many novel biologically active compounds, although very few have been thoroughly investigated for their medicinal properties (Heinrich and Gibbons, 2001).

Apart of the 30% and 40% used in today's conventional drugs, other plants are used as herbal supplements, botanicals and teas (Kirby, 1996; Hostettmann and Marston, 2002). The World Health Organization (WHO) estimates that 4 billion people, or 80% of the world population, presently use herbal medicine for some aspect of primary health care. Herbal medicine is a major component in all indigenous peoples' traditional medicine and is a common element in ayurvedic, homeopathic, naturopathic, traditional Oriental and Native American Indian medicines. WHO notes that of the 119 plant-derived pharmaceutical medicines, about 74% are used in modern medicine in ways that correlated directly with their traditional uses as plant medicines by native cultures (Shulz *et al.*, 2001). The uses of some medicinal plants vary a lot according to regional and cultural aspects. Their use is often associated with witchcraft and superstition, because people do not have the scientific insight to explain or predict the curative action of plants. One example of such an irrational concept is the Doctrine of Signatures (elements of which are found in many of the healing cultures of the world), which is based on the assumption that the appearance of plants may give clues to their medicinal properties (van Wyk and Wink, 2004).

Medicinal plants typically contain mixtures of different chemical compounds that may act individually, additively or synergistically to improve health. A single plant may contain bitter substances that stimulate digestion, anti-inflammatory compounds that reduce swelling and pain, phenolic compounds that act as antioxidants and venotonics, antibacterial and antifungal tannins that act as natural antibiotics, diuretic substances that enhance the elimination of waste product and toxins and alkaloids that enhance mood and give a sense of well-being (van Wyk and Wink, 2004). The importance of plants lies not only on their chemotherapeutic effect, but also in their role as a source of model compounds for drug development. In addition to plant constituents being used directly as therapeutic agents, they can be utilized as starting material or templates for drug synthesis (Eloff, 1998). In addition to active ingredients, the plant's bioflavanoids and other substances are important in supporting its medicinal properties. These elements also provide an important natural safeguard. Isolated or synthesized active compounds can become toxic in relatively small doses; unlike whole plant which reaches a toxic level only when taken in large quantities.

Medicinal plants are also important for pharmacological research and drug development, not only when plant constituents are used directly as therapeutic agents, but also as starting materials for the synthesis of drugs or as models for pharmacologically active compounds (Mukherjee, 2003). Major pharmaceutical companies are currently conducting extensive research on plant materials, gathered from forests and other habitats, for their potential medicinal value. Rather than using a whole plant, scientists identify, isolate, extract, and synthesize individual components, thus capturing the active compounds. There are over 750,000 plant species on earth, but relatively speaking, only a very few of the healing plants have been studied scientifically. Because modern pharmacology looks for one active ingredient and seeks to isolate it to the exclusion of all the others, most of the research that is done on plants continues to focus on identifying and isolating active ingredients, rather than studying the medicinal properties of the whole plants. Herbalists, however, consider that the power of a plant lies in the interaction of all its ingredients. Plants used as medicines offer synergistic interactions between ingredients both known and unknown (Mabogo, 1990). Despite the remarkable progress in synthetic organic chemistry of the twentieth century, over 25% of prescribed medicines in industrialized countries are derived directly or indirectly from plants (Newman *et al.*, 2003).

Medicinal Plants with Antimycobacterial Activity

Over the past decade there has been a proliferation of literature on the antibacterial, antituberculosis, antifungal and antiviral properties of plant extracts. Screening plant extracts for antimycobacterial activity is usually carried out using mycobacteria cultured in various types of broth and agar based media (Newton *et al.*, 2000). There are several reports on *in vitro* inhibition of mycobacterium species by medicinal plants and the bioassay-guided research for antimycobacterial properties from plants has shown signs of success. Major review articles have appeared on antimycobacterial natural products in the last eight years. Although no marketable products for the treatment of tuberculosis have been isolated from plants, some lead compounds have been identified (Cantrell *et al.*, 1999). Cantrell *et al.*, (2001) isolated norditerpenoid, '12 demethylmulticauline', from the roots of *Salvia multicaulis*, which was more active than the first line tuberculosis (TB) drugs ethambutol (EB) and nearly as active as rifampicin (RIF) *in vitro*. Mitscher and Baker discussed plant-derived compounds (berberine, lichoisoflavone, erygibisoflavone, phaseollidin, erythrabyssin II and tryptanthrin) as potential antituberculosis agents (Mitscher and Baker, 1998). Newton *et al.*, 2000 reviewed plant-derived antimycobacterial natural products, describing the activity of extracts and compounds from 123 plants species (Newton *et al.*, 2000).

Reports of 88 naturally occurring compounds and synthetic analogues from plants, fungi and marine organisms, that demonstrated significant activity in the *in vitro* bioassays against *M. tuberculosis* and other mycobacterial species, have been described (Okunade *et al.*, 2004). Recent developments in mycobacteriology and innovative natural products chemistry tools and their potential to impact on the early steps of the TB drug discovery process have been reviewed (Pauli *et al.*, 2005). Gautam *et al.*, 2007 described 70% (255 of 365) of Indian medicinal plant species, from a wide range of families, which have shown antimycobacterial activity. Interestingly, when tested preliminary in the *in vitro* screening, 149 species have shown positive ethnomedicinal uses in correlation with the traditional knowledge for TB or related diseases (Gautam *et al.*, 2007). Ten of the 408 ethanolic extracts of plants such as *Actaea spicata*, *Angustura vera*, *Cinnamonium camphora*, *Piper cubeba*, *Guauacum officinale*, *Ipomea purga*, *Rhamnus cathartica* inhibited growth of *M. tuberculosis* H37Rv at dilutions of 1 in 160 to 1280 and a high proportion of the other extracts inhibited growth at lower dilutions (Grange and Dawey, 1990). It was found that *M. tuberculosis* was also sensitive towards *Pentas longifolia*, *Tetradenia riparia* and *Bidens pilosa*, medicinal plants used in Rwanda. The active compound isolated from the leaves of *T. riparia* was tested against *M. tuberculosis* which showed activity at 100 μg/ml (van Puyvelde *et al.*, 1994). *Hydrocotyle asiaticum* inhibited growth of *M. tuberculosis* at a dilution of 1:20 (Grange and Davey, 1990). Organic extracts of *Helichrysum crispum* inhibited the growth of *M. tuberculosis* (Salie et al., 1996). Lall and Meyer (2001) demonstrated the inhibition of drug-sensitive and drug-resistant strains of *M. tuberculosis* by diospyrin isolated from the roots of *Euclea natalensis* AD. The phytochemical and biological studies of *E. natalensis* and isolated compounds from this plant indicated *in vitro* activity against *M. tuberculosis*.

In structure-activity related studies against *M. tuberculosis* different research groups have found activity using a variety of natural products with no definite trend towards a specific group of compounds (Houghton *et al.*, 1999). In South Africa, it has been reported that people smoke dried flower and seed of *Helichrysum krausii* in a pipe for the relief of coughs and as a remedy for pulmonary tuberculosis (Watt and Breyer-Brandwijk, 1962). Chelerythrine isolated from methanolic root extracts of *Sanguinaria canadensis* was found to be the most active isolated compound against *M. smegmatis* at 29.0 μg /ml (Newton *et al.*, 2002).

Plants have been endowed with therapeutic virtues both in legend and in scientific literature and are being used in treating various ailments such as coughs, colds, other pathogenic bacterial and viral infections. The use of antimicrobials from the natural vegetation has a great impact in human health care in undeveloped countries. Herbal medicine has been used for centuries in rural areas by local healers and has been improved in industrialized countries.

THE EPIDEMIOLOGY, PREVENTION AND TREATMENT OF TUBERCULOSIS

The Natural History of Tuberculosis

Tuberculosis (TB) is a disease known since antiquity and evidence of spinal TB in the form of fossil bones dates back to around 8000 BC (Ayyazian, 1993; Basel, 1998). TB occurred as an endemic disease among animals long before it affected humans (Steele and Ranney, 1958). The first confirmed instance of TB in humans was noted in the deformities of the skeletal and muscular remains of the Egyptian mummies of around 2400 BC (Haas, 1996). However, it could not be determined whether the disease was due to *M. bovis* or *M. tuberculosis*. In the 1700s and early 1800s, TB prevalence peaked in Western Europe and the United States and was undoubtedly the largest cause of death. Hundred to 200 years later, it had spread in full force to Eastern Europe, Asia, Africa and South America (Bloom and Murray, 1992).

Epidemiology

In the late 1980s, TB began re-emerging and now globally, kills more than 2 million people each year. It is thought that as many as 2 billion people have been exposed to the TB bacillus and are therefore at risk of developing the active disease (Gutierrez-Lugo et al., 2005). According to WHO (1999), TB is known to be the largest cause of death of the human species. There has been a resurgence of the disease over the last two decades with currently eight million new cases and about 200,000 deaths annually. It is estimated that between 2000 and 2020, nearly one billion people will become infected, 200 million will acquire the disease and 35 million will die from TB (WHO, 2006), in contrast to the 1.6 million deaths from TB in 2005. Both the highest number of deaths and the highest mortality rate are in the Africa region. The two essential factors for the rapid spread of TB are; crowded living conditions, which favour airborne transmission and a population with little natural resistance. TB in populations can be attributed to three distinct factors:

- Infection of an individual in the community with tubercle bacilli within a given time period.
- Development of the disease shortly after such infection.
- The disease developing long after the original infection, owing to the reactivation of latent bacilli (Raviglone *et al.*, 1995; Bloom, 1994).

Today, TB is the leading cause of death worldwide from a single human pathogen, claiming more lives than diseases such as Human Immunodeficiency Virus / Acquired Immune deficiency Syndrome (HIV/AIDS), malaria, diarrhoea, leprosy and all the other tropical diseases combined (Zumla and Grange, 1998). The pandemic of HIV/AIDS infection and the evidence of an association with TB, have caused marked increases in the incidence of the disease in some countries (Bloom, 1994). Because of its ability to destroy the immune system, HIV has emerged as the most significant risk factor for progression of dormant

TB infection to clinical disease (Selwyn *et al.*, 1989). The Global Programme on AIDS of the WHO estimated that in 1992 at least 13 million adults and 1 million children had been infected with HIV worldwide (WHO, 1999). The impact of HIV/AIDS infection on the TB situation is greatest in those populations where the prevalence of TB infection in young adults is very high (Bloom, 1994).

The number of cases worldwide is now increasing rapidly due to multi-drug resistant strains of *M. tuberculosis* as a result of patient non-compliance and also due to an increase in patients with HIV/AIDS (Collins, 1998; Zumla and Grange, 1998). About 450 000 multi-drug resistant tuberculosis (MDR-TB) cases are estimated to occur every year; the highest rates are in countries of the former Soviet Union and China (WHO, 2006). There are a number of countries that have made remarkable progress in expanding population coverage with cure rates, whereas South Africa battles with more than 188 000 new TB cases per year (Bloom, 2002). South Africa is burdened by one of the worst TB epidemics in the world, with the disease rates more than double of those observed in other developing countries and up to 60 times higher than those currently seen in developed countries (Bapela, 2005).

Current strategies for the control of TB centres around treatment with multi-drug regimes based on the very effective combination of isoniazid (INH., Fig. 6.1a) and rifampicin (RIF., Fig. 6.1b). In endemic areas, the diagnosis and treatment of smear positive patients are emphasized in order to interrupt the spread of the disease within the community. Obstacles to the success of this strategy are the difficulties of early diagnosis and operational problems associated with delivery of a treatment that involves administration of multiple drugs over a period of at least six months (Young and Duncan, 1995).

Transmission of Tuberculosis

The principal risk method of being infected with TB is by inhaling contaminated air containing microbes that cause this disease (Rom and Garay, 1996). TB microbes can be present in sufficient concentrations in the air to cause infections and the disease. Once in air, water evaporates from the surface of a particle, decreasing its size and concentrating its contents of microbes. These particle forms a droplet nuclei in which evaporation continues until the vapour pressure of the droplet equals to the atmospheric pressure. The droplet nuclei are very stable, settle very slowly and remain suspended in the air for very long periods. Droplet nuclei are produced when a patient with active pulmonary or laryngeal tuberculosis coughs, speaks, sneezes or sings. Coughing can produce 3000 infectious droplet nuclei, talking for 5 minutes an equal number and sneezing can produce over a million particles with a diameter of less than 100 nm (Bloom, 1994). When inhaled, droplet nuclei usually travel through the airway until they reach the alveoli. Larger particles that are deposited on the way are removed through normal mechanism of airway clearance (Dannenberg, 1989).

Immunology of Tuberculosis

TB is a prototype infection that requires control by the cellular immune response. In the first few weeks the host has almost no immune defence against infection by the bacteria causing TB. Small inhalation inocula multiply freely in the alveolar space or within alveolar macrophages. Unrestrained bacterial multiplication proceeds until the development of tissue hypersensitivity and cellular immunity intervene. The organism causing TB adheres to alveolar macrophages via multiple complements and might be destroyed in the phagosome (Beyers, 1999). The intracellular mechanisms for killing or inhibiting the growth of the bacteria in alveolar macrophages include the production of nitric oxide and reactive oxygen intermediates. Alveolar macrophages can also participate, in a broader context of cellular immunity, through the process of antigen presentation and recruitment of T-lymphocytes, which are the white blood cells produced in the bone marrow but which mature in the thymus. These cells are important in the body's defence against certain bacteria and fungi (Beyers, 1999).

Macrophages which are antigens are processed in phagosomes via Major Histocompatibility Complex (MHC) class II molecules to CD4 T-lymphocytes which are the major effector cells in cell-mediated immunity. The antigens bind to T-cell receptors on the surface of the T-lymphocytes. These CD4 T-lymphocytes tend to polarize into either Th1 cells (these are essential in controlling intracellular pathogens), producing predominantly interferon gamma (IFN-γ) and interleukin 2 (IL-2) or Th2 cells producing predominantly cytokines interleukin 4 (IL-4), interleukin 5 (IL-5), interleukin 6 (IL-6), interleukin 10 (IL-10) and interleukin 13 (IL-13). In mice, immunity correlates with a Th1 response. Macrophages infected with *M. tuberculosis* secrete interleukin 12 (IL-12), which induces the secretion of IFN-γ by CD4 cells and natural killer cells. The IFN-γ enhances the activation of macrophages and improves their ability to prevent the spread of *M. tuberculosis* (Orme, 1993). However, *M. tuberculosis* is not defenceless. It can produce ammonia to counteract phagosomal acidification. Its lypogly can actively scavenge toxic radicals reduced against it by the macrophage (Orme, 1993; Bapela, 2005).

Prevention of Tuberculosis

The outcome of mycobacterial infection depends on the host immune response. In most individuals, infection with *M. tuberculosis* induces an immune response sufficient for the protection against progression to the primary disease (Bapela, 2005). Bacille Calmette-Guérin (BCG) vaccine reproduces minimal infection but does not impose a disease risk. BCG vaccine, which is derived from a strain of *M. bovis* attenuated through years of serial passage in culture, was first used in 1921 to protect against tuberculosis in humans (Young and Duncan, 1995). Many BCG vaccines are currently administered to 100 million young children each year throughout the world. These vaccines are derived from the original strain but vary in cultural characteristics and ability to induce sensitization to tuberculin. There are differences in techniques and methods of producing them as well as various routes of vaccine administration (Young, 1994).

Treatment of Tuberculosis

Before effective drugs were available, half of the patients with active pulmonary TB died within 2 years, and only a quarter were cured. With the advent of anti-TB chemotherapy, protracted bed rest and lengthy isolation became unnecessary, and in theory at least, successful treatment was a reasonable goal in all adults (Bartmann, 1988). *Mycobacterium* is naturally resistant to most common antibiotics and chemotherapy agents. This is probably due to their highly hydrophobic cell envelope acting as an efficient permeability barrier. Due to the discovery of the effective antimycobacetrial agents ethambutol (EMB., Fig. 6.1c), INH, pyrazinamide (PZA., Fig. 6.1d), RIF and streptomycin (STR., Fig. 6.1e) between 1950 and 1970s, and reduction in poverty, there was a drastic decrease in the number of TB cases especially in developed countries. However, since 1980s, the number of TB cases throughout the world has been increasing rapidly due to the emergence of MDR-

TB (Chan and Iseman, 2002). The MDR forms of the disease, defined as forms resistant to two or more existing TB-drugs, are often fatal and are difficult and expensive to treat (Basso and Blanchard, 1998; Bastian and Colebunders, 1999). The situation has recently been complicated by the association of TB with HIV in sub-Saharan Africa and many developing countries (Corbett *et al.*, 2003; Lurie *et al.*, 2004). The situation is exacerbated by the increasing emergence of extensively drug-resistant (XDR) TB (Lurie *et al.*, 2004).

Reliable treatment therapy for TB treatment takes a period of 6 - 9 months with first line drugs (EMB, INH, PZA, RIF and STR). In the case of acquired drug resistance only second-line drugs (capreomycin, cycloserine, kanamycin and ethionamide) can be used and these have significant side effects with approximately 50% cure rate (Gautam *et al.*, 2007; Heym and Cole, 1997). The current therapies reduce the pulmonary bacterial burden but the treatment periods of 6 months for non-immune suppressed individuals and at least 9 months for immune suppressed patients are required for reliable treatment efficacy (Bapela, 2005; Quenelle *et al.*, 2001). However, floroquinolones such as ofloxacin, norfloxacin can be used which are safer than the above-mentioned second-line drugs but have the disadvantage of being very expensive (Tripathi *et al.*, 2005). Emergence of drug-resistant mycobacterial strains is alarming these days. This occurs when a single drug is given alone and when the viable bacterial population in the lesions is large. The occurrence of drug resistance is widely thought to be due to the overgrowth of sensitive organisms by mutant resistant bacilli present in wild strains before they were ever in contact with the drug concerned (Mitchison, 1984). There have been no new anti-TB drugs introduced in the past 30 years. Thus, there is an urgent need to search for and develop new effective and affordable anti-TB drugs (Gautam *et al.*, 2007).

TARGETS, MODE OF ACTION OF FIRST-LINE TB DRUGS

Current chemotherapy for TB largely relies on drugs that inhibit bacterial metabolism with a heavy emphasis on inhibitors of the cell wall synthesis (Zhang, 2005). According to their mode of action, first and second line drugs can be grouped as cell wall inhibitors (INH, EMB, ethionamide, cycloserine), nucleic acid synthesis inhibitors (RIF, quinolones), protein synthesis inhibitors (STR, kanamycin) and inhibitors of membrane energy metabolism (PZA) (Mitchison, 1980). Targets and mechanisms of action of current TB drugs are summarised in Table 6.1.

Existing TB drugs are therefore only able to target actively growing bacteria through the inhibition of cell processes such as cell wall biogenesis and DNA replication. This implies that current chemotherapy is characterised by an efficient bactericidal activity but an extremely weak sterilising activity (defined as the ability to kill the slowly growing or metabolising bacteria that persist after most of the growing bacteria have been killed by bactericidal drug). Sterilising activity also describes the ability to eliminate latent or dormant bacteria that survive inside the host macrophages (Mitchison, 1980). Although achieving a clinical cure, the current TB chemotherapy does not achieve a bacteriological-eradication of all bacilli in the lesions (McCune and Tompsett, 1956).

Isoniazid (INH)

INH (Fig. 6.1a) is the synthetic hydrazide of isonicotic acid discovered in 1952 and the first-line antituberculosis medication used in the prevention and treatment of TB. INH is the cornerstone of the therapy and should be included in all regimens unless a high degree of INH resistance exists. This drug is never used on its own to treat TB because resistance develops quickly. INH is

Table 6.1: Commonly used first and second line TB drugs and their targets (Zhang, 2005)

Drug (year of discovery)	*MIC (µg/mL)*	*Effect on bacterial cell*	*Mechanisms of action*	*Targets*	*Genes involved in resistance*
Isoniazid (1952)	0.01 - 0.2	Bactericidal	Inhibition of cell wall mycolic acid and other multiple effects on DNA, lipids, carbohydrates and NAD metabolism	Primarily acyl carrier protein reductase (inhA)	*katG*; *inhA*, *ndh*
Rifampicin (1966)	0.05 - 0.5	Bactericidal	Inhibition of RNA synthesis	RNA polymerase β subunit	*rpoB*
Pyrazinamide (1952)	20.0 - 100.0	Bactericidal	Disruption of membrane transport and energy depletion	Membrane energy metabolism	*pncA*
Ethambutol (1961)	1.0 - 5.0	Bactericidal	Inhibition of cell wall arabinogalactan synthesis	Arabinosyl transferase	*emb*CAB
Streptomycin (1944)	2.0 - 8.0	Bacteriostatic	Inhibition of protein synthesis	Ribosomal S12 protein and 16S rRNA	*rps*L; *rrs* (operon)
Kanamycin (1957)	1.0 - 8.0	Bactericidal	Inhibition of protein synthesis	Ribosomal S12 protein and 16S rRNA	*rps*L; *rrs* (operon)
Quinolones (1963)	0.2 - 4.0	Bactericidal	Inhibition of DNA replication and transcription	DNA gyrase	*gyrA*; *gyr*B
Ethionammide (1956)	0.6 - 2.5	Bacteriostatic	Inhibition of mycolic acid synthesis	Acyl carrier protein reductase (inhA)	*inh*A; *etaA/ethA*
Para-aminosalicylic acid (1946)	1.0 - 8.0	Bacteriostatic	Inhibition of folic acid and iron metabolism	Unknown	Unknown
Cycloserine (1952)	5.0 - 20.0	Bacteriostatic	Inhibition of peptidoglycan synthesis	D-alanine racemase	*alr*A; *Ddl*

highly selective and acts almost exclusively against *M. tuberculosis*, *M. bovis* and *M. africanum*. This remarkable selectivity in its action is thought to be mediated by the bacterial enzyme catalase peroxidase which catalyses the reaction converting INH to a potent bactericidal derivative. INH is bactericidal at MIC levels of less than 0.1 μg/ml for 80% of susceptible strains of *M. tuberculosis* (Reichman and Hershfield, 2000).

Mechanism of Action

The exact mechanism of the action of INH has not been fully elucidated, but several mechanisms including interference with the metabolism of bacterial proteins, nucleic acids, carbohydrates and lipids have been proposed. INH is a prodrug and must be activated by bacterial catalase. It is activated by catalase-peroxidase enzyme katG to form isonicotinic acyl anion or radical. These forms will then react with a NADH radical to form isonicotinic acyl-NADH complex. This complex will then binds tightly to ketoenoylreductase known as InhA and prevent access of the natural enoyl-AcpM substrate. This mechanism inhibits the synthesis of mycolic acid in the mycobacterial cell wall. INH combines with an enzyme which interferes with the cell metabolism of the bacteria. As a result of the disruption in its metabolism and without a cell wall the bacteria die (Bapela, 2005). INH reaches therapeutic concentration in serum, cerebrospinal fluid (CSF) and within caseous granulomas and metabolised in the liver via acetylation. INH is bactericidal to rapidly-dividing mycobacteria, but is bacteriostatic if the *Mycobacterium* is slow-growing. Susceptible bacteria may undergo 1 or 2 divisions before multiplication is arrested (Bartmann, 1988).

Resistance to INH

INH inhibits the biosynthesis of mycolic acids present in the cell wall of *M. tuberculosis*. This renders the mycobacterial cell wall defective, thereby penetratable to toxic oxygen. KatG is the only enzyme in *M. tuberculosis* capable of activating INH. Expression of either the KatG or an alkyl hydroperoxidase AhpC is considered sufficient to protect the bacilli against toxic peroxides (Wilson and Collins, 1996).

Side Effects and Toxicity

Adverse reactions include rash, abnormal liver functions, hepatitis, sideroblastic anemia, peripheral neuropathy, mild central nervous system (CNS) effects and drug interactions resulting in increased phenytoin (dilantin) or disulfiran (antabuse) levels. Peripheral neuropathy and CNS effects are associated with the use of INH and are due to pyridoxine (vitamin B6) depletion. Headache, poor concentration, poor memory and depression have all been associated with INH use. The frequency of these side effects is not known and the association with INH is not well validated. The presence of these symptoms is not frequently disabling and is not a reason to stop treatment with INH and the patients are strongly encouraged to continue treatment despite these symptoms (Holdiness, 1984).

The hepatoxicity associated with INH results from the toxic effect of an intermediate product produced by N-hydroxylation of monoacetylhydrazine, one of the metabolites of INH, by the liver cytochrome P-450 mixed function oxidase system. Hepatoxicity, nausea, vomiting, abdominal pains and appetite loss can be avoided with close clinical monitoring of the patient (Holdiness, 1984).

Rifampicin (RIF)

RIF (Fig. 6.1b) is the second major antituberculosis agent which is used in conjunction with other antituberulosis agents in the treatment of TB. RIF is a semi synthetic derivative of one of a group of structurally similar, complex macrocyclic antibiotics produced by *Streptomyces mediterranei* (Bartmann, 1988). RIF inhibits the growth of most Gram-positive bacteria as well as many Gram-negative bacteria. RIF inhibits *M. tuberculosis* at concentrations ranging from 0.005 – 0.2 μg/mL *in vitro* (Bapela, 2005; Duman *et al.*, 2004). RIF is soluble in organic solvents and in water at acidic pH (Bapela, 2005).

Mechanism of Action

RIF may be bacteriostatic or bactericidal in action, depending on the concentration of the drug attained at the site of infection and the susceptibility of the infecting organism. RIF inhibits dioxyribonucleic acid (DNA)-dependent ribonucleic acid (RNA)-polymerase of the *Mycobacterium* by forming a stable drug-enzyme complex, leading to the suppression of the initiation of chain formation in RNA synthesis (Bapela, 2005). More specifically, the β–subunit of this complex enzyme is the site of the action of the drug, although RIF binds only to the holoenzyme (Bartmann, 1988).

Resistance to RIF

Mutation in RNA polymerase beta subunit gene (rpoB) is the major mechanism of resistance to RIF with high frequencies of 90% or more (Taniguchi, 2000). Evaluation of the relationship between RIF's susceptibility and genetic alteration in rpoB gene also showed that 95% of the RIF-resistant *M. tuberculosis* isolates involved genetic alterations in an 81-base pair core region of rpoB gene. This region is called the rifampicin resistance-determining region (Ramaswammy and Musser, 1998). Moreover, these genetic alterations in the rpoB gene are suspected as being the resistance mechanisms to RIF (Taniguchi, 2000).

Side Effects and Toxicity

In humans, acute overdose with RIF, i.e. up to 12 g has not been fatal, however one fatality has been reported following ingestion of a single 60 g dose of the drug (AHFS Drug Information, 2000). The lethal dose (LD_{50}) of RIF in mice is 0.885 g/kg. The most important complication of RIF is liver toxicity, which occurs 4 times more frequently in regimens containing both INH and RIF than in those containing INH alone (Bartmann, 1988., Bapela, 2005).

Ethambutol (EMB)

EMB (Fig. 6.1c) is a synthetic antituberculosis agent prescribed to treat TB. It is active *in vitro* and *in vivo* against *M. tuberculosis, M. bovis, M. marinum, M. avium* and *M. intracellular*. EMB is usually given in combination with other drugs such as INH, RIF and PZA, at a daily dose of 25 mg/kg to humans during the first 2 months of well-supervised therapy and at 15 mg/kg for longer, often less well supervised periods (Bartmann, 1988).

Mechanism of Action

EMB may be bacteriostatic or bactericidal in action, depending on the concentration of the drug attained at the site of infection and the susceptibility of the organism. Although the exact mechanism has not yet been fully determined, the drug appears to inhibit the synthesis of one or more metabolites in susceptible bacteria resulting in the impairment of cellular metabolism, arrest of multiplication, and cell death. EMB is active against susceptible bacteria only when they are undergoing cell division (AHFS Drug Information, 2000).

Resistance to EMB

EMB has been shown to inhibit the incorporation of mycolic acids into the cell wall. It has also been shown to inhibit the transfer of arabinogalactan into the cell wall of mycobacteria (Ramaswamy and Musser, 1998). Only the dextroisomer of EMB is biologically active, an observation consistent with the idea that the drug binds to a specific drug target, which is assumed to be arabinosyl transferase (Ramaswammy and Musser, 1998). The EmbB gene, encoding arabinosyl transferase which catalyses cell wall synthesis, is mutated in EMB-resistant strains (Taniguchi, 2000).

Side Effects and Toxicity

A single administration of EMB has low toxicity in mice (Diermeier *et al.*, 1966). In humans the adverse effects of EMB include dermatitis, pruritis, headache, dizziness, fever and mental confusion.

Pyrazinamide (PZA)

PZA (Fig. 6.1d) is a derivative of niacinamide and is a synthetic antituberculosis drug used to treat TB in patients (AHFS Drug Information, 2000). Currently, PZA is considered as a first line drug, and only used in combination with other drugs such as INH and RIF in the treatment of *M. tuberculosis*.

PZA has no other medical uses and is not used to treat other mycobacteria (*M. bovis* and *M. leprae*) which are resistant to the drug. PZA is used in the first two to four months of treatment to reduce the duration of treatment required.

Mechanism of Action

PZA may be bacteriostatic or bactericidal in action, depending on the concentration of the drug attained at the site of infection and the susceptibility of the organism (Bapela, 2005). The drug is active *in vitro* and *in vivo* at a slightly acidic pH. PZA stops the growth of *M. tuberculosis*, which has an enzyme pyrazinamidase that is only active at acidic pH. PZA converts the enzyme to the active form, pyrazinoic acid (POA). POA inhibits the enzyme fatty acid synthetase 1, which is required by the bacterium to synthesise fatty acids.

In addition, POA lowers the pH of the environment below a certain level which is optimal for *M. tuberculosis* growth. Mutations of the pyrazinamidase gene (*pncA*), are responsible for PZA resistance in *M. tuberculosis*. This appears to contribute to the drug's antimycobacterial activity *in vitro* (Bartmann, 1988).

Resistance to PZA

The mechanism of action and the resistance of *M. tuberculosis* to PZA have also been partially identified. PZA is crucial for achieving sterilization by killing persisting semi-dormant bacilli in the lungs. Its activity depends on the presence of a bacterial amidase, which converts PZA to POA, which is the active antibacterial molecule (Mitchison and Selkon, 1996). PZA-resistant bacilli lack this amidase activity. The pncA gene encoding for this has been identified and the mutation to this pncA gene has been associated with resistance to PZA (Scopio and Zhang, 1996).

Side Effects and Toxicity

The most frequent adverse effect of PZA is hepatoxicity. Hepatoxicity becomes a problem when PZA is given in large doses and for long periods. Hepatoxicity may appear at any time during therapy. When PZA is used in short-course therapy no increase in the incidence of hepatotoxicity is noted (Bapela, 2005). The original dose for PZA was 40 – 70 mg/kg and the incidence of drug-induced hepatoxicity has fallen significantly since the recommended dose has been reduced. In the standard four-drug regime (INH, RIF, PZA and EMB), PZA is the most common cause of drug-induced hepatitis. It is not possible to clinically distinguish pyrazinamide-induced hepatitis from hepatitis caused by INH or RIF. Another common side effect of PZA is joint pains (arthralgia), which can be distressing to patients, but never harmful. Other side effects include nausea and vomiting, anorexia, sideroblastic anemia, skin rash, urticaria, pruritus, hyperuricemia, dysuria, interstitial nephritis, malaise, rarely porphyria and fever (British Thoracic Society, 1984). In mice, PZA has a LD_{50} of 3.4 g/kg when administered orally (Robinson *et al.*, 1954).

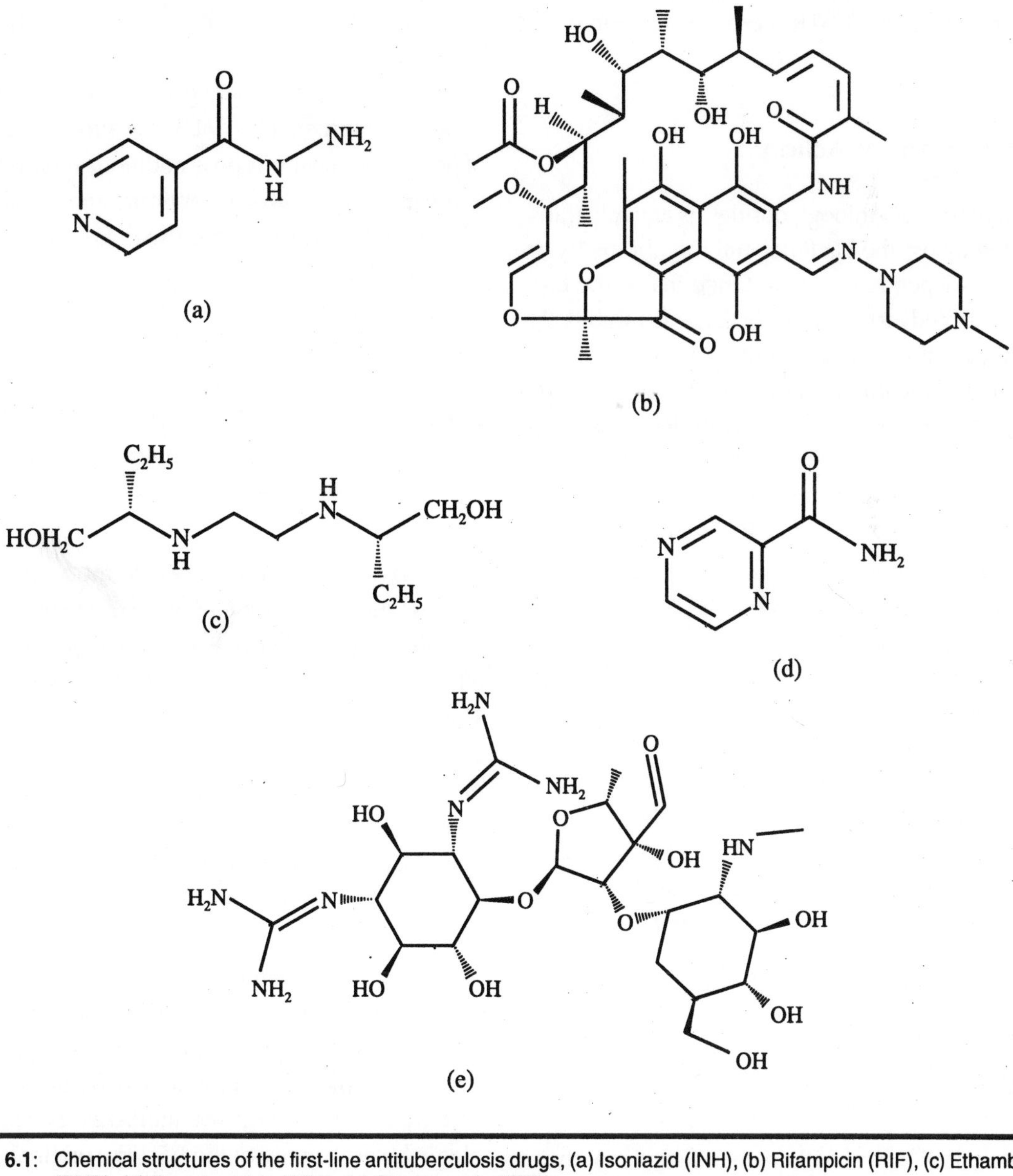

Fig. 6.1: Chemical structures of the first-line antituberculosis drugs, (a) Isoniazid (INH), (b) Rifampicin (RIF), (c) Ethambutol (EMB), (d) Pyrazinamide (PZA), (e) Streptomycin (STR)

Streptomycin (STR)

STR (Fig. 6.1e) is an aminoglycoside antibiotic which is particularly active against *M. tuberculosis* as well as against many Gram-negative bacteria. STR is bactericidal for the tubercle bacillus *in vitro*. Concentrations as low as 0.4 μg/mL inhibit growth of the tubercle bacillus *in vitro*. STR is an alternative to EMB in the four-drug protocols for the treatment of TB. STR is easily soluble in water (Bapela, 2005).

Mechanism of Action

STR, like other aminoglycosides, is actively transported across the bacterial cell membrane by an oxygen-dependent system. Once inside the bacteria, it binds to the polysomes and inhibits the synthesis of proteins. The drug binds to the 30S subunit of the bacterial ribosome which consists of 21 proteins and a single 16S molecule of RNA. Protein synthesis in the bacteria is blocked by inhibiting the movement of the peptidyl-Trna associated with translocation and this stimulates tRNA errors (Bapela, 2005).

Resistance to STR

Most STR resistance strains have a mutation on the rrs and rspL genes encoding a 16S rRNA and a 12S ribosomal subunit protein respectively (Taniguchi, 2000). In contrast to other bacteria, which have multiple copies of rRNA genes, *M. tuberculosis* complex members have only one copy. Hence, single nucleotide changes can potentially produce antibiotic resistance (Ramaswammy and Musser, 1998).

Side Effects and Toxicity

The toxic effects of STR are manifested mainly on vestibular rather than auditory function in human beings. An acute toxic effect following intracisternal injection in animals is clonic-convulsion. Other acute toxic effects following cutaneous or intravenous injections are nausea, vomiting and ataxia (Holdiness, 1984).

Why are New TB Drugs Needed?

HIV/AIDS has dramatically increased the risk of developing active TB and HIV co-infection makes TB more difficult to diagnose and treat. The increasing emergence of MDR-TB and the nature of persistent infections pose additional challenges to the treatment with conventional anti-TB drugs. Although TB can be treated with current drugs, treatment is complex and long involving 4 drugs for 2 months and 2 more drugs for at least another 4 months. Direct Observed Treatment (DOT) as promoted by the WHO to improve compliance for the difficult and long regimen can improve cure rates, but is demanding for patients and labour intensive for health staff (O'Brien and Nunn, 2001).

In pioneering studies McDermott and colleagues showed that the efficacy of drugs against *M. tuberculosis in vitro* was not matched by their efficiency *in vivo* (McCune and Tompsett, 1956). The exponentially growing cultures of *M. tuberculosis* can be sterilised using frontline bactericidal drugs such as INH and RIF, yet the same drug combination requires months to achieve similar effects against bacteria living in host tissues. This is because of the failure of the drugs to achieve optimal levels within TB lesions, but there is evidence that drug availability is not a limiting factor (Barclay *et al.*, 1953; Clark, 1985). It has been proposed that persistence of tubercle bacilli, which consists of 4 different populations, in the chemotherapy treatment might be attributable to physiologic heterogeneity of the bacteria in the tissues (Mitchison, 1979).

These populations are:

- Bacteria that are actively growing are killed primarily by INH.
- Bacteria that have spurts of metabolism are killed by RIF.
- Bacteria that are characterised by low metabolic activity and reside in acid pH environment are killed by PZA.
- Bacteria that are dormant or persisters are not killed by any current TB drug.

This idea was supported by the long established observation that slow and non-growing bacteria are phenotypically resistant or tolerant to killing by antimicrobials (Handwerger and Tomasz, 1985).

During the initial phase of chemotherapy treatment, which lasts about 2 days, the bacilli are killed exponentially at a rapid rate, followed by a further lengthy period of much slower exponential killing. It is assumed that those bacilli that are killed in the first 2 days are actively multiplying, while those in the succeeding period are persisters killed by the slower sterilising activities of the drugs (Jindani *et al.*, 2003). In an *in vitro* model of drug action, a 30-day static culture has been extensively used for the last 60 years and has been taken to resemble the persister population in its response to the drugs (Mitchison and Selkon, 1956; Mitchison, 1992; Herbert *et al.*, 1996). The drugs added to this static culture have the same slow sterilising actions that are responsible for the prolongation of therapy. This evidence suggests that activity against the population of persistent bacilli ultimately determines the duration of therapy necessary to provide a stable cure of the host (Grosset and Ji, 1998). Evidently there is an urgent need to develop new and more effective TB drugs that are not only active against MDR-TB but also shorten the length of treatment and target the non-replicating persistent bacilli.

New TB Drugs in the Pipeline

Drug development for TB and other diseases has been at a standstill for decades. Today thanks to, the Global Alliance for TB Drug Development (TB Alliance), which was created in 2000 and funded by the Bill and Melinda Gates Foundation, the TB drug pipeline is richer than it has been in the last 40 years. This TB alliance focuses on both preclinical and clinical development of candidate compounds for TB chemotherapy and is associated with projects aimed to identify compounds currently being developed. In addition to this, increased public awareness on the lack of research and development for neglected diseases have led in recent years to some multinational pharmaceutical companies up setting Research and Development (R&D) institutes on a 'no-profit-no-loss' basis for drug development for TB, malaria and leishmaniasis. Among the multinational pharmaceutical companies currently involved in anti-TB drug R&D are: Novartis, AstraZeneca and GlaxoSmithKline (GSK). Smaller pharmaceutical companies have also engaged in neglected disease R&D on a commercial basis and with some success as two of the anti-TB candidate drugs currently in clinical trials have been developed by medium-size pharmaceutical companies such as Lupin Limited (India) and Otsuka Pharmaceuticals (Japan., Moran *et al.*, 2005).

The Global TB drug pipeline as reported by the Stop TB partnership working group on new TB drugs is summarised in Table 6.1. This is an overview of all drug candidates in the pipeline, belonging to different entities and not only the TB Alliance. In order to analyse the pipeline, the drug candidates are grouped in two main categories: novel chemical entities and compounds originating from existing families of drugs where novel chemistry is used to optimise the compounds.

NOVEL CHEMICAL ENTITIES

Diarylquinoline TMC_{207}

The diarylquinoline TMC_{207} (Fig. 6.1a, Table 6.1), an extremely promising member of a new class of anti-mycobacterial agents, has a potent early and late bactericidal activity in the non-established infection in murine TB model exceeding that of INH. The substitution of RIF, INH or PZA with diarylquinoline TMC_{207} accelerated activity leading to complete culture conversion after 2 months of treatment in some combinations. The diarylquinoline-isoniazid-pyrazinamide with diarylquinoline-rifampicin-pyrazinamide combinations cleared the lungs of TB in all mice after 2 months. Diarylquinoline TMC_{207} also has been tested in various combinations with the second line drugs such as amikacin, PZA, moxifloxacin and ethionamide in mice infected with the drug-susceptible virulent *M. tuberculosis* $H_{37}RV$ strain (Adries et al., 2005). The target and mechanism of action of diarylquinoline TMC_{207} is different from those of other anti-TB agents implying low probability of cross-resistance with existing TB drugs (Adries et al., 2005). It is further suggested that diarylquinoline TMC_{207} is able to inhibit bacterial growth, when tested on MDR-TB isolates, by inhibiting ATP synthase leading to ATP depletion and pH Imbalance (Adries *et al.*, 2005., Petrella *et al.*, 2006). About 20 molecules of this agent have been shown to have an MIC of below 0.5 µg/mL against *M. tuberculosis* $H_{37}RV$ strain. Antimicrobial activity was confirmed *in vivo* for three of these molecules. A thorough assessment of diarylquinoline activity against MDR-TB *in vivo* would however require testing of animal models infected with multi-drug resistant bacterial strains rather than with drug-susceptible strains (Lounis *et al.*, 2006). Diarylquinoline TMC_{207} is currently in Phase II Clinical Trials (Table 5.1)

Nitroimidazole PA-8_{24}

Nitroimidazole PA-8_{24} (Fig. 6.1), is a new nitroimidazole derivative developed by PathoGenesis-Chiron in 1995 and currently being developed by the TB Alliance. The TB Alliance received worldwide exclusive rights to PA-8_{24} and its analogs for the treatment of TB. PA-8_{24} entered Phase I clinical trials in June 2005 (Casenghi, 2006). *In vitro*, PA-8_{24} showed high activity against drug-sensitive and drug-resistant *M. tuberculosis* strains, indicating that there is no cross-resistance with current TB drugs (Stover et al., 2000). Experiments performed on mice showed that the administration of PA-8_{24} at doses ranging from 25.0 - 100.0 mg/mL produced reductions in the bacterial burden in the spleen and lungs when compared to that produced by INH at 25 mg/mL (Stover *et al.*, 2000., Tyagi *et al.*, 2005). Further investigations are required to assess the potentiality of PA-8_{24} to improve the treatment of both drug-susceptible and multi-drug resistant tuberculosis when used in novel combinations with new drug candidates in addition to existing antituberculosis drugs. Nitroimidazole PA-8_{24} is currently in Phase II Clinical Trials (Table 6.1).

Nitroimidazole OPC-$6_7 68_3$

Nitroimidazole OPC-$6_7 68_3$ (Fig. 6.1c) belongs to a subclass of mycolic acid inhibitors, which interferes with the biosynthesis of the mycobacterial cell wall. MIC's of this compound were determined using standard and clinical isolated *M. tuberculosis* strains, including MDR strains. *In vitro*, OPC-$6_7 68_3$ showed high activity against drug-sensitive as well as drug-resistant strains with MIC's ranging from 6.0 - 24.0 mg/mL and also strong intracellular activity against *M. tuberculosis* $H_{37}RV$ strain residing within human macrophages (Casenghi, 2006). Studies in animal models showed that OPC-$6_7 68_3$ is effective against sensitive $H_{37}RV$ and

MDR-TB strains *in vivo* starting from a concentration of 0.03125 mg/body (Casenghi, 2006). The TB Alliance is currently negotiating with Otsuka Pharmaceuticals concerning the further joint development of this compound. OPC-$6_7 68_3$ is in Phase II Clinical Trials (Casenghi, 2006., Table 6.1).

Pyrrole LL-$_3 8_5 8$

Very little information on the development of pyrroles as anti-mycobacterial agents is currently available (Casenghi, 2006). Pyrroles derivatives were found to be active against standard and drug-sensitive *M. tuberculosis* strains *in vitro* (Deidda et al., 1998., Ragno *et al.*, 2000). Lupim Limited reported the identification of a pyrrole derivative (LL-$_3 8_5 8$) that showed higher bactericidal activity than INH when administered as monotherapy to infected mice. In mice models, a 12 weeks treatment with LL-$_3 8_5 8$ plus INH and RIF, or LL-$_3 8_5 8$ plus INH-RIF-PZA, sterilized the lungs of all infected mice. Experiments conducted in mice and dogs showed that the compound is well absorbed, with levels in serum above the MIC. No information is available concerning the molecular mechanisms that mediate LL-$_3 8_5 8$'s bacterial activity (Casenghi, 2006). Pyrrole LL- $_3 8_5 8$ is in Phase II Clinical Trial (Table 6.1).

Pleuromutilins

The pleuromutilins represent a novel class of antibiotics derived from a natural product. They interfere with protein synthesis by binding to the $_{23}$S rRNA and therefore inhibiting the peptide bond formation (Schlunzen *et al.*, 2004). Recent studies showed that cross-resistance might occur among pleuromutilins and oxazolidinones (Long et al., 2006). Pleuromutilins have also showed to inhibit the growth of *M. tuberculosis in vitro* (Casenghi, 2006)

Dipiperidine SQ-6_{09}

Dipiperidine SQ-6_{09} is a novel compound structurally unrelated to existing anti-TB drugs. It kills *M. tuberculosis* by interfering with cell wall biosynthesise. Antimicrobial activity has been demonstrated *in vivo* in mice models (Nikonenko *et al.*, 2004).

ATP Synthase Inhibitor FAS_{20013}

FAS_{20013} is a novel compound identified by Fasgen. It belongs to the class of â-sulphonylcarboxamides. Fasgen claims that FAS_{20013} will kill more organisms in a 4 hour exposure that INH or RIF can during a 12-14 day exposure (Casenghi, 2006). The compound is very effective in killing MDR-TB organisms that are resistant to the multiple drugs currently in use. A series of recent laboratory experiments indicate the superior effect of FAS_{20013} as compared to current drugs in terms of its ability to sterilize TB lesions and kill latent TB. Therapeutic evaluation of FAS_{20013} has repeatedly shown its effectiveness in mice, but it appears to or has no serious side effects. The compound is up to 100% bio-available when administered orally. To date no dose-limiting toxicity has been encountered, even when doses are 10 times administered. The compound is thought to act through inhibition of ATP synthase, however the available publications assessing the efficacy of this compound are of poor quality (Casenghi, 2006., Jones *et al.*, 2000., Parrish *et al.*, 2004).

Translocase I inhibitor

These are compounds which specifically inhibit mycobacterial translocase I, an enzyme required for bacterial cell wall. Preclinical evaluations of the compounds are planned (Casenghi, 2006).

InhA Inhibitors

Frontline drugs such as INH target the enoyl reductase enzyme InhA, found in *M. tuberculosis* which catalyses the last step in the fatty acid synthase pathway (FAS II). Drug resistance to INH results primarily from KatG (the enzyme that activates INH), therefore the InhA inhibitors that do not require activation by KatG are attractive candidates in the search for new drugs. The main purpose is to bypass the activation step and directly inhibit InhA. A possible limitation for this kind of compound is that cross-resistance with INH may easily occur (Casenghi, 2006., Banerjee *et al.*, 1994).

Isocitrate Lyse Inhibitors

The isocitrate lyase (ICL) enzyme has been shown to be essential for long-term persistence of *M. tuberculosis* in mice, but not required for bacilli viability in normal culture (McKinney *et al.*, 2000). McKinney and collaborators have shown that inhibition of ICL1 and ICL2 (the two isoforms of isocytrate lyase present in *M. tuberculosis*), blocks the growth and survival of *M. tuberculosis* in macrophages and in mice at an early and late stage of infection (McKinney *et al.*, 2000). GSK planned in 2000 to screen 400 000 ICL inhibitors as potential therapeutic drugs. Up to now 900 000 compounds have been screened but no successful inhibitors have been identified (Casenghi, 2006). The structure of the ICL active site makes the screening of inhibitors lengthy and the active site of this enzyme appears not to be easily reached by compounds (Casenghi, 2006).

CHEMICALS ORIGINATING FROM EXISTING FAMILIES OF DRUGS

Fluoroquinolones

Fluoroquinolones were introduced into clinical practice in the 1980's. They are characterised by broad spectrum antimicrobial activity and are recommended and widely used for the treatment of bacterial infection of the respiratory, gastrointestinal and urinary tracts (Bartlett *et al.*, 2000. Neu, 1987). Fluoroquinolones have been also found to have activity against *M. tuberculosis* and are currently part of the recommended regimen as second line drugs (Grosset, 1998., Tsukamura et al., 1985). Since fluoroquinolones share the same molecular targets, it is highly probable that they will trigger the same mechanisms of resistance. The major concern is that widespread use of fluoroquinolones for treatment of other bacteria infections may select for resistant strains of *M. tuberculosis*. In a study conducted in USA and Canada, among referral samples isolates between 1996 and 2000, resistance to ciprofloxacin was assessed and was found to occur in 1.8% of isolates and 75.8% were also MDR. The authors concluded that despite the widespread use of fluoroquinolones for treatment of common bacterial infection in USA and Canada, resistance to fluoroquinolones remains rare and occurs mainly in MDR strains (Bozeman *et al.*, 2005). In contrast, in a different study conducted by Ginsburg and collaborators between 1998 and 2002, the incidence of *M. tuberculosis* fluoroquinolone resistance in a small sample of patients with newly diagnosed TB was found to be high among patients with prior fluoroquinolone exposure (Ginsburg *et al.*, 2003b). The risk of selecting fluoroquinolones-resistant *M. tuberculosis* strains by empirically treating with fluoroquinolones for presumed infections before a diagnosis of TB established is of great concern. For this reason, some investigators in the TB field argue that the use of fluoroquinolones might be better reserved for specific serious infection such as TB rather than becoming the workhorse of antimicrobial treatment, however given the current widespread use of quinolones this might not be realistic (Bozeman *et al.*, 2005).

The interest in fluoroquinolones as antituberculosis agents has focused on the new fluoroquinolones moxifloxacin and gatifloxacin. Despite a lack of a comprehensive work comparing the activities of old and new classes of fluoroquinolones in *M. tuberculosis*, what can be inferred from published sources are that moxifloxacin and gatifloxacin are characterised by a higher activity against *M. tuberculosis in vitro* when compared to the old fluoroquinolones ofloxacin and ciprofloxacin (Hu *et al.*, 2003; Paramasivan *et al.*, 2005; Rodriguez *et al.*, 2001; Sulochana *et al.*, 2005).

Gatifloxacin

Gatifloxacin (GAT, Fig. 6.1d) is a new fluoroquinolone marketed in the U.S. by Bristol-Myers Squibb as Tequin. GAT has been found to have *in vitro* and *in vivo* bactericidal activity against *M. tuberculosis* (Hu *et al.*, 2003). In an *in vivo* study, GAT showed the highest bactericidal activity during the first 2 days but not thereafter (Paramasivan *et al.*, 2005). Similar results were obtained when GAT was used in combination with INH or RIF, GAT was able to slightly increase the bactericidal activity of INH or RIF only during the first 2 days (Paramasivan *et al.*, 2005). One paper reported that when tested in mice in combination with ethionamide and PZA (high doses: 450 mg/kg, 5 days per week) GAT was able to clear lungs of infected mice after 2 months of treatment (Cynamon and Sklaney, 2003).

Current available data on GAT does not support the hypothesis that introduction of GAT with first-line drugs will·impressively contribute to shorten TB treatment. Further investigation should be done to properly assess the activity of GAT *in vitro* and in animal models. GAT is currently in Phase II Clinical Trials (Table 6.1), conducted under the supervision of the European Commission Oflotub Consortium (Hu *et al.*, 2003). The aim of the trial is to evaluate the efficacy and safety of a four months gatifloxacin-containing regimen for treatment of pulmonary TB (Hu *et al.*, 2003).

Moxifloxacin

Moxifloxacin (MXF, Fig. 6.1e) is produced by Bayer Pharmaceuticals and marketed as Avelox in the USA. MXF is the most promising of the new fluroquinolones being tested against *M. tuberculosis* (Miyazaki *et al.*, 1999). *In vitro*, MXF appeared to kill a subpopulation of tubercle bacilli not killed by RIF, i.e. rifampicin-tolerant persisters, while other fluoroquinoles ciprofloxacin and ofloxacin did not have any significant bactericidal effect on the same subpopulation (Hu *et al.*, 2003). One possibility is that MXF interferes with protein synthesis in slowly metabolising bacteria, through a mechanism that differs from that used by RIF.

In mice models, the activity of MXF against tubercle bacilli was comparable to that of INH (Miyazaki *et al.*, 1999).When used in combination with MXF and PZA, MXF has been reported to kill the bacilli more effectively that the INH+RIF+PZA combination. In conclusion, *in vitro* and *in vivo* studies suggest that MXF might be a promising candidate drug to shorten TB treatment (Grosset *et al.*, 1992). MXF is currently in Phase III Clinical Trials (Table 6.1). A trial substituting EMB with MXF during intensive phase was initiated before the animal models and showed no advantage over EMB (Miyazaki *et al.*, 1999).

New Quinolones

In 2003, the TB Alliance launched a project in collaboration with the Korean Research Institute of Chemical Technology (KRCT) and the Yonsei University aimed to synthesise and evaluate novel and more effective quinolone compounds that could shorten first-line treatment. To date, 450 compounds have been synthesised and tested for their antituberculosis activity (Flamm *et al.*, 1995). During the research, the sub-class termed 2-pyridones was identified as being the one showing the most potent activity against *M. tuberculosis* in both its growing and persistent states. This sub-class of compounds was already identified by Abbott in 1998 and found to have activity against drug-susceptible and drug-resistant *M. tuberculosis*. The lead compounds identified so far, showed better activity than GZF and MXF (Oleksijew *et al.*, 1998).

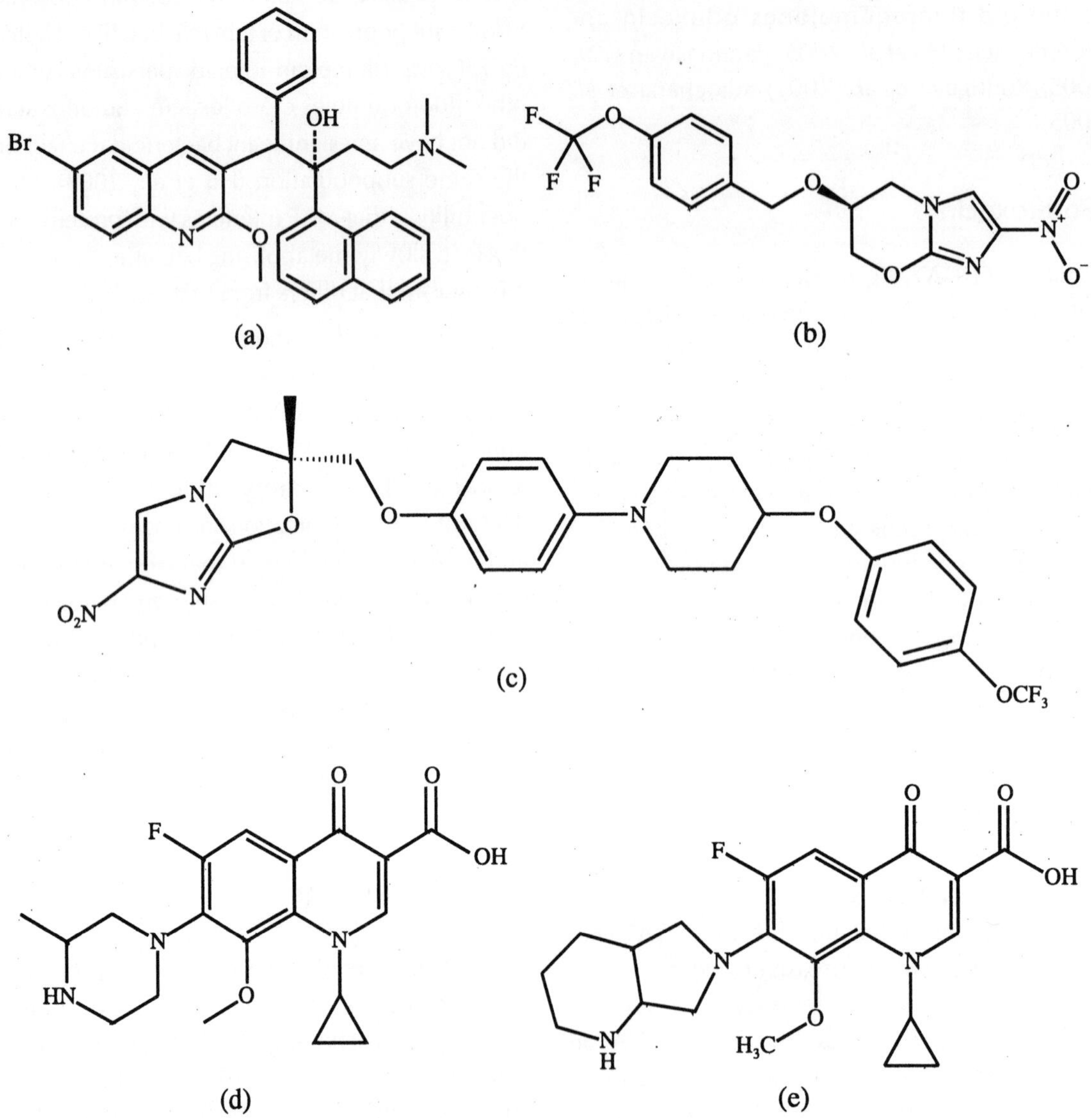

Fig. 6.2: Chemical structures of new antituberculosis drugs—(a) Diarylquinoline TMC$_{207}$, (b) Nitroimidazole PA-8$_{24}$, (c) Nitroimidazole OPC-6$_{7}$68$_{3}$, (d) Gatifloxacin (GAT), (e) Moxifloxacin (MXF)

Table 6.2: Global TB drug pipeline, March 2006 (provided by Stop TB Partnership working on new TB drugs)

Discovery		*Preclinical*	*Clinical*
Thiolectomycin Analog NIAID, NIH	*Nitrofuranylamides* NIAID, University of Tennessee	*Diamine SQ-109* Sequella Inc	*Diarylquinoline TMC207* Johnson & Johnson
Cell Wall Inhibitors Colorado State University, NIAID	*Nitroamidazole Analogs* NIAID, Novartis Institute for Tropical Diseases TR Alliance (University of Auckland)	*Dipiperidines SQ-609* Sequella Inc.	*Gatifloxacin* OFLOTUB Consortium, Lupin, NIAID TBRU, Tuberculosis Research Centre, WHO-TDR
Dihydrolipoamide Acyltransferase Inhibitors Cornell University, IAID	*Focused Screening* GlaxoSmithKline, TB Alliance	*Nitroimidazo-oxazole* Otsuka	*Moxifloxacin* Bayer Pharmaceuticals,CDC TBTC, Johns Hopkins University, NIAID TBRU, TB Alliance
InhA Inhibitors GlaxoSmithKline, TB Alliance	*Picolinamide Imidazoles* NIAID, TAACF	*Synthase Inhibitor FAS20013* FasGEN Inc.	*Nitroimidazole PA-824* Chiron Corporation, TB Alliance
Isocitrate Lyase Inhibitors (ICL) GlaxoSmithKline, TB Alliance	*Pleuromutilins* GlaxoSmithKline, TB Alliance	*Translocaase Inhibitors* Sequella Inc. Sankyo	*Nitroimidazo-axazole OPC-67883* Otsuka
Macrolides TB Alliance, University of Illinois	*Quinolones* KRICT/Yonsel University, NIAID, TAACF, TB Alliance	*Non-Fluorinated Quinolones* TaiGen	*Pyrrole LL-3858* Lupin Limited
Methyltransferase Inhibitors Anacor Pharmaceuticals	*Screening and Target identification* AstraZeneeca		
Natural Products Exploration BIOTEC, California State University, ITR, NIAID			

Mycobacterium Tuberculosis

M. tuberculosis belongs to the family Mycobacteriaceae and the genus *Mycobacterium*. This bacterium was described on the 24th of March 1882 by Robert Koch, who in 1905 received the Novel Prize in physiology or medicine for this discovery (Newton *et al.*, 2000). Many non-pathogenic mycobacteria are components of the normal flora of humans and are found most often in dry and oily locales. *M. tuberculosis* is also known as Koch's bacillus and it is a member of the "tuberculosis complex", a group of closely related mycobacterial pathogens, which include *M. bovis* (which infects cattle and may also infect humans), *M. microti*, *M. africanum* (which causes TB in West Africa) and *M. avium*, *M. intracellulare* and *M. scrofulaceum* (causing opportunistic infectious disease in patients with AIDS, Horne, 1996).

M. tuberculosis the causative agent of TB in humans is a fairly large nonmotile rod-shaped bacterium distantly related to the actinomycetes. The rods are 2-4 um in length and 0.2-0.5 um in width (Fig. 6.3a). The major components of the cell wall structure of the bacteria consist of peptidoglycan and lipids. Mycolic acids, which are á-branched lipids in cell walls, make up 50% of the dry weight of the mycobacterium cell envelope and are very strong hydrophobic molecules that form a lipid shell around the organism (Goren, 1990). Cord factor is a glycolipid (trehalose dimycolate) found in the cell wall that induces replication *in vitro*, resulting in serpentine cords of organisms. The role of the cord factor in the pathogenesis of tuberculosis is still under investigation, however, it is thought to be important because it inhibits and induces secretion of TNF-alpha by macrophages (Brennan, 1998).

M. tuberculosis is not classified as either a Gram-negative or Gram-positive bacteria because it does not have the biochemical characteristics of either (Camus *et al.*, 2002). If a Gram stain is performed on *M. tuberculosis*, it stains very weakly Gram-positive or not at all. *Mycobacterium* species, along with members of a related genus *Norcardia*, are classified as acid-fast bacteria due to their impermeability by certain dyes and stains. One acid-fast staining method for *M. tuberculosis* is staining with carbon-fuchsin (a pink dye) and decolourising with acid alcohol. The smear is counterstained with methylene blue or certain other dyes on different media such as Lowenstein-Jensen (Fig. 6.3b; Fadda and Roe, 1984).

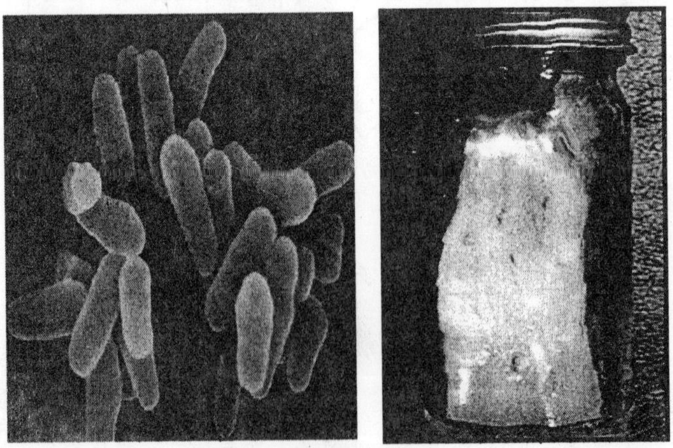

Fig. 6.3: *M. tuberculosis*—
(a) Rods of *M. tuberculosis*, magnification x 6.250 (based on a 35 mm slide *image* of 24 mm in the narrow dimension (Courtesy: SEM/ 97229A).
(b) Colonies of *M. tuberculosis* on Lowenstein-Jensen medium.

Infection with *M. tuberculosis* occurs by inhalation of small (1 – 10 microns) droplets containing only a few live tubercle bacilli. The primary focus of infection is usually the middle or lower zones of the lung. The bacilli are readily taken up by lung macrophages but can survive and grow to form the primary focus of infection and from there, enter the local lymphatic system and then move throughout the body via the blood and lymphatic system. This stage (the local lymphatic system), of disease is usually clinically silent or associated with mild fever and in most cases immunity develops within a few weeks and the patient becomes tuberculin positive (Girling, 1989). A key characteristic of *M. tuberculosis* infection is that the bacterium multiplies intracellularly, primarily in macrophages and in this way evading many host defence mechanisms (Velasco-Velazquez *et al.*, 2003). *M. tuberculosis* infects about 32% of the world's population. Every year, approximately 8 million of these infected people develop active tuberculosis and almost 2 million of these will die from the disease (WHO, 2008).

CONCLUSION

Herbal medicine is the oldest form of healthcare known to mankind. The use of herbs, which for most of history had been mainstream medical practice, began to be considered unscientific, or at least unconventional, and to fall into relative obscurity.

Many drugs that are commonly used today are of herbal origin. The World Health Organization (WHO, 2007 Fact Sheet 104) estimates that 4 billion people, or 80% of the world population, presently use herbal medicine for some aspect of primary health care. About 25% of the prescription drugs dispensed in the United States contain at least one active ingredient derived from plant material. Some are made from plant extracts; others are synthesized to mimic a natural plant compound. These herbal drugs provide strength to the body organs and stimulate normal functioning. The herbal drugs act selectively and gently without disturbing other systems, whereas modern medicine affects several metabolic activities in the human system and has side effects which make the body more susceptible to other diseases.

According to the WHO Global TB Report of 2006, South Africa has an estimated number of nearly 340,000 new TB cases per year with an incidence rate of 718 cases per 100,000. The TB epidemic in South Africa is exacerbated due to HIV/AIDS with an estimated 60% of adult TB patients being HIV positive. MDR-TB is further exacerbating the epidemic (WHO, 2007 Fact Sheet 104). Early stage drug discovery is a key in the pipeline to find novel drugs for tuberculosis. While the existence of a TB drug pipeline, after decades of virtually no new TB drug, is welcome, there are still far too few compounds that represent new chemical classes with novel mechanisms of action and a low probability of encountering pre-existing drug resistance. Of the approximately 40 compounds in the current pipeline, it is unlikely that a useful therapy will emerge, given that only about 1 compound in 20 successfully emerges from an anti-infective drug discovery program. Since new drugs for TB should only be used in combination, to prevent resistance, it would be a responsible act of global leadership to take whatever steps are necessary to attract as many new lead compounds into the pipeline as quickly as possible.

Another possible approach for generating a significant scale-up of TB drug discovery is to improve public sector capacity for running drug discovery programs. Government funding agencies could establish a medicinal chemistry resource center that would work as a core facility offering free lead optimization and ADMET (absorption, distribution, metabolism, excretion, and toxicology) studies in animal models. Such a facility would be directed by scientists with experience in drug discovery, and could also carry out training activities in order to ensure medicinal chemistry expertise in academia. A major challenge, though, would be attracting talented scientists to the not-for-profit medicinal chemistry sector and retaining them in competition with industry. Moreover, to invest in medicinal chemistry for the public sector without the other technologies, resources, and expertise that go into drug development might result in limited success or strategic failure (Casenghi *et al.*, 2007).

REFERENCES

American Hospital Formulatory Services (AHFS) Drug Information. American Society of Health-System Pharmacists, pp 485-506, (2000).

Andries K, Verhasselt P, Guillemont J, Gohlmann HW, Neef JM, Winkler H, Van Gestel J, Timmerman P, Zhu M, Lee E. A diarylquinoline drug active on the ATP synthase of *Mycobacterium tuberculosis*. *Science*; 307, 223-227, (2005).

Arnold HJ, Gulumian M. Pharmacopoeia of traditional medicine in Venda. *J Ethnopharmacol*, 12, 35-74, (1984).

Ayyazian LF. History of tuberculosis. In: Reichman LB. Hershfield (eds) Tuberculosis. Dekker, New York, pp 293-238, (1993).

Barclay WR, Ebert RH, Le Roy GV, Manthei RW, Roth LJ. Distribution and excretion of radioactive isoniazid in tuberculosis patients. *J Amer Med Assoc*; 151, 1384-1388, (1953).

Balick MJ. Ethnobotany and the identification of therapeutic agents from the rainforest. *Institute Economic Bot*, 154, 22-39, (1990).

Banerjee A, Dubnau E, Quemard A, Balasubramanian V, Um KS, Wilson T, Collins D, de Lisle G, Jacobs WR. InhA, a gene encoding a target for isoniazid and ethionamide in *M. tuberculosis*. *Science*, 263, 227-230, (1994).

Bapela NB. Isolation of naphthoquinones from the roots of *Euclea natalensis* and their *in vitro* antimycobacterial activity and toxicity. Dissertation, University of Pretoria, (2005).

Bartlett JG, Dowell SF, Mandell LA, File TM, Musher DM, Fine MJ. Practice guidelines for the management of community-acquired pneumonia in adults. Infectious Diseases Society of America. *Clin Infect Dis*, 31, 347-382, (2000).

Bartmann K. Anti-tuberculosis drugs. Handbook of experimental pharmacology. Springer-Verlag, Berlin Heidelberg Germany, 84, (1988).

Basel HH. History of Tuberculosis. *Respiration*, 65, 5-15, (1998).

Basso LA, Blanchard JS. Resistance to anti-tubercular drugs. *Adv Exp Med Biol*, 456, 115-144, (1998).

Bastian I, Colebunders R. Treatment and prevention of multidrug resistant tuberculosis. *Drugs*, 58, 633-666, (1999).

Beyers N. Tuberculosis. Wellcome Trust Workshop on Immunology, University of Cape Town, (1999).

Bloom BR, Murray CJL. Tuberculosis: commentary on a re-emergent killer. *Science*, 257, 1055-1064, (1992).

Bloom BR. Tuberculosis: pathogenesis, protection and control. *Americ Soc Microbiol*, Washington, DC, (1994).

Bloom BR. Tuberculosis - The Global view. *J Med*, 346, 1434-1435, (2002).

Bozeman L, Burman W, Metchock B, Welch L, Weiner M. Fluoroquinolone susceptibility among *Mycobacterium tuberculosis* isolates from the United States and Canada. *Clin Infect Dis*, 40, 386-391, (2005).

Brennan PJ. *Mycobacterium* and other actinomycetes, in *Microbial lipids*, 1. Ed. Academic Press, London, pp 203-298, (1988).

British Thoracic Society. A controlled trial of 6 months chemotherapy in pulmonary tuberculosis, final report: results during the 36 months after the end of chemotherapy and beyond. *Br J Dis Chest*, 78, 330-336, (1984).

Camus JC, Pryor MJ, Medigue C, Cole ST. Re-annotation of the genome sequence of *Mycobacterium tuberculosis* H37Rv. *Microbiology*, 148, 2967-2973 (2002).

Casenghi M. Development of new drugs for TB chemotherapy: Analysis of the current drug pipeline. Medecin Sans Frontieres, (2006).

Casenghi M, Cole ST, Nathan CF. New approaches to filling the gap in tuberculosis drug discovery. P*LoS Med*, 4, 293, (2007).

Cantrell CL, Abate L, Fronczek FR, Franzblau SG, Quijano L, Fischer NH. Antimycobacterial eudesmanolides from *Inula helenium* and *Rudbeckia subtomentosa. Planta Med*, 65, 351-355, (1999).

Cantrell CL, Franzblau SG, Fischer NH. Antimycobacterial plant terpenoids. *Planta Med*, 67, 685-694, (2001).

Chan ED, Iseman MD. Current medical treatment for tuberculosis. *Br Med J*. 325,1282-1286, (2002)

Clark DW. Genetically determined variability in acetylation and oxidation: Therapeutic implications. *Drugs*, 29, 342-375, (1985).

Collins FM. *Mycobacterium* pathogenesis: a historical perspective. *Front Biosci*, 3, 123-132, (1998).

Corbett EL, Watt CJ, Walker N, Maher D, Williams BG, Raviglione MC, Dye C. The growing burden of tuberculosis. Global trends and interactions with the HIV epidemic. *Arch Intern Med*, 163, 1009-1021, (2003).

Cragg GM, Newman DJ. Plants as a source of anticancer agents. *J Ethnopharmacol*, 100, 72-79, (2005).

Cynamon MH, Sklaney M. Gatifloxacin and ethionamide as the foundation for therapy of tuberculosis. *Antimicrob Agents Chemother*, 47, 2442-2444, (2003).

Dannenberg AM. Immune mechanisms in the pathogenesis of pulmonary tuberculosis. *Rev Infect Dis*, 11, S369-S377, (1989).

Davis SD, Heywood VH, Hamilton AC (eds.) Centres of Plant Diversity:A Guide and Strategy for their Conservation. Cambridge, pp 136-139, (1995).

Deidda D, Lampis G, Fioravanti R, Biava M, Porretta GC, Zanetti S, Pompei R. Bactericidal activities of the pyrrole derivative BM212 against multidrug-resistant and intra-macrophagic *Mycobacterium tuberculosis* strains. *Antimicrob Agents Chemother*, 42, 3035-3037, (1998).

De Smet PAGM. The role of plant derived drugs and herbal medicines in healthcare. *Drugs*, 54, 801-840, (1997).

Diermeier HF, Kaiser JA, Yuda N. Safety evaluation of ethambutol. *Ann NY Acad Sci*, 135, 735-746, (1966).

Duman N, Cevikbas A, Johansson C. The effects of rifampicin and fluoroquinolones on tubercle bacilli within human macrophages. *Int J Antimicrob Agents*, 23, 84-87, (2004).

Eloff JN. A sensitive and quick microplate method to determine the minimal inhibitory concentration of plant extracts for bacteria. *Planta Med*, 64, 711-713, (1998).

Fadda G, Roe SL. Recovery and susceptibility testing of *Mycobacterium tuberculosis* from extra pulmonary specimens by the BACTEC radiometric method. *J Clin Microbiol*, 19, 720-721, (1984).

Farnsworth NR. The role of medicinal plants in drug development. In: Natural Products and Drug development. Bailliere, Tindal and Cox. London, pp 8-98, (1984).

Flamm RK, Vojtko C, Chu DT, Li Q, Beyer J, Hensey D, Ramer N, Clement JJ, Tanaka SK. *In vitro* evaluation of ABT-719, a novel DNA gyrase inhibitor. *Antimicrob Agents Chemother*, 39, 964-970, (1995).

Fourie B, Weyer K. TB and HIV-the deadly duo. *MRC News*, 31, 21-22, (2000).

Gautam R, Saklani A, Jachak SA. Indian medicinal plants as a source of antimycobacterial agents. *J Ethnopharmacol*; 110, 200-234, (2007).

Ginsburg AS, Hooper N, Parrish N, Dooley KE, Dorman SE, Booth J, Diener West M, Merz WG, Bishai WR, Sterling TR. Fluoroquinolone resistance in patients with newly diagnosed tuberculosis. *Clin Infect Dis*, 37, 1448-1452, (2003).

Girling DJ. The chemotherapy of tuberculosis. In: Ratledge C, Stanford JL, Grange JM (eds.) Biology of the *Mycobacterium tuberculosis*, 3, 43-47, (1989).

Goren MB. Mycobacterial fatty esters of sugars and sulfosugars. In: Glycolipids, Phospholipids and Sulfoglycolipids. *Handbook Lipid Res.* 6. Plenum Press, pp 363-461, (1990).

Grosset J, Ji B. (Experimental chemotherapy of mycobacterial diseases, 51-97. In: Gangadharam P.R.J, Jenkins P.A. *Mycobacteria, II chemotherapy*, Chapman and Hall, New York, (1998).

Grange JM, Davey RW. Detection of antituberculosis activity of plant extracts. *J Appl Bacteriol*, 68, 587-591, (1990).

Gutierrez-Lugo MT, Wang Y, Franzblau SG, Timmermann BN. Antitubercular sterols from *Thalia multiflora* Horkel ex Koernicke. *Phytother Res*, 19, 876-880, (2005).

Haas W. The history of human tuberculosis. Dissertation, University of Witwatersrand, (1996).

Handwerger S, Tomasz A. Antibiotic tolerance among clinical isolates of bacteria. *Rev Infect Dis*, 7, 368-386, (1985).

Heinrich M, Gibbons S. Ethnopharmacology in drug discovery: an analysis of its role and potential contribution. *J Pharm Pharmacol*, 53, 425-432, (2001).

Herbert D, Paramasivan CN, Venkatesan P, Kubendiran G, Prabhakar R, Mitchison DA. Bactericidal action of ofloxacin, sulbactamampicilin, rifampin and isoniazid on logarithmic and stationary phase cultures of *Mycobacterium tuberculosis. Antimicrob Agents Ch*, 40, 2296-2299, (1996).

Heym B, Cole ST. Multidrug resistance in *Mycobacterium tuberculosis. International J Antimicrob Agents*, 8, 61-70, (1997).

Holdiness MR. Clinical pharmacokinetics of the antituberculosis drugs. *Clinic Pharmacokinet*, 9, 511-544, (1984).

Horne N. Tuberculosis and other mycobacterial diseases. In: Cook G.C (eds) Manson's Tropical Diseases. Saunders, London, pp 971-1015, (1996).

Hostettmann K, Marston A. Twenty years of research into medicinal plants: results and perspectives. *Phytochem Rev*, 1, 275-285, (2002).

Houghton PJ, Woldermarian TZ, Watanabe Y, Yates M. Activity against *Mycobacterium tuberculosis* of alkaloid constituents of Angosturab a r k , *Galipea officinalis. Planta Med*, 65, 250-254, (1999).

Hu Y, Coates AR, Mitchison DA. Sterilizing activities of fluoroquinolesagainst rifampin-tolerant populations of *Mycobacterium tuberculosis. Antimicrob Agents Chemother*, 47, 653-657, (2003).

Kirby GC. Medicinal plants and the control of protozoal diseases, with particular reference to malaria. *Trans R Soc Trop Med Hyg*, 90, 605-609, (1996).

Klopper RR, Smith GF, Van Rooy J. The biodiversity of Africa. In: Baijnath H, Singh Y (eds) Rebirth of Science in Africa. A Shared Vision for Life and Environmental Sciences. Umdaus Press, Hatfield, pp 60-86, (2002).

Jindani A, Dore CJ, Mitchison DA. Bactericidal and sterilizing activities of antituberculosis drugs during the first 14 days. *Am J Respir Crit Care Med*, 167, 1348-1354, (2003).

Jones PB, Parrish NM, Houston TA, Stapon A, Bansal NR, Dick JD, Townsend CA. A new class of antituberculosis agents. *J Med Chem*, 43, 3304-3314, (2000).

Lall N, Meyer JJM. *In vitro* inhibition of drug-resistant and drug sensitive strains of *Mycobacterium tuberculosis* by ethnobotanically selected South African plants. *J Ethnopharmacol*, 66, 347-354, (1999).

Lall N, Meyer JJM. Inhibition of drug-sensitive and drug-resistant strains of *Mycobacterium tuberculosis* by diospyrin, isolated from *Euclea natalensis*. *J Ethnopharmacol*, 78, 213-216, (2001).

Lounis N, Veziris N, Chauffour A, Truffot-Pernot C, Andries K, Jarlier V. Combinations of R_{207910} with drugs used to treat MDR-TB have the potential to shorten treatment duration. *Antimicrob Agents Chemother*, 50, 3543-3547, (2006).

Lurie MN, Carter EJ, Cohen J, Flanigan TP. Directly observed therapy for HIV/tuberculosis co-infection. *Lancet Infect Dis*, 4, 137-138, (2004).

Mabogo DEN. The ethnobotany of Vhavenda. Dissertation, University of Pretoria, (1990).

Megehee J, Lundrigan M. Temporal expression of *Mycobacterium smegmatis* respiratory terminal oxidase. *Can J Microbiol*, 53, 459-460, (2007).

McCune RM, Tompsett R. Fate of *Mycobacterium tuberculosis* in mouse tissues as determined by the microbial enumeration technique. The persistence of drug-susceptible tubercle bacilli in the tissues despite prolonged antimicrobial therapy. *J Exp Med*, 104, 737-762, (1956).

McKinney JD. *In vivo* veritas: the search for TB drug targets goes live. *Nat Med*, 6, 1330-1333, (2000).

McGaw LJ, Jager AK, van Steden J. Antibacterial, antihelmintic and anti amoebic activity in South African medicinal plants. *J Ethnopharmacol*, 72, 247-263, (2000).

Mitchison DA. Basic mechanisms of chemotherapy. *Chest*, 76, 771-781, (1979).

Mitchison DA. Treatment of tuberculosis. The Mitchell lecture 1979. *J Roy Coll Physic Lon*, 14, 91-99, (1980).

Mitchison DA. Drug resistance in mycobacteria. *Brit Med Bull*, 40, 84-90, (1984).

Mitchison DA. The Garrod Lecture. Understanding the chemotherapy of tuberculosis-current problems. *J Antimicrob Chemother*, 29, 477-493, (1992).

Mitchison DA, Selkon JB. The bactericidal activities of antituberculosis drugs. *Am Rev Tuberc*, 74, 109-116, (1996).

Miyazaki E, Miyazaki M, Chen JM, Chaisson RE, Bishai WR. Moxifloxacin (BAY12-8039), a new 8-methoxyquinolone, is active in a mouse model of tuberculosis. *Antimicrob Agents Chemother*, 43, 85-89, (1999).

Moran M, Ropars AL, Guzman J, Diaz J, Garrison C. The new landscape of neglected disease drug development. London School of Economics and The Wellcome Trust. (2005).

Mukherjee PK. GMP for Indian Systems of Medicine. In: Mukherjee PK, Verpoorte R (eds) *GMP for Botanicals: Regulatory and Quality Issues on Phytomedicines*, Business Horizons, New Delhi, pp 99-112, (2003).

Neu HC. Clinical use of the quinolones. *Lancet Infect Dis*, 2, 1319-1322, (1987).

Newman DJ, Cragg GM, Snader KM. Natural products as sources of new drugs over the period 1981-2002. *J Nat Prod*, 66, 1022-1037, (2003).

Newton SM, Lau C, Wright CW. A review of antimycobacterial natural products. *Phytother Res*, 14, 302-322, (2000).

Newton SM, Lau C, Gurcha SS, Besra GS, Wright CW. Theevaluation of forty-three plant species for *in vitro* antimycobacterial activities; isolation of active constituents from *Psoralea corylifolia* and *Sanguinaria canadensis*. *J Ethnopharmacol*, 79, 57-67, (2002).

Niederweis M, Ehrt S, Heinz C, Klöcker U, Swiderek KM, Riley LW Benz R. Cloning of the *mspA* gene encoding the porin from *Mycobacterium smegmatis*. *Mol Microbiol*, 33, 933-945, (1999).

Nigro SA, Makunga NP, Grace OM. Medicinal plants at the ethnobotany biotechnology interface in Africa. *S Afr J Bot*, 70, 89-95, (2004).

Nikonenko BV, Samala R, Eincck L, Nacy CA. Rapid, simple *in vivo* screen for new drugs active against *Mycobacterium tuberculosis*. *Antimicrob Agents Chemother*, 48, 4550-4555, (2004).

O'Brien RJ, Nunn PP. The need for new drugs against tuberculosis. Obstacles, opportunities and next steps. *Am J Resp Crit Care Med*, 163, 1055-1058, (2001).

Okunade AL, Elvin-Lewis MP, Lewis WH. Natural antimycobacterial metabolites: current status. *Phytochem*, 65, 1017-1032, (2004).

Oleksijew A, Meulbroek J, Ewing P, Jarvis K, Mitten M, Paige L, Tovcimak A, Nukkula M, Chu D, Alder JD. *In vivo* efficacy of ABT 255 against drug-sensitive and resistant *Mycobacterium tuberculosis* strains. *Antimicrob Agents Chemother*, 42, 2674-2677, (1998).

Orme I. Immunity to mycobacteria. *Curr Opin Immunol*, 5, 497-502, (1993).

Paramasivan CN, Sulochana S, Kubendiran G, Vnekatesan P, Mitchison DA. Bactericidal action of gatifloxacin, rifampicin and isoniazid on logarithmic and stationary-phase cultures of *Mycobacterium tuberculosis*. *Antimicrob Agents Chemother*, 49, 627-631, (2005).

Parrish NM, Ko CG, Hughes MA, Towsend CA, Dick JD. Effect ofN-octanesulphonylacetamide (OSA) on ATP and protein expression in *Mycobacterium bovis* BCG. *J Antimicrob Chemother*, 54, 722-729, (2004).

Pauli GF, Case RJ, Inui T, Wang Y, Cho S, Fischer NH, Franzblau SG. New perspectives on natural products in TB drug research. *Life Sci*, 9, 88-91, (2005).

Petrella S, Cambau E, Chauffour A, Adries K, Jarlier V, Sougakoff W. Genetic basis for natural and acquired resistance to the diarlyquinoline R207910 in mycobacteria. *Antimicrob Agents Chemother*, 50, 2853-2856, (2006).

Phillpson JD. Phytochemistry and medicinal plants. *Phytochemistry*, 56, 237-243, (2001).

Quenelle DC, Winchester GA, Staas JK. Treatment of tuberculosis using a combination of sustained-release Rifampin-loaded microspheres and oral dosing with Isoniazid. *Antimicrob Agents Chemother*, 45, 1637-1644, (2001).

Ragno R, Marshall GR, Di Santo R, Costi R, Massa S, Rompei R, Artico M. Antimycobacterial pyrroles: synthesis, *antimycobacterium tuberculosis* activity and QSAR studies. *Bioorgan Med Chem*, 8, 1423-1432, (2000).

Ramaswammy S, Musser JM. Molecular genetic basis of antimycobacterial agent resistance in *Mycobacterium tuberculosis*. *Tubercle Lung Dis*, 79, 3-29, (1998).

Raviglone MC, Snider DE, Kochi A. Global epidemiology of tuberculosis. *J Am Med Assoc*; 273, 220-226, (1995).

Robinson HJ, Siegel H, Pietrowski JJ. Toxicity of pyrazinamide. *Am Rev Tuberc*, 70, 423-429, (1954).

Rodriguez JC, Ruiz M, Climent A, Royo G. *In vitro* activity of four fluoroquinoles against *Mycobacterium tuberculosis*. *Int J Antimicrob Agents*, 17, 229-231, (2001).

Reichman LB, Hersfield ES. Tuberculosis. A comprehensive international approach. Marcel Dekker, New York. (2000).

Salie F, Eagles PFK, Leng HMJ. Preliminary antimicrobial screening of four South African Asteraceae species. *J Ethnopharmacol*, 52, 27-37, (1996).

Selwyn PA, Sckell BM, Alcabes P. High risk of active tuberculosis in HIV infected drug users with cutaneous energy. *J Am Med Assoc*, 268, 504, 509, (1992).

Schlunzen F, Pyeten E, Fucini P, Yonath A, Harms JM. Inhibition of peptide bond formation by pleuromutilins: the structure of the ribosomal subunit from *Delnococcus radiodurans*. *Mol Microbiol*, 54, 1287-1294, (2004).

Scopio A, Zheng Y. Mutation in pncA, a gene encoding pyrazinamide ornicotinamide cause resistance to the antituberculosis drug PZA in tubercle bacillus. *Nat Med*, 2, 266-267, (1996).

Smith GF, Van Wyk AE 2002. Regions of Floristic Endemism in Southern Africa: A Review with Emphasis on Succulents. Umdaus Press, Pretoria.

Steele JH, Rammey AF. Animal tuberculosis. *Ann Int Med*, 116, 937-994, (1958).

Stover CK, Warrener P, Van Devanter DR, Sherman DR, Arain TM, Langhorne MH, Anderson SW, Towell JA, Yuan Y, McMurray DN. A small molecule nitroimidazopyran drug candidate for the treatment of tuberculosis. *Nat*, 405, 962-966, (2000).

Sulochana S, Rahman F, Paramasivan CN. *In vitro* activity of fluoroquinolones against *Mycobacterium tuberculosis*. *J Chemotherapy*, 17, 169-173, (2005).

Taniguchi H. Molecular mechanisms of multidrug resistance in *Mycobacterium tuberculosis*. *J Occup Health*, 27, 269-282, (2000).

Theunis FG, Isabel I, Snyckers FO. Folk Medicine: a viable starting point for pharmaceutical research. *S Afri J Sci*, 88, 190-192, (1992).

Tripathi RP, Tewari N, Dwivedi N, Tiwari VK. Fighting tuberculosis: an old disease with new challenges. *Med Res Rev*, 25, 93-131, (2005).

Tsukamura M, Nakamura E, Yoshii S, Amano H. Therapeutic effect of a new antibacterial substance ofloxacin ($DL8_28_0$) on pulmonary tuberculosis. *Am Rev Res Dis*, 131, 352-356, (1985).

Tyagi S, Nuermberger E, Yoshimatsu T, Williams K, Rosenthal I, Lounis N, Bishai W, Grosset J. Bactericidal activity of the nitroimidazopyran PA 8_{24} in a murine model of tuberculosis. *Antimicrob Agents Ch*, 49, 2289-2293, (2005).

Van Puyvelde L, Ntawukiliyaya JD, Portaels F. *In vitro* inhibition of mycobacteria by Rwandese medicinal plants. *Phytother Res*, 8, 65-69, (1994).

Van Wyk BE, Van Oudtshoorn B, Gericke N. Medicinal plants of South Africa. Briza Publications. South Africa (1997).

Van Wyk BE, Wink M. Medicinal plants of the world. Briza Publications. South Africa. (2004).

Velasco-Velazquez MA, Barrera D, Gonzalez-Arenaz A, Agramonte HJ. Macrophage-*Mycobacterium tuberculosis* interactions: role of complement receptor 3. *Microb Pathogenesis*, 35, 125-131, (2003).

Watt C, Breyer-Brandwyk MG. The medicinal and poisonous plants of Southern and Eastern Africa. Edinburgh, London, pp 449-451 (1962).

Wilson TM, Collins DM. AhpC, a gene involved in isoniazid resistance of the *Mycobacterium tuberculosis* complex. *Mol Microbiol*, 19, 1025-1034, (1996).

World Health Organisation. World Report 1999. Office of World Health Reporting. Geneva, Switzerland. Cited 11 May (2005).

World Health Organisation. Tuberculosis Facts. Cited 11 May (2006).

World Health Organisation. *Tuberculosis.* Fact Sheet number 104, revised March 2007. World Health Organization: Geneva, Switzerland. Cited 21 Aug. (2007).

World Health Organisation. *Global Tuberculosis Control.* WorldHealthOrganization: Geneva, Switzerland. Cited 21 Aug. (2008).

Yelne MB, Sharma PC, Dennis TJ. Database on medicinal plants used in Ayurvede. New Delhi, pp 124-135, (2001).

Young DB. Tuberculosis. Beating the bacillus. *Curr Biol*, 4, 351-353, (1994).

Young DB, Duncan K. Prospects for new interventions in the treatment and prevention of mycobacterial disease. *Ann Rev Microbiol*, 49, 641-673, (1995).

Zhang Y. The magic bullets and tuberculosis drug targets. *Ann RevPharmacol*, 45, 529-564, (2005).

Zumla A, Grange J. Clinical review: tuberculosis. *Brit Med J*, 316 1962-1964, (1998).

chapter 7

PHYTO-PHARMACOLOGY OF ANTI-ASTHMATIC MEDICINAL PLANTS

Vimal Kumar, Mohammad Yaseen Khan and Amit Nayak

INTRODUCTION

Asthma has emerged as a major public health problem worldwide; it continues to be a significant cause of morbidity and mortality. Despite impressive advances in our knowledge, it is still a major health care problem and, in the past two decades, incidences have steadily risen worldwide along with costs related to drugs and medical care. Around 275 million people around the globe suffer from asthma and these numbers have been rising worldwide, mortality from this condition has reached 18 million annually. On 3rd May of every year, the World Health Organization (WHO), together with its partners around the world, is observing World Asthma Day for many million asthmatic sufferers. Asthma is a one of the most common chronic disease of lower respiratory system characterized by increased responsiveness of trachea and bronchi to various stimuli and manifested by widespread narrowing of the airways (Bills and Soderberg, 1998). These symptoms are due to the liberation of endogens and intrinsic mediators like histamine, leukotrienes(LTs), bradykinin, prostaglandins (PGs), nitric oxide, platelet-activating factor (PAF), chemokines and endothelin from mast cells during the allergic reactions and inflammation of the air passages in the lungs (Spina, 2000), which affect the sensitivity of nerve endings in the airways and render them easily irritable (Nagarajan and Naik, 1996). Allergic asthma is characterized by airway hyperresponsiveness associated with elevated serum IgE and bronchial inflammation. Although corticosteroids are effective nonspecific anti-inflammatory agents, the side effects of corticosteroid treatment are a significant concern, particularly for children, in whom the morbidity and mortality of asthma have been increasing (Akinbami and Schoendorf, 2002). Till today, world's population is about 5 billion and with this rate of growth likely to touch 7.5 billion by the year 2020. The global estimate indicate that over 5 billion world population mostly from Asia and Africa cannot afford the products of the western pharmaceutical industries and have to rely upon the use of traditional medicines, which mainly derived from plants. Medicinal plants continue to be an important resource material for phytomedicinal agents in developing countries like India and China. The need for safe, effective and cheap treatments of this disease is greater than ever. Complementary and alternative medicine approaches are increasingly being considered by patients, and the use of complementary and alternative medicine has grown substantially during the last 10 years in Western countries as well as through out the world (MacLennan et al., 1996; Kesseler et al., 2001). A recent study reported that up to 50% of asthmatic patients were using some form of complementary and alternative medicine, and that a growing number of asthma patients wish to use complementary and alternative medicine (Steurer-Stey et al., 2002). However, a role for complementary and alternative medicine in asthma therapy is uncertain because there are few well-controlled scientific studies demonstrating efficacy, and any beneficial actions of these materials on allergic processes are largely unknown (Steurer-Stey et al. 2002). Traditional medicine has played a central role in treating diseases including asthma for centuries and is still widely used in modern medical practice throughout the world. Still there is a great potential in traditional medicine for development of herbal interventions to treat asthma and allergy (Steurer-Stey et al., 2002).

MEDICINAL PLANTS IN TREATMENT OF ASTHMATIC DISORDERS

Many Ayurvedic plants have been described to be useful in the treatment of various bronchial disorders including bronchial asthma. Plant drugs are considered as safe and effective since they are natural products. Most widely used traditional anti-asthmatic plants are growing in India and Asian subcontinents. In the ayurvedic medical tradition, the leaves of Datura were smoked for the relief of respiratory ailments and this was the form and purpose for which it became widely used in the West. (Indeed "stramonium cigarettes" continued to be used well into the 20th century in both Europe and North America.) Atropine was isolated and discovered to be the active ingredient in such plants by German chemists in the middle of the 19th century, from which time atropine became the standard treatment for "Asthma" (Courty, 1859).

Many studies on herbal drugs have been reported to be useful in the treatment of asthma and allergy. Various compounds from specific medicinal plants have also been identified as the anti-asthmatic components with their mechanisms of action throughout the history of medicine. Since plants may contain hundred of metabolites, there is currently a resurgence of interest in secondary metabolites of plants as a possible source of new lead compounds.

The infusion of the seeds of the *Ammi visnaga* was used in the treatment of respiratory disorders for many years. Later the bronchodilator principle 'khellin' was isolated from this plant, the structural modification of khellin, led to the development of disodium cromoglycate (Cox et al., 1970), which is the most successful anti-allergic drug developed from natural products and ephedrine alkaloid was also isolated from *Ephedra vulgaris,* which has been used in the treatment of respiratory disorders since long time. *Ephedra* consists of the dried aerial parts of xerophytic *Ephedra* species belonging to the family *Ephedraceae.* The plant is a shrub, 0.5-1 m high with scale-like leaves that clasp the stem. Nowadays the *Ephedra* species are mainly used for extraction of the active ingredient, the alkaloid (–) ephedrine. Not only the classical Chinese species *E. sinica* Stapf. is used, but mainly the species *E. gerardiana.* Wall ex. Stapf and *E. major* Host. (*E. nebrodensis* Finco), which both grow in India and Pakistan, and *E. distachya* L., which grows in Southern France. The alkaloid ephedrine was isolated in 1885 by the Japanese chemist W. N. Nagai. Two pharmacologists, the Chinese K.K. Chen and the American G. F. Schmidt, showed in the 1920s that ephedrine is a sympathomimetic, i.e. it has an adrenaline-like effect with two important modifications: it is much less active, but the effect has a longer duration and it is effective by oral administration. Owing to the vasoconstrictor effect explains its use in allergic nasal catarrh and for pretreatment prior to spinal anaesthesia.

A large number of medicinal plants have been used traditionally in the Ayurveda, other complementary and alternative systems of medicine for the management of asthma and allergic disorders. Some of them have been confirmed experimentally are shown in Table 1. Structures of some the pharmacologically active anti-asthamatic phyto-constituents is shown in Figure 1.

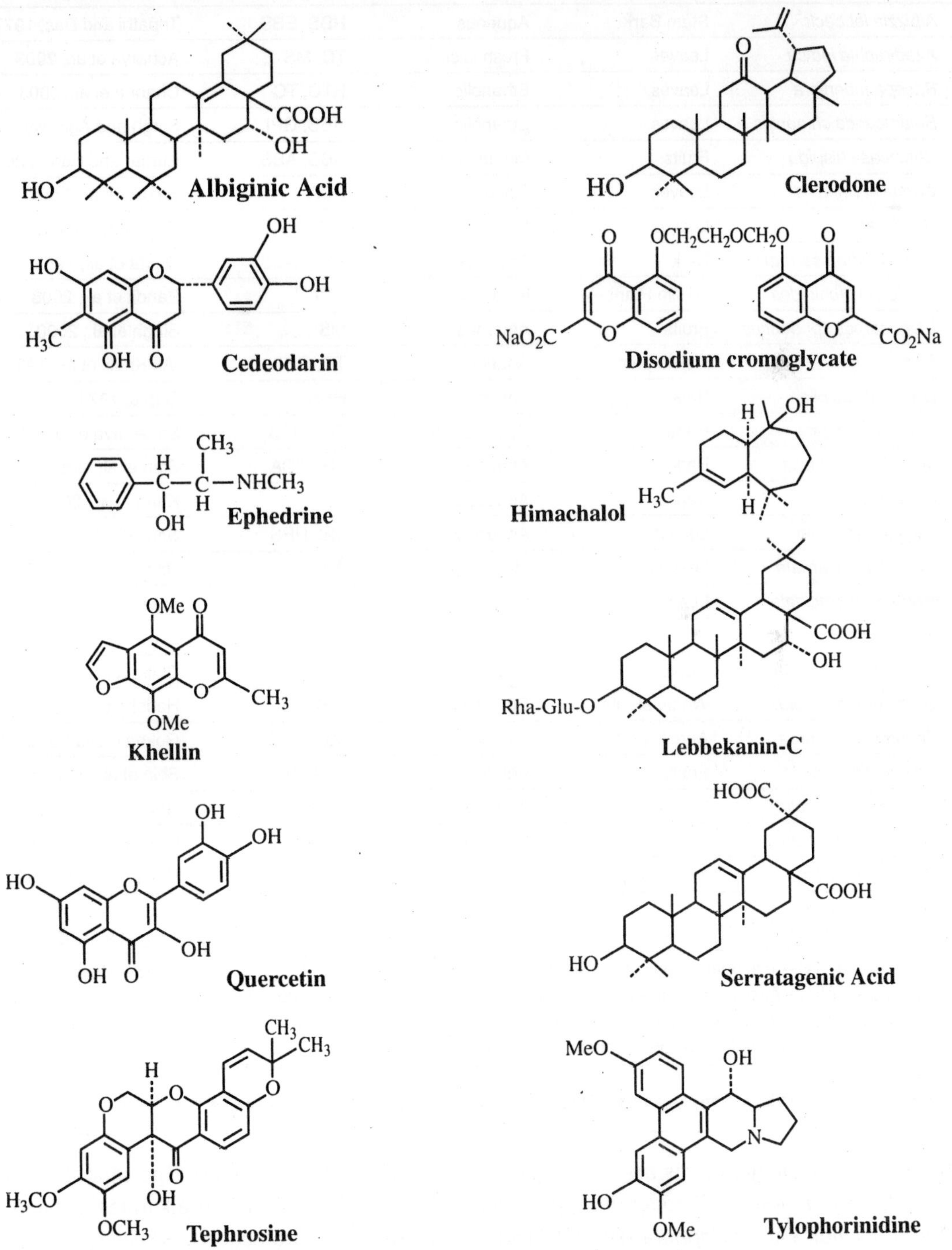

Table 7.1 Medicinal Plants Experimentally Investigated for Asthmatic Disorder

Plants	*Part Used*	*Extract / Fraction*	*Models studied**	*References*
Achyranthes aspera	Whole plant	Aqueous	MS	Agrawal et al., 2003
Aegle marmelos	Leaves	Ethanolic	TC, GPI	Arul et al., 2004
Albizzia lebbeck	Stem Bark	Aqueous	HBS, EBS	Tripathi and Das, 1977
Azadirachta indica	Leaves	Fresh juice	TC, MS	Acharya et al., 2003
Bacopa monniera	Leaves	Ethanolic	RTC, TC	Channa et al., 2003
Belamcanda chinensis	Leaves	Ethanolic	HBS, GPI	Singh and Agrawal, 1990
Benincasa hispida	Fruits	Methanolic	HBS, ABS	Kumar and Ramu, 2002
Camellia sinensis	Leaves	Flavonoids	PCA	Suzuki et al., 2000
Cassia alata	Leaves	Ethanolic	MS	Palanichamy et al.,1991
Clerodendron serratum	Bark	Aqueous	HBS, ABS	Gupta et al., 1968
Curculigo orchioides	Whole Plant	Ethanolic	GPI	Pandit et al., 2008
Elaeocarpus sphaericus	Fruits	Aqueous	MS	Singh et al., 2000
Ferula ovina	Whole plant	Aqueous	TC, GPI	Al- Khalil et al., 1990
Gardenia latifolia	Bark	Saponins	HBS	Gupta, 1974
Inula racemosa	Roots	Hydro-alcoholic	PCA, MS	Srivastava et al., 1999
Magnolia officinalis	Bark	Aqueous	MS, PCA	Shin et al., 2001b
Nigella sativa	Seeds	Aqueous	TC	Khan et al., 2000
Ocimum sanctum	Leaves	Aqueous	MS, HBS	Sen, 1993
Passiflora incarnate	Leaves	Methanolic	ABS	Dhawan et al., 2003
Romarinus officinale	Leaves	Volatile oil	TC	Aqel, 1991
Saururus chinensis	Whole plant	Ethanolic	MS	Lee et al., 2006
Solanum xanthocarpum	*Roots*	Alkaloidal	PCA, MS	Chitravanshi et al., 1990
Striga orobanchioids	Whole plants	Ethanolic	GPI, MS	Harish et al., 2001
Tephrosia purpurea	Aerials parts	Ethanolic	48/80 PO,	Gokhale and Saraf, 2000
Terminalia chebula	Fruits	Aqueous	PCA, MS	Shin et al., 2001a
Tinospora cordifolia	Stems	Aqueous	TC, MS	Nayampalli et al., 1986
Tylophora asthmatica	Leaves	Ethanolic	48/80 PO	Gokhale and Saraf, 2000
Tylophora indica	Whole plant	Alkaloidal	GPI, TC	Nayampalli et al., 1979
Rutin, Quercetin (Pure Compounds)	—	—	BALF	Jung et al., 2007

***Abbreviation: TC**—Tracheal chain, **MS**—Mast cell stabilization, **GPI**—Guinea pig ileum, **HBS**—Histamine induced brochospasm, **ABS**—Acetyl choline induced brochospasm, **EBS**—Egg albumin induced brochospasm, **PCA**—Passive cutaneous anaphylaxis, 48/80, **PO**—48/80 induced paw oedema , **BAL**—Bronchoalveolar lavage, **PAF**—Platelets activating factor, **INF**—Anti-Inflammatory, **BALF**—Bronchoalveolar lavage fluid.

MECHANISM OF ACTION OF SOME IMPORTANT ANTI-ASTHMATIC PLANTS

The several medicinal plants are investigated for the anti-asthmatic effects. The saponins isolated from *Albizzia lebbeck, Clerodendron serratum and Gardenia latifolia* and alkaloids isolated from *Tylophora indica* and *Tylophora asthmatica* were found to accord protection to sensitized guinea pigs against histamine and egg albumin micro-aerosols (Gupta, 1994).

Albizzia lebbeck

The effect of *Albizzia lebbeck* bark decoction has been reported on sensitized peritoneal mast cells of rats, when challenged with antigen (horse serum and triple antigen). The drug has also been reported to have significant cromoglycate like action on the mast cells. The isolated saponins of drug are protecting the guinea pigs against histamine and acetylcholine induced bronchospasm (Tripathi et al., 1979). The anti-asthmatic and anti-anaphylatic activity of *Albizzia lebbeck* was mainly due to smooth muscle relaxation and anti-histaminic activity (Tripathi and Das, 1977).

Tylophora indica

The effect of the alkaloidal fraction of *Tylophora indica* has been investigated against the constrictor responses of histamine on isolated guinea pig ileum and tracheal chain. The inhibition responses of drug alkaloids are found to be significant and dose dependent. The drug has been reported for several pharmacodynamic effects due to inhibition of histamine, potentiation of adrenergic response on tracheo-bronchial muscles and bronchodilator response of in perfused lung experiment. (Gupta and Tripathi, 1973). The aqueous extract of *Tylophora indica* also significantly increased the rate of air flow from 7.65 to 19.55 ml /minute during the perfusion of sensitized rat lung. This action of drug may be due to direct bronchodilator property (Nayampalli and Sheth 1979). The mast cell stabilizing effect of drug has been reported in comparison with disodium cromoglycate by challenging against three different mast cell degranulators, diazoxide, carbachol and polymixin-B *in-vitro.* The Tylophora alkaloids significantly prevented mast cell degranulation induced by diazoxide alone, it suggests by Geetha et al., 1981 that alkaloids are able to antagonize the fall in intra cellular cyclic-AMP level due to inhibition of phosphodiesterase enzymes in mast cells.

Cedrus deodara

The volatile oil of *Cedrus deodara* and himacholol an active constituent of drug has been reported to inhibit the pedal edema volume induced by compound 48/80 in rats. The drug extract at a concentration of 200 μg/ml has also been reported to possess significant mast cell stabilization activity against compound 48/80 induced mast cell degranulations (Shinde et al., 1999)

Vitex negundo

The ethanolic extract of *Vitex negundo* leaves has been reported for significant mast cells stabilization activity against compound 48/80 and egg albumin induced mast cell degranulations (Nair et al., 1994). The ethanolic extract is also reported to have significant inhibition of contracted spirally cut trachea of guinea pig induced by compound 48/80 and histamine. This effect was attributed due to either inhibition of the synthesis of PEG_2 or the diversion of the arachidonic acid metabolism in to the synthesis lipoxygenase agents (Nair and Saraf, 1995).

Clerodendron serratum

The saponins isolated from root bark of *Clerodendron serratum* has been offered significant protection against anaphylactic shock in sensitized guinea pigs exposed to egg albumin (antigen) aerosol. The drug also possesses significant delay in onset of dyspnea in guinea pigs, exposed to 1% egg albumin aerosol as compared to the control. The anti asthmatic effect of drug was may be due to significant depletion of the amine from lungs of rats (Gupta 1968).

Tephrosia purpurea

The ethanolic extract of aerial parts of drug has been offered dose dependent protection to guinea pigs, against histamine-induced bronchospasm. The broncho-protective effect of *Tephrosia purpurea* could be due to its H_1 recepter blocking activity or due to a direct bronchodilator effect. The ehanolic extract at a concentration of 25-100 µg/ml also reported to possess a dose-depended inhibition in rat mast cell degranulation induced by compound 48/80 and egg albumin (Gokhale et al., 2000). The drug has also been significantly inhibiting the eosinophils infiltration without any change in the mononuclear cell population (Gokhale and Saraf, 2000).

CONCLUSION

More than 400 medicinal plant species have been used ethnopharmacologically and traditionally to treat the symptoms of asthmatic and allergic disorders world wide, such medicinal plants represent to more than 86 families. Many plant-derived novel molecules used in modern medicine are developed by ethno-medical lead and subsequent detailed pharmacological studies. There are more than 100 drugs of known structure that are extracted from medicinal plants and used in modern medicine. A proper ethno-pharmacological and various ancient Ayurvedic text search can lead to many more promising phyto-chemicals (drugs) for asthmatic disorders.

In future the various types of phyto-pharmaceuticals from medicinal plants could serve as a cheap and steady source for varied range of novel therapeutic agent like anti-asthmatic, anti-allergic, anti-oxidants, anti-bacterial, anti-inflammatory and immuno-stimulant with great significance in the modern system of medicine. Even as we commence the new century with its exciting prospect of gene therapy, herbal medicine and phyto-pharmaceuticals remains common forms of therapy available to a great extent of world's population.

REFERENCES

Acharya SB, Yanpallewar SU, Singh RK. A preliminary study on the effect of *Azadiracchta indica* on bronchial smooth muscles and mast cells. *J Nat Remed,* 3(1), 78-82, (2003).

Agrawal BB, Paranjape AN, Metha AA. A study on mast cell stabilizing activity of *Achyranthes aspera.* National convention on current trend in herbal dugs and annual conference of Indian Society of Pharmacognosy, KBIPER, Gandhinagar, India, 23-24th February, (2003).

Al-Khalil S, Aqel, M, Afifi, F, Al-Eisawi D. Effects of an aqueous extract of *Ferula ovina* on rabbit and guinea pig smooth muscle. *J. Ethnopharmacol.*, 30(1), 35-42 (1990).

Akinbami LJ, Schoendorf KC. Trends in childhood asthma: prevalence, health care utilization, and mortality. *Pediatrics*, 110, 315-22 (2002).

Aqel MB. Relexant effect of the volatile oil of *Romarinus officinalis* on tracheal smooth muscle. *J Ethnopharmacol,* 33 (1-2), 57-62, (1991).

Arul V, Miyazaki S, Dhananjayan R. Mechanisms of the contractile effect of the alcoholic extract of *Aegle marmelos* Corr. on isolated guinea pig ileum and tracheal chain. *Phytomedicine,* 11(7-8), 679-83, (2004).

Bills GW, Soderberg RC. *Principle of Pharmacology for Respiratory Care*. Delmar, New York, pp. 278-292 (1998).

Channa S, Dar A, Yaqoob M, Anjum S, Sultani Z. Atta-ur-Rahman. Broncho-vasodilatory activity of fractions and pure constituents isolated from *Bacopa monniera. J Ethnopharmacol,* 86(1), 27-35, (2003).

Courty MA. Treatment of asthma. *Edin Med J*, 5, 665, (1859).

Chitravanshi VC, Gupta PP, Kulshrestha DK, Kar K, Dhawan BN. Anti-allergic activity of *Solanum xanthocarpum. Indian J Pharmacol,* 22, 23-24, (1990).

Cox JSG, Beach JE, Blair, AM, Clark AJ, King J, Lee TB, Loveday DE, Moss GE, Orr TS, Richie JT, Sheard P. Disodium cromoglycate (Intal). *Adv Drug Res,* 5, 115-26, (1970).

Dhawan K, Kumar S, Sharma A. Anti-asthmatic activity of the methanol extract of leaves of *Passiflora incarnata. Phytother Res,* 17(7), 821-22, (2003).

Geetha VS, Viswanathan S, Kameswaran L. Comparision of total alkaloids of *Tylophora indica* and disodium cromoglycate on mast cell stabilization. *Indian J Pharmacol,* 13 (2), 199-201, (1981).

Gokhale AB, Dikshit VJ, Damre AS, Kulkarni KR, Saraf MN. Influence of ethanolic extract of *Tephrosia purpurea* Linn. on mast cells and erythrocytes membrane integrity. *Indian J. of exp boi.,* 38(8), 837-40 (2000).

Gokhale A, Saraf MN. Influence of ethanolic extract of Tephrosia purpurea Linn. on the late-phase of allergic reaction. *Indian J. of Pharm. Sci,* 62(5), 356-359, (2000).

Gupta SS. Development of antihistamine and antiallergic activity after prolonged administration of a plant saponin from *Clerodendron serratum. J. Pharm. Pharmacol.* 20 (10):801-802, (1968).

Gupta SS, Tripathi RM. Experimental studies on *Tylophora indica. Aspect Aller. Appl. Immunol.* 6: 93-99 (1973).

Gupta SS, Prospect and perspectives of natural products in medicine. *Indian J. Pharmacol.*26 (1): 1-12 (1994).

Harish MS, Nagur M, Badami S. Antihistaminic and mast cell stabilizing activity of *Striga orobanchioides. J. Ethnopharmacol.*76 (2): 197-200 (2001).

Jung CH, Lee JY, Cho CH, Kim CJ, Anti-asthmatic Action of Quercetin and Rutin in Conscious Guinea-pigs Challenged with Aerosolized Ovalbumin. *Arch Pharm Res,* 30(12), 1599-1607, (2007).

Kessler RC, Davis RB, Foster DF, VanRompay MI, Walters, E.E., Wilkey, S.A. Long-term trends in the use of complementary and alternative medical therapies in the United States. *Ann Intern Med,* 135, 262-8 (2001).

Khan MTH, Jabbar S, Choudhari MSK, Gafur MA. Effect of crude extract of *Nigella sativa* Linn. on isolated guinea pig tracheal chain preparations. *Hamdard Medicus,* 43 (4), 30-32, (2000).

Kumar DA, Ramu P. Effect of methanolic extract of *Benincasa hispida* against histamine and acetylcholine induced bronchospasm in guinea pigs. *Indian J Pharmacol,* 34, 365-66, (2002).

Lee E, Haa K, Yook JM, Jin MH, Seo CS, Son KH, Kim HP, Bae KH, Kang SS, Son JK, Chang HW. Anti-asthmatic activity of an ethanol extracts from *Saururus chinensis. Biol Pharm Bull,* 29(2), 211-5, (2006).

MacLennan AH, Wilson DH, Taylor AW. Prevalence and cost of alternative medicine in Australia. *Lancet,* 347, 569-73 (1996).

Nagaragan R, Naik SR. Recent development on anti-asthmatic agents-an overview. *Indian drugs,* 33 (7), 303-12, (1996).

Nair AM, Saraf MN. Inhibition of antigen and compound 48/80 induced contractions of guinea pig trachea by the ethanolic extract of the leaves of *Vitex negundo* Linn. *Indian J Pharmacol,* 27, 230-33, (1995).

Nair AM, Tamhankar CP, Saraf MN. Studies on the mast cell stabilizing activity of *Vitex negundo* Linn. *Indian Drugs,* 32 (6), 277-82, (1994).

Nayampalli S, Desai NK, Ainapure SS. Anti-allergic properties of *Tinospora cordifolia* in animal models. *Indian J Pharmacol,* 18, 250-52, (1986).

Nayampalli S, Sheth UK. Evaluation of antiallergic activity of *Tylophora indica* using rat lung perfusion. *Indian J Pharmacol,* 11 (3), 229-32, (1979).

Pandit P, Singh A, Bafna AR, Kadam PV, Patil MJ. Evaluation of antiasthmatic activity of *Curculigo orchioides gaertn*. rhizomes. *Indian J Pharm Sc*, 70 (4), 440-444, (2008).

Palanichamy S, Amala Bhaskar E, Nagarajan S. Effect of *Cassia alata* leaf extract on mast cell stabilization. *Indian J Pharmacol,* 23, 189-91, (1991).

Sen P. Therapeutic potential of Tulsi (*Ocimum sanctum*) from experience to fact. *Drug and Views,* 1, 15-18, (1993).

Shin TY, Jeong HJ,.Kim DK, Kim SH, Lee JK, Chae BS, Kim JH, Kang HW, Lee CM. Inhibitory action of water-soluble fraction of *Terminalia chebula* on systemic and local anaphylaxis. *J Ethnopharmaco,*.74 (2), 133-40, (2001a).

Shin TY, Kim DK, Chae BS, Lee EJ. Antiallergic action of *Magnolia officinalis* on immediate hypersensitivity reaction. *Arch Pharm Res,* 24 (3), 249-55, (2001b).

Shinde UA, Phadke AS, Kulkarni KR, Nair AM, Mungantiwar AA, Dikshit VJ, Saraf MN. Mast cell stabilizing and lipoxygenase inhibitory activity of *Cedrus deodara* (Roxb.) wood oil. *Indian J Exp Biol,* 37 (3), 258-61, (1999).

Singh RK, Acharya SB, Bhattachaya SK. Studies on extract of *Elaeocarpus sphaericus* fruits on in vitro rat mast cells. *Phytomedicine,* 7 (3), 205-07, (2000).

Singh S, Agrawal SS. Bronchorelextant activity of *Belamcanda chinensis*. *Indian J Pharmacol,* 22, 107-09, (1990).

Spina D. Asthma mediators: Current views. *J Pharm Pharmacol,* 52, 125-45, (2000).

Srivastava S, Gupta PP, Prasad R, Dixit KS, Palit G, Ali B, Mishra G, Saxena RC. Evaluation of antiallergic activity (Type I hypersensitivity) of *Inula racemosa* in rats. *Indian J Physiol Pharmacol,* 43 (2), 235-41, (1999).

Steurer-Stey C, Russi EW, Steurer J. Complementary and alternative medicine in asthma: do they work? *Swiss Med Wkly*, 132, 338-44 (2002).

Suzuki M, Yoshino K, Yamamoto MM, Miyase T, Sano M. Inhibitory effect of *Tea* catechins and o-methylated derivatives of (-) – epigallocatechin –3-O-gallate on mouse type IV allergy. *J Agri Food Chem,* 48 (11), 5649-53, (2000).

Tripathi RM, Das PK. Studies on anti-asthmatic and anti-anaphylactic activity of *Albizzia lebbeck*. *Indian J Pharmacol,* 9(3), 189-94, (1977).

Tripathi RM, Sen PC, Das PK. Studies on the mechanism of action of *Albizzia lebbeck,* an Indian indigenous drug used in the treatment of atopic allergy. *J Ethnopharmacol,* 1, 385-86, (1979).

chapter 8

Pathogenesis of Rheumatoid Arthritis and its Treatment by Traditional Herbal Medicines

Mahaboob Khan Rasool and Evan Prince Sabina

INTRODUCTION

Rheumatoid arthritis (RA) is a systemic autoimmune disease characterized by chronic inflammation of the synovial joints, ultimately leading to joint destruction and permanent disability. It is a chronic disease of unknown cause affecting over 2 million adults in the USA and 1% of world population. It may be accompanied by the development of other disorders, including anemia, osteoplasia and muscular atrophy, as well as abnormal changes in the skin, eyes, lungs, blood vessels, and heart. RA usually begins with a symmetrical attack on the joints. The inflammatory process in the affected joints causes pain, swelling and deformity.

DISTRIBUTION AND PREVALENCE

RA is found in all climatic zones world-wide. Several studies have shown that the mean age at which the disease debute is somewhat above 50 years. It occurs in all racial groups and affects females 2 to 4 times more frequently than males. Approximately 50% of patients are unable to work within 10 years of onset and the lifetime costs of the disease rival those of coronary heart disease or stroke (William, 2001). Mortality rates among persons with RA are increased atleast 2-fold and correlate with the extent and severity of disease (Felson, 2001).

Genetic predisposition

There is an increased frequency of RA among first degree relatives and an approximately 30% concordance rate in monozygous twins. A complex association exists between RA and HLA (human leukocyte antigens) genes. Also it is observed that particular amino acid sequence in the third variable region of the HLA-D4 molecule may be the element causing susceptibility to RA (Lipsky, 1994).

Etiopathogenesis

RA is essentially an idiopathic disease that is characterized by immune mediated destruction of joints. The etiology of the disease is not well understood, but many factors have been implicated, including altered immune regulation, hormonal influences, infectious triggers and other environmental influences (Schuna and Megeff, 2000). Some evidences suggest that the antigens are introduced by an infection, with suspicion falling on the *Epistein-Barr virus, Paro viruses* and *Mycobacteria*. A peptidoglycan component of bacterial cell walls has been reported to be arthritogenic in rats and in man (Bennet, 1978).

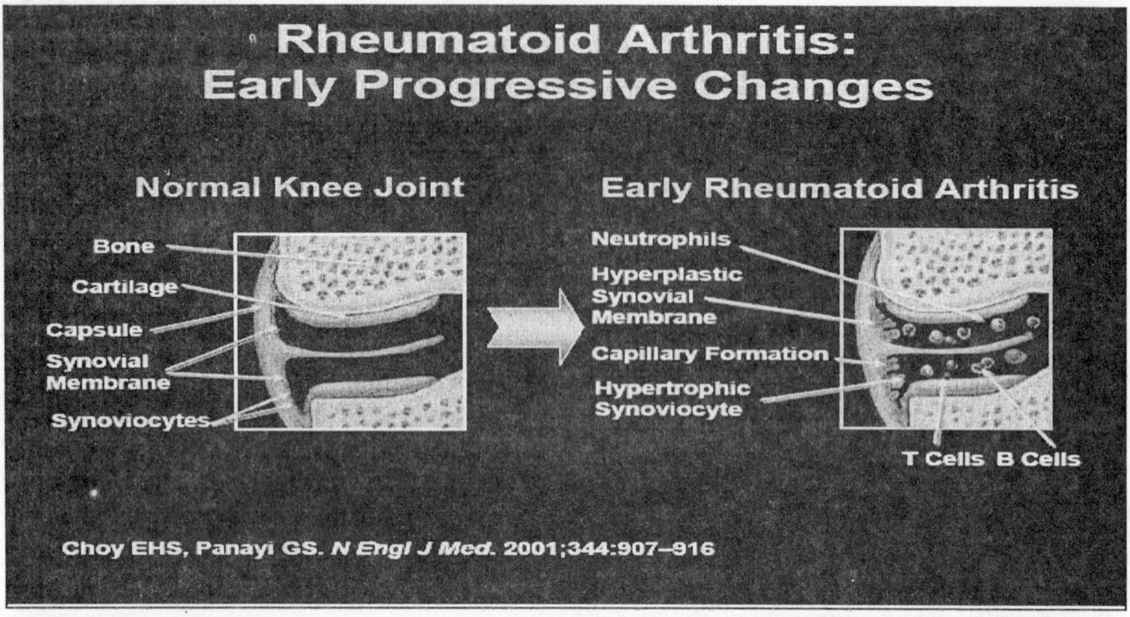

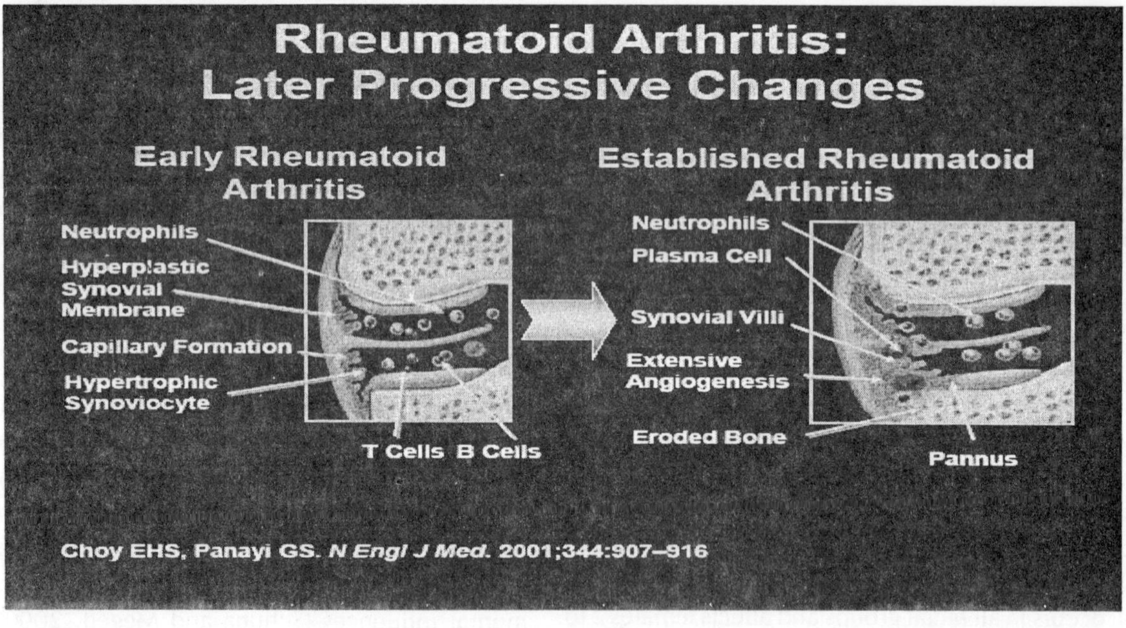

Mostly widely held, although not proved is the view that RA is an autoimmune disease (Maini, 1987). About 80% of patients with RA have a circulating auto-anti-body called rheumatoid factor (RF) against the FC portion of the autologous IgG antibody. Most of the RF is IgM but some is IgG, IgA or IgE. All types of RF form immune complexes with autologous IgG. The IgG-RF immune complexes synthesized within joints and articular spaces activate complement with the resultant accumulation of neutrophils. Leucocytes are attracted to the immune complexes which, along with the fibrin, form on the surface of the inflamed synovium. These cells, filled with particles of ingested fibrin and immune complex, may be found in the synovial fluid and are called "RA cells" or "rhagocytes". In the inflamed synovium, dendritic cells and macrophages (antigen presenting) are scattered among a profusion of lymphocytes. The proximity of T cells and antigen presenting cells speaks in favour of a cell mediated immune reaction. Circulating immune complexes are thought to underlie the wide ranging extra-articular manifestations of RA. The levels of circulating immune complexes are very high in patients with RA. These immune complexes are not cleared rapidly from the system but accumulate in the joints (Theofilopoulous and Dixon, 1979). This inturn triggers an inflammatory response at the joints, causing the erosion and destruction of the synovial membrane and underlying cartilage.

The pathogenic events occurring in RA can be defined in four phases: an initiation phase (with no clinical evidence of disease), an early inflammatory phase (which leads to clinical manifestations), a destructive phase (in which, the switch to erosive disease has occurred and RA starts to progress) and a perpetuating phase (in which, the consequences of the disease becomes more severe) (Smolen et al., 1996). The destructive phase of the disease is associated with production of the chronic granulation tissue or pannus, which spreads over the articular cartilage surface. Neutral proteolytic enzymes (matrix metallo proteinases) secreted by activated macrophages in the pannus and acidic lysosomal enzymes secreted by polymorphonuclear leucocytes in the synovial fluid, both play a part in bone and cartilage destruction (Barrett & Saklatvala, 1981).

The potential mediators of the destruction of the cartilage and subadjacent bone in RA are summarized as follows:

Neutrophils in the synovial fluid release reactive free radicals and lysosomal enzymes, mitigating the inflammation, while released proteinase and proteoglycanases degrade the cartilage (Mainardi, 1987).

Synovial lining cells, activated by inflammation or phagocytosis of immune complexes, elaborate collagenase and large amount of prostaglandin E2 and Interleukin-1

Lymphocytes (T4 cell) play an important role, the activated T cells produce a variety of lymphokines such as interleukin-2, gamma-interferon, macrophage migration inhibition factor and macrophage activating factor. Activated macrophages elaborate in addition to lytic enzymes and prostaglandins, a variety of monokines, including interleukin-1 and tumour necrosis factor (TNF).

Currently interleukin-1 and tumour necrosis factor are accorded a central role, as they are capable of

(a) Stimulating synthesis and release of collagenase by dendritic cells and synovial fibroblasts.

(b) Inhibiting the synthesis of proteoglycans by chondrocytes.

(c) Acting as a chemoattractant for neutrophils and lymphocytes.

Therapy for Rheumatoid arthritis

Modern therapeutic approaches with non-steroidal anti-inflammatory drugs (NSAIDs- eg. indomethaccin, phenyl butazone, and ibuprofen), steroidal (cortisone, and prednisolone), immunosuppressive drugs (methotrexate, azathioprine, cyclophosphamide, and cyclosporine) and disease modifying anti-rheumatic drugs (gold salts, pencillamine and sulfasalazine) are used to alleviate the agonizing symptoms due to arthritis. None of the existing above treatments can be considered to be curative or definitive therapies for the RA and they offer only temporary relief accompanying with various side effects like weight loss, diarrhea, skin rash and alopecia. Although the recent years have brought new information for the researchers and clinicians, but the treatment of RA still remains a challenge. Cytokine research has led to idea for the use of anti-cytokine therapy for the treatment of RA. Etanercept (recombinant form of the p75 TNFR-II) and infliximab (monoclonal antibody directed against TNF-alpha) were the first biological response modifiers approval for the treatment of RA (Lipsky et al., 2000). Both drugs have been designed to bind with TNF-alpha and decrease its bioavailability. Apart from all the above described treatment approaches, scientists are now trying to cure RA using gene therapy, but it is still not fully explored. Despite early detection, current treatment medications are limited in their efficacy and are frequently toxic.

Many patients look for complementary and alternative medicine (CAM) options in coping with this debilitating disease. Research has indicated that people suffering from pain, as in RA, and those dissatisfied with current treatment are very likely to seek alternative treatment, and an estimated 60-90% of persons with arthritis use CAM (Cesar Ramos and Ashwini Kumar, 2008).

Herbal remedies

Medicinal herbs are moving from the fringes to mainstream use with greater number of people seeking remedies and health approaches free from side effects caused by synthetic chemicals. Recently, considerable attention has been paid to utilize eco-friendly and biofriendly plant-based products for the prevention and cure of different human diseases. Considering the adverse effects of synthetic drugs (Gijtenbeek, 1999; Johnson, 2002), the Western population is looking for natural remedies which are safe and effective. It is documented that 80% of the world's population has faith in traditional medicine, particularly plant drugs for their primary healthcare. More than 2000 plants of medicinal value are mentioned in Indian ancient Ayurvedic, Unani and Tibbi systems of medicine.

Withania somnifera, popularly known as Ashwagandha is widely considered as the Indian ginseng. It is a green shrub distributed through out the drier parts of India, Baluchistan, Pakistan, Afghanistan, Sri lanka, Congo, South Africa, Egypt, Morocco and Jordan. Various parts of this plant have been used for centuries to treat variety of ailments (Bhattacharya et al, 2001; Kulkarni et al, 1998). The major biochemical constituents of *Withania somnifera* are steroidal alkaloids and lactones, a class of constituents together known as withanolides (Elaskka et al, 1990). Withanolides, which are extracted from *Withania somnifera,* are employed in the treatment of arthritis and are known to be potent inhibitor of angiogenesis, inflammation and oxidative stress. Begum and Sadique (1988), for the first time reported the long term effects of *Withania somnifera* on adjuvant-induced arthritis in rats. Studies carried out in our laboratory have demonstrated that oral administration of *Withania somnifera* root powder reversed the biochemical and immunological changes observed in adjuvant-induced arthritis, an experimental model of RA (Rasool et al, 2007). More recently Ichikawa et al (2006) showed that withanolides can indeed inhibit the activation of transcription factor nuclear factor-KB (NF-KB) and NF-KB-regulated gene expression.

Ginger (*Zinger officinale* Roscoe, Zingiberacae) is a medicinal plant that has been widely used in Chinese, Ayurvedic and Unani herbal medicines all over the world, since antiquity for arthritis and rheumatism. The anti-inflammatory properties of ginger have been known for centuries. Ginger and its constituents like gingerdiones have been reported to have pharmacological properties mimicking dual–acting non-steroidal anti-inflammatory drugs in intact human leukocytes in vitro (Flynn et al., 1986). More recently, it has been shown that ginger and its constituents are effective against arthritis through suppression of pro-inflammatory cytokines and chemokines produced by synoviocytes, chondrocytes, and leukocytes. Ginger was also found to modulate some biochemical pathways activated in chronic inflammation (Grzanna et al., 2005). It is established that neither ginger nor its constituents produce the gastrointestinal damage that are usually produced by the non-steroidal anti-inflammatory drugs (Konturek et al., 2005). Therefore, ginger appears to be a relatively safe and effective supplement to reduce symptoms of rheumatoid arthritis.

Triphala is the most commonly used Indian ayurveda herbal formulation, comprising the fruits of three trees, Indian goose berry (*Emblica officinalis* Gaertn, family-Euphobiaceae), Belleric myrobalan (*Terminalia belerica* Linn. family-Combretaceae) and Chebulic myrobalan (*Terminalia chebula* Retzr. family-Combretaceae). In ayurveda, it is an important medicine of the rasayana group and is believed to promote health, immunity and longevity (Sandhyaa et al., 2006). Recent studies indicate that this triphala might play a role in the prevention and treatment of arthritis through by the inhibition of lysosomal enzymes, glycoproteins, lipid peroxidation and inflammatory mediator TNF-alpha in adjuvant-induced arthritic rats (Rasool et al., 2007). Triphala was also found to be effective against monosodium urate crystal-induced inflammation, an experimental model for gouty arthritis (Sabina et al., 2007). Moreover, triphala constituent *Emblica officinalis,* is already well established against arthritis by reducing it biochemical and immunological symptoms (Asmawi et al., 1993).

Curcumin is the principal curcuminoid of the popular Indian curry spice turmeric that has commonly used in Chinese and Indian medicine system for centuries. The curcuminoids are polyphenols and are responsible for the yellow color of turmeric. Curcumin in several lines of evidence, both in vitro and in vivo, has been well documented as an anti-inflammatory agent. The cyclo-oxygenase 2 (COX-2) inducible and nitric oxide synthase (iNOS) are important enzymes that mediate inflammatory responses. Improper up-regulation of COX-2 and iNOS has been associated with pathophysiology of certain types of human cancers as well as inflammatory disorders. Recent studies have demonstrated that eukaryotic transcription factor nuclear factor kB (NF-KB) was involved in regulation of COX-2 and iNOS expression. The work from the laboratory of Aggarwal et al (2006) and others have shown that curcumin can downregulate activation of the transcription of the expression of the transcription factor NF-ÊB, thus leading the downregulation of TNF-alpha, adhesion molecules, matrixmetallo proteinases, COX-2 and other inflammatory intermediates all of which are associated with arthritis. Jackson et al (2006) reported that curcumin inhibited neutrophil activation, synoviocyte proliferation, angiogenesis, and collagenase, thus suggesting that curcumin has therápeutic potential in arthritis.

Boswellia serrata (Salai guggul) commonly called as Frankincense is a moderate tree widely distributed in India and the Middle East. Several researches in the past 30 years identified the principal component boswellic acid and its derivatives from the gum resin of *Boswellia serrata*. Boswellic acid has demonstrated the anti-inflammatory as well as anti-arthritic activity against serum albumin-induced arthritis and osteoarthritis. Boswellic acid derivative (acetyl-11-keto-beta-boswellic acid) is also reported to contribute antiarthritic action through the inhibition of NF-KB, COX-2 and 5-lipo-oxygenase (Jolad et al, 2005).

Traditional Chinese Medicines (TCM) have been used for centuries in China to treat various immune-mediated disorders like rheumatoid arthritis. The "thunder god" vine, Tripterygium wilfordii Hook F (TWHf), has been extensively used in China to treat RA. TWHf not only found to inhibit mitogen-stimulated lymphoproliferation, but its active derivatives have also been shown to inhibit production of proinflammatory cytokines by monocytes and lymphocytes, as well as prostaglandin E2 production via the cyclooxygenase, COX-2, pathway, a potential mechanism of action in patients with RA (Ramgolam et al., 2000). Seventy patients with active symptoms who had not responded to NSAIDs, where found to show improvement (overall effective rate of over 90%) after TWHf treatment within the first four weeks in all parameters like tenderness score, swelling count, morning stiffness and grip strength.

Ulmus davidiana Planch (Ulmaceae) (UD) and ***Clematis mandshurica Rupr*** (Ranunculaceae) roots have long been known to be anti-inflammatory in traditional Korean medicine. UD demonstrated a strong growth inhibition in tested mouse osteoblasts in vitro, and suppressed proliferating cell nuclear antigen (PCNA) expression, COX-2 expression and PGE2 synthesis in osteoblasts (Seok-Jung Suh et al., 2006). Inhibition of PGE2 synthesis via suppression of COX-2 expression may be responsible for its anti-inflammatory activity. The ethanolic extract of *Clematis mandshurica* at 100mug/ml was found to significantly block the production of the pro-inflammatory mediators, nitric oxide (NO) and prostaglandin E(2) (PGE(2)), in lipopolysaccharide (LPS)/interferon(IFN)-gamma-stimulated mouse peritoneal macrophages, by up to 77% and 59%, respectively. In addition, it significantly inhibited cell proliferation and cytokine production (interleukin (IL)-2 and IFN-gamma) in splenocytes stimulated with Con A (concanavalin A; 5 mug/ml).

CONCLUSION

RA is a systemic autoimmune disease characterized by chronic inflammation of the synovial joints, ultimately leading to joint destruction and permanent disability. Although the pathogenesis of RA remains incompletely understood, the treatment for various forms of arthritis like NSAIDs, diseases modifying anti-rheumatic drugs are available in the market, but they suffer from various drawbacks, such as lack of efficacy, excessive side effects and high cost. Nowadays, with increasing awareness on traditional medicines, many patients look for complementary and alternative medicine options in coping with this disease, however this growing interest in alternative medical practices requires extensive investigation into their safety and efficacy to prove their usefulness against RA.

REFERENCES

Aggarwal BB, Sundaram C, Malani N, Ichikawa H. Curcumin: the Indian solid gold. *Adv Exp Med Biol*, 595, 1-75, (2007).

Aggarwal S, Ichikawa H, Takada Y, Sandur SK, Shishodia S. Curcumin (Diferuloylmethane) Down-regulates Expression of Cell Proliferation, Anti-apoptotic and Metastatic Gene Products Through Suppression of IkBa Kinase and AKT Activation. Mol Pharmacol, 69, 195-206, (2006).

Asmawi MZ, Kankaanranta H, Moilanen E, Vapaatalo H. Anti-inflammatory activities of *Emblica officinalis* Gaerth leaf extract. *J Pharm Pharmacol* 45 (6), 581-584, (1993).

Barrett AJ, Saklatvala J. Proteinases in joint disease. In: Kelley, WN, Harris Jr, ED, Ruddy, S and Sledge, CB, Editors, *Textbook of Rheumatology*, Saunders, Philadelphia, pp. 195-209 (1981).

Begum VH, Sadique J. Long term effect of herbal drug *Withania somnifera* on adjuvant-induced arthritis in rats. *Indian J Exp Biol*, 26(11), 877-882, (1988).

Bennett JC. The infectious etiology of rheumatoid arthritis. New considerations. *Arthritis Rheum.* 21(5), 531-538, (1978).

Bhattacharya A, Ghosal S, Bhattacharya SK. Anti-oxidant effect of *Withania somnifera* glycowithanolides in chronic footshock stress-induced perturbations of oxidative free radical scavenging enzymes and lipid peroxidation in rat frontal cortex and striatum, *J Ethnopharmacol* 74, 1-6, (2001).

Cesar Ramos-Remus, Ashwinikumar Raut Complementary and alternative practices in rheumatology *Best Practice & Research Clinical Rheumatology*, 22 (4), 741-757, (2008).

Choy EHS, Panayi GS, Cytokine pathways and joint inflammation in rheumatoid arthritis. *New Engl J Med,* 334, 907-916, (2001).

Elaskka M, Grigorescu E, Stanescu U, Dorneanu. V. New data referring to chemistry of *Withania somnifera* species, *Rev. Med. Chir. Soc. Med. Nat. Iasi,* 94 (2), 385-387, (1990).

Felson DT. Epidemology of the rheumatic diseases, In:Arthritis and Allied conditions, Koopman WJ, ed.14 th ed.philadelphia, Pa: Lippincott Willams & Wilkins, pp. 3-38, (2001).

Flynn DL, Rafferty MF, Boctor AM. Inhibition of human neutrophil 5-lipoxygenase activity by gingerdione, sh ogaol, capsaicin and related pungent compounds. *Prostaglandins .Leukot. Med.* 24, 195, (1986).

Gijtenbeek JMM, Vanden Bent MJ, Vecht CJ. Cyclosporine neurotoxicity. *J. Neurol,* 246, 339-346, (1999).

Grzanna, R, Phan, P, Polotsky, A, Lindmark, L, Frondoza, C.G. Ginger-an herbal medicinal product with broad anti-inflammatory actions. *J. Med. Food.* 8, 125-132, (2005).

Ichikawa H, Takada Y, Shishodia S, Jayaprakasam B, Nair MG, Aggarwal BB. Withanolides potentiate apoptosis, inhibit invasion, and abolish osteoclastogenesis through suppression of nuclear factor-kappaB (NF-kappaB) activation and NF-kappaB-regulated gene expression. *Mol Cancer Ther,* 5(6),1434-45, (2006).

Jackson JK, Higo T, Hunter WL, Burt HM. The antioxidants curcumin and quercetin inhibit inflammatory processes associated with arthritis *Inflamm Res.* 55(4), 168-75, (2006).

Johnson WC, William OW. Warfarin toxicity. *J. Vasc. Surg.* 35, 413-421, (2002).

Jolad SD, Lantz RC, Chen GJ, Bates RB, Timmermann BN. Commercially processed dry ginger (Zingiber officinale): composition and effects on LPS-induced PGE2 production. *Phytochemistry,* 66, 1614-1635, (2005).

Konturek SJ, Konturek PC, Brzozowski T. Prostaglandins and ulcer healing, *J. Physiol. Pharmacol.* 56 (5), 5-31, (2005).

Kulkarni SK, George B, Mathur R, Neuroprotection by *Withania somnifera* root extract against lithium-pilocarpine-induced seizures, *Indian Drugs,* 35, 208-215, (1998).

Lipsky PE, van der Heijde DM, St Clair EW, Furst DE, Breedveld FC, Kalden JR, Smolen JS, Weisman M, Emery P, Feldmann M, Harriman GR, Maini RN. Infliximab and methotrexate in the treatment of rheumatoid arthritis. Anti-Tumor Necrosis Factor Trial in Rheumatoid Arthritis with Concomitant Therapy Study Group. *N Engl J Med,* 343(22), 1594-1602, (2000).

Mainardi CL, Hasty KA, Hibbs MS. Collagen degradation by inflammatory phagocytes. *The Journal of rheumatology*, 14, 59-60, (1987).

Maini RN, Plater-Zyberk C, Andrew E. Autoimmunity in rheumatoid arthritis. An approach via a study of B lymphocytes. *Rheum Dis Clin North Am,* 13(2), 319-33, (1987).

Ramgolam V, Ang SG, Lai YH, Loh CS, Yap HK. Traditional Chinese medicines as immunosuppressive agents. Ann Acad Med Singapore, 29(1), 11-6, (2000).

Rasool M, Varalakshmi P. Protective effect of *Withania somnifera* root powder in relation to lipid peroxidation, antioxidant status, glycoproteins and bone collagen on adjuvant-induced arthritis. *Fund. Clin.pharmacol,* 21, 157-164, (2007).

Sabina EP, Rasool M. An in vivo and in vitro potential of Indian ayurvedic herbal formulation Triphala on experimental gouty arthritis in mice. *Vas pharmacol,* 48, 4-20, (2008).

Sandhya T, Lathika KM, Pandey BN, Mishra KP. Potential of traditional ayurvedic formulation, Triphala, as a novel anticancer drug. *Cancer Letters,* 231(2), 206-214, (2006).

Schuna A, Megeff C. New drugs for the treatment of rheumatoid arthritis, *Am J Health Syst Pharm,* 57, 225-234, (2000).

Seok-Jong Suh, Woo-Sik Yun, Kap-Sung Kim, Un-Ho Jin, June-Ki Kim, Myung-Sunny Kim, Dae Young Kwon, Cheorl-Ho Kim. Stimulative effects of *Ulmus davidiana* Planch (Ulmaceae) on osteoblastic MC3T3-E1 cells. *J Ethnopharmacol*, 109(3), 480-485, (2007).

Theofilopoulos AN, Dixon FJ. The biology and detection of immune complexes. *Adv Immunol,* 28, 89-220, (1979).

William J, Koopman MD. Research advances in rheumatoid arthritis, *JAMA*, 285, 648-650, (2001).

chapter 9

Ethnomedicinal Grasses of the Indian Desert, (Rajasthan) India

S.S. Katewa, Anita Jain and Praveen Kumar Galav

INTRODUCTION

The searing heat and inhospitality of the Indian desert belies its remarkable ability to harvest nature resources in the most creative and efficient manner imaginable. Adaptability and survival are inextricably linked in this austere wonderland. In the Indian subcontinent, deserts, with an area of about 2,25,000 sq. km. account for just under seven per cent of the total land area. Better known as the Great Indian Desert, this arid, extreme habitat spreads over western Rajasthan and the Great Rann of Kutchh in Gujarat.

Many tribes are scattered in different parts of Indian desert. These aboriginal people still depend largely on nature for their essential requirements. The traditional botanical knowledge of indigenous people of Indian desert contains a fund of knowledge about the properties of plants, an oral heritage that has accrued over ages, after generations of observations and experience. Unfortunately, much of this knowledge and many of the cultures are becoming fast eroded in most regions. It is, therefore, essential to rescue the disappearing knowledge and to revitalize and return it to the local communities. With this objective in mind, some ethnobotanical investigations were carried out by the author and his associates in the tribal-dominated areas of Indian desert (Katewa, 2003; Katewa et.al., 2001; Katewa and Jain, 2006; Chaudhary et. al., 2008; Jain et. al., 2004)

The traditional healthcare practice of indigenous people pertaining to human health is known as ethnomedicine. Indian civilization has played a pioneer role from time immemorial in utilizing plants such as indigenous drugs. Ethnomedicine practices are the mother of all other traditional systems of medicine such as Ayurveda, Siddha, Unani and Nature cures and even today's most popular modern therapeutic system or allopathic system (Jain, 1991). Herbal medicine is not just a poor man's substitute for conventional medicine but a valuable form of treatment in its own right.

It has been estimated that approx. 80% of the population of developing countries is partially or fully dependent upon herbal drugs for primary healthcare, and higher plants are known to be the main source of drug therapy in traditional medicine (Fransworth, 1990; Ramawat et. al., 2004; Ramawat and Goyal, 2008). The World Health Organization (WHO) estimated that 80 to 90% of the world's population relies mainly on local herbal practitioners (Fransworth, 1990). The WHO in its 29th and 30th assemblies (1976–77) gave formal recognition to traditional medicine and recommended the association of traditional healers in the national healthcare programme (Trivedi and Nehra, 2004). The major classical systems of medicine used on the Indian subcontinent like Ayurveda, Siddha and Unani together use about 1200 plant species to treat human ailments, but the tribals of India are using over more than 7500 plant species (Pushpangadan, 1994). India is one of the world's 12 hotspots, having the largest plant biodiversity, and it has almost 45,000 plant species of which 15,000 to 20,000 are used for medicinal purposes (Krishna Kumar, 1996).

Grasses–a natural homogenous group of plants belongs to the family Poaceae, undoubtedly forms one of the most fascinating families of flowering plants with a wide range of diversity and is playing a significant role in the lives of animals and human beings. The value of grasses to mankind has been recognized since the dawn of the human civilization and the culture of the cereal grasses dates back to a period, when man was emerging from wild beast stage. The members of this group are present in all the conceivable habitats suitable for the growth of the plant communities. In India, the Poaceae is one of the dominant families both on the basis of its number of genera and species. Like dicots, some grasses are also used in medicine, more especially in indigenous system of medicine. In Indian desert, a lot of work has been done on ethnomedicinal plants used for various ailments by tribal community (Joshi, 1995; Singh and Pandey, 1998; Katewa et. al., 2001; 2003; 2004; 2006; Katewa and Galav, 2005; 2006; Jain et. al., 2005; 2007; Katewa and Jain, 2006).

Perusal of the literature indicates that no comprehensive ethnobotanical work has been published yet on grasses as compared to other wild dicotyledonous plants. Therefore in the present chapter an attempt has been made to record ethnomedicinal grasses of Indian desert.

OBSERVATIONS

Healthcare

The art of herbal healing is deeply rooted in Indian culture and folklore. Even today in most rural areas, people depend on the local traditional healing system for their primary healthcare. For tribals, the ambient vegetation is the main source of drugs for their ailments. Their expertise is vast and they have cures for all ailments, including the deadly diseases. But it is very difficult to extract information from them, because some tribes strongly believe that the efficacy of the drug would be lost if details were divulged.

Ethnoveterinary medicines are of specific value in developing countries where allopathic veterinary medicines are often beyond the reach of livestock producers. It can play an important role in grassroot development, which seeks to empower people by enhancing the use of their own knowledge and resources. The present paper is also intended to contribute to this growing body of knowledge by supplying information on the grass based ethnoveterinary curative techniques found in tribal areas of Rajasthan.

The traditional healers of Indian desert have a commendable knowledge of the medicinal virtues of the plants that grow around them. A few important medicinal grasses of the tribals, along with their local name, flowering and fruiting, ecology, plant part/s used, and mode of administration for effective control in different ailments are given as follows:

Alloteropsis cimicina (Linn.) Stapf.

Erect or ascending annual, upto 1 m high with hairy nodes; leaves ovate-lanceolate, amplexicaul at base; inflorescence made up of 2-10 spike-like racemes seated on the top of peduncle; caryopsis sub orbicular to elliptic-oblong.

Ecology: Sporadic grass found on the hills and in the wastelands.

Ethnomedicinal uses: Roots are aromatic. Paste of roots is massaged on teeth and gums to treat toothache.

Apluda mutica Linn.

Annuals; leaves linear–lanceolate, long acuminate, base narrowed; ligule membranous, rounded; panicles of 2 to many, simple racemes terminating the culms, enclosed in a peduncled spathe; spikelets three, one sessile and two pedicelled; seeds caryopsis.

Ecology: Common on the hills, among hedges of cultivated field and bushes in wastelands preferring moist places.

Ethnomedicinal uses: Herbal bath of whole plant is taken by the tribals to treat jaundice.

Ethnoveterinary medicinal uses: Paste of whole plant is used to treat mouth sores of cattle.

Aristida adscensionis Linn.

Erect or ascending, annual or perennial grass upto 60 cm high; leaves filiform; ligule a ridge of short hair; panicles 5-30 cm long, contracted, unequally branched; rachis filiform; spikelets 6- 8 mm long, single flowered; fruit caryopsis, linear-oblong.

Ecology: Commonly found in sandy to rocky habitats, sometimes forming pure formations in the plains.

Ethnomedicinal uses: Decoction of 100 g inflorescence is taken as diuretic twice a day for three days.

Arundo donax Linn.

Erect, stout, tall, perennial grass, upto 2.5 m high, with creeping woody rhizome; culms fistular; leaves 15-50 × 2-5 cm, distichous, linear- lanceolate; spikelets 1-1.5 cm long, light brown, 2-flowered, fruits caryopsis with linear hilum.

Ecology: Commonly found in marshy habitats along the rivers and streams, particularly in dried up beds.

Ethnomedicinal uses: Decoction of rhizome is taken by the tribals to treat fever. Decoction is also to women as anticoagulant and stimulates the menstrual cycle.

Brachiaria ramosa (Linn.) Staff

Tufted, ascending annuals, often rooting at the base; leaves linear–lanceolate, acuminate, base rounded, glabrescent; ligule a line of hairs; racemes 3 or more, each upto 5 cm long; spikelets 3 mm long, ovoid, apiculate; caryopsis 1.5 - 2.0 mm long, broadly elliptic, flattened.

Ecology: Fairly common throughout Rajasthan in mixed habitats. It is a good fodder grass and highly polymeric.

Ethnomedicinal uses: The chapatti (bread) prepared from the flour of grains of this grass is eaten to treat digestive disorders. "Ladoo" (local sweet) prepared from flour of grains of this millet is given to women after delivery. The ash of the plant is used as an ointment on burns.

Chloris virgata SW.

Tufted, erect annuals, 60 cm high, sometimes rooting at lower nodes; leaves flat, linear, acute, glabrous; sheaths beared; ligule a narrow, membranous ridges; spikes erect, crowded, digitate; spikelets 3-flowered, 2-awned.

Ecology: Common throughout Rajasthan in mixed habitats.

Ethnomedicinal uses: Decoction of roots is used to treat of cold and rheumatism.

Coix lacryma-jobi Linn.

Erect, perennial herb, upto 1.5 m high with basal rooting nodes; leaves linear lanceolate, midrib stout, ligule narrow, membranous, racemes nodding or drooping from long peduncles carrying male / female peduncles; fruits subglobose.

Ecology: Growing in water logged conditions along road side.

Ethnomedicinal uses: The boiled involucres (fruits) are eaten by the tribals as antidysenteric and extract of involucres is used as a drink for invalids. The leaf juice is taken orally by the tribals to treat urinary complaints. The paste of involucres is applied externally as well as taken orally to treat cancerous tumors. The extract of involucres is given to get relief from bodyache.

Capillipedium huegelii (Hack.) Stapf.

Suffrutescent, branched perennial, leaves flat, linear-lanceolate, acuminate; ligule membranous, ciliate; panicles 5-12 cm long; joints and pedicels bearded, sessile spikelets 3- 4 mm long, green with purplish tinge, awned; callus densely villous.

Ecology: Commonly found near the water courses in shaded localities. The plant often emits odour.

Ethnomedicinal uses: Essential oil extracted from inflorescence of this grass is used for massage in rheumatism. Essential oil is also applied locally for easy expulsion of guinea-worm.

Cymbopogon martinii (Roxb.) Wats.

Perennial, sweet-scented grass, 1.5-2.5 m high; leaves linear-lanceolate, sub - cordate, amplexicaul and finely cordate; flowers in panicled spikelets, turning reddish brown when mature, glumes channelled corresponding to a midrib on the inner side, awned.

Ecology: Prefers drier soils.

Ethnomedicinal uses: Decoction of leaves is taken orally twice a day for 7 days to treat jaundice. Herbal bath of the plant is also taken to treat jaundice. Paste of leaves is warmed with mustard oil (*Brassica campestris*) and used for massage in rheumatic pain. Juice of crushed leaves and stem is given to children to treat stomachache while decoction is given to treat cough, cold and fever. The flowers of this grass are smelled by the tribals several times in a day to treat cough and cold. The oil extracted from leaves acts as antiseptic and used to treat various skin diseases. Two drops of leaf extract is poured in ear to remove insect from the ear. The smoke of plant is used by the tribals as rodent and mosquito repellent.

Cymbopogon schoenanthus (Linn.) Spreng.

Perennial, compactly caespitose, with numerous intravaginal innovation, culms erect, slender, few to 4-noded; leaf-blade semiterete, filiform, wiry, flexuous, very firm and often circinate upwards, rounded on the back; inflorescence terete, glabrous.

Ecology: Commonly found in sandy habitats in the desertic zone.

Ethnomedicinal uses: The oil is massaged in rheumatism and neuralgia. The decoction of grass is used as febrifuge.

Cynodon dactylon (Linn.) Pers.

A perennial grass, stem creeping, spreading widely; culms decumbented, often creeping at the base, finally erect in tufts, shortly branched; leaves narrowly linear or lanceolate, flat, glaucous, soft, sheaths short below, elongated above, ligule represented by a narrow ciliaterim.

Ecology: A common perennial grass along the banks of ponds and other damp places.

Ethnomedicinal uses: Aqueous extract of plant with sugar is taken by the tribals to treat nostril haemorrage. Leaf juice along with a pinch of common salt is taken orally in stomachache. Decoction of whole plant is given orally to treat menstrual disorders. Tribals cure dysentery by giving extract of whole plants to adults (one fourth cup) and children (one tea spoon only). The grass is chewed by the tribals and the paste so formed is applied locally on the skin to treat scars and cured within one or two days. Whole plant is crushed and dipped in mustard oil. The oil becomes viscous. This oil is given to patient to treat jaundice. Half cup extract of whole plant is taken orally by the tribals to treat of dysuria.

Dactyloctenium aegyptium (Linn.) Willd.

Erect or geniculately ascending, hispid annuals, 15-70 cm high, often rooting at lower nodes; leaves linear; ligule a ring of white hairs; spikelets 3 to 5 flowered, 3.5-4.25 mm long; caryopsis, compressed, subglobose, reddish.

Ecology: Commonly found in moist places.

Ethnomedicinal uses: Powder of grains and leaves is taken orally with water to treat stomachache whereas decoction of seeds is used as an alleviator of kidney pain. Porridge made from seeds is taken by the tribals to treat diarrhoea.

Dactyloctenium sindicum Boiss

A prostrate perennial grass, branched profusely; stem glabrous, rooting at leafy nodes and sending erect slender branches which bear the inflorescence.

Ecology: A common grass of rainy season found growing in cultivated field.

Ethnomedicinal uses: Whole plant extract is taken orally to treat rheumatism.

Dendrocalamus strictus (Roxb.) Nees

Densely tufted, arborescent bamboos, upto 10 m tall, with swollen nodes; lower stem-sheaths covered on the back with golden-brown stiff hairs; internodes upto 50 cm long; ligules narrow, serrate; inflorescence a panicle of dense, globular heads; caryopsis subglobose, brown.

Ecology: Fairly common in dry deciduous forests on the top of hills forming distant patches.

Ethnomedicinal uses: One tender culm about 25-30 cm in length is crushed and given orally 2-3 times a day to expel the intestinal worms. Inner portion of the culm is given to patients suffering from the tuberculosis.

Ethnoveterinary medicinal uses: Infusion of tender shoot is given to animals by the tribals once in a day for three days to treat the fractured bone. Decoction prepared from the mixture of jaggery, shoots of *Dendrocalamus strictus*, milk, roots of *Tephrosia purpurea* and Ajwain (*Trachyspermum ammi*) is given to buffaloes for dispossession of placenta after delivery.

Desmostachya bipinnata (Linn.) Stapf.

Tufted, stout, erect, rhizomatous perennial, upto 1.25 m tall; with creeping root-stocks; leaves acuminate, sheaths glabrous, densely flagellate; inflorescence 25-50 cm long, spikes 1.5-3.5 cm long, cluster bearing 20-30 spikelets, spikelets 2.5-3.5 mm long, linear, oblong, glumes unequal, lemmas 2.5 mm long, straw coloured.

Ecology: Commonly found near moist places particularly in sandy and clayey soils.

Ethnomedicinal uses: Paste of whole plant is taken orally by the tribals to treat dysentery. Leaf paste is used to cure cuts and wounds. Half cup of root decoction is taken orally twice a day for 5 days to treat asthma and for 7 days to treat jaundice.

Echinochloa crus-galli (Linn.) P. Beauv.

Erect or ascending, stout annual, rooting at the nodes; leaves linear; racemes either solitary or 2 to 3 together; pedicels with prominent bulbous based white setae; caryopsis 1.5-1.75 mm long, elliptic.

Ecology: Common in moist marshy habitats.

Ethnomedicinal uses: Juice of whole plant is taken orally to treat nostril haemorrhage.

Eleusine coracana (Linn.) Gaertn.

Tall erect, stout annuals; leaves distichous, acute, sparsely hairy; ligule of hairs; spikes suberect; rachis often 3-gonous; spikelet awnless; caryopsis smooth or rugose.

Ecology: Mostly for its edible grains; often escape from cultivation.

Ethnomedicinal uses: Flour of grains is used as nourishing food for infant by the tribal women.

Ethnoveterinary medicinal uses: Bread made up of 500 g grain flour is fed to the animal once a day for 5 days to treat diarrhoea. Paste made from the grains is applied locally to treat mastitis.

Eleusine indica (Linn.) Gaertn.

Erect or geniculately ascending annuals; leaves distichous, flat, linear, acute; ligule a hairy membrane; spikes digitate; rachis flattened; caryopsis obliquely striated.

Ecology: Commonly found along road-sides in open wastelands.

Ethnomedicinal uses: Paste of whole plant is taken orally by the tribals to treat fever.

Hemarthria compressa (L.f.) R. Br.

Prostrate, spreading, stoloniferous perennial rooting at the lower nodes; leaves folded when dry, linear, acute; racemes 3-8 cm long; internodes obliquely articulate.

Ecology: Common in moist and marshy habitats

Ethnomedicinal uses: Root paste is taken orally with a pinch of common salt to treat digestive disorder.

Heteropogon contortus (Linn.) P. Beauv.

Erect, tufted perennial; leaves, linear, acuminate, sheaths compressed, keeled, glabrous; ligule a ciliate, scarious rim; racemes solitary; spikelets closely imbricate; lower glumes of sessile spikelets long, elliptic-oblong, hispedulous awn long, hirtellous.

Ecology: Fairly in open wastelands, fallow fields, along roadsides etc.

Ethnomedicinal uses: Crushed seeds are taken orally by the tribals to treat dysuria. Root paste is taken orally as well as applied locally in snake bite and dog bite as an antidote. The tribals use the root extract of this grass to treat dysentery.

Ethnoveterinary medicinal uses: The whole plant is crushed and given orally to animals to treat constipation.

Imperata cylindrica (Linn.) Raeuschel.

Erect, rhizomatous perennial, with bearded nodes; leaves tapering at both ends, villous at the base; panicles spiciform, cylindrical, silky white hairy; spikelets in pairs, one sessile and other pedicelled, arranged in racemose panicles.

Ecology: Fairly common in moist and marshy habitats.

Ethnomedicinal uses: Root paste is applied locally in scorpion sting.

Panicum antidotale Retz.

Stout grass, with creeping, woody rootstock; leaves linear, acute; ligule short, membranous, ciliate;

spikelets in panicles; lower florets neuter; lower glume 5 nerved.

Ecology: Found in sandy habitats.

Ethnomedicinal uses: Poultice of whole plant is tied to treat wounds.

Panicum miliaceum Linn.

Tufted, tall annual, 50-150 cm high, leaves linear-lanceolate, often covered with tubercle based hairs; ligule a narrow ciliate rim; panicle long lax.

Ecology: Often found as a weed in irrigated fields.

Ethnoveterinary medicinal uses: Either grains or whole plant is fed to the animals as lactogogues.

Paspalum scrobiculatum Linn.

Erect or ascending, perennial grass, often rooting at the lower nodes; leaves tapering to fine point; racemes digitate, with 2 ranked spikelets; caryopsis subglobose.

Ecology: Commonly found near ponds, tanks etc. in marshy habitats.

Ethnomedicinal uses: Paste of whole plant is applied externally in various skin diseases like boils, sores etc. The chapatties (bread) prepared from the grains of this grass are eaten with curd to treat dysentery.

Ethnoveterinary medicinal uses: Grains are given to milch cattle as lactogogues.

Perotis indica (Linn.) O. Ktze.

Geniculately ascending grass, with hairy sheaths and slender, spike-like, upto 15 cm long racemes; callus definite; caryopsis cylindrical.

Ecology: Common in open, dry waste places and fellow fields.

Ethnomedicinal uses: Decoction of dried inflorescence is taken orally by the tribal ladies to stop bleeding after delivery.

Phragmites karka (Retz.) Trin. ex Steud.

Densely tufted, erect, perennial; leaves bifarious, linear-lanceolate, scabrid beneath; panicles long with filiform and spreading branches; rachilla-hair 7-12 mm long, silky brown; caryopsis terete.

Ecology: Found near marshy habitats like ditches, tanks, ponds and streams.

Ethnomedicinal uses: The leaf juice along with water is taken orally by the tribals as astringent during the summer.

Saccharum bengalense Retz.

Erect perennial, upto 3.5 m tall and with solid stem; leaves flat, linear; ligule membranous; panicles upto 80 cm long, silvery-white, wolly; glumes equal, lower glume of sessile spikelets hairy on the back.

Ecology: Common in river-beds and other damp places.

Ethnomedicinal uses: Decoction of 100 g fresh leaves is taken orally by the tribal women for 3 days to treat menstrual disorder. It is also used for abortion. The extract of leaves is taken orally to treat fever.

Saccharum officinarum Linn.

Tall, perennial, rhizomatous plant, with juicy culms; leaves wide and laminated right to the base; spikelets awnless, glumes glabrous.

Ecology: Cultivated for culm-juice which is used for making jaggery.

Ethnomedicinal uses: Semisolid jaggery made from stem juice is eaten to purify the blood whereas stem juice is taken orally to treat jaundice.

Ethnoveterinary medicinal uses: Sugarcane (7-8 kg) is given to animal to facilitate dispossession of placenta after delivery.

Sehima nervosum (Rottl.) Staff

Densely tufted, erect grass; leaves flat, linear, acuminate, glabrous; sheaths terete, striated, glabrescent; raceme terminal, solitary; sessile spikelets laterally compressed, acuminate; pedicelled spikelets lanceolate, acuminate, awnless.

Ecology: Fairly common on low hillocks and alluvial plains. It is a common fodder grass.

Ethnomedicinal uses: The powder of the dried leaves of this grass is smelt twice a day for two days to treat jaundice.

Setaria glauca (Linn.) P. Beauv.

Decumbent –ascending or erect annual, with glabrous nodes; leaves linear, acuminate, base round, with scabrid margins; sheaths compressed, smooth; ligules a ridge of hairs; inflorescence dense, cylindrical, spike–like raceme.

Ecology: Common weed in sandy and rocky habitats; sometimes cultivated. It is a useful fodder grass and grains are eaten during scarcity.

Ethnomedicinal uses: Powder of grain is mixed in urine of goat and about two teaspoon of this powder is taken orally with water for about a week to treat syphilis.

Setaria tomentosa (Roxb.) Kunth

Weak ascending annuals, often rooting at the lower nodes; leaves narrowly linear-lanceolate, acuminate, sparsely hairy; sheaths loose, keeled, ciliate at the margin; ligule shortly ciliate; panicle lax, more or less cylindrical, interrupted, branched, spikelets solitary, enclosed in an involucre; caryopsis plano-convex, rotundate-ovate, with punctiform hilum.

Ecology: Found in rocky habitats in open wastelands, roadsides etc. It is used as fodder.

Ethnomedicinal uses: One drop of extract of leaves is poured in eyes to treat conjunctivitis.

Setaria intermedia Roem. & Schult.

Weak ascending annual; leaves sparsely hairy; panicles upto 18 cm long, lax, cylindrical; spikelets solitary, enclosed in an involucer; caryopsis plano - convex, rotundate-ovate, with punctiform hilum.

Ecology: Found in rocky habitats in open wastelands and roadsides. It is used as a fodder grass.

Ethnomedicinal uses: 1-2 drop of leaf juice is poured in the eyes to treat conjunctivitis.

Setaria italica (Linn.) P. Beauv.

Tufted erect grass; leaves linear-lanceolate, acute, mouth of the sheath beared; panicles dense, cylindric, lobed; lemmas quite smooth or minutely rugulose.

Ecology: Occasionally escapes from cultivation; found in sandy loam soils.

Ethnomedicinal uses: Crushed grains are taken with water to treat dysuria.

Sorghum halepense (Linn.) Pers.

Stout, erect perennial; with creeping, stoloniferous root-stock; leaves broadly linear- lanceolate, acuminate, base rounded or subamplexicaul; panicles lax, open; spikelets 2-nate in pairs.

Ecology: Common in wastelands and in fallow fields.

Ethnomedicinal uses: Juice of whole plant is taken orally with a pinch of common salt to treat fever. The flowers are dried and boiled in water. The steam obtained is inhaled once in a day for 2-3 days to treat typhoid.

Themeda quadrivalvis (Linn.) O. Ktze.

Tall, erect, geniculately branched perennial grass; leaves linear, acute; ligule long, membranous; panicle dense.

Ecology: Common along the bank of rivers, streams, at the foot of hills and in open grassy plains.

Ethnomedicinal uses: Warmed paste of whole plant is applied locally to treat psoriasis.

Ethnoveterinary medicinal uses: Small fishes molded in this grass are fed to cattle to treat flatulence.

Vetiveria zizanioides (Linn.) Nash

Tufted, erect, perennial, aromatic grass; spikelets in panicles; sessile spikelets awnless; lower glumes spinosely muricated.

Ecology: Common in low-lying areas.

Ethnomedicinal uses: Extract of roots is used as stimulant, cooling, febrifuge and as a tonic whereas paste is taken with water as anthelmintic.

Zea mays Linn.

Monoecious annual; male spikelets usually in terminal racemes; female inflorescence consists of many spikelets seated on a spongy axis.

Ecology: Cultivated during rainy season for its grains.

Ethnomedicinal uses: Extract of leaves is taken orally to treat renal disorders. The root decoction is taken orally to treat ulcer. Half cup decoction of mixture of style of female inflorescence of *Zea mays* and seeds of *Dolichos lobatus* is taken orally once a day for three days early in the morning for removal of calculi from kidney.

Result and Discussion

Ethnomedicinal studies on the grasses of Indian desert are of considerable interest as the economy of the arid region mostly depends on the grasses. Although much ethnomedicinal studies on plants other than the grasses has been carried out, such properties of grasses is restricted to a limited number of people of the study.

As a result of present study the ethnomedicinal uses of 37 grass species belonging to 28 genera and have been documented for their interesting therapeutic properties for curing various ailments such as sexual diseases, blood cancer, rickets, urinary diseases, skin diseases and ailments related to digestive system, respiratory system and liver complaints have been reported. Most of remedies reported in the present article are not reported in available literature notable among these are inflorescence of ***Aristida adscensionis*** which is used as diuretic while roots of ***Chloris virgata*** are used to treat cold and rheumatism; inflorescence of ***Capillipedium huegelii*** is used by the tribals to treat rheumatism and essential oil is applied locally for easy expulsion of guinea-worm. Hence, the role of ethnomedicinal surveys and field work is of crucial importance as some miraculous medicines are known to the tribes and aboriginal and much acquired knowledge through the ages is usually passed on from generation-to-generation as a guarded secret of certain families. Therefore, it is necessary to popularize the identity and utility of the grasses. More efforts should be done for identification of such medicinal grasses through ethnobotany. As population and demand for agriculture land by modern man increases the forest area are gradually cleared and converted into townships, agriculture land and plantation. This process of encroachment on the rich forest of Rajasthan has been steadily increasing, with the result that today we are face with the possibility of total extermination of the forest and the floristic wealth they contain. Also, as the domain of civilized man extends into the forest lands the tribal culture is gradually lost. This process has already led to our loosing forever a wealth of empirical knowledge the forest tribe have had, particularly with respect to the medicinal plants. It is therefore, pertinent that ethnobotanical studies be undertaken so that we may preserve and record the knowledge about useful plants and conserve the plants themselves before both are lost in society's quest for land to raise cash and plantation crops.

An extensive survey of tribal and rural area of Indian desert yielded ethnoveterinary uses of 8 grass species. The ethnoveterinary medicinal plants listed here are locally available and easily accessible and thus provide a cheaper treatment as compared to western drugs. The only limitation is the seasonal availability of certain plants, for which tribals have acquired different ways to preserve them for off-season uses. Most common way of preserving is sun-drying.

Ethnoveterinary medicine can provide an opportunity of new drug research for human use also. For example, Rwandan cattle raisers used a preparation made from *Neorautanenia mitis* to treat mange, a disease caused by mites that burrow under the animal's skin. Scientists found that this plant contained an ingredient that kills the mites. They were able to make an ointment for humans as an alternative providing low cost alternative to imported drugs (Wanzala et al., 2005). Therefore, the plants reported here may be clinically tested for their possible use in human medicine also.

CONCLUSION

The list of folk medicinal plants from the tribal area of Indian desert and their utilization will provide basic data for further studies aimed at conservation, cultivation, traditional medicine and economic welfare of rural and tribal population of the region.

REFERENCES

Chaudhary BL, Katewa SS, Galav PK. Plants in material culture of tribals and rural communities of Rajsamand district of Rajasthan. *Indian Journal of traditional knowledge*, 7(1), 11-22, (2008).

Fransworth NR. The role of ethnopharmacology in drug development. In: Chandwick, DJ and Marsh J (eds) Bioactive Compounds from Plants. Wiley, Chichester (Ciba Foundation Symposium), pp. 2-21, (1990).

Jain SK. Dictionary of Indian Folk Medicine and Ethnobotany. Deep Publication, New Delhi, (1991).

Jain A, Katewa SS, Choudhary BL, Galav P. Folk Herbal medicines used in birth control and Sexual diseases by tribals of Southern Rajasthan, India. *J Ethnopharmacol.* 90 (1), 171-177, (2003).

Jain A, Katewa SS, Choudhary BL, Galav P. Folk Herbal medicines used in birth control and Sexual diseases by tribals of Southern Rajasthan, India. J Ethnopharmacol. 90 (1): 171-177, (2004).

Jain A, Katewa SS, Galav PK, Sharma P. Medicinal plant diversity from the Sitamata wild life sanctuary, Chittorgarh district India. *J of Ethnopharmacology,* 102 (3): 543-557, (2005).

Jain A, Katewa SS, Galav PK, Nag A. Unrecorded ethnomedicinal uses of biodiversity from Tadgarh-Raoli Wildlife sanctuary, Rajasthan, India. *Acta botanica Yunnanica.* 29 (03):337-344, (2007).

Joshi P. Ethnobotany of primitive tribes in Rajasthan. Printwell, Jaipur, India, (1995).

Katewa SS, Guria BD, Jain A. Ethnomedicinal and Obnoxious grasses of Rajasthan, India. *J Ethnopharmacol.* 76 (3): 293-297, (2001).

Katewa SS, Chaudhary BL, Jain A, Galav PK. Traditional uses of plant biodiversity from Aravalli hills of Rajasthan. *Indian J Tradit knowl.* 2(1): 27-39, (2003).

Katewa SS. Contribution of some wild food plants from forestry in the diet of tribals of Southern Rajasthan. *The Indian Forester* 129 (8): 1117-1131, (2003).

Katewa SS, Chaudhary BL, Jain A. Folk herbal medicines from Tribal area of Rajasthan. *J Ethnopharmacol.* 92: 41-46, (2004)

Katewa SS, Galav PK. Traditional Folk Herbal Medicines from Shekhawati Region of Rajasthan. *Indian Journal of traditional knowledge.* 4(3): 237-245, (2005).

Katewa SS, Jain A, Chaudhary BL, Galav PK. Some unreported medicinal uses of plants from the tribal area of Southern Rajasthan. *Bull. Bot. Surv. India.* 47 (1-4): 121-136, (2006).

Katewa SS, Galav PK. Additions to traditional Folk Herbal Medicines from Shekhawati Region of Rajasthan. *Indian Journal of traditional knowledge.* 5(4): 494-500, (2006).

Katewa SS, Jain A. Traditional Folk Herbal Medicines. Apex Publishing House, Udaipur (Rajasthan), India, (2006).

Krishna Kumar PR. Indian medicine industry and the emerging patent regimes. *Ancient Sci Life* 15(3), 161, (1996).

Pushpangadan P. Ethnobiology in India—a status report, All India Coordinated Research project on Ethnobiology (AICRPE), Ministry of Environment and Forests, Government of India, New Delhi, (1994).

Ramawat KG, Sonie KC, Sharma MC. Therapeutic potential of medicinal plants. In: Ramawat KG (ed) Biotechnology: Medicinal Plants. Science Publishers, Enfield, CT, pp. 1, (2004).

Ramawat KG, Goyal S, Indian herbal drugs scenario in global perspectives. In: Ramawat KG, Merillon JM (eds) Biotechnology: Bioactive Molecules. Springer, Berlin Heidelberg New York, p. 323. (2008).

Singh V, Pandey RP. Ethnobotany of Rajasthan. Scientific Publishers, Jodhpur (1998).

Trived PC, Nehra S. Traditional herbal medicines for health care and management of human diseases. In: Trivedi PC. (ed) Herbal Drugs and Biotechnology. Pointer Publishers, Jaipur, India, pp. 1 (2004).

chapter 10

NATURAL ANTIOXIDANTS AND THEIR POTENTIAL HEALTH BENEFITS

Manoranjan Adak

INTRODUCTION

Antoine Lavoisier, noble laureate and a pioneer oxygen chemist had pointed out that animals somehow transform chemical fuels (foods) into heat energy through the process of respiration, which is essential to life. He observed that in general, respiration is nothing but a slow combustion of carbon and hydrogen in presence of oxygen (Lehninger et al., 1990). Therefore, oxygen is an element indispensable for life and oxidation is a natural process that occurs anytime a substance combines with oxygen to form oxidized molecules, then it becomes a highly active free radical that may damage other molecules while it is trying to neutralize itself (Sies, 1991; 1993; 1997). Free radicals are simply defined as any species capable of independent existence that contains one or more unpaired electrons, an unpaired electrons being one that is alone in an orbital. These active by-products are generally reactive oxygen species (ROS) as well as reactive nitrogen species (RNS) that outcome from the cellular redox process (Halliwell, 2007). These compounds play a dual role as both toxic and beneficial to health. The delicate balance between their two antagonistic effects is clearly an important aspect of life. At low or moderate levels, ROS and RNS exert beneficial effects on cellular responses and immune function. At high concentrations, they generate oxidative stress, a destructive process that can damage all cell structures (Young and Woodside, 2001; Willcox et al., 2004; Bahorun et al., 2006; Valko et al., 2007). A certain level of free radicals is essential for good health as they are involved in fighting infection and in the contraction of smooth muscles in the blood vessels. Cells have a number of ways of dealing with excess free radicals including the use of enzyme systems and specific antioxidants (Matill, 1947; Droge, 2002). Endogenous and exogenous antioxidants act as "free radical scavengers" by preventing and repairing damages caused by ROS and RNS, and therefore can enhance the immune defense and lower the risk of cancer and degenerative diseases (Valko et al., 2005; 2006; Parthasarathy et al., 1999; Chatterjee et al., 2007). Antioxidants neutralize free radicals before they attack healthy cells (Davies, 1995).

Reactive oxygen species (ROS) include superoxide ($O_2^{\bullet -}$), thiyl ($RS^{\bullet}$), trichloromethyl ($CCl_3^{\bullet}$) or nitric oxide ($NO^{\bullet}$) in which the unpaired electron is delocalized between both atoms. The $O_2^{\bullet -}$, hydroxyl radicals ($^{\bullet}OH$) and other reactive oxygen species such as H_2O_2 are continuously produced *in vivo*. Non-radical oxidants include hydrogen peroxide, singlet oxygen and ozone, which form free radicals in tissues through various chemical reactions (Briviba et al., 1996). Most of the ROS produced by cells come from the following four sources: (1) normal aerobic respiration in mitochondria, which generates superoxide radical ($O_2^{\bullet -}$) and the ensuing toxic products, hydrogen peroxide (H_2O_2) and the highly reactive hydroxyl radical ($^{\bullet}OH$); (2) stimulated macrophages and polymorph nuclear leukocytes, which release superoxide and the nitric oxide radical ($NO^{\bullet}$), which in turn can interact to form the non radical destructive peroxynitrite; (3) peroxisomes, cell organelles that produce H_2O_2 as a by-product of degrading fatty acid and other molecules; and (4) oxidant by-products that occur during the induction of cytochrome P_{450} enzymes (Valko et al., 2007).

Exogenous sources of ROS include the following: tobacco smoke, which has a broad spectrum of oxidant-ionizing radiation, which generates free radicals in exposed tissues, notably the highly reactive $OH^{\bullet}$ radical; UV light, which produces singlet oxygen ($1O_2$) and OH; ozone (O_3) and oxides of nitrogen in polluted air; industrial toxins such as carbon-tetrachloride; drugs such as phenobarbital, which is a known tumor promoter in liver; and charcoal-broiled foods, which form a variety of carcinogens, notably benzo(a)pyrene (Tiwari, 2001). These exogenous pollutants generating free radicals have become part of our daily inhaling/ingesting life and in fact, there appears no escape from them. Continuous interaction of the animal physiological systems with these free radicals either generated indigenously or inhaled/ingested from exogenous sources which lead to excess load of free radicals and cause cumulative damage of protein, lipid, DNA, carbohydrates and membrane, resulting in so-called oxidative stress. Therefore, living creatures have evolved a highly complicated defence system with antioxidants composed of enzymes and vitamins against oxidative stress in the course of their evolution. These defence systems are mainly classified (Noguchi et al., 2000) as (i) suppression of generation of ROS, (ii) scavenging of ROS, (iii) clearance, repairing and reconstitution of damage and (iv) induction of antioxidant proteins and enzymes.

However, amounts of these protective devices present under normal physiological conditions are sufficient only to cope with the normal threshold of physiological rate of free-radical generation. Therefore, any additional burden of free radicals, either from an indigenous or exogenous source on the animal (human) physiological system can tip free radical (pro-oxidant) and anti-free radical (antioxidant) balance leading to oxidative stress (Tiwari, 2001). The oxidative stress, defined as the imbalance between oxidants and antioxidants in favour of the former potentially leading to damage has been suggested to be the cause of aging and various human diseases (Sies, 1982). Therefore, in modern Western medicine, the balance between antioxidation and oxidation is believed to be a critical concept for maintaining a healthy biological system (Finkel, 2000; Davies, 2000). Any vitiation therefore, is understood to give rise to chaos in the physiological system leading to a variety of diseases depending upon the sensitivity and susceptibility of the organ. Thus, the status of protective mechanism against oxidants, the antioxidants in humans reflect the dynamic balance between antioxidant defence and pro-oxidant conditions and have been suggested as a useful tool in estimating the risk of oxidative damage (Tiwari, 2001; Nose, 2000; Papas,1996 ; Polidori et al., 2001).

Oxidative modification of DNA, proteins, lipids and small cellular molecules by reactive oxygen species (ROS) plays a role in a wide range of common diseases and age-related degenerative conditions (Halliwell and Gutreridge, 1989; Vertuani et al., 2004). This stress is responsible to contribute to the development of a diseases like Alzheimer's disease (Christen, 2000; Nunomura et al., 2006), Parkinson's disease (Wood-Kaczmar et al., 2006), diabetes (Davi et.al., 2005; Giugliano et al., 1996), rheumatoid arthritis (Hitchon and El-Gabalawy, 2004) and neurodegeneration in motor neuron diseases (Cookson and Shaw, 1999). Low-density lipoprotein (LDL) oxidation appears to trigger the process of atherogenesis, which results in atherosclerosis, and finally cardiovascular disease and prevent apoptosis and neurological damage (Aviram, 2000; Van Gaal et al., 2006). Oxidant damage by ROS is linked to photo aging, radiation toxicity, cataract formation and macular degeneration; it is implicated in ischemia/reperfusion tissue injury and thought to play a role in decreased function of some immune cells (Opie, 1989; Kilgore and Lucchesi, 1993).

Antioxidants are also being investigated as possible treatments for neurodegenerative diseases such as Alzheimer's disease, Parkinson's disease, and amyotrophic lateral sclerosis, (Di Matteo and Esposito, 2003; Rao and Balachandran, 2002) and as a way to prevent noise-induced hearing loss (Kopke et al., 2007). Antioxidants can cancel out the cell-damaging effects of free radicals (Hitchon and El-Gabalawy, 2004). Furthermore, people who eat fruits and vegetables, which are good sources of antioxidants, have a lower risk of heart disease and some neurological diseases, (Stanner et al., 2004) and there is evidence that some types of vegetables, and fruits in general, probably protect against a number of cancers. Some evidence that antioxidants might help prevent diseases such as macular degeneration (Bartlett and Eperjesi, 2003) suppressed immunity due to poor nutrition, (Wintergerst et al., 2006) and neurodegeneration (Wang et al., 2006). Other substances like fruit and vegetables (possibly flavonoids) may contribute to the better cardiovascular health of those who consume more fruit and vegetables (Cherubini et al., 2005; Lotito and Frei, 2006). It is thought that oxidation of low-density lipoprotein in the blood contributes to heart disease, and initial observational studies found that people taking Vitamin E supplements had a lower risk of developing heart disease (Rimm et al., 1993).

Vitamin C (Ascorbic acid) is a reducing agent and can reduce and thereby neutralize reactive oxygen species such as hydrogen peroxide (Padayatty et al., 2003) and antioxidant enzyme ascorbate peroxidase (Shigeoka et al., 2002). Its other beneficial effects are anti-atherogenic, anti-carcinogenic, immune modulator (Li and Schellhorn, 2007) and sperm motality (Abel et al., 1982). Carotenoid are fat soluble pigments which are found in fruits and vegetables like carrots, green plants, squash, spinach etc. (Willcox et al., 2004). They have a wide range of protective properties against disease including cancer (Omaye et al., 1997) and cardiovascular disease (Goulinet and Chapman, 1997). Lycopene, another fat-soluble carotenoid has been found to be very protective, particularly for prostate cancer (Dahan al., 2008).The antioxidant properties of the tea are generally attributed to its flavonoids components acids (Rice-Evans, 1999) and these compounds are all potent antioxidant *in vitro*. Aged garlic extract (AGE) is a concentrated form of organic garlic that provides the health benefits of fresh garlic, without its unpleasant side-effects (Borek, 2001; Kasuga et al., 2001; Imai et al., 1994; Nagae et al., 1994). It contains mostly stable water-soluble organosulfur compounds like *S*-allylcysteine (SAC) and *S*-allylmercaptocysteine (SAMC), which have potent antioxidant activity (Amagase, 1987; Ide and Lau, 1997; Imai et al., 1994; Wei and Lau, 1998). Some levels of antioxidant vitamins and minerals in the diet are required for good health, there is considerable doubt as to whether antioxidant supplementation is beneficial, and if so, which antioxidant(s) are beneficial and in what amounts (Stanner et al., 2004; Shenkin, 2006; Woodside et al., 2005). This article deals with the catabolism of the free radicals, examines their beneficial effects on cellular activities, and discusses the potential role of the antioxidants in preventing and/or repairing damages caused by oxidative stress.

HISTORY

The term antioxidant originally was used to refer specifically to a chemical that prevented the consumption of oxygen. In the late 19th and early 20th century, extensive study was devoted to the uses of antioxidants in important industrial processes, such as the prevention of metal corrosion, the vulcanization of rubber, and the polymerization of fuels in the fouling of internal combustion engines (Matill, 1947). Early research on the role of antioxidants in biology focused on their use in preventing the oxidation of unsaturated fats, which is the cause of rancidity (German, 1999).

Antioxidant activity could be measured simply by placing the fat in a closed container with oxygen and measuring the rate of oxygen consumption. However, it was the identification of vitamins A, C, and E as antioxidants that revolutionized the field and led to the realization of the importance of antioxidants in the biochemistry of living organisms (Jacob, 1996; Knight, 1998). Research into how vitamin E prevents the process of lipid peroxidation led to the identification of antioxidants as reducing agents that prevent oxidative reactions, often by scavenging reactive oxygen species before they can damage cells (Wolf, 2005).

Characteristics of free radicals

ROS and RNS are the terms collectively describing free radicals and other non-radical reactive derivatives called oxidants. A molecule with one or more unpaired electron in its outer shell is called a free radical (Bahorun et al., 2006; Valko et al., 2007; 2004). Free radicals are formed from molecules via the breakage of a chemical bond such that each fragment keeps one electron, by cleavage of a radical to give another radical and via redox reactions (Bahorun et al., 2006; Halliwell, 2007). These radicals are hydroxyl ($OH^\bullet$), superoxide ($O_2^{\bullet-}$), nitric oxide ($NO^\bullet$), nitrogen dioxide (NO_2), peroxyl ($ROO^\bullet$) and lipid peroxyl ($LOO^\bullet$). Also, hydrogen peroxide (H_2O_2), ozone (O_3), singlet oxygen ($1O_2$), hypochlorous acid (HOCl), nitrous acid (HNO_2), peroxynitrite ($ONOO^-$), dinitrogen trioxide (N_2O_3), lipid peroxide(LOOH), are not free radicals and generally called oxidants, but can easily lead to free radical reactions in living organisms (Genestra, 2007). Biological free radicals are thus highly unstable molecules that have electrons available to react with various organic substrates such as lipids, proteins, DNA (Vertuani et al., 2004; Sies,1997). These oxidants can damage cells by starting chemical chain reactions such as lipid peroxidation, or by oxidizing DNA or proteins. (Sies, 1997). Damage to DNA can cause mutations and possibly cancer, if not reversed by DNA repair mechanisms, (Nakabeppu et al., 2006; Valko et al., 2004) while damage to proteins causes enzyme inhibition, denaturation and protein degradation (Stadtman, 1992).

Generation of free radicals

Formation of ROS and RNS can occur in the cells by two ways: enzymatic and non-enzymatic reactions. Enzymatic reactions generating free radicals include those involved in the respiratory chain, the phagocytosis, the prostaglandin synthesis and the cytochrome P_{450} system (Bahorun et al.,2006; Halliwell,2007; Valko et al.,2007; Willcox et al.,2004; Pacher et al.,2007). The superoxide anion radical ($O_2^{\bullet-}$) is generated via several cellular oxidase systems such as NADPH oxidase, xanthine oxidase, peroxidases and then it participates in several reactions yielding various ROS and RNS which are hydrogen peroxide, hydroxyl radical ($OH^\bullet$), peroxynitrite ($ONOO^-$), hypochlorous acid (HOCl), etc. Non-radical H_20_2 is produced by the action of several oxidase enzymes, including amino acid oxidase and xanthine oxidase. Hydroxyl radical ($OH^\bullet$), the most reactive free radical *in vivo*, is formed by the reaction of $O_2^{\bullet-}$ with H_2O_2 in the presence of Fe^{2+} or Cu^{++} (catalyst). This reaction is known as the Fenton reaction (Stohs and Bagchi, 1995; Valko et al., 2007; 2004, Droge, 2002; Willcox et al., 2004).

$$2Fe^{3+} + \text{Ascorbate} \rightarrow 2Fe^{2+} + \text{Dehydroascorbate}$$

$$2Fe^{2+} + 2H_2O_2 \rightarrow 2Fe^{3+} + 2OH^{\bullet} + 2OH^{+}$$

The neutrophil-derived enzyme, myeloperoxidase, which oxidizes chloride ions in the presence of H_2O_2, produces hypochlorous acid (HOCl). Nitric oxide radical ($NO^{\bullet}$) is formed in biological tissues from the oxidation of L-arginine to citrulline by nitric oxide synthase (Pacher et al., 2007; Genestra, 2007). Free radicals can be produced from non-enzymatic reactions of oxygen with organic compounds as well as those initiated by ionizing radiations. The non-enzymatic process can also occur during oxidative phosphorylation (i.e. aerobic respiration) in the mitochondria (Genestra, 2007; Valko et al., 2007; Droge, 2002).

ROS and RNS are generated from either endogenous or exogenous sources. Endogenous free radicals are generated from immune cell activation, inflammation, mental stress, excessive exercise, ischemia, infection, cancer, aging. Exogenous ROS/RNS result from air and water pollution, cigarette smoke, alcohol, heavy or transition metals (Cd, Hg, Pb, Fe, As), certain drugs (cyclosporine, tacrolimus, gentamycin, bleomycin), industrial solvents, cooking (smoked meat, used oil, fat), radiation (Droge, 2002, Valko et al., 2006; 2005; Parthasarathy et al., 1999).

Beneficial activities of free radicals

At low or moderate concentrations, ROS and RNS are necessary for the maturation process of cellular structures and can act as weapons for the host defense system. Indeed, phagocytes (neutrophils, macrophages, monocytes) release free radicals to destroy invading pathogenic microbes as part of the body's defense mechanism against disease (Droge, 2002; Young and Woodside, 2001). The importance of ROS production by the immune system is clearly exemplified by patients with granulomatous disease due to defective membrane-bound NADPH oxidase system which makes them unable to produce the superoxide anion radical ($O_2^{\bullet -}$), thereby resulting in multiple and persistent infection (Valko et al., 2007; Droge, 2002). Other beneficial effects of ROS and RNS involve their physiological roles in the function of a number of cellular signaling systems (Pacher et al., 2007, Genestra, 2007). Their production by nonphagocytic NADPH oxidase isoforms plays a key role in the regulation of intracellular signaling cascades in various types of nonphagocytic cells including fibroblasts, endothelial cells, vascular smooth muscle cells, cardiac myocytes, and thyroid tissue. For example, nitric oxide (NO) is an intercellular messenger for modulating blood flow, thrombosis, and neural activity (Pacher et al., 2007). In brief, ROS/RNS at low or moderate levels are vital to human health cytic NADPH oxidase isoforms plays a key role in the regulation of intracellular signaling cascades in various types of nonphagocytic cells including fibroblasts, endothelial cells, vascular smooth muscle cells, cardiac myocytes, and thyroid tissue (Pacher et al., 2007).

Harmful activities of free radicals and Pathogenesis

An oxidative stress, a deleterious process that can seriously alter the cell membranes and other structures such as proteins, lipids, lipoproteins, and deoxyribonucleic acid (DNA) due to generation of excess free radicals and oxidants (Bruckdorfer, 1996; Nose, 2000;Young and Woodside, 2001, Droge, 2002, Willcox et al., 2004). Oxidative stress can arise when cells cannot adequately destroy the excess of free radicals formed. In other words, oxidative stress results from an imbalance between formation and neutralization of ROS/RNS. For example, hydroxyl radical and peroxynitrite in excess can damage cell membranes and lipoproteins by a process called lipid peroxidation. This reaction leads to the formation of malondialdehyde (MDA) and conjugated diene compounds, which are cytotoxic and mutagenic (Frei, 1997). Proteins may also be damaged by ROS/RNS, leading to structural changes and loss of enzyme activity (Halliwell and Gutteridge, 2007; Frei, 1997). Oxidative damage to DNA leads to the formation of different oxidative DNA lesions, which can cause mutations. The body has several mechanisms to counteract these attacks by using DNA repair enzymes and/or antioxidants (Willcox et al., 2004; Genestra, 2007). If not regulated properly, oxidative stress can induce a variety of chronic and degenerative diseases as well as the aging process and some acute pathologies like stroke, atherosclerosis, cancer, cardiovascular disease etc.

Cardiovascular disease

Cardiovascular disease (CVD) is of multifactorial etiology associated with a variety of risk factors for its development including hypercholesterolemia, hypertension, smoking, diabetes, poor diet, stress and physical inactivity amongst others (Bahorun et al., 2006; Chatterjee et al.,2007; Ceriello,2008). Recently, research data has raised a passionate debate as to whether oxidative stress is a primary or secondary cause of many cardiovascular diseases (Ceriello, 2008). Evidence supporting ROS as a culprit of myocardial damage due to ischemia-reperfusion (Opie, 1989; Kilgore and Lucchesi, 1993).

There have been reports showing a close correlation between the production of ROS and simultaneous consumption of endogenous antioxidants (Godin and Garnett, 1989; Pyles et al., 1995; Ko et al., 1990; Leichtweis and Ji, 2001). Indirect evidence consistent with this view is the cardioprotective effects of free radical scavengers and antioxidant supplements (Steare and Yellon, 1995; Nishinaka et al., 1992). In addition, direct genetic manipulations to overexpress or underexpress genes participating in the antioxidant defense also exhibit profound influence on the outcome of ischemia-reperfusion (IR) injury (Li et al., 1997; Chen et al., 1998; Jones et al., 2003). In addition to IR injuries, ROS have also been implicated in many clinical conditions including atherosclerosis, autoimmune diseases, alcoholic liver disease, and various inflammation related disorders. Accumulated evidence has shown that ROS production is a key event in reperfusion injury when oxygen is reintroduced to ischemic tissues (Park and Lucchesi, 1999; Ambrosio and Tritto, 1999; Weisfeldt et al., 1988).

Oxygen radicals ($O_2^{\bullet-}$) are also produced by the electron transport system of the mitochondria and nicotinamide adenine dinucleotide phosphate (NADPH) oxidase. The highly toxic ROS are converted to hydrogen peroxide (H_2O_2) by superoxide dismutase (SOD), and then to H_2O by catalase and/or glutathione oxidase. However, under ischemic conditions, the endogenous antioxidant system is eroded and the tendency for metal ion assisted conversion of H_2O_2 into the destructive hydroxyl radical ($OH^{\bullet-}$) is increased (Hess and Manson, 1984).

Atherosclerosis

Atherosclerosis is a condition that results from the gradual build-up of fatty substances, including cholesterol, on the walls of the arteries. This build-up, called plaque, reduces the blood flow to the heart, brain and other tissues and can progress to cause a heart attack or stroke. This process is commonly referred to as hardening of the arteries. An elevated plasma low-density lipoprotein (LDL) concentration is a primary risk factor for the development of atherosclerosis and coronary artery disease. Reactive oxygen species generated through lipid peroxidation can oxidatively modify i.e. oxidize the amino acid residues of LDL and this can initiate the atherosclerotic process. Antioxidants thought to be able to inhibit oxidative modification of LDL that leads to the accumulation of cholesterol in the atherosclerotic lesion (Brown and Goldstein, 1983; Steinberg et al., 1989; Tiwari, 1996).

Many therapeutic agents have been developed to counteract major risk factors for cardiovascular disease like hyperlipidemia and hypertension. However, no therapy is available to address the root cause of atherosclerosis. Recently, two groups have emerged with success in designing, developing and taking antioxidant-based antiatherosclerotic candidates to the level of clinical-trials (Cynshi et al., 1998; Wasserman et al., 2003). Japanese study reported an inverse correlation between flavonoid (antioxidant) intake and total plasma cholesterol concentrations, other clinical studies, as mentioned earlier, stated that flavonoid intakes protect against coronary heart disease (Hertog et al., 1993; 1995).

Stroke

Stroke is the third leading cause of death and the major cause of disability in USA. In the general population, incidence of stroke is 1/1000 individuals, however, incidence doubles in individuals who are 80 years of age (Sorbera et al., 2002). Stroke is defined as an abrupt impairment of brain function resulting from occlusion or rupture of intra or extra cranial blood vessels. There are several types of stroke: cerebral thrombosis and cerebral embolism, also classified as ischaemic stroke and subarachnoid haemorrhage, and intra cerebral haemorrhage also classified as haemorrhagic stroke.

In atherogenesis, fat-laden cream gradually builds up on the surface of passive artery walls and when the deposit (plaque) grows large enough, it eventually closes off an affected 'pipe', preventing blood from reaching its intended tissue; after a while, the blood starved tissue dies. As a result, when a part of the cardiac muscle succumbs, it leads to heart attack and when it affects the brain, it is called a stroke. Many strokes stem instead from less obstructive plaques that rupture suddenly, triggering the emergence of a blood clot, or thrombus, which blocks blood flow (Libby, 2002).

Cerebral thrombosis is the most common type of stroke and occurs when a thrombus develops on the wall of a cerebral artery, usually damaged by atherosclerosis (Sorbera et al., 2002). Therefore, therapeutics developed for atherosclerosis, based on imbalance between oxidant and antioxidant homeostasis appears to be important in treating stroke provided it reaches the brain-tissue sites. Extensive research generated in the recent past has disclosed that free radicals play a major role in the damage caused by hypoxia and reperfusion during cerebral ischaemia, affecting a late stage of the ischaemic process. These developments also support views that agents that scavenge free radicals or prevent their production may be able to prolong the therapeutic time window (Sorbera et al., 2002). Several antioxidants and free radical scavenging-based therapeutics have been recently launched and are under development for treatment of stroke (Sorbera et al., 2002).

Cancer

Cancer is emerging as a major problem globally; both in more developed and in less developed countries. The recent world cancer report released by WHO observes that world cancer rates are set to double by 2020 (Eaton, 2003). The development of cancer in humans is a complex process including cellular and molecular changes mediated by diverse endogenous and exogenous stimuli. It is well established that oxidative DNA damage is responsible for cancer development (Poulsen et al., 1998; Valko et al., 2004; 2006). Cancer initiation and promotion are associated with chromosomal defects and oncogene activation induced by free radicals. A common form of damage is the formation of hydroxyled bases of DNA, which are considered an important event in chemical carcinogenesis (Halliwell and Gutteridge, 2007; Steenken and Jovanovic, 1997). This adduct formation interferes with normal cell growth by causing genetic mutations and altering normal gene transcription. Oxidative DNA damage also produces a multiplicity of modifications in the DNA structure including base and sugar lesions, strand breaks, DNA-protein cross-links and base-free sites (Steenken and Jovanovic, 1997). DNA damage that can contribute to the development of lung cancer and other tumors (Willcox et al., 2004; Valko et al., 2004). The highly significant correlation between consumption of fats and death rates from leukemia and breast, ovary, rectum cancers among elderly people may be a reflection of greater lipid peroxidation (Young, 2001).

Carcinogenesis is a multistage disease process that has been classified into initiation, promotion and progression stages; and each stage probably involves both genetic and epigenetic changes (Bishop, 1991). These observations have been substantiated experimentally by external administration of carcinogens (Wattenberg, 1995). Metabolic activation of carcinogen is a free-radical-dependent reaction. DNA damage mediated by free radicals plays a critical role in carcinogenesis (Guyton and Kensler, 1993: Feig et al., 1994).

In biological systems, damaged DNA is repaired enzymatically and cells regain their normal functions. However, disrepair of DNA damage may result in mutations such as base substitution and deletion, leading to carcinogenesis (Poulsen et al., 1998). Sequence specificity of DNA damage plays a key role in the mutagenic process. Endogenous DNA damage arises from a variety of intermediates of oxygen reduction and several free radicals have been reviewed to take part in this process by various mechanisms (Kawanishi et al., 2001). These reactive species have different redox potentials and redox potentials of these free-radical species may play an important role in sequence- specific DNA damage (Wright, 2003).

Apart from a variety of free radicals, non-radical oxidant like H_2O_2 also plays an important role in DNA damage. In biological systems, H_2O_2 is generated through spontaneous and/or superoxide dismutase (SOD) catalysed dismutation of $O_2^{\bullet}$. The $O_2^{\bullet}$ is produced by one electron reduction of molecular oxygen through reaction with free radicals and enzymatic reaction catalysed by xanthine oxidase. H_2O_2 has emerged as a critical molecule not only for cancer cell proliferation, but also in determining the fate of cancer cells exposed to phenolic phytochemicals. Higher amounts of ROS and H_2O_2 are produced in some cancer cells. The cumulative production of free radicals and H_2O_2 in human melanoma, neuroblastoma, colon carcinoma and ovarian carcinoma cell lines are comparable to that in phorbol ester-stimulated human blood neutrophils (Szatrowski and Nathan, 1991).

Since cancer cells constitutively produce high amounts of H_2O_2, the concept of constant oxidative stress in cancer originated (Toyokuni et al., 1995), which provides possible explanation for some of the abnormal characteristics of cancer cells (Loo, 2003). It has also been reviewed that phytochemicals (particularly antioxidant polyphenols) mediated inhibition of cancer cell proliferation take place through redox-sensitive mechanisms (Loo, 2003). Cancer cells, particularly those that are highly persistent or metastatic, require a certain level of oxidative stress to maintain a balance between undergoing either proliferation or apoptosis. They constitutively generate large but tolerable amounts of H_2O_2 that apparently function as signalling molecules in mitogen-activated protein kinase (MAPK) pathway to constantly activate redox-sensitive transcription factors and responsive genes that are involved in survival of cancer cells as well as their proliferation (Loo, 2003).

Antioxidants have also been advocated to impart anticancer activities by several other mechanisms (Smith et al.,1995) : (i) Trapping the ultimate carcinogen, (ii) blocking the metabolic activation of carcinogens, (iii) modulating xenobiotic metabolizing enzymes, (iv) scavenging free radicals, (v) inhibiting generation of free radicals, (vi) inhibiting promotion stage of carcinogenesis by inhibiting cell proliferation through blocking lipoxygenase/cycloxygenase pathway or by lowering ornithine decarboxylase activity, and (vii) by decreasing the bioavailability of ultimate carcinogen, etc.

Diabetes

There is considerable evidence that hyperglycemia results in the generation of ROS, ultimately leading to increased oxidative stress in a variety of tissues. In the absence of an appropriate compensatory response from indigenous antioxidant network, the system becomes overwhelmed (redox imbalance), leading to the activation of stress sensitive intracellular signalling pathways. One major consequence of this is the expression of gene products that cause cellular damage and are ultimately responsible for late diabetic complications. Apart from playing a key role in late diabetic complications, activation of it or similar signalling pathways also appears to play a role in mediating insulin resistance and impaired insulin secretion. The ability of antioxidant/free-radical scavengers to protect against the effects of hyperglycemia and free fatty acids along with clinical benefits following antioxidant therapy supports the causative role of oxidative stress in mediating and/or worsening these abnormalities (Evans et al., 2002). A number of reviews have appeared recently, stressing the role of oxidative stress in pathogenesis of cellular dysfunction leading to cardiovascular, hepatic and other complications of diabetes (Strowing and Raskin, 1995; Baynes and Thrope, 1996).

Similarly, supplementation with antioxidants has also been shown to decrease oxidative stress and complications in animal models of diabetes (Karasu et al., 1997; Kocak et al., 2000) and diabetic patients (Jain et al., 2000). Diabetes-induced defects in the homeostasis and the transport of intracellular calcium have been shown to decrease or recover by treatment of diabetic animals with some antioxidants (Pekiner et al., 2002). Several studies have demonstrated that antioxidants supplementation prevents lipid peroxidation, haemoglobin glycation and inhibition of Na^+, K^+- ATPase and/or Ca^{+2}-ATPase activity caused by hyperglycemia in various cells (Kowluru et al., 2000; Jain et al., 2001).

Multiple activities of phytochemicals present in traditional medicines and their preparations have been reviewed recently (Tiwari and Rao, 2002). There are several medicinal plants the world over used in traditional medicine, which possess rich antioxidant principles and strong antioxidant activities. It has been argued that major antidiabetic activities from these plants might originate from their antioxidant principles (Scartezzini and Speroni, 2000; McCune and Johns, 2002).

Neurodegenerative Diseases

Oxidative stress has been investigated in neurodegenerative diseases including Alzheimer's disease (AD), Parkinson's disease (PD), multiple sclerosis, amyotrophic lateral sclerosis, memory loss depression (Halliwell, 2001; Singh et al., 2004; Christen, 2000; Butterfield, 2002). A large body of evidence indicates that oxidative stress is involved in the pathogenesis of AD and PD. Simultaneously, increasing number of studies show that nutritional antioxidants can block neuronal death and may have therapeutic properties in animal models of these neurodegenerative diseases (Esposito et al., 2002; Behl, 1999).

Alzheimer's Disease

The risk of acquiring AD is considerable in countries with long life expectancies. In USA alone, the current estimate of 3.6 lakh new cases of AD each year is expected to triple in the next 40 years (Foley and White, 2003). AD is the commonest form of dementia with a prevalence of 0.4% in women and 0.3% in men aged 60–69 years (Rocca1991). Estimated prevalence of senile dementia in Europe increases with age from 1% in man and women of age 60 years to 44.7% in a population of 90–95 years age (Hofman et al., 1991).

Selective sensitivity and susceptibility of neurons are the most important characteristics of this disorder. Free radical theory of aging suggests that oxidative damage is a major player in degeneration of cells (Harman and Eddy, 1976). The role of oxidative stress in the etiology of AD has long been hypothesized, described and supported by a variety of experimental and clinical studies. This research has also promoted interest in assessing antioxidants for their possible benefits in modifying the course, reducing the risk, or delaying the onset of AD. Recent research reveals that dietary antioxidants may have promising therapeutic potential in delaying the onset as well as preventing the aging population with AD and its related complications (Engelhart et al., 2003).

Characteristic histopathological alterations in AD are neutristic plaques composed largely of amyloid *b*-peptides and neuronal aggregates of abnormally phosphorylated cyctoskeletal proteins due to over production of ROS (Esposito et al., 2002; Behl, 1999). Vitamin E has been proposed to impart beneficial effect in this connection by quenching the ROS formed, and selegiline protects neurons by preventing the formation of ROS and by inhibiting oxidative metabolism of catecholamines (Azzi, 2007). These advances provide a sound basis for search, design and development of targeted antioxidants for prevention and treatment of AD.

Parkinson's Disease

PD is a neurological syndrome manifested by any combination of tremble at rest, rigidity, bradykinesia and loss of postural reflexes. Neuropathalogical hallmark of PD is selective degeneration of dopaminergic neurons in the nigrostriatal system (Scherman et al., 1989). These neurons synthesize and release dopamine, and loss of dopaminergic influence on other structures in the basal ganglia leads to classical Parkinsionian symptoms (Esposito et al., 2002).

Epidemiological studies indicate that a number of factors like exposure to herbicides, industrial chemicals, trace metals, cyanide, organic solvents, carbon monoxide and carbon disulphide may increase the risk of developing PD (Olanow and Tatton, 1999). Majority of them are known to increase ROS and oxidative stress (Jenner et al., 1992). Alterations in pro-antioxidant molecules have also been observed in post-mortem tissues from individuals with PD (Esposito et al., 2002). Activated microglias are thought to contribute to neuronal damage using the release of pro-inflammatory and neurotoxic factors like TNF*a*, IL-1, RNS, and ROS, etc. Markers of elevated accumulation of NO, ROS, TNF*a*, IL-1*b*, INF-*g* in substantia nigra of PD patients have been demonstrated (Gao et al., 2003). Esposito et al (2003) suggested that there are many alternative antioxidative approaches that may be considered in prospect of clinical trials, including free radical scavengers, indigenous antioxidant enzyme boosters, iron chelators and drugs that interfere with oxidative metabolism of dopamine in Parkinsonism.

Pulmonary Disease

There is now considerable evidence that inflammatory lung diseases such as asthma and chronic obstructive pulmonary disease (COPD) are characterized by systemic and local chronic inflammation and oxidative stress (Guo and Ward, 2003; Caramori and Papi, 2004). Oxidants may play a role in enhancing inflammation through the activation of different kinases and redox transcription factors such as NF-kappa B and AP-1 (Hoshino and Mishima, 2008; MacNee, 2001).

Rheumatoid Arthritis

Rheumatoid arthritis is an autoimmune disease characterized by chronic inflammation of the joints and tissue around the joints with infiltration of macrophages and activated T cells (Walston et al., 2006; Valko et al., 2007). The pathogenesis of this disease is due to the generation of ROS and RNS at the site of inflammation. Oxidative damage and inflammation in various rheumatic diseases were proved by increased levels of isoprostanes and prostaglandins in serum and synovial fluid compared to controls (Mahajan and Tandon, 2006).

Renal Disease

Oxidative stress theater a role in a variety of renal diseases such as glomerulonephritis and tubulointerstitial nephritis, chronic renal failure, proteinuria, uremia (Droge, 2002; Galle, 2001). The nephrotoxicity is developed due to certain drugs such as cyclosporine, tacrolimus (FK506), gentamycin, bleomycin, vinblastine which is mainly due to oxidative stress via lipid peroxidation (Sadeg et al.,1993; Massicot et al.,1997). Heavy metals (Cd, Hg, Pb, As) and transition metals (Fe, Cu, Co, Cr)-induced different forms of nephropathy and carcinogenicity are strong free radical inducers in the body (Valko et al., 2005; 2006).

Ocular Disease

Oxidative stress is concerned in age-related macular degeneration and cataracts by altering various cell types in the eye either photochemically or nonphotochemically (Santosa and Jones, 2005). Under the action of free radicals, the crystalline proteins in the lens can cross-link and aggregate, leading to the formation of cataracts (Meyer and Sekundo, 2005). In the retina, long-term exposure to radiation can inhibit mitosis in the retinal pigment epithelium and choroid, damage the photoreceptor outer segments, and has been associated with lipid peroxidation (Beatty et al., 2000).

Reproductive Disease

Infertility

Infertility affects of all couples trying to conceive. Male factor infertility is a major contributing factor in reproductive biology (Sharlip et al., 2002). Excessive production of free radicals or reactive oxygen species (ROS) can damage sperm, and ROS have been extensively studied as one of the mechanisms of infertility. Superoxide anion, hydroxyl radical and hydrogen peroxide are some of the major ROS present in seminal plasma. Cells living under aerobic conditions constantly face the oxygen (O_2) paradox: O_2 is required to support life, but its metabolites such as ROS can modify cell functions, endanger cell survival, or both (Agarwal et al.,2003).Hence, any excess ROS must be continuously inactivated in order to maintain normal cell function. This function is taken up by the antioxidants present in the seminal plasma. Oxidative damage can cause base degradation, DNA fragmentation and cross-linking of proteins (Sharma et al., 2004). Spermatozoa with damaged DNA lose their ability to fertilize the oocyte (Sun et al., 1997).

Fetus

Oxidative stress is involved in many mechanisms in the development of fetal growth restriction and pre- eclampsia in prenatal medicine (Myatt, 2006; Hracsko et al., 2008). Some reports indicate that blood levels of lipid peroxidation products (F2-isoprostanes, MDA) are elevated in pre-eclamptic pregnancy and intra-uterine growth retardation and it has been suggested that ROS/RNS play a role in the etiology of these diseases (Biri et al.,2007; Hracsko et al.,2008). In pregnancies complicated by pre-eclampsia due to increased expression of NADPH oxidase-1 and 5 isoforms, that is the major enzymatic sources of superoxide in the placenta (Braekke et al., 2006). Finally, Figure 10.1 summarizes oxidative stress-induced diseases in humans.

Antioxidants

It is a compound that help prevent free-radical damage is known as antioxidant or "free-radical scavenger". In foods, antioxidants (see Table 10.1) have been defined as a substance that in small quantities is able to prevent or greatly retard the oxidation of easily oxidizable materials such as fats (Chipault, 2001). However, in biological systems the definition for antioxidants has been extended to any substance that when present at low concentrations compared to those of an oxidizable substrate significantly delays or prevents oxidation of that substrate like lipids, proteins, DNA, and carbohydrates (Halliwel,1990). Currently however, biological antioxidants have further assumed a broad definition to include repair systems such as iron transport proteins (e.g. transferrin, albumin, ferritin and caeruloplasmin), antioxidant enzymes, and factors affecting vascular homeostasis, signal transduction and gene expression (Frankel and Meyer, 2000).

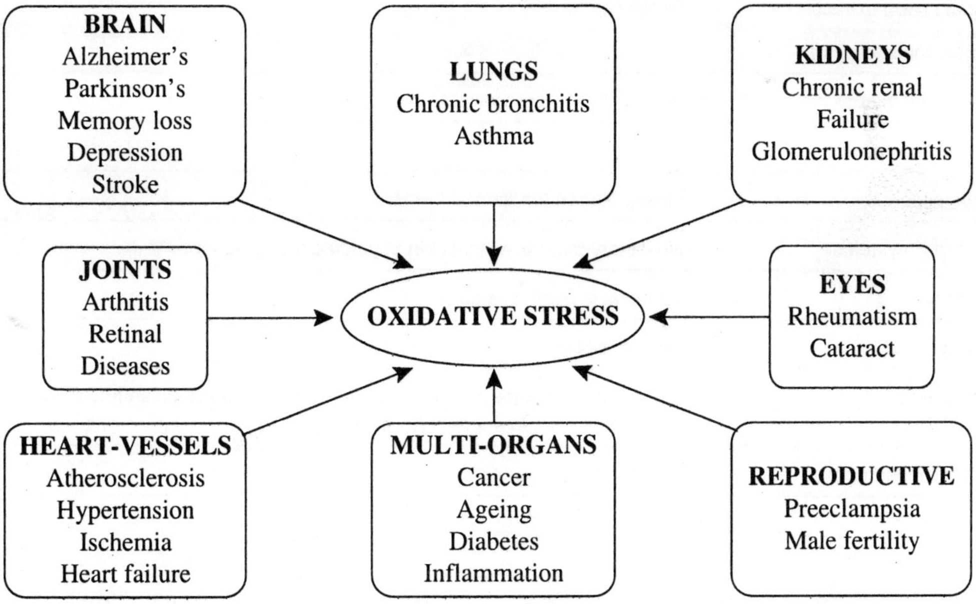

Fig. 10.1: Oxidative stress-induced diseases in humans

Table 10.1: Name and source of some antioxidants

Antioxidant	*Food Sources*
Vitamin C	Citrus fruits (oranges, grapefruits, tangerines), berries, broccoli, Brussels sprouts, collards, guava, kale, turnip greens, sweet peppers, cabbage, cauliflower, spinach, watercress, melons.
Vitamin E	Unprocessed vegetable oils. Smaller amounts are found in whole grains, dark-green leafy vegetables, nuts, legumes.
Beta-carotene	Yellow-orange or green fruits and vegetables such as carrots, kale, kohlrabi, parsley, spinach, turnip greens, apricots
Lycopene	Tomatoes and tomato-based products (tomato sauce, etc.), watermelon, papaya, pink Grape fruit and pink guava. Processed tomato products contain more lycopene than fresh Tomatoes.
Lutein and zeaxanthin	Corn, egg yolks, and green vegetables and fruits (broccoli, Brussels sprouts, kale, cabbage, green beans, green peas, spinach, kiwi, and honeydew melon).
Selenium	Seafood, meat, and organ meats. Content of selenium in plant sources (whole grains and seeds) depends on selenium content of the soil.
Coenzyme Q10	Heart meats are the richest sources. Beef and chicken contain smaller amounts.
Alpha-lipoic acid	Red meat, yeast, and liver.
Grape seed extract (proanthocyanidins)	Grape seeds
Pine bark extract	No dietary source; available in supplement form.
Green tea	Green tea.
Quercetin	Onions, green tea, and red wine.
N-acetyl cysteine	No dietary source; available in supplement or drug form.
Turmeric	Turmeric is used as a spice.
Ellagic acid	Berries, pecans, walnuts, pomegranates.
Hesperidin	Citrus fruits. Oranges, tangelos, and lemons are the richest sources. Peel and pulp of fruit contain the highest amount.
Reishi mushroom	Reishi mushroom.

Antioxidants may exert their effects by different mechanisms, such as suppressing the formation of active species by reducing hydroperoxides ($ROO^{\bullet}$) and H_2O_2 and by sequestering metal ions, scavenging active free radicals, repairing and/or clearing damage. Antioxidant works by retarding the oxidation. In biology, oxidation is often started by free radicals. The role of an antioxidant is to intercept a free radical before it can react with the substrate. For example, phenol (AOH), the reaction of interest with $ROO^{\bullet}$ is:

$$AOH + ROO^{\bullet} \longrightarrow AO^{\bullet} + ROOH.$$

This H-atom transfer reaction effectively stops chain reaction. Therefore, antioxidants of biological/therapeutic importance should have the property that they will react/trap the free radical before it reacts with the susceptible substrate and initiate chain reaction. Based on several theoretical models and complex calculations, Wright (2003) concluded that bond dissociation enthalpy (BDE) gives excellent correlation for this requirement with many known families of antioxidants that have been extensively studied in biological systems, like vitamins E and C, resveratrol, gallocatechins, ubiquinol, etc. He suggested that lower the BDE, the more reactive the antioxidant. However, it should not be too low to reduce the molecular oxygen, forming $HO_2^{\bullet}$ the process of autoxidation (Wright, 2003). Major understanding of beneficial therapeutic activities of antioxidants has arisen with studies on vitamins E and C and ubiquinol Q10 that serve as excellent reference material (Tiwari,1999).

Progress in sciences is providing crucial insights in the understanding mechanisms of disease pathogenesis and is opening up rich field of potential targets for pharmaceutical intervention. The broader and clearer understanding of the molecular basis of disease processes therefore is paving a way to develop more effective and targeted treatment. Over the past three decades, free-radical theory has greatly stimulated interest in the role of dietary antioxidants in preventing many human diseases, including cancer, atherosclerosis, stroke, rheumatoid arthritis, neurodegeneration and diabetes etc. (Fang et al., 2002). These wide varieties of chronic inflammatory diseases form the basis for development of antioxidant based therapeutics. Regardless of their initiating pathological events, these diseases share a series of steps that lead to a common mechanistic pathway of oxidative stress through regulatory oxidative signals (Figure 10.1) (Morganti et al., 2002).

Chemistry of Antioxidant Phenolic Phytochemicals

Phenolic phytochemicals are one of the most abundant groups of natural metabolites and form an important part of both human and animal diets (Mann, 1978; Bravo, 1998; Crozier et al., 2000). These phenolic metabolites function to protect the plants against biological and environmental stresses and therefore are synthesized in response to pathogenic attack such as fungal or bacterial infection or high-energy radiation exposure such as prolonged UV exposure (Shetty, 1997; Briskin, 2000). Common fruits such as apples, cranberries, grapes, raspberries, and strawberries and their beverages like red wine, apple and orange juices are rich sources of phenolic phytochemicals. In addition to fruits, vegetables such as cabbage, tomato, garlic, onion etc.; food grains such as sorghum, millet, barley, peas, and other legumes are also described as important sources of phenolic phytochemicals (Urquiaga and Leighton, 2000).

There are numerous different types of phenolic phytochemicals which are classified according to their ring structure and the number of carbon atoms substituting the ring and linking them together (Table 10.2). Metabolic processing of phenolic phytochemicals in plants for their final biological function has led to chemical variations in basic phenolic structure. They vary structurally from being simple molecules (e.g. phenolic acids with a single ring structure), biphenyls and flavanoids having 2-3 phenolic rings. Another abundant group of phenolic phytochemicals in fruits and vegetables often referred to as polyphenols contain 12-16 phenolic groups. These polyphenols are classified as condensed proanthocyanidins, tannins which include galloyl and hexahydroxydiphenoyl (or ellagoyl) esters and their derivatives, or phlorotannins (Harborne, 1980; Haslam, 1988). Some common phenolic structures are cited in Fig. 10.2.

Table 10.2 : The major classes of phenolic compounds in plants

Number of Carbon atoms	*Basic skeleton*	*Class*
6	C6	Simple phenols Benzoquinones
7	C6-C1	Phenolic acids
8	C6-C2	Acetophenones Tyrosine derivatives Phenylacetic acids
9	C6-C3	Hydroxycinnamic acids Phenylpropenes Coumarins Isocoumarins Chromones
10	C6-C4	Naphthoquinones
13	C6-C1-C6	Xanthones
14	C6-C2-C6	Stilbenes Anthraquinones
15	C6-C3-C6 Isoflavonoids	Flavonoids
18	(C6-C3)2	Lignans
30	(C6-C3-C6)2	Biflavonoids
N	(C6-C3)n	Lignins
	(C6)n	Catechol
	(C6-C3-C6)n	Flavolans (Condensed Tannins)

Flavanoids

The flavonoids are a diverse group of polyphenolic compounds widely distributed in the plant kingdom and over 4000 structurally unique flavonoids have been identified in plant sources. These are primarily recognized as the pigments responsible for the many shades of yellow, orange, and red ink of flowers, fruit, and leaves. These natural products were known for their beneficial effects on health long before they were isolated as the effective compounds (Hertog et al., 1993; Peluso, 2006). Flavonoids may be divided into six different major classes (flavonols, flavanones, flavones, isoflavones, flavonols and anthocyanidins) based on differences in molecular backbone structure (Harborne, 1974; Beecher, 2003). The major classes of flavonoids consist of two fused six-membered rings (an aromatic A-ring and a heterocyclic C ring) connected through a carbon-carbon bridge to an aromatic B-ring. The specific C ring functional groups, unsaturation of C ring, and other details are given in Figure 10.3 and Table 10.3. The flavonol quer-

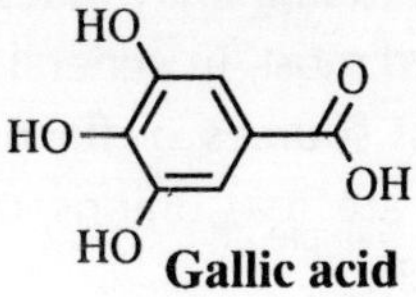

Gallic acid

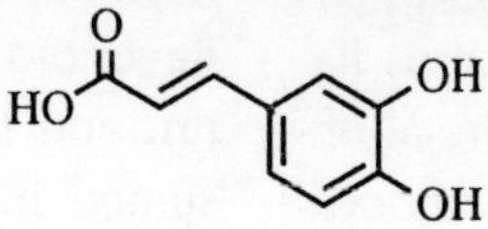

Caffeic acid

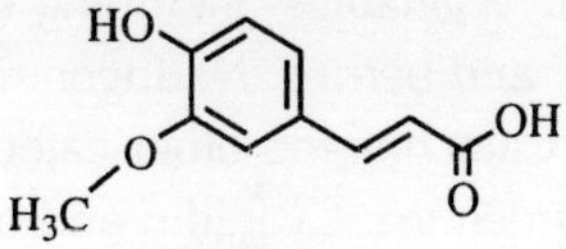

Ferulic acid

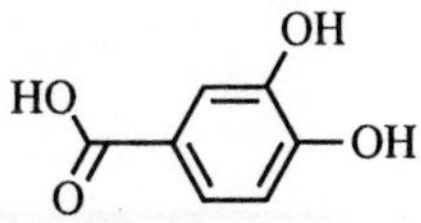

Protocatechuic acid

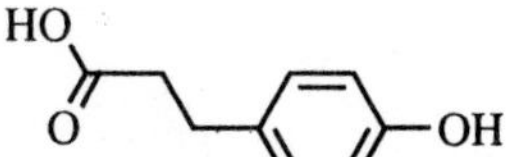

Coumaric acid

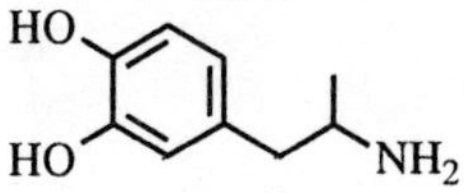

L-DOPA

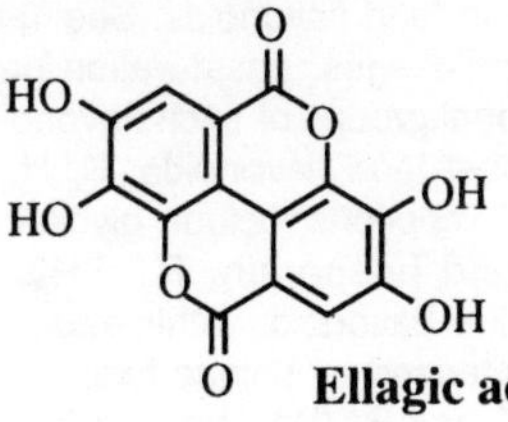

Ellagic acid

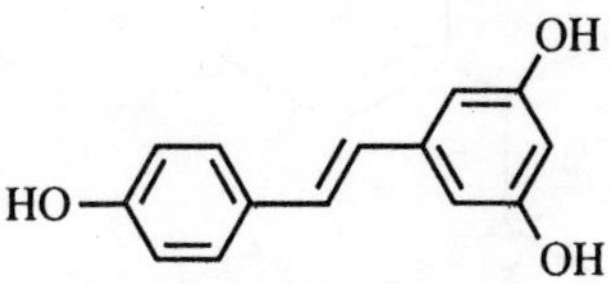

Resveratrol

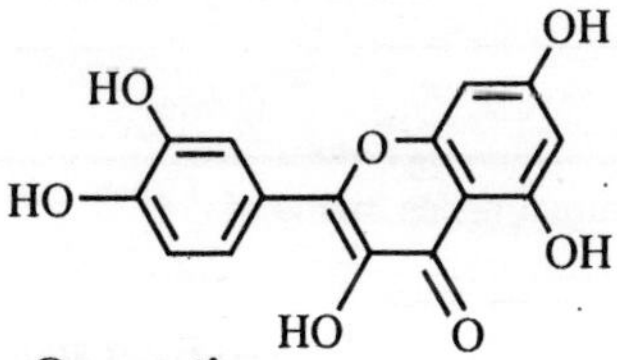

Quercetin

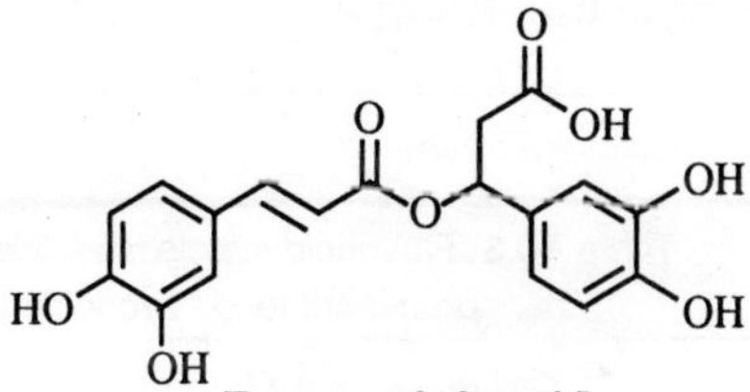

Rosemarinic acid

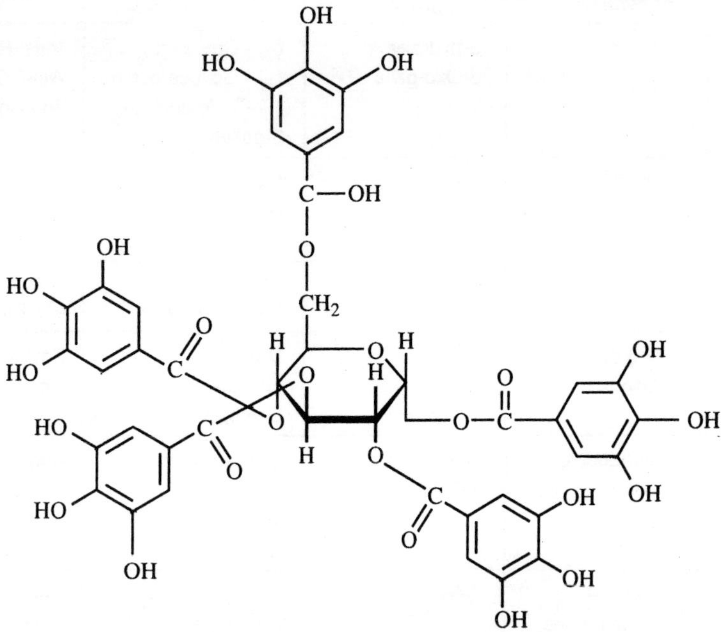

Fig. 10.2: Common simple phenol, biphenyls, flavanoids and tannins in plants

cetin and the flavone apigenin are found in many fruits and vegetables, including onions, apples, broccoli, and berries. Naringenin is a citrus flavanone. Catechin and other catechins are abundant in green tea. Cyanidin and other anthocyanidins are largely responsible for the deep colors of berries, grapes, and red wine. Genistein is an isoflavone found predominantly in legumes. The flavonoid consumed most, in general, is quercetin, and the richest sources of flavonoids consumed in general are tea, onions, and apples (Hertog et al., 1993).

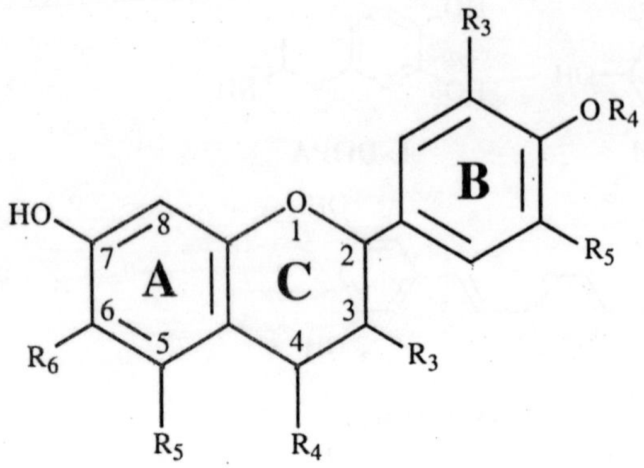

Fig. 10.3: General structure and numbering pattern for common food flavonoids. See Table 10.3 for unique linkages, unsaturation positions and functional groups of each flavonoid subclass. For most food flavonoids, R_4' H, R_5OH and R_6H. Exceptions include glycitein, R_5 H, R_6 OH; and hesperitin, R_4' CH_3. Additional individual flavonoids within each subclass are characterized by unique functional groups at R_3, R_3', and R_5' (Beecher, 2003).

Table 10.3: Flavonoid subclasses, their chemical characteristics,.name of prominent food flavonoids and typical food sources.

Flavonoid sub classes	*C ring unsaturation*	*C ring functional group*	*Prominent foodflavonoid*	*Food source*
Flavanol	None	3-hydroxy 3-Oxo-gallate	(+) - Catechin (+) - Gallocatechin (–) - Epicatechin-3-gallate	Teas, Red grapes, Red Wine, Cococa beverages And Chocolate
Flavanones	None	4-Oxo	Eriodictyol Hesperetin Naringenin	Citrus food like Orange, Lemmon etc.
Flavones	2-3 double bond	4-Oxo	Apigenin Lutcolin	Green leafy vegetables e.g. Parsley
Isoflavones	2-3 double bond	4-Oxo	Daidzein Genistein Glycitein	Soybeans, soy foods and legumes
Flavanols	2-3 double bond	3-hydroxy, 4-Oxo	Isorhamnetin Kaempferol Myricetin Quercetin	Apple, tomato, cherry, Broccoli, onion etc.
Anthocyanidins	1-2, 3-4 double bond	3-hydroxy	Cyanidin Delphinidin Petunidin	Red, blue, purple berries, Plum, strawberry etc.

Note: position of B ring on C ring is 2 in all cases except isoflavones where it is 3

The health benefits of flavonoids are related to their antioxidant capacity apart from their many other interactions. They are capable to neutralize reactive oxygen species (ROS), to chelate metal ions and to form complexes with bioactive proteins such as the enzymes, especially those involved in generation of free radicals (Majzisova and Kuchta, 2001).

Flavonoids inhibit the oxidation of LDLs involving multiplicity of mechanisms such as the direct scavenging of ROS and inhibiting peroxynitrite formation that may affect cellular integrity by reversible oxidation of LDLs. Peroxynitrite is formed because of the reaction of nitric oxide (NO) and the free radicals. However, flavonoids like silibin inhibit NO reaction with free radicals. The flavonoids also interfere in the conversion of xanthene to uric acid by inhibiting xanthene oxidase (Nijveldt et al., 2001).

The polyphenols of green tea are found as (-) epicatechin, (-) epicatechin-3-gallate, (-) epigallocatechin and (-) epigallocatechin-3-gallate while theaflavin and thearubigin are found in black tea, which are able to reduce the risk of cancer, CHD and inflammations (Aneja et al., 2004; Mukhtar and Ahmed, 2002). A review has recently been published on nutritional protection ability of flavornoids against oxidative burst and UV induced cellular damage (Saraf et al., 2007).

Measurement of antioxidants

Measurement of antioxidants is not a clear-cut process, as this is a diverse group of compounds with different reactivities to different reactive oxygen species. In food science, the oxygen radical absorbance capacity (ORAC) has become the current industry standard for assessing antioxidant strength of whole foods, juices and food additives (Cao et al., 1993; Ou et al., 2001). Other measurement tests include the Folin- Ciocalteu reagent, and the Trolox equivalent antioxidant capacity assay(Prior et al.,2005).

Antioxidants are found in varying amounts in foods such as vegetables, fruits, grain cereals, legumes and nuts. Some antioxidants such as lycopene and ascorbic acid can be destroyed by long-term storage or prolonged cooking (Xianquan et al., 2005; Rodriguez-Amaya, 2003). The polyphenolic antioxidants in foods such as whole-wheat cereals and tea are more stable (Baublis et al., 2000; Rietveld and Wiseman, 2003). In general, processed foods contain fewer antioxidants than fresh and uncooked foods, since the preparation processes may expose the food to oxygen (Henry and Heppell, 2002). The CAP-e assay measures antioxidants that are available to enter and protect live cells (Honzel et al., 2008).

Antioxidant capacity

Total antioxidant capacity was based on ORAC assays. The fruits, nuts, rice bran and vegetables were freeze-dried before analysis. Brunette potato, broccoli, carrot and tomato, which were in their cooked form used for analysis. Total antioxidant capacity is summarized in Table 10.4.

Table 10.4 : Source and total capacity of antioxidants

Antioxidant sources	Total antioxidant capacity (μmol TE/g)	Antioxidant sources	Total antioxidant capacity (μmol TE/g)
Fruits		**Vegetables**	
Plum	62.4	Broccoli	15.9
Blueberry	62.2	Potato, Russet	13.2
Raspberry	49.3	Carrot	12.2
Strawberry	35.8	Radish	9.5
Avocado	19.3	Celery	5.7
Navel orange	18.1	Lettuce, Iceberg	4.5
Grapefruit	15.5	Baby carrot	4.4
Kiwi	9.2	Tomato	3.4
Cantaloupe	3.1		

Contd. to next page.

Honeydew	2.4		
Watermelon	1.4		
Nuts		**Other foodstuffs**	
Pecan	179	Rice bran	242.9
Pistachio	79.8	Prune	85.4
Almond	44.5	Date	39.1
Cashew	20	Raisin	30.4
Macadamia	17		

Classification of antioxidant

The body has several mechanisms to counteract oxidative stress by producing antioxidants, either naturally generated in situ (endogenous antioxidants), or externally supplied through foods (exogenous antioxidants). The roles of antioxidants are to neutralize the excess of free radicals, to protect the cells against their toxic effects and to contribute to disease prevention (Willcox et al., 2004; Young and Woodside, 2001; Valko et al., 2005).Endogenous compounds in cells can be classified as enzymatic and non-enzymatic antioxidants.

Enzymatic Antioxidants

The major enzymatic antioxidants directly involved in the neutralization of ROS and RNS are superoxide dismutase (SOD), catalase (CAT), glutathione peroxidase (GPx) and glutathione reductase (GRx).

Superoxide Dismutase

Superoxide dismutase (SOD) scavenges both extracellular and intracellular superoxide anion and prevents lipid peroxidation of the plasma membrane (Nozik-Grayck et al., 2005). It is first line enzyme of defense against free radicals, catalyzes the dismutation of superoxide anion radical ($O_2^{\bullet -}$) into hydrogen peroxide (H_2O_2) by reduction (Johnson and Giulivi, 2005). The oxidant formed (H_2O_2) is transformed into water and oxygen (O_2) by catalase or glutathione peroxidase (Jeulin et al., 1989). SOD also prevents premature hyperactivation and capacitation induced by superoxide radicals before ejaculation (de Lamirande and Gagnon, 1995).

Glutathione Peroxidase/Reductase System

This system forms an excellent protection against lipid peroxidation of plasma membrane of spermatozoa. It scavenges lipid peroxides thereby arresting the progressive chain reaction of lipid peroxidation. It also scavenges hydrogen peroxide (H_2O_2), which is responsible for the initiation of lipid peroxidation. Glutathione reductase (GRx) stimulates the reduction of glutathione disulfide to reduced glutathione. Glutathione reductase, a flavoprotein enzyme, regenerates reduced glutathione (GSH) from oxidized glutathione (GSSG), with NADPH as a source of reducing power. Besides hydrogen peroxide, GPx also reduces lipid or non lipid hydroperoxides while oxidizing glutathione (GSH). This ensures a steady supply of the reductive substrate (NADPH) to glutathione peroxidase (Young and Woodside, 2001).

Catalase

Catalase detoxifies both intracellular and extracellular H_2O_2 to water and oxygen (Baker et al., 1996). In addition, catalase activates NO-induced sperm capacitation, which is a complex mechanism involving H_2O_2 (de Lamirande et al., 1997).

Non-enzymatic Antioxidants

The non-enzymatic antioxidants are also divided into metabolic and nutrient antioxidants. Metabolic antioxidants belonging to endogenous antioxidants, are produced by metabolism in the body, such as lipoid acid, glutathione, L-arginine, coenzyme Q10, melatonin, uric acid, bilirubin, metal-chelating proteins, transferrin, etc. (Droge,2002; Willcox et al.,2004). While nutrient antioxidants belonging to exogenous antioxidants, are compounds which cannot be produced in the body and must be provided through foods or supplements, such as vitamin E, vitamin C, carotenoids, trace metals (selenium, manganese, zinc), flavonoids, omega-3 and omega-6 fatty acids, etc. copper and iron (Donaldson, 2004).

Nutrient Antioxidants

Antioxidants from our diet play an important role in helping endogenous antioxidants for the neutralization of oxidative stress. The nutrient antioxidant deficiency is one of the causes of numerous chronic and degenerative pathologies. Each nutrient is unique in terms of its structure and antioxidant function (Donaldson, 2004; Willcox et al., 2004) which are discusses in below:

Vitamin E

Vitamin E is a chiral compound with eight stereoisomers: α, β, γ, δ- tocopherol and α, β, γ, δ- tocotrienol, which are fat-soluble vitamins with antioxidant properties (Herrera and Barbas, 2001; Packer et al., 2001). Among these stereoisomers, only α-tocopherol is the most bioactive and easily absorbing and metabolising this form in the human body (Brigelius-Flohé and Traber, 1999). Studies in both animals and humans indicate that natural dextrorotatory *d*-α-tocopherol is nearly twice as effective as synthetic racemic dl-α-tocopherol (Nguyen et al., 2006). It has also been claimed that the α-tocopherol form is the most important lipid soluble antioxidant, and that it protects membranes from oxidation by reacting with lipid radicals produced in the lipid peroxidation chain reaction (Herrera and Barbas,2001; Traber and Atkinson,2007). This reaction produces oxidized α-tocopheroxyl radicals that can be recycled back to the active reduced form through reduction by other antioxidants, such as ascorbate, retinol or ubiquinol (Wang and Quinn, 1999).

Vitamin E has also been claimed for the prevention against colon, prostate and breast cancers, cardiovascular diseases, ischemia, cataract, arthritis and certain neurological disorders (Mayo, 2005). In vitro studies show that vitamin E is a major chain-breaking antioxidant in the sperm membranes and it appears to have a dose dependent protective effect (Hull et al., 2000). However, the roles and importance of the various forms of vitamin E are presently unclear (Brigelius-Flohé et al., 2007 ; Atkinson, 2007) and it has even been suggested that the most important function of á-tocopherol is as a signalling molecule, with this molecule having no significant role in antioxidant metabolism (Azzi, 2007; Zingg and Azzi, 2004). The functions of the other forms of vitamin E are even less well-understood, although α-tocopherol is a nucleophile that may react with electrophilic mutagens (Brigelius-Flohé and Traber,1999) and tocotrienols may be important in protecting neurons from damage (Sen et al., 2006).

Vitamin C

Vitamin C chemically known as ascorbic acid and is a water-soluble vitamin. It is a monosaccharide antioxidant found in both plants and animals. Animals except humans are able to produce this compound in their bodies and do not require it in their diets (Linster and Van Schaftingen, 2007). In cells, it is maintained in its reduced form by reaction with glutathione, which can be catalysed by protein disulfide isomerase and glutaredoxins (Meister, 1994; Wells et al., 1990). Ascorbic acid is a reducing agent and it reduce the reactive oxygen species like hydrogen peroxide (Padayatty et al., 2003). In addition to its direct antioxidant effects, ascorbic acid is also a substrate for the antioxidant enzyme ascorbate peroxidase, a function that is particularly important in stress resistance in plants (Shigeoka et al., 2002).

Vitamin C is essential for collagen, carnitine and neurotransmitters biosynthesis and its beneficial effects are antioxidant, anti-atherogenic, anticarcinogenic, immune modulator (Li and Schellhorn, 2007). A dose dependent effect of vitamin C on sperm motility has been demonstrated that at a dose of 1000 microgram/L, vitamin C positively influenced the motility of the spermatozoa. However, above that level, vitamin C reduced the motility of the spermatozoa. On the other hand, doses fewer than 200 mg of vitamin C did not provide any benefit (Abel et al., 1982). Dawson et al. (1992) reported that smokers receiving 1000 mg/day vitamin C showed improvement in sperm quality. Natural sources of vitamin C are acid fruits, green vegetables, tomatoes and it is a labile molecule, therefore it may be lost from during cooking (Naidu, 2003).

Carotenoids

Carotenoid and retinyl ester are two major provitamins because they can be converted to active vitamin A (Stipanuk, 2000). There are more than 600 carotenoid in nature of which six can be measured in blood (Britton, 1995). Carotenoid are fat soluble pigments which are found in fruits and vegetables like carrots, green plants, squash, spinach etc. (Willcox et al., 2004). Carotenoids cannot be synthesized in animals or humans and therefore needs to be part of the dietary intake. α and β-carotene are the major carotenoids which are mainly composed of carbon and hydrogen atoms. In humans and animals, carotenoids play an important role in protection against photooxidative processes by acting as oxygen and peroxyl radical scavengers (Demming-Adams and Adams 2003). Their synergistic action with other anti-oxidants makes them an even more potent compound (Pastori et al., 1998).

Several studies have shown that less plant derived carotenoids is absorbed, cleaved, reduced and finally available as retinyl esters (HetHof et al., 2000). Therefore, bioequivalence is less than predicted and factors such as food preparation, matrix properties, co-ingestion of fat, diseases of the gastrointestinal tract and malnutrition may be contributors (Von Lintig et al., 2004).

Carotenoids have a wide range of protective properties against disease and aging and can act as a modulator for cellular processes and function (Stahl and Sies, 2005). Some other studies have shown that carotenoids can protect against cancer (Omaye et al., 1997; Omenn et al., 1996) and cardiovascular disease (Peng et al., 1995; Goulinet et al., 1997). Furthermore, dietary carotenoids can protect the skin against sun exposure (Berneburg and Krutmann, 2000; Krutmann, 2000), whilst antioxidant and cellular signalling effects have been shown in a number of studies (Young and Lowe, 2001; Karas et al., 2000). However, beta-carotene supplement in doses of 20mg daily for 5-8 years has been associated with an increased risk of lung and prostate cancer and increased cardiovascular mortality in cigarette smokers (Mayo, 2005).

Beta-carotene

Beta-carotene is a fat-soluble member of the carotenoids, which are considered provitamins because they can be converted to active vitamin A. Beta-carotene is converted to retinol, which is essential for vision. It is a strong antioxidant and is the best quencher of singlet oxygen. However, beta-carotene supplement in doses of 20 mg daily for 5-8 years has been associated with an increased risk of lung and prostate cancer and increased total mortality in cigarette smokers (Mayo Clinic Medical Information, 2005). Beta-carotene 20-30 mg daily in smokers may also increase cardiovascular mortality by 12% to 26% (Mayo, 2005). These adverse effects do not appear to occur in people who eat foods high in beta-carotene content. Beta-carotene is present in many fruits, grains, oil and vegetables (carrots, green plants, squash, spinach) (Willcox et al., 2004).

Curcumin

Curcumin [1,7-bis (4-hydroxy-3-methoxy phenyl)-1-6- hepatadine-3-5-dione] a member of curcuminoid family represents one of the yellow pigments isolated from turmeric. Turmeric is the dried rhizome of plant *Curcuma longa* and apart from its culinary appeal and common use as the spice, it is well known for its medicinal properties in Egyptian and Indian culture for more than 6000 year ago. Its immunomodulatory properties including anti-oxidant, anti-inflammatory and anti-tumor properties are well-documented (Gao et al., 2004). The curcumin reduces nitric oxide (NO) and exerts beneficial effects in experimental colitis. Ukil et al. (2003) reported that the yellow pigment treats inflammatory bowl diseases due to the oxidative and nitrosative stresses. Recently the immuno-nutritional ability of curcumin demonstrating its active role in treatment of the allergic response has been highlighted in a review (Kurup and Barrios, 2008).

Lycopene

Lycopene, a member of the carotenoid family, is a fat-soluble pigment responsible for the red color of certain fruits and vegetables. Its pigment protects the plant from damage by oxygen and light. Lycopene possesses antioxidant and anti proliferative properties in animal (Seren et al., 2008). Lycopene has been found to be very protective, particularly for prostate cancer (Dahan et al., 2008). Several prospective cohort studies have found associations between high intake of lycopene and reduced incidence of prostate cancer, though not all studies have produced consistent results (Seren et al., 2008). The major dietary source of lycopene is tomatoes, with the lycopene in cooked tomatoes, tomato juice and tomato sauce included, being more bioavailable than that in raw tomatoes (Donaldson, 2004). The dietary antioxidant lycopene reduces oxidative stress and the levels of bone turnover markers in postmenopausal women, and may be beneficial in reducing the risk of osteoporosis (Rao et al., 2007).

Green Tea

Tea is one of the most consumed beverages of the world after water. Tea beverage is an infusion of the dried leaves of *Camellia sinesis*, a member of Theaceae family. Freshly harvested tea leaf is processed differently in different parts of the world to give oolong tea (2%), green tea (20%) or black tea (78%) (Kuroda Hara, 1999). Green tea is prepared from the fresh tea leaf and widely consumed in Japan and China. Western cultures favour black tea, which is prepared through the oxidation, curing process of maceration and exposure to atmospheric oxygen (Graham, 1992; Langley-Evans, 2000). Tea is linked to beneficial effects on human health with the polyphenols as the responsible constituents (Riemersma et al., 2001; Mukhtar and Ahmad, 2000).

Fresh tea leaf is rich in water soluble polyphenols, particularly flavanols, flavanol gallate and flavanol glycosides (Willson and Clifford, 1992; Bors et al., 1996). The major tea catechins: α-epigallocatechin-3-gallate (EGCG), α-epigallocatechin (EGC), α- epicatechin-3-gallate (ECG), α-epicatechin (EC), α-epicatechin-3-gallate (ECG), α-epicatechin (EC), α-gallocatechin and β-catechin; constitutes 30% to 42% of the green tea solids by weight (Chung et al., 2005). These compounds are all potent antioxidant *in vitro* and, when consumed, may act as the free radical scavengers, which remove endogenously generated superoxide, peroxyl and hydroxyl radicals. Many *in vitro* and *in vivo* effects of tea polyphenols have been reported (Vinson et al., 1995; 1999; Rice-Evans and Miller, 1996) including antioxidant, anticarcinogenic and hypolipidemic properties.

The powerful antioxidant properties of the tea are generally attributed to its flavonoids components; theaflavins, bisflavanols and theaflavic acids (Rice-Evans and Miller, 1999). The antioxidant property of tea is coupled with several mechanisms e.g. depolarization of electrons, formation of intramolecular hydrogen bonds (Van Acker et al., 1996), rearrangement of the molecular structure (Salah et al., 1995; Jovanovic et al., 1994). The bioactive flavanol compounds of tea may also prevent oxidative reactions by chelating free copper and iron, which may catalyze the formation of reactive oxygen species *in vitro* (Halliwell, 1997; Weisburger, 1999).

Garlic

Garlic (*Allium sativum*) is used universally as a traditional medicine, and a functional food to enhance physical and mental health (Linnaeus, 1957). It is used for flavoring in cooking and is unique because of its high sulfur content. In addition to sulfur, garlic also contains arginine, oligosaccharides, flavonoids, and selenium, all of which may be beneficial to health (Amagase et al., 2001; Milner, 1996). The medicinal uses of garlic has a long history (Block, 1985). Recent studies have validated many of the medicinal properties attributed to garlic and its potential to lower the risk of disease. Cancer-preventive actions of garlic, garlic extracts and its components have been demonstrated in animals (Amagase and Milner 1993; Milner 1996; Nishino et al., 1990). Epidemiologic studies show an inverse correlation between garlic consumption and reduced risk of gastric and colon cancer (Steinmetz et al., 1994). Garlic has been shown to have antithrombotic activity (Block, 1985), lower blood lipids and have a cardioprotective effect (Neil and Sigali, 1994). The mechanisms of garlic have been endorsed to its potent antioxidant action, (Wei and Lau, 1998; Yang et al., 1993) its ability to stimulate immunological responsiveness (Reeve et al., 1993) and its modulation of prostanoid synthesis (Belman et al., 1989; Dimitrov and Bennink, 1997).

Aged garlic extract (AGE) is an odorless product resulting from prolonged extraction of fresh garlic at room temperature; it is highly bioavailable and has biological activity in vitro in both animals and humans (Moriguchi et al., 1997). AGE contains water-soluble allyl amino acid derivatives, which account for most of its organosulfur content, stable lipid-soluble allyl sulfides, flavonoids, saponins and essential macro- and micronutrients (Amagase, 1998). The lipid-soluble volatile organosulfur compound allicin, which is produced enzymatically when garlic is cut or chopped, is absent in AGE. Allicin is an unstable and transient compound with oxidant activity (Freeman and Kodera, 1995); it is virtually undetectable in blood circulation after garlic ingestion (Lawson et al., 1992) because it decomposes to form other organosulfur compounds (Freeman and Kodera, 1995). The major unique organosulfur compounds in AGE are water-soluble *S*-allylcysteine (SAC) and *S*-allylmercaptocysteine (SAMC), which have potent antioxidant activity (Amagase, 1997; Ide and Lau, 1997; Imai et al., 1994; Wei and Lau, 1998). The content of SAC and SAMC in AGE is high because they are produced during the process of aging, thus providing AGE with higher antioxidant activity than fresh garlic and other commercial garlic supplements (Imai et al., 1994).

The antioxidative actions of AGE and its components are determined by their ability to scavenge ROS and inhibit the formation of lipid peroxides. These effects are determined by measuring the decrease in ROS-induced chemiluminescence, inhibition of thiobarbituric acid reactive substances (lipid peroxides) (TBARS assay), and in vitro inhibition of the release of pentane, a product of oxidized lipids, in the breath of an animal exposed to oxidative stress (Amagase, 1997; Awazu and Horie, 1997; Horie et al., 1989; Ide et al., 1996; Imai et al., 1994).

Oxidation of lipids, notably oxidative modification of LDL, is implicated in the development of cardiovascular and cerebrovascular disease (Cox and Cohen, 1996; Witztum, 1993). Lipid oxidation products, including peroxides and toxic aldehydes such as malondialdehyde (Horie et al., 1989), can damage proteins and DNA and have been implicated in carcinogenesis (Borek, 1993). AGE inhibits lipid oxidation and oxidative modification of LDL (Ide and Lau, 1997). Other protective actions of AGE include inhibition of platelet aggregation (Steiner, 1996) and suppression of prostanoid synthesis with subsequent anti-inflammatory, antiathrogenic and antithrombotic effects (Dimitrov and Bennink, 1997). The protection of endothelial cell integrity by inhibition of lipid peroxidation–induced injury (Geng and Lau, 1997) and reduction in serum cholesterol and other lipids by AGE (Lau et al., 1987; Steiner, 1996) further add to its potential in helping prevent heart disease and stroke.

Cytosolic nuclear factor- B (NF-B) is a transcription factor that is regulated by the redox state of the cell and can be activated by mitogens, bacteria and viruses and by ROS-producing agents such as UV, ionizing radiation, hydrogen peroxide and tumor necrosis factor (TNF). The major clinical significance of NF-B activation is its involvement in human immunodeficiency virus (HIV) gene expression (Griffin et al., 1989). AGE and SAC inhibit TNF- and hydrogen peroxide–induced activation of NF-B in human T-cells (Geng et al., 1997), indicating their potent antioxidant function and suggesting a potential role for AGE in modulating HIV replication.

Oxidant-induced DNA damage and mutagenesis are determinants in the multistage process of cancer in animals and in vitro (Borek, 1993). Allixin, an active component in AGE, which has been shown to inhibits aflatoxin-induced DNA damage and mutagenesis in *Salmonella typhimurium*, in part by inhibiting cytochrome P450 activity (Yamasaki et al., 1991). Several group of workers reported that AGE inhibits both early and late stages of carcinogenesis of tumor growth in many tissues like colon, mammary glands, skin, stomach and esophagus (Amagase and Milner, 1993; Amagase et al., 1996; Liu et al., 1992; Milner, 1996; Nishino et al., 1989, 1990; Reeve et al., 1993).

Supplementation with AGE may have an important protective role against liver toxicity caused by a variety of medicinal and environmental substances (Wang et al., 1998). Tadi et al. (1991) reported that AGE protects against liver toxicity by benzo (a) pyrene and aflatoxin B_1, two potent free radical–producing environmental carcinogens (Borek, 1993; 1997). Studies in mice showed that SAC and SAMC were potent inhibitors of liver toxicity induced by the industrial oxidant carbon tetrachloride and by the commonly used analgesic agent, acetaminophen (Nakagawa et al., 1988).

CONCLUSION

The present age is facing stress, pollution, hyperactivity and tension. The allegation of oxidative stress in the etiology of several chronic and degenerative diseases suggests that antioxidant therapy represents a promising avenue for treatment. It is well documented now that lack of neutral bioactive components in our every day diet leads to variety of diseases. In the future, a therapeutic strategy to increase the antioxidant capacity of cells may be used to strengthen the long-term effective treatment. Therefore, opinions are divided over whether or not antioxidant supplements offer the same health benefits as antioxidants in foods. Although many epidemiological data suggest that antioxidants may have a beneficial effect on many chronic diseases, the systematic use of supplements is hindered by several factors: the lack of prospective and controlled studies, the long-term effects and the dosages necessary for each type of disease. However, many questions about antioxidant supplements in disease prevention remain unsolved. Further research is needed before this supplementation could be officially recommended as an adjuvant therapy. In the meantime, it is reminded that avoiding oxidant sources (cigarette, alcohol, bad food, stress, etc.) must be considered as important as taking diet rich in antioxidants.

REFERENCES

Abel BJ, Carswell G, Elton R, Hargreave TB, Kyle K. Randomized trial of clomiphene citrate treatment and vitamin C for male infertility. *Br. J Urol.* 54, 780-784, (1982).

Agarwal A, Saleh RA, Bedaiwy MA. Role of reactive oxygen species in the pathophysiology of human reproduction. *Fertil. Steril.*79, 829-843, (2003).

Amagase H, Petesch BL, Matsura H, Kasuga S, Itakura Y. Intake of garlic and its bioactive compounds. *J Nut.* 131, 955S-962S, (2001).

Amagase H. Antioxidant and radical scavenging effects of aged garlic extract and its constituents. Antioxidants and Disease, 6th Congress on Clinical Nutrition, 28 Banff Alberta, Canada, (1987).

Amagase H. Intake of garlic and its components, 4th Nutritional and Health Benefits of Garlic as a Supplement Conference Newport Beach, Canada, (1998).

Amagase H. Antioxidant and radical scavenging effects of aged garlic extract and its constituents. Antioxidants and Disease, 6th Congress on Clinical Nutrition. Banff Alberta, Canada, (1997).

Amagase H, Milner JA. Impact of various sources of garlic and their constituents on 7, 12-DMBA binding to mammary cell DNA. *Carcinogenesis* 14, 1627-1631, (1993).

Amagase H, Schaffer EM, Milner J. Dietary components modify the ability of garlic to suppress 7, 12,-dimethyl (a) anthracene induced DNA adducts. *J. Nutr.*126, 817-824, (1996).

Ambrosio G, Tritto I. Reperfusion injury: experimental evidence and clinical implications. *Am. Heart J.*138, 69-75, (1999).

Aneja R, Hake PW, Burroughs TJ, Denenberg AG, Wong HR, Zingarelli B. Epigallocatechin, a green tea polyphenol, attenuates myocardial ischemia reperfusion injury in rats. *Mol. Med.* 10, 1-6, (2004).

Atkinson J, Epand RF, Epand RM. Tocopherols and tocotrienols in membranes: A critical review. *Free Radic. Biol. Med.* 44 (5): 739-764, (2007).

Aviram M. Review of human studies on oxidative damage and antioxidant protection related to cardiovascular diseases. *Free Radic. Res.* 33, S85-97, (2000).

Awazu S, Horie T. Antioxidants in garlic. II. Protection of heart mitochondria by garlic extract and diallyl polysulfide from the doxorubicin-induced lipid peroxidation. Lanchance PP(eds) Nutraceuticals Designer Foods III Garlic, Soy and Licorice. Food and Nutrition Press Trumbull, CT. pp. 131-138, (1997).

Azzi A. Molecular mechanism of alpha-tocopherol action. *Free Radic. Biol. Med.* 43 (1): 16-21, (2007).

Bahorun T, Soobrattee MA, Luximon-Ramma V, Aruoma OI. Free radicals and antioxidants in cardiovascular health and disease. *Inter.J Med. Update.*1, 1-17, (2006).

Baker HW, Brindle J, Irvine DS, Aitken RJ. Protective effect of antioxidants on the impairment of sperm motility by activated polymorphonuclear leukocytes. *Fertil. Steril.* 65, 411-419, (1996).

Bartlett H, Eperjesi F. Age-related macular degeneration and nutritional supplementation: a review of randomized controlled trials. *Ophthalmic Physiol. Opt.* 23 (5): 383-399, (2003).

Baublis A, Lu C, Clydesdale F, Decker E. Potential of wheat based breakfast cereals as a source of dietary antioxidants. *J Am. Coll. Nutr.* 19 (3): 308S-311S, (2000).

Baynes JW, Thrope SR. The role of oxidative stress in diabetic complications. *Curr. Opin. Endocrinol.* 3, 277-284, (1996).

Beatty S, Koh HH, Phil M, Henson D, Boulton M. The Role of oxidative stress in the pathogenesis of age-related macular degeneration. *Surv Ophthalmol.* 45, 115-134, (2000).

Beecher GR. 'Overview of Dietary Flavonoids: Nomenclature, Occurrence and Intake', *J Nutr*, 133, 3248-3254, (2003).

Behl C. Alzheimer's disease and oxidative stress: implications for novel therapeutic approach. *Prog. Neurobiol.* 57, 301-323, (1999).

Belman S, Solomon J, Segal, A. Inhibition of soybean lipoxygenase and mouse skin tumor promotion by onion and garlic compounds. *J. Biochem. Toxicol.*4, 151-160, (1989).

Berneburg M, Krutmann J. Photoimmunology, DNA repair and photocarcinogenesis. *J Photochem Photobiol.*54, 87-93, (2000).

Biri A, Bozkurt N, Turp A, Kavutcu M, Himmetoglu OI, Durak I. Role of oxidative stress in intrauterine growth restriction. *Gynecol. Obstet. Invest.* 64, 187-192, (2007).

Bishop JM. Molecular themes in oncogenesis. *Cell* 64,235-248, (1991).

Block E. The chemistry of garlic and onion. *Sci. Am.* 252,114-119, (1985).

Borek C. Antioxidant health effects of aged garlic extract. *J Nutr.* 131, 1010S-1015S, (2001).

Borek C. Antioxidants and cancer. *Sci. Med.*4, 51-62, (1997).

Borek C. Molecular mechanisms in cancer induction and prevention. Environ. *Health Perspect.* 101, 237-245, (1993).

Bors W, Heller W, Michel C, Stettmaier K. Flavonoids and polyphenols: Chemistry and biology. In. Cadenas E, Des PL (eds). Handbook of Antioxidants. New York: Marcel Dekker, Inc. pp, 409-466, (1996).

Braekke K, Harsem NK, Staff AC. Oxidative stress and antioxidant status in fetal circulation in preeclampsia. *Pediatr Res.*60, 560-564, (2006).

Bravo L. Phenolic phytochemicals: chemistry, dietary sources, metabolism, and nutritional significance. *Nutr. Rev.* 56, 317-333, (1998).

Brigelius-Flohé R, Davies KJ. "Is vitamin E an antioxidant, a regulator of signal transduction and gene expression, or a 'junk' food? Comments on the two accompanying papers: "Molecular mechanism of alpha-tocopherol action" by A. Azzi and "Vitamin E, antioxidant and nothing more" by M. Traber and J. Atkinson". *Free Radic. Biol. Med.* 43(1): 2-3, (2007).

Brigelius-Flohé, R, Traber M. Vitamin E: function and metabolism. *Faseb J.* 13 (10), 1145-1155, (1999).

Briskin DP. Medicinal plants and Phytomedicines. Linking plant biochemistry and physiology to human health. *Plant Physiol.*124, 507-514, (2000).

Britton G. Structure and properties of carotenoid in relation to function. *Faseb J.* 9, 1551-1558, (1995).

Briviba K, Roussyn I, Sharov VS, Sies H. Attenuation of oxidation and nitration reactions of peroxynitrite by selenomethionine, selenocystine and Ebselen. *Biochem. J.* 319, 13-15, (1996).

Brown MS, Goldstein JL. Lipoprotein metabolism in the macrophage: implication of cholesterol deposition in atherosclerosis. *Annu. Rev. Biochem.* 52, 223-261, (1983).

Bruckdorfer RK, Antioxidants, lipoprotein oxidation, and arterial function. *Lipids*, 31, S83-S85, (1996).

Butterfield DA. Amyloid beta-peptide (1-42)-induced oxidative stress and neurotoxicity: implications for neurodegeneration in Alzheimer's disease brain. A review. *Free Radic. Res.* 36, 1307-1313, (2002).

Cao G, Alessio H, Cutler R. Oxygen-radical absorbance capacity assay for antioxidants. *Free Radic. Biol. Med.* 14 (3), 303-311, (1993).

Caramori G, Papi A. Oxidants and asthma. Review. *Thora.x* 59, 170-173, (2004).

Ceriello A. Possible role of oxidative stress in the pathogenesis of hypertension. Review. *Diabetes Care.* 31(Suppl 2), S181-184, (2008).

Chatterjee M, Saluja R, Kanneganti S, Chinta S, Dikshit, M. Biochemical and molecular evaluation of neutrophil NOS in spontaneously hypertensive rats. *Cell Mol. Biol.*53, 84-93, (2007).

Chen EP, Bittner HB, Davis RD, Van-Trigt P, Folz RJ. Physiologic effects of extracellular superoxide dismutase trans gene over expression on myocardial function after ischemia and reperfusion injury. *J Thorac. Cardiovasc .Surg.* 115(2), 450-458, (1998).

Cherubini A, Vigna G, Zuliani G, Ruggiero C, Senin U, Fellin R . "Role of antioxidants in atherosclerosis: epidemiological and clinical update". *Curr. Pharm. Des.* 11 (16), 2017-2032, (2005).

Chipault JR. Antioxidants for use in food. In Auto oxidation and Antioxidants. Lundberg WO (eds) Inter science, New York, vol. II, pp, 477-542, (1962).

Christen Y. Oxidative stress and Alzheimer disease. *Am. J Clin. Nutr.* 71 (2), 621S–629S, (2000).

Chung S, Liao YJ, Yang GY, Lu G. Inhibition of lung tumor genesis by tea. *Exp.Lung Res.* 31, 135-144, (2005).

Cookson M, Shaw P. Oxidative stress and motor neuron disease. *Brain Pathol.* 9 (1), 165-186, (1999).

Cox DA, Cohen ML. Effects of oxidized low-density lipoproteins on vascular contraction and relaxation: clinical and pharmacological implications in atherosclerosis. *Pharmacol. Rev.* 48, 3-9, (1996).

Crozier A, Burns J, Aziz AA, Stewart AJ, Rabiasz HS, Jenkins GI, Edwards CA, Lean MEJ. Antioxidant flavonols from fruits, vegetables and beverages: measurements and bioavailability. *Biol. Res.* 33, 79-88, (2000).

Cynshi O, Kawabe Y, Suzuki T, Takashima Y, Kaise H, Nakamura M, Ohba NE, Kodama T. Antiatherogenic effects of antioxidant BO-653 in three different animal models. *Proc. Natl. Acad. Sci. USA*, 95, 10123-10128, (1998).

Dahan K, Fennal M, Kumar NB. Lycopene in the prevention of prostate cancer. *J Soc. Integr. Oncol.*6, 29-36, (2008).

Davi G, Falco A, Patrono C. Lipid peroxidation in diabetes mellitus. *Antioxid. Redox. Signal.* 7, (1-2): 256-268, (2005).

Davies KJA. Oxidative stress, antioxidant defenses and damage removal, repair, and replacement system. *IUBMB Life* 50, 279-289, (2000).

Davies K. Oxidative stress: the paradox of aerobic life. *Biochem. Soc. Symp.* 61, 1-31, (1995).

Dawson EB, Harris WA, Teter MC, Powell LC. Effect of ascorbic acid supplementation on the sperm quality of smokers. *Fertil. Steril.* 58, 1034-1039, (1992).

de Lamirande E, Gagnon C. Capacitation-associated production of superoxide anion by human spermatozoa. *Free Radic. Biol. Med.* 18, 487-495, (1995).

de Lamirande E, Leclerc P, Gagnon C. Capacitation as a regulatory event that primes spermatozoa for the acrosome reaction and fertilization. *Mol. Hum. Reprod.* 3, 175-194, (1997).

Demming-Adams B, Adams III WW. Antioxidants in photosynthesis and human nutrition. *Science.* 298, 2149-2153, (2002).

Di Matteo V, Esposito E. Biochemical and therapeutic effects of antioxidants in the treatment of Alzheimer's disease, Parkinson's disease, and amyotrophic lateral sclerosis. *Curr Drug Targets CNS Neurol. Disord.* 2 (2): 95-107, (2003).

Dimitrov NV, Bennink MR. Modulation of arachidonic-acid metabolism by garlic extract. Lanchance PP (eds). Nutraceuticals: Designer Foods III Garlic, Soy and Licorice. Food and Nutrition Press Trumbull, CT. pp, 199-120, (1997).

Donaldson MS. Nutrition and cancer: A review of the evidence for an anti-cancer diet. *Nutr J.* 3, 19-25, (2004).

Droge W. Free radicals in the physiological control of cell function. Review. *Physiol. Rev.*82, 47-95, (2002).

Eaton L. World cancer rates set to double by 2020. *Br. Med. J.* 326, 728, (2003).

Engelhart MJ, van Swieten JC, Hofman A, Witteman JC, Breteler MM. Dietary intake of antioxidants and risk of Alzheimer's disease. *JAMA*, 287, 3223-3229, (2003).

Esposito E, Ratilio D, Di Matteo V, Di Glulia C, Cacchio M, Algeri S, A review of specific dietary antioxidants and the effects on biochemical mechanisms related to neurodegenerative processes. *Neurobiol. Aging*. 23, 719-735, (2002).

Evans JL, Goldfine ID, Maddux BA, Grodsky GM, Oxidative stress and stress activated signalling pathways: a unifying hypothesis of type-2 diabetes. *Endocr. Rev*. 23, 599-622, (2002).

Fang YZ, Yang S, Wu G. Free radicals, antioxidants and nutrition. *Nut. J.* 18, 872-879, (2002).

Feig DI, Reid TM, Loeb LA. Reactive oxygen species in tumor genesis. *Cancer Res*. (*Suppl.* 7). 54, 1890-1894, (1994).

Finkel T. Oxidants, oxidative stress and the biology of aging. *Nature*, 408, 239-248, (2000).

Foley DJ, White LR. Dietary intake of antioxidants and risk of Alzheimer disease: food for thought. *J Am. Med .Assoc*. 287, 3261-3263, (2003).

Frankel EN, Meyer AS. The problems of using one-dimensional methods to evaluate multifunctional food and biological antioxidants. *J. Sci. Food Agric*. 80, 1925-1941, (2000).

Freeman F, Kodera Y. Garlic chemistry: stability of *S*-(2-propenyl) 2-propene-1-sulfinothioate (allicin) in blood, solvents and simulated physiological fluids. *J. Agric. Food Chem.* 43, 2332-2338, (1995).

Frei B. Reactive oxygen species and antioxidant vitamins. Linus Pauling Institute. Oregon State University. http://lpi.oregonstate.edu/ f-w97/ reactive.htm, (1997).

Galle J. Oxidative stress in chronic renal failure. *Nephrol. Dial. Transplant*16, 2135-2142, (2001).

Gao HM, Liu B, Zhang W, Hong JS, Novel anti-inflammatory therapy for Parkinson' disease. *Trends in Pharmacol. Sci.* 24, 395-401, (2003).

Gao X, Kuo J, Jiang H, Deeb D, Liu Y, Divine, G, Chapman, R.A., Dulchavsky, S.A., Gautam, S.C. Immuno-modulatory activity of curcumin: suppression of lymphocyte proliferation, development of cell-mediated cytotoxicity and cytokine production *in vitro*. *Biochem. Pharmacol.* 68, 51-61, (2004).

Genestra M. Oxyl radicals, redox-sensitive signalling cascades and antioxidants. Review. *Cell Signal.* 19, 1807-1819, (2007).

Geng Z, Lau BHS. Aged garlic extracts modulate glutathione redox cycle and superoxide dismutase activity in vascular endothelial cells. *Phytother. Res.* 11, 54-56, (1997).

Geng Z, Rong Y, Lau BHS. S-Allyl cysteine inhibits activation of nuclear factor kappa B in human T cells. *Free Radic. Biol. Med.* 23, 345-350, (1997).

German J. Food processing and lipid oxidation. *Adv. Exp. Med. Biol.* 459, 23-50, (1999).

Giugliano D, Ceriello A, Paolisso G. Oxidative stress and diabetic vascular complications. *Diabetes Care* 19 (3), 257-67, (1996).

Godin DV, Garnett ME. Altered antioxidant status in the ischemic/reperfused rabbit myocardium: effects of allopurinol. *Can. J Cardiol.*5 (7), 365-371, (1989).

Goulinet S, Chapman MJ. Plasma LDL and HDL subspecies are heterogeneous in particle content of tocopherols and oxygenated and hydrocarbon carotenoids. Relevance to oxidative resistance and atherogenesis. *Arterioscler. Thromb. Vasc. Biol.*17, 786-796, (1997).

Graham HN. Green tea composition, consumption and polyphenol chemistry. *Preventive Med.*21, 334-350, (1992).

Griffin GE, Leung K, Folks TM, Kunkel S, Nabel GJ. Activation of HIV gene expression during monocyte differentiation by induction of NF-B. *Nature* 339, 70-73, (1989).

Guo RF, Ward PA. Role of oxidants in lung injury during sepsis. *Antioxid. Redox Signal.* 29, 1991-2002, (2007).

Guyton KZ, Kensler TW. Oxidative mechanisms in carcinogenesis. *Br. Med. Bull.* 49, 523-544, (1993).

Halliwell B. Antioxidants and human disease: a general introduction. *Nutr Rev.* 55, S44-S52, (1997).

Halliwell B. Role of free radicals in neurodegenerative diseases: therapeutic implications for antioxidant treatment. Drugs Aging 18, 685-716, (2001).

Halliwell B. Biochemistry of oxidative stress. *Biochem. Soc. Trans.*35, 1147 1150, (2007).

Halliwell B, Gutreridge JMC. Free Radicals in Biology and Medicine. 2nd (edn), Clarendon Press, Oxford, UK, (1989).

Halliwell B, Gutteridge JMC. Free radicals in biology and medicine. 4th edn. Clarendon Press Oxford, UK, (2007).

Halliwell B. How to characterize biological antioxidants. *Free Radic. Res. Commun.* 9, 1-32, (1990).

Harborne JB, Mabry TJ, Mabry H. The Flavonoids, London, Chapman and Hall, (1974).

Harborne JB. Plant phenolic. In: Bella EA, Charlwood BV (eds) Encyclopedia of Plant Physiology, Springer-Verlag 8, pp. 329-395,(1980).

Harman D, Eddy DE, Naffsinger J. Free radical theory of aging: inhibition of amyloidosis in mice by antioxidants; possible mechanism. *J. Am. Geriatr. Soc.* 24, 203-210, (1976).

Haslam E. Practical polyphenolic: from structure to molecular recognition and physiological action. Cambridge University Press: Cambridge UK, (1998).

Henry C, Heppell N. Nutritional losses and gains during processing: future problems and issues. *Proc. Nutr. Soc.* 61 (1), 145-148, (2002).

Herrera E, Barbas C. Vitamin E: action, metabolism and perspectives. *J Physiol. Biochem.* 57 (2), 43-56, (2001).

Hertog MG, Feskens EJ, Hollman PC, Katan MB, Kromhout D. 'Dietary antioxidant flavonoids and risk of coronary heart disease: the Zutphen Elderly Study'. *Lancet* 342, 1007-1011, (1993).

Hertog MG, Kromhout D, Aravanis C, Blackburn H, Buzina R, Fi-danza F, Giampaoli S, Jansen A. Flavonoid intake and long-term risk of coronary heart disease and cancer in the seven countries study', *Arch. Intern. Med.* 155, 381-386, (1995).

Hess ML, Manson NH. Molecular oxygen: friend and foe. The role of the oxygen free radical system in the calcium paradox, the oxygen paradox and ischemia / reperfusion injury. *J Mol. Cell. Cardiol.* 16(11), 969-985, (1984).

HetHof KH, West CE, Weststrate JA, Hautvest JG. Dietary factors that affect the bioavailability of carotenoid. *J Nutr.* 130, 503-506, (2000).

Hitchon C, El-Gabalawy H. Oxidation in rheumatoid arthritis. *Arthritis Res. Ther.* 6 (6), 265-278, (2004).

Hofman A, Grobbee DE, de Jong PT, van den Ouweland FA. The prevalence of dementia in Europe: a collaborative study of 1980–1990 findings. *Int. J. Epidemiol.* 20, 736-748, (1991).

Honzel D, Carter, S.G., Redman, K.A., Schauss, A.G., Endres, J.R., Jensen, G.S. Comparison of chemical and cell-based antioxidant methods for evaluation of foods and natural products: generating multifaceted data by parallel testing using erythrocytes and polymorphonuclear cells. *J Agric. Food Chem.* 56 (18): 8319-8325, (2008).

Horie T, Murayama T, Mishima T, Fumiyaki I, Minamide Y, Fuwa T, Awaxu S. Protection of liver microsomal membranes from lipid peroxidation by garlic extract. *Planta Med.* 55, 506-508, (1989).

Hoshino Y, Mishima M. Antioxidants & redox signaling redox-based therapeutics for lung diseases. *Antioxid. Redox Signal.*10, 701-714, (2008).

Hracsko Z, Orvos H, Novak Z, Pal A, Varga, I.S. Evaluation of oxidative stress markers in neonates with intra-uterine growth retardation. *Redox Rep.*13, 11-6, (2008).

Hull MG, North K, Taylor H, Farrow A, Ford WC. Delayed conception and active and passive smoking. The Avon Longitudinal Study of Pregnancy and Childhood Study Team. *Fertil Steril.*74, 725-733, (2000).

Ide N, Lau BHS. Garlic compounds protect vascular endothelial cells from oxidized low-density lipoprotein-induced injury. *J. Pharm. Pharmacol.*49, 908-911, (1997).

Imai J, Ide N, Nagae S, Moriguchi T, Matsuura H, Itakura Y. Antioxidants and free radical scavenging effects of aged garlic extract and its constituents. *Planta Med.*60, 417-420, (1994).

Jacob R. "Three eras of vitamin C discovery". *Subcell Biochem.* 25, 1-16, (1996).

Jain SK, Lim G. Pyridoxine and pyridoxamine inhibits superoxide radicals and prevents lipid peroxidation, protein glycation, and ($Na^+ + K^+$)-ATPase activity reduction in high glucose treated human erythrocytes. *Free Radic. Biol. Med.* 30, 232-237, (2001).

Jain SK, McVie R, Smith T. Vitamin E supplementation restores glutathione and malonaldehyde to normal concentrations in erythrocytes of type-1 diabetic children. *Diabetes Care.* 23, 1389-1394, (2000).

Jenner P, Dexter DT, Sian J, Schapira AHV, Marsolen CD. Oxidative stress as a cause of nigral cell death in Parkinson's disease and incident Lewy body disease. *Ann. Neurol.* 32, 582-587, (1992).

Jeulin C, Soufir JC, Weber P, Laval-Martin D, Calvayrac R. Catalase activity in human spermatozoa and seminal plasma. *Gamete Res.* 24, 185-196, (1989).

Johnson F, Giulivi C. Superoxide dismutases and their impact upon human health. *Mol. Aspects Med.* 26 (4-5): 340-352, (2005).

Jones SP, Hoffmeyer MR, Sharp BR, Ho YS, Lefer DJ. Role of intracellular antioxidant enzymes after *in vivo* myocardial ischemia and reperfusion. *Am. J Physiol. Heart Circ. Physiol.* 284(1), H277-282, (2003).

Jovanovic S, Steenken S, Tosic M, Marjanovic B, Simic MG. Flavonoids as antioxidants. *J Am. Chem. Soc.* 116, 4846-4851, (1994).

Karas M, Amir H, Fishman D, Danilenko M, Segal S, Nahum A, Koifmann A, Giat Y, Levy J, Sharoni Y. Lycopene interferes with cell cycle progression and insulin-like growth factor I signaling in mammary cancer cells. *Nutr. Cancer.* 36, 101-111, (2000).

Karasu C, Ozansoy G, Bozkurt O, Erdogan D, Omeroglu S. Antioxidant and triglyceride lowering effect of vitamin E associate with the prevention of abnormalities in the reactivity and morphology of aorta from streptozotocin-diabetic rats. *Metabolism* 46, 872-879, (1997).

Kasuga S, Uda N, Kyo E, Ushijima M, Morihara N, Itakura Y. Pharmacological activities of aged garlic extract in comparison with other garlic preparations. *J. Nutr.* 131, 1080S-1084S (2001).

Kawanishi S, Hiraku Y, Oikawa S. Mechanism of guanine specific DNA damage by oxidative stress and its role in carcinogenesis and aging. *Mutat. Res.* 488, 65-76, (2001).

Kilgore KS, Lucchesi BR. Reperfusion injury after myocardial infarction: the role of free radicals and the inflammatory response. *Clin. Biochem.* 26(5), 359-370, (1993).

Knight J. Free radicals: their history and current status in aging and disease. *Ann. Clin. Lab. Sci.* 28 (6), 331-346, (1998).

Ko KM, Garnett ME, Godin DV. Altered antioxidant status in ischemic/reperfused rabbit myocardium: reperfusion time-course study. *Can. J Cardiol.*6 (7), 299-304, (1990).

Kocak G, Aktan F, Canbolat O, Özo⌣gul C, Elbe⌣g S, Yildizo⌣glu-Ari, N, and Karasu Ç. Alpha lipoic acid treatment ameliorates metabolic parameters, blood pressure, vascular reactivity and morphology of vessels already damaged by streptozotocin-diabetes (The ADIC Study group). *Diabetes Nutr. Metab.* 13, 308-319, (2000).

Kopke RD, Jackson RL, Coleman JK, Liu J, Bielefeld EC, Balough BJ. "NAC for noise: from the bench top to the clinic". *Hear. Res.* 226 (1-2), 114-125, (2007).

Kowluru RA, Engerman RL, Kern TS. Diabetes induced metabolic abnormalities in myocardium: effect of antioxidant therapy. *Free Radic. Res.* 32, 67-74, (2000).

Krutmann. Ultraviolet: A radiation-induced biological effects in human skin: relevance for photo aging and photodermatosis. *J Dermatol. Sci.* 23, S22-S26, (2000).

Kuroda Y, Hara Y. Anti-mutagenic and anticarcinogenic activity of tea polyphenols. *Mutat. Res.* 436, 69-97, (1999).

Kurup VP, Barrios CS. Immuno-modulatory effects of curcumin in allergy. *Mole. Nutr. Food Res.* 52, 1031-1039, (2008).

Langley-Evans SC. Antioxidant potential of green and black tea determined using the ferric reducing power assay (FRAP). *Int. J. Food Sci. Nutr.* 51, 181-188, (2000).

Lau BHS, Lam F, Wang-Ceng R. Effect of an odor modified garlic preparation on blood lipids. *Nutr. Res.* 7, 139-149, (1987).

Lawson LD, Ransom DK, Hughs BG. Inhibition of whole blood platelet aggregation by compounds in garlic clove extracts and commercial garlic products. *Thromb. Res.* 65, 141-156, (1992).

Lehninger AL, Nelson DL, Cox MM. Principle of Biochemistry. Worth Publishers, 2nd edn. New York, pp 359, (1990).

Leichtweis S, Ji LL. Glutathione deficiency intensifies ischaemia-reperfusion induced cardiac dysfunction and oxidative stress. *Acta Physiol. Scand.* 172(1), 1-10, (2001).

Li G, Chen Y, Saari JT, Kang YJ. Catalase-over expressing transgenic mouse heart is resistant to ischemia-reperfusion injury. *Am. J Physiol.* 273(3 Pt 2), H1090-1095, (1997).

Li Y, Schellhorn HE. New developments and novel therapeutic perspectives for vitamin C. Critical Review. *J Nutr.*137, 2171-2184, (2007).

Libby P. Atherosclerosis: The new view. *Sci. Am.* 286, 28–37, (2002).

Linnaeus C. Species Plantanum: a facsimile of the first edition. London, (1957).

Linster CL, Van Schaftingen E. Vitamin C. Biosynthesis, recycling and degradation in mammals. *Febs. J.* 274 (1), 1-22, (2007).

Liu JZ, Lin XY, Milner JA. Dietary garlic powder increases glutathione content and glutathione *S*-transferase activity in rat liver and mammary tissues. *Faseb J* 6, A3230, (1992).

Loo G. Redox sensitive mechanisms of photochemical-mediated inhibition of cancer cell proliferation. *J. Nutr. Biochem.* 14, 64-73, (2003).

Lotito SB, FreiB. Consumption of flavonoid-rich foods and increased plasma antioxidant capacity in humans: cause, consequence, or epiphenomenon? *Free Radic. Biol. Med.* 41 (12), 1727-1746, (2006).

MacNee W. Oxidative stress and lung inflammation in airways disease. *Eur. J Pharmacol.*429, 195-207, (2001).

Mahajan A, Tandon VR. Antioxidants and rheumatoid arthritis. *J Ind. Rheumatol. Ass.*12, 139-142, (2004).

Majzisova G, Kuchta M. Dietary flavonoids and risk of coronary heart disease. *Physiol. Res.* 50, 529-535, (2001).

Mann J. Secondary Metabolism. Oxford Chemistry Series, Clarendon Press: Oxford, (1978).

Massicot F, Martin C, Dutertre-Catella H, Ellouk-Achard S, Pham-Huy C. Modulation of energy status and cytotoxicity induced by FK506 and cyclosporine A in a renal epithelial cell line. *Arch Toxicol.* 71, 529-531, (1997).

Matill HA. Antioxidants. *Annu. Rev. Biochem.* 16, 177-192, (1947).

Mayo Clinic Medical Information. Drugsand supplements.VitaminE.

http://www.mayoclinic.com/health/vitamin-e/NS_patientvitamin-e, (2005).

McCune LM, Johns T. Antioxidant activity in medicinal plants associated with the symptoms of diabetes mellitus used by the indigenous people of the North American boreal forest. *J. Ethnopharmacol.* 82, 197-205, (2002).

Meister A. Glutathione-ascorbic acid antioxidant system in animals. *J Biol Chem* 269 (13), 9397–9400, (1994).

Meyer CH, Sekundo W. Nutritional supplementation to prevent cataract formation. *Dev. Ophthalmol.* 38, 103-119, (2005).

Milner JA. Garlic: Its anticarcinogenic and antitumorigenic properties. *Nutr. Rev.* 54, S82-S86, (1996).

Morganti M, Carpi A, Nicolini A, Gorini I, Glaviano B, Fini M. Atherosclerosis and cancer: common pathways on vascular endothelium. *Biomed. Pharmacother.* 56, 317-324, (2002).

Moriguchi T, Saito H, Nishiyama N. Anti-aging effect of aged garlic extract in the inbred brain atrophy mouse model. *Clin. Exp. Pharmacol. Physiol.* 24:235-242, (1997).

Mukhtar H, Ahmad N. Tea polyphenols: prevention of cancer and optimizing health. *Am. J. Clin. Nutr.* 71, 1698S–1704S, (2000).

Myatt L. Placental adaptive responses and fetal programming. *J Physiol.*572, 25-30, (2006).

Nagae S, Ushijima M, S Hatono S, Imai J, Kasuga S, Matsuura H, Itakura Y, Higashi Y. Pharmacokinetics of the garlic compound S-allyl cysteine. *Planta Med.* 60, 214-217 (1994).

Naidu AK. Vitamin C in human health and disease is still a mystery. An overview. *Nutr. J* 2, 1-10, (2003).

Nakabeppu Y, Sakumi K, Sakamoto K, Tsuchimoto D, Tsuzuki T, Nakatsu Y. Mutagenesis and carcinogenesis caused by the oxidation of nucleic acids. *Biol. Chem.* 387 (4): 373-379, (2006).

Nakagawa S, Kasuga S, Matsuura H. Prevention of liver damage by aged garlic extract and its components in mice. *Phytother. Res.*1, 1-4, (1988).

Neil H, Sigali C. Garlic, its cardioprotective properties. *Curr. Top. Lipidol.* 5, 6-10, (1994)

Nguyen LA, He H, Pham-Huy C. Chiral drugs. An overview. *Int. J Biomed. Sci.* 2, 85-100, (2006)

Nijveldt RJ, Nood E, Hoorn DEC, Boelens PG, Norren K, Leeuwen PAM. Flavonoids: a review of probable mechanism of action and potential applications. *Am. J. Clin. Nutr.* 74, 418-425, (2001).

Nishinaka Y, Sugiyama S, Yokota M, Saito H, Ozawa T. The effects of a high dose of ascorbate on ischemia-reperfusion-induced mitochondrial dysfunction in canine hearts. *Heart Vessels* 7(1), 18-23, (1992).

Nishino H, Iwashima A, Itakura H, Matsuura T, Fuwa T. Antitumor promoting activity of garlic extracts. *Oncology* 46, 277-280, (1989).

Nishino H, Nishino A, Takayasu A, Iwashima Y, Itakura Y, Kodera Y, Matsuura H, Fuwa T. Antitumor promoting activity of allixin, a stress compound produced by garlic. *Cancer J.* 3, 20-21, (1990).

Noguchi N, Watanabe A, Shi H. Diverse functions of antioxidants. *Free Radic. Res.*33, 809-817, (2000).

Nose K. Role of reactive oxygen species in the regulation of physiological functions. *Biol. Pharm. Bull.* 23, 897-903, (2000).

Nozik-Grayck E, Suliman H, Piantadosi C. Extracellular superoxide dismutase. *Int. J Biochem. Cell Biol.* 37 (12), 2466-2471, (2005).

Nunomura A, Castellani R, Zhu X, Moreira P, Perry G, Smith M. Involvement of oxidative stress in Alzheimer disease. *J Neuropathol. Exp. Neurol.* 65 (7), 631-41, (2006).

Olanow CW, Tatton WG. Etiology and pathogenesis of Parkinson's disease. *Annu. Rev. Neurosci.*, 22, 123-144, (1999).

Omaye ST, Krinsky NI, Kagan VE, Mayne ST, Liebler DC, Bidlack WR. Âeta-Carotene: friend or foe? *Fundam Appl Toxicol.* 40, 163-174, (1997).

Omenn GS, Goodman GE, Thornquist MD, Balmes J, Cullen MR, Glass A, Keogh JP, Meyskens FL, Valanis B, Williams JH, Barnhart S, Hammar S. Effects of a combination of beta-carotene and vitamin A on lung cancer and cardiovascular disease. *N. Engl. J Med.* 334, 1150-1155, (1996).

Opie LH. Reperfusion injury and its pharmacologic modification. *Circulation* 80(4), 1049-1062, (1989).

Ou B, Hampsch-Woodill M, Prior R. Development and validation of an improved oxygen radical absorbance capacity assay using fluorescein as the fluorescent probe. *J Agric Food Chem* 49 (10), 4619-2466, (2001).

Pacher P, Beckman JS, Liaudet L. Nitric oxide and peroxynitrite in health and disease. *Physiol Rev.* 87, 315-424, (2007).

Packer L, Weber SU, Rimbach G. Molecular aspects of alpha tocotrienol antioxidant action and cell signalling. *J. Nutr.* 131 (2), 369S-3673S, (2001).

Padayatty S, Katz A, Wang Y, Eck P, Kwon O, Lee J, Chen S, Corpe C, Dutta A, Dutta S, Levine M. Vitamin C as an antioxidant: evaluation of its role in disease prevention. *J Am. Coll. Nutr.* 22 (1), 18-35, (2003).

Papas AM. Determinants of antioxidants status in humans. *Lipids* 31, S77-S82, (1996).

Park JL, Lucchesi BR. Mechanisms of myocardial reperfusion injury. *Ann. Thorac. Surg.* 68(5), 1905-1912, (1999).

Parthasarathy S, Santanam N, Ramachandran S, Meilhac O. Oxidants and antioxidants in atherogenesis: an appraisal. *J Lipid Res.*40, 2143-2157, (1999).

Pastori M, Pfander H, Boscoboinik D, Azzi A. Lycopene in association with α-tocopherol inhibits at physiological concentrations proliferation of prostate carcinoma cells. *Biochem. Res. Commun.* 250, 282-585, (1998).

Pekiner B, Ulusu NN, Das Evcimen N. *In vivo* treatment with stobadine prevents lipid peroxidation, protein glycation and calcium overload but does not ameliorate Ca^{+2}-ATPase activity in heart and liver of streptozotocin- diabetic rats: comparison with vitamin E. *Biochim. Biophys.Acta*, 1588, 71-78, (2002).

Peluso MR. Flavonoids Attenuate Cardiovascular Disease, Inhibit Phosphodiesterase, and Modulate Lipid Homeostasis in Adipose Tissue and Liver. *Exp. Biol. Med.* 231, 1287-1299, (2006).

Peng YM, Peng YS, Lin Y, Moon T, Roe DJ, Ritenbaugh C. Concentrations and plasma tissue diet relationships of carotenoid, retinoids and tocopherols in humans. *Nutr. Cancer.* 23, 233-246, (1995).

Polidori MC, Stahl W, Eichler O, Niestroj N, Sies H. Profiles of antioxidants in human plasma. *Free Radic. Biol. Med.* 30, 456-462, (2001).

Poulsen HE, Prieme H, Loft S. Role of oxidative DNA damage in cancer initiation and promotion. *Eur. J. Cancer Prev.* 7, 9-16, (1998).

Prior R, Wu X, Schaich K. Standardized methods for the determination of antioxidant capacity and phenolics in foods and dietary supplements. *J Agric. Food Chem.* 53 (10), 4290-4302, (2005).

Pyles LA, Fortney JE, Kudlak JJ, Gustafson RA, Einzig S. Plasma antioxidant depletion after cardiopulmonary bypass in operations for congenital heart disease. *J Thorac. Cardiovasc. Surg.* 110 (1), 165-171, (1995).

Rao A, Balachandran B. Role of oxidative stress and antioxidants in neurodegenerative diseases. *Nutr Neurosci* 5 (5), 291-309, (2002).

Rao LG, Mackinnon ES, Josse RG, Murray TM, Strauss A, Rao AV. Lycopene consumption decreases oxidative stress and bone resorption markers in postmenopausal women. *Osteop. Intern.* 18, 109-115, (2007).

Reeve VE, Bosnic M, Rosinova E, Boehm-Wilcox C. A garlic extract protects from ultraviolet B (280–320 nm) radiation induced suppression of contact hypersensitivity. *Photochem. Photobiol.* 58, 813-817, (1993).

Rice-Evans C. Implications of the mechanisms of action of tea polyphenols as antioxidants in vitro for chemoprevention in humans. *Proc. Soc. Exp. Biol. Med.* 220, 262-266, (1999).

Rice-Evans CA, Miller MN, Paganga G. Structure antioxidant activity relationships of flavonoids and phenolic acids: *Free Radic. Biol. Med.* 20, 933-956, (1996).

Riemersma RA, Rice-Evans CA, Tyrrell RM, Clifford MN, Lean ME. Tea flavonoids and cardiovascular health. *Q. J. Med.* 2001; 94: 277-282, (2001).

Rietveld A, Wiseman S. "Antioxidant effects of tea: evidence from human clinical trials". *J Nutr.* 133 (10), 3285S-3292S, (2003).

Rimm EB, Stampfer MJ, Ascherio A, Giovannucci E, Colditz GA, Willett WC (1993). Vitamin E consumption and the risk of coronary heart disease in men. *N Engl. J Med.* 328 (20), 1450-1456, (1993).

Rodriguez-Amaya D. Food carotenoids: analysis, composition and alterations during storage and processing of foods. *Forum Nutr.* 56, 35-37, (2003).

Sadeg N, Pham-Huy C, Martin C, Warnet JM, Claude, J.R. Effect of cyclosporine A and its metabolites and analogs on lipid peroxidation in rabbit renal microsomes. *Drug Chem. Toxicol.* 16, 165-174, (1993).

Salah N, Miller NJ, Paganga G, Tijburg L, Bolwell GP, Rice-Evans CA. Polyphenolic flavanols as scavengers of aqueous phase radicals and as chain-breaking antioxidants. *Arch. Biochem. Biophys.* 322, 339-346, (1995).

Santosa S, Jones PJ. Oxidative stress in ocular disease: does lutein play a protective role? *Can. Med. Ass. J* 173, 861-862, (2005).

Saraf S, Ashwat MS, Saraf S. Flavonoids: a nutritional protection against oxidative and UV induced cellular damages. *Pharmacog. Rev.* 1, 30-40, (2007).

Scartezzini P, Speroni E. Review of some plants of Indian traditional medicine with antioxidant activity. *J. Ethnopharmacol.* 71, 23-43, (2000).

Scherman D, Desnos C, Darchen F, Pollak P, Javoy-Agid F, Agid Y. Striatal dopamine deficiency in Parkinson's disease; role of aging. *Ann. Neurol.* 26, 551-557, (2989).

Sen C, Khanna S, Roy S. Tocotrienols: Vitamin E beyond tocopherols. *Life Sci.* 78 (18), 2088-2098, (2006).

Seren S, Lieberman R, Bayraktar UD, Heath E, Sahin K, Andic F, Kucuk O. Lycopene in cancer prevention and treatment. Review. *Am. J Ther.* 15, 66-81, (2008).

Sharlip ID, Jarow JP, Belker AM, Lipshultz LI, Sigman M, Thomas AJ, Schlegel PN, Howards SS, Overstreet JW, Sadovsky R. Best practice policies for male infertility. *Fertil Steril* 77, 873-882, (2002).

Sharma RK, Said T, Agarwal A. Sperm DNA damage and its clinical relevance in assessing reproductive outcome. *Asian J Androl.* 6, 139-148, (2004).

Shenkin A. The key role of micronutrients. *Clin. Nutr.* 25 (1), 1-13, (2006).

Shetty K. Biotechnology to harness the benefits of dietary phenolics; Focus on Lamiaceae. *Asia Pac. J Clin. Nutr.* 6, 162-171, (1997).

Shigeoka S, Ishikawa T, Tamoi M, Miyagawa Y, Takeda T, Yabuta Y, Yoshimura K. Regulation and function of ascorbate peroxidase isoenzymes. *J Exp. Bot.* 53 (372), 1305-1319, (2002).

Sies H. Oxidative stress introduction. In Oxidative Stress: Oxidants and Antioxidants. Sies H (eds) Academic Press, London, pp xv-xxii, (1991)

Sies H. Oxidative stress oxidants and antioxidants. *Exp. Physiol.* 82 (2), 291, (1997).

Sies H. Oxidative stress; introductory remarks. In Oxidative Stress. Sies H (eds). Academic Press, London, pp, 1-8, (1982).

Sies H. Strategies of antioxidant defense. *Eur. J Bio,* 215, 213-219, (1993).

Singh RP, Sharad S, Kapoor S. Free radicals and oxidative stress in neurodegenerative diseases: Relevance of Dietary Antioxidants. *J Ind. Acd. Clin. Med.*5, 218-225, (2004).

Smith TJ, Hong J Y, Wong Z Y and Yang CS. How can carcinogenesis be inhibited. *Ann. N.Y. Acad. Sci.* 768, 82-90, (1995).

Sorbera LA, Leeson PA, Castaner J, del Frenso, M. NXY-059 Treatment of ischaemic stroke, Free radical scavenger. *Drugs Future.* 27, 240-247, (2002).

Stadtman E. Protein oxidation and aging. *Science* 257 (5074), 1220-1224, (1992).

Stahl W, Sies H. Bioactivity and protective effects of natural carotenoid. *Biochemica. Biophysica. Acta.* 1740, 101-107, (2005).

Stanner SA, Hughes J, Kelly CN, Buttriss J. A review of the epidemiological evidence for the antioxidant hypothesis. *Public Health Nutr.* 7 (3), 407-422, (2004).

Steare SE, Yellon DM. The potential for endogenous myocardial antioxidants to protect the myocardium against ischaemia-reperfusion injury: refreshing the parts exogenous antioxidants cannot reach? *J Mol. Cell. Cardiol.*27 (1), 65-74, (1995).

Steenken S, Jovanovic S. How easily oxidizable is DNA? One electron reduction potential of adenosine and guanosine radicalsin aqueous solution. *J. Am. Chem. Soc.* 119, 617-618, (1997).

Steinberg D, Parthasarathy S, Carew TE, Khoo JC, Witztum JL. Beyond cholesterol: modification of low-density lipoprotein that increases its atherogenesity. *N. Engl. J. Med.* 320, 915-924, (1989).

Steiner M. A double blind crossover study in moderately hypercholesterolemic men that compares the effect of aged garlic extract and placebo administration on blood lipids and platelet function. *J. Clin. Nutr.* 64, 866-870, (1996).

Stipanuk MH. Biochemical and physiological aspects of human nutrition. Philadelphia: WB Saunders Company, (2000).

Stohs S, Bagchi D. "Oxidative mechanisms in the toxicity of metal ions". *Free Radic. Biol. Med.* 18 (2), 321-36, (1995).

Strowing SM, Raskin P. Glycemic control and the complications of diabetes: after the diabetes control and complication trial. *Diabetes Rev.* 3, 237-257, (1995).

Sun JG, Jurisicova A, Casper RF. Detection of deoxyribonucleic acid fragmentation in human sperm: correlation with fertilization in vitro. *Biol. Reprod.*56, 602-607, (1997).

Szatrowski TP, Nathan CF. Production of large amounts of hydrogen peroxide by human tumor cells. *Cancer Res.*51, 794-798, (1991).

Tadi PP, Teel RW, Lau BHS. Organosulfur compounds of garlic modulate mutagenesis, metabolism and DNA binding of aflatoxin B1. Nutr. Cancer15, 87-95, (1991).

Tiwari AK, Rao JM, Diabetes mellitus and multiple therapeutic approaches of phytochemicals: present status and future prospects. *Curr. Sci.*83, 30-38, (2002).

Tiwari AK. Imbalance in antioxidant defence and human disease: multiple approach of natural antioxidants therapy. *Curr. Sci.* 81, 1179-1187, (2001).

Tiwari AK, Natural product antioxidants and their therapeutic potential in mitigating per oxidative modification of lipoproteins and atherosclerosis: recent developments. *J. Med. Aromat. Plant Sci.* 21, 730-741, (1999).

Tiwari AK. Pathogenesis of atherosclerosis: peroxidation of lipoprotein lipids and use of antioxidants; current developments. *Ann. Natl. Acad. Med. Sci. (India)*, 32, 87-95, (1996).

Tiwari AK. Antioxidant: New–generation therapeutic base for treatment of polygenic disorder. *Cur. Sci.* 86(8), 1092-1102, (2004).

Toyokuni S, Okamoto K, Yodoi J, Hiai H. Persistent oxidative stress in cancer. *Febs Lett.* 1995, 358, 1-3, (1995).

Traber MG, Atkinson J. Vitamin E, antioxidant and nothing more. *Free Radic. Biol. Med.* 43 (1), 4-15, (2007).

Ukil A, Maity S, Karmakar S, Datta N, Vedasiromoni JR, Das PK. Curcumin, the major component of food flavor turmeric, reduces mucosal injury in trinitrobenzene sulphonic acid-induced colitis. *Br. J. Pharmacol.* 139, 209-218, (2003).

Urquiaga I, Leighton F. Plant Polyphenol Antioxidants and Oxidative Stress. *Biol. Res.* 33, 55-64, (2000).

Valko M, Izakovic M, Mazur M, Rhodes CJ, Telser J. Role of oxygen radicals in DNA damage and cancer incidence. *Mol. Cell Biochem.* 266, 37-56, (2004).

Valko M, Morris H, Cronin MTD. Metals, toxicity and oxidative stress. *Curr. Med. Chem.*12, 1161-1208, (2005).

Valko M, Leibfritz D, Moncol J, Cronin M, Mazur M, Telser J. Free radicals and antioxidants in normal physiological functions and human disease. *Int. J Biochem. Cell Biol.* 39 (1), 44-84, (2007).

Valko M, Rhodes CJ, Moncol J, Izakovic M, Mazur M. Free radicals, metals and antioxidants in oxidative stress-induced cancer. Mini-review. *Chem Biol Interact.*160, 1-40, (2006).

Van Acker, SABE, Van Den Berg DJ, Tromp MNJL, Griffioen DH, Van Bennekom WP, Van Der Vijgh WJF, Bast A. Structural aspects of antioxidant activity of flavonoids. *Free Rad. Biol. Med.* 20, 331-342, (1996).

Van Gaal L, Mertens I, De Block C. Mechanisms linking obesity with cardiovascular disease. *Nature* 444 (7121): 875-880, (2006).

Vertuani S, Angusti A, Manfredini S. The antioxidants and pro-antioxidants network: an overview. *Curr. Pharm. Des,* 10 (14), 1677-94, (2004).

Vinson JA, Dabbagh YA, Serry MM, Jang J. Plant flavonoids, especially tea flavonols, are powerful antioxidants using an in vitro oxidation model for heart disease. *J. Agric. Food Chem.* 43, 2800-2802, (1995).

Vinson JA, Jang J, Yang J, Dabbagh Y, Liang X, Serry M, Proch J, Cai S. Vitamins and especially flavonoids in common beverages are powerful in vitro antioxidants which enrich low-density lipoproteins and increase their oxidative resistance after ex vivo spiking in human plasma. *J. Agric. Food Chem.* 47, 2502-2504, (1999).

Von Lintig J, Vogt K. Vitamin A formation in animals: molecular identification and functional characterization of carotene cleaving enzymes. *J Nutr.* 134, 251S-256S, (2004).

Walston J, Xue Q, Semba RD, Ferrucci L, Cappola AR, Ricks M, Guralnik J, Fried LP. Serum antioxidants, inflammation, and total mortality in older women. *Am. J Epidemiol.*163, 18-26, (2006).

Wang BH, Zuel KA, Rahaman K, Billington D. Protective effects of aged garlic extract against bromo benzene toxicity to precision cut rat liver slices. *Toxicology* 126, 213-222, (1998).

WangJ, Wen L, Huang Y, Chen Y, Ku M. Dual effects of antioxidants in neurodegeneration: direct neuroprotection against oxidative stress and indirect protection via suppression of glia-mediated inflammation. *Curr. Pharm. Des.* 12 (27), 3521-3533, (2006).

Wang X, Quinn P. Vitamin E and its function in membranes. *Prog. Lipid Res.* 38 (4), 309-36, (1999).

Wasserman MA, Sundell CL, Kunsch C, Edwards D. Chemistry and biology of vascular protactants: a novel approach to the treatment of atherosclerosis and coronary artery disease. *Am. J. Cardiol. (Suppl.).* 91, 34A-40A, (2003).

Wattenberg LW. What are the clinical attributes for cancer chemotherapy? *Ann. N.Y. Acad. Sci.* 768, 73-81, (1995).

Wei Z, Lau BHS. Garlic inhibits free radical generation and augments antioxidant enzyme activity in vascular endothelial cells. *Nutr. Res.* 18, 61-70, (1998).

Weisburger JH. Tea and Health: The underlying Mechanisms. *Proc. Soc. Exp. Biol Med.* 220,203-209, (1999).

Weisfeldt ML, Zweier J, Ambrosio G, Becker LC, Flaherty JT. Evidence that free radicals result in reperfusion injury in heart muscle. *Basic Life Sci.* 49, 911-999, (1988).

Wells W, Xu D, Yang Y, Rocque P. Mammalian thioltransferase (glutaredoxin) and protein disulfide isomerase have dehydroascorbate reductase activity. *J Biol. Chem.* 265 (26), 15361-15364, (1990).

Willcox JK, Ash SL, Catignani GL. Antioxidants and prevention of chronic disease. Review. *Crit. Rev. Food. Sci. Nutr.* 44, 275-295, (2004).

Willson KC, Clifford MN. Tea: Cultivation to Consumption. Chapman and Hall, London, (1992).

Wintergerst E, Maggini S, Hornig D. Immune-enhancing role of vitamin C and zinc and effect on clinical conditions. *Ann. Nutr. Metab.* 50 (2), 85–94, (2006).

Witztum JL. The role of oxidized low-density lipoproteins in atherogenesis.*Br. Heart J.* 69, 12-14, (1993).

Wolf G. The discovery of the antioxidant function of vitamin E: the contribution of Henry A. Mattill. *J Nutr.* 135 (3), 363-366, (2005).

Wood-Kaczmar A, Gandhi S, Wood N. Understanding the molecular causes of Parkinson's disease. *Trends Mol. Med.* 12 (11), 521-528, (2006).

Woodside J, McCall D, McGartland C, Young I (2005). "Micronutrients: dietary intake v. supplement use". *Proc. Nutr. Soc.* 64 (4), 543-53, (2005).

Wright JS. Searching for fountain of youth. *Chem. Br.* 39, 25-27, (2003).

Xianquan S, Shi J, Kakuda Y, Yueming J. Stability of lycopene during food processing and storage. *J Med. Food* 8 (4), 413-422, (2005).

Yamasaki T, Teel RW, Lau BHS. Effect of allixin, a phytoalexin produced by garlic, on mutagenesis, DNA-binding and metabolism of aflatoxin B1. *Cancer Lett.* 59, 89-94, (1991).

Yang GC, Yasaei MP, Page SW. Garlic as anti-oxidant and free radical scavenger. *J. Food Drug Anal.*1, 357-364, (1993).

Young AJ, Lowe GM. Antioxidant and prooxidant properties of carotenoids. *Arch Biochem Biophys.* 385, 20-27, (2001).

Young I, Woodside J. Antioxidants in health and disease. *J Clin Pathol.*54, 176-186, (2001).

Zingg JM, Azzi A. "Non-antioxidant activities of vitamin E". *Curr.Med. Chem.* 11 (9): 1113–1133, (2004).

chapter 11

Plant Drugs are a Good Tool to Fight against Cancer and AIDS

Joseph Adetunji Aladesanmi

INTRODUCTION

The necessity to feed, protect and conserve health, resulting from the fear of illness and death, led men of all times, under all the skies, to resort to anything that nature can offer them. It could be rightly said that natural products with medicinal properties, formed the beginning of science and the art of healing. Egyptians and Jews of old used a lot of organic and inorganic materials in soft mushy forms as poultice and their extracts as preservatives e.g. embalming the bodies of their dead (Wambebe, 1995).

Natural products from plants in human history have been used as medicines, fragrances, food additives and pesticides. Through the use of plants, human beings have taken advantages of the defensive, attractive and medicinal compounds present in leaves, flowers, roots, sap and bark of species around the World. The first record of the use of plant in human medicine was in an Egyptian papyrus of about 1500 B.C. It recorded extracts from ancient Egypt, Assyria, China and India for medicinal purposes (Evans, 1989).

ANTIMITOTIC, ANTITUMOR, ANTICANCER

Cancer is a general term applied to a series of malignant diseases which may affect many different parts of the body. These diseases are characterized by a rapid and uncontrolled formation of abnormal cells which may mass together to form a growth or tumors, or proliferate throughout the body, initiating abnormal growth at other sites. If the process is not arrested, it may progress until it causes the death of the organism, hence the search for plant drugs amongst others, which should kill or incapacitate cancer cells without causing excessive damage to normal host cells. In 2000, there were an estimated 170,000 new cases of prostate cancer and 31,000 deaths in the United States. Cancer is therefore the second cause of death worldwide.

Research focused on discovery of plant anticancer constituents become increasingly productive, and agents discovered include the amoorastatins, aphanastatin, bauhinia-statins, combretastatin (of which CA-4 and CA-1 are in clinical trials), the lychno-statins, the meliastatins, multigilin, multistatin, narcistatin, the nootkastatins, palstatin, pancratistatin (in advanced preclinical development), pedilstatin, the phyllantostatins (1 and 2 completed phase I clinical trials), radiatin, rolliniastatins, the sansevistatins, and the schleicherastatins. Pettit et al., 1998, 2000 isolated the first cancer cell growth inhibitor, (–)-combretastatin from African tree Combretum caffrum, a representative of the tropical and subtropical trees of the family Combretaceae (about 600 species in

20 genera) with a reserve of constituents with potentially useful biological properties, as up to 25 species are used in the traditional medicine of Africa and India. This research subsequently led to discovery of 20 cancer cell growth inhibitory stilbenes, bibenzyls, dihydrophenanthrenes, and phenanthrenes which had resulted in the development of the first well established antiangiogenic/vascular-disrupting anticancer drug, sodium combretastatin A-4 phosphate (CA4P), which is in broad human cancer clinical trials.

The combretastatins, despite their relative simple chemical structures are characterized by remarkable biological activity as inhibitors of tubulin polymerization, while some exhibit potent in vitro inhibition against human cancer lines, in vivo efficacy as vascular disrupting agents, and act as antiangiogenesis agents. Tumors receive their nutrients through existing vasculature using newly formed neovascularization (angiogenesis), and the combretastatin A-4 (CA4) and A-1 (CA1) phosphate prodrugs (CA4P and CA1P) selectively damage tumor neovasculature with induction of extensive blood flow shutdown in the metastatic tumor compared to normal tissues, thereby causing hypoxia and necrosis of the tumor. This led to four Phase I human cancer clinical trials of CA4P while later clinical trials have incorporated combination with other anticancer drugs such as paclitaxel (Taxol), Carboplatin, Avastin (antiangiogenic monoclonal), and/or fractionated external beam radiotherapy. In July of 2003, the US FDA awarded orphan drug status to CA4P for treatment of advanced anaplastic thyroid cancer and in May of 2006 orphan drug status to CA4P for treatment of ovarian cancer in combination with Carboplatin.

Highlights of parallel studies of microorganism anticancer constituents include the isolation and structural elucidations of carminomycin (in clinical use), kitastatin 1, the labradorins, montanastatin and the streptomyces antitumor antibiotic 593A (clinical trials by the NCI), as well as convenient syntheses of the Streptomyces anticancer drugs, DON and azotomycin.

Doskotch et al., 1983 and El Naggar et al., 1980 had also worked independently, particularly on the constituents of local North American flora, with cytotoxic (antitumor) activity and insect stimulants (for the elm bark beetle) and insect antifeedants (for gypsy moth larvae). Of importance are the work of Sun et al., 1998 and Xue et al., 2001 on anticancer and chemopreventive agents from plants.

The efforts in discovering antitumor agents are based on bioactivity-directed fractionation and isolation from medicinal plants, especially those used in traditional Chinese medicine, followed by rational drug design-based methods to produce the most promising lead for development. Isolated therapeutic agents from plants can also serve as leads in the development of better and more effective drugs. From podophyllotoxin, a lignan isolated from Podophyllum peltatum (American mandrake, which was previously used as cathartics in folklore medicine) was developed etopside and teniposide as potent drugs used in the treatment of small-cell lung cancer, testicular cancer, lymphomas and leukeamia (Stahelin et al., 1991). Podophyllotoxin and derivatives are from Podophyllum plants, including the American P. peltatum L. and Tibetan P. emodi, were long prized as medicines by the native populations of North America and the Himalayas. The complex path from the plan (Podophyllum) to bioactive lead compound (podophyllotoxin) to clinically used drugs (etoposide and teniposide) and forward to new generation anticancer candidates illustrates the successful development of clinically useful drugs from natural (plant) sources.

In 1942, studies found that podophyllin, the alcoholic extract of Podophyllum rhizome, exhibited curative effects on the benign tumor Condylomata accuminata (Kaplan, 1942). Further research showed that its major constituent, podophyllotoxin, inhibits assembly of the mitotic spindle (Sullivan et al., 1947) and was effective against tumors in mice (Hartwell et al., 1947). Mechanistically, podophyllotoxin binds reversibly to cellular tubulin, inhibits mitotic spindle formation, disturbs the dynamic equilibrium between microtubule assembly/disassembly, and eventually causes mitotic arrest.

Studies on Podophyllum glycosides in the 1950s led to the opportune discovery of etoposide and teniposide in the late 1960s. These two compounds displayed significant antineoplastic effects (Stahelin et al., 1991). In 1983, the FDA approved etoposide for the treatment of testicular cancer and in 1992 teniposide was brought into the US market. These drugs are currently used against many cancers, including small cell tung cancer, testicular cancer, lymphoma, leukemia, and Kaposi's sarcoma (Zhang & Lee, 1994). Therefore, the synthetic etoposide analog, GL-331, derived from podophyllotoxin (Lee et al., 2005), was designed successfully to combat solubility, drug resistance, and other detrimental issues of the anticancer drug etoposide, which has been developed to Phase II clinical trials. In addition JC-9, discovered based on the curcumin model, has been licensed and developed by Androscience (San Diego, CA) also against prostate cancer (Lin et al., 2006).

The work of Potier et al., 1989 has produced two major anticancer drugs, Navelbine (vinorelbine), an analog of vinblastine isolated from the Madagascan periwinkle and Taxotere (docetaxel), an analog of Taxol (paclitaxel) extracted from the bark of the yew tree (Guenard et al., 1993). Pierre Fabre Laboratories and Sanofi-Aventis manufacture these two drugs, respectively. The diterpenoid taxol has become one of the most promising lead compounds to emerge from the anti-tumour screening of natural products in recent years. Isolated from the stem bark of the Pacific yew Taxus brevifolia Nutt. (Taxaceae) and Taxus baccata L. Taxol possesses an original, highly functionalized diterpene steleton. The mode of action of taxol is also unique. In contrast to other antimitotic drugs, it enhances both the rate and yield of microtubule assembly.

The major obstacle in the development of taxol to the clinical stage has been its very limited supply from natural sources. The compound occurs only in the stem bark at low concentrations. In order to supply 2.5 kg of taxol for clinical trial, the National Cancer Institute contracted for 27 tons of T. brevifolia bark, requiring the sacrifice of some 12,000 trees. With the current demand for taxol, it has been estimated that yew population worldwide would soon become extinct if no alternative source of taxol could be developed. A diterpenoid alkaloid, Paclitaxel (Taxol Reg.), a natural product with major anticancer activity against breast and lung cancers was developed (Furia, 1997).

However, an economically or technically realistic approach to the supply problem has been devised by French researchers with the partial synthesis of taxol from a congener found in the leaves in appreciable amounts. The side-chain analog RP 56976 has reportedly greater chemotherapeutic potential than taxol itself and it has been developed and registered as Paclitel. A side chain analog of taxol (Taxus baccata), known as taxotere, has also been developed by semi-synthesis from 10-deacetylbaccatin III. It has improved water solubility and better activity than taxol in some assays, and is also currently available for drug use against resistant breast cancer. Similarly, elucidation of the structure of Ellipticine, an alkaloid extracted from Ochrosia sp., led to the synthesis of Celiptium, used for a few years in the treatment of breast cancer. Acronycine, another alkaloid found in an Australian Acronychia led Francois Tillequin to develop very active synthetic analogs, (Tillequin, 2007). Shohat et al., 1967 isolated the anticancer withanolides from Withania somnifera, which was, among other uses, used as an antidepressant.

Throughout the 1990s the NCI Laboratory of Drug Discovery Research and Development natural products efforts focused primarily on extracts with selective cytotoxicity profiles in the 60-cell anticancer screen or extracts with HIV inhibiting properties in the anti-HIV screen. The significant anticancer schweinfurthins (Beutler et al., 1998) are notable terrestrial plant anticancer agents.

Another notable natural products work are those of Crews et al., 2004, and Ireland et al., 2003 which include four marketed agents, one of them is topotecan, a camptothecin analog with superior properties to the parent compound that was dropped from clinical trial due to unacceptable toxicity, and is marketed by SmithKline Beecham (now GlaxoSmithKline). Twenty-one more agents have entered clinical trials including four derived from natural products.

Anticancer natural product (plant) drugs introduced into major markets (US, Europe, Japan) in the last 25 years are Epirubicin (1984), Leuprolide (1984), Vinorelbine (1989), Idarubicin (1990), Paclitaxel (1993), Irinotecan (1994) (Cragg et al., 2009).

Dictyostatin-1 was originally reported by Pettit et al., 1994 as a potent cytotoxic agent. Further studies showed that it is a potent microtubule-stabilizing agent with very significant activity against paclitaxel and multi-drug resistant cancer cell lines.

Neopeltolide also demonstrated potent cytotoxicity, and cell cycle analysis of tumor cells showed arrest at the G1/S transition. The discoveries of camptothecin in 1966 (Wall et al., 1966) and taxol in 1971 (Wani et al., 1971) have had a huge impact on cancer chemotherapy, and as just one indicator, in 2002, the global market place for antineoplastic agents was estimated at $9 billion annually with the combined sales of taxol and the camptothecin analogs totalling at least a third of that market (Oberlies et al., 2004). Camptothecin and derivatives from Camptotheca acuminata showed broad-spectrum activity with some limitations. The natural 10-hydroxycamptothecin is more active than camptothecin, and is used in China against cancers of the neck and head. The synthetic analogs 9-aminocamptothecin and particularly the water-soluble derivatives topotecan and irinotecan showed good responses in a number of cancers, topotecan and irinotecan are available for the treatment of ovarian cancer and colorectal cancer respectively. Thanks to the relentless efforts of Drs. Cordell, Farnsworth, Kinghorn, Pezzuto, and Soejarto among others (Kinghorn et al., 1999, 2003).

By 1970 the cephalotaxine esters harringtonine, isoharringtonine and homoharringtonine were identified by Powell et al., 1970, 1972 as the anticancer principles of Cephalotaxus harringtonia, a small tree native to Japan and China. Homoharringtonine has shown encoura-ging activity in preclinical and Phase I-II trials in patients with hematologic and some solid tumors. Early studies in China reported high response rates in patients with leukemia (Kantarjian et al., 2001), and studies in the United States and England have shown promising results in patients with chronic myeloid leukemia (O'Brien et al., 1995; Marin et al., 2005). This has been granted orphan drug status by the US FDA, which is being promoted by ChemGenex Pharmaceuticals under the trademark Ceflatonin. These actions have encoura-ged expanded clinical trials and evaluation of the potential of this drug for treatment of various malignant diseases.

Maytansinoids/Ansamitocins have been implicated in anticancer therapy. Maytansine, the parent compound of this group of potent antitumor agents was discovered in 1972 by Kupchan et al., 1972 by bioassay-guided fractionation of the extracts of the Ethiopian shrub Maytenus serrata. Since this report, about 50 additional members of this group of compounds have been isolated by several investigators from the same and closely related plants and from members of two unrelated plant families (Cassady et al., 2004). The mode of action of the maytansinoids has been traced to inhibition of tubulin–polymerization by binding to the β-subunit at a site overlapping the vincristine binding site, and different from the colchicines binding site (Yu et al., 2005).

After biological testing showed that the extract obtained from the Western (or Pacific) yew, Taxus brevifolia had activity against the 9KB cell line, led to the isolation of taxol (Wani et al., 1971) with in vivo activity against P388 lymphocytic leukemia, which was found to act by promoting the assembly of tubulin into microtubules (Schiff et al., 1979). Taxol entered Phase I clinical trials in 1983 while the first positive Phase II clinical results showed activity against ovarian cancer (McGuire et al., 1989) and the result turned taxol from an obscure lead compound into an instant celebrity, and also found against breast cancer in 1991 (Holmes et al., 1991). Taxol is presently marketed as paclitaxel and together with its relative docetaxel, the worldwide sales totaled approximately US $4 billion in 2005.

The research efforts on the Southeast Asian Catharanthus roseus led to the isolation of vincristine and vinblastine with activity against the P-1534 leukemia (Svoboda et al., 1959, 1961).They have been developed as commercial drugs. Vincristine was approved by FDA and marketed in 1963. A major importance of the discovery of vincristine was its novel mechanism of action (at the time); blocking mitosis with metaphase arrest and specifically binding with tubulin and preventing its polymerization. Because of this, vincristine became an important component of combination chemotherapy. The major use of vinblastine is the treatment of patients with Hodgkin's disease, non-Hodgkin's lymphomas, and renal, testicular, head and neck cancer.

Two additional semi-synthetic alkaloids related to vincristine and vinblastine, vinorelbine and vindesine were marketed (Johnson et al., 1996; Gueritte and Fahy, 2005).

The types of anticancer agents isolated from plants was also presented by the review of Hartwell in 1976 in which the active compounds isolated from twenty-five plants were tannins, sterols (including simple glycosides but not saponins), quinines, terpenes, lignans, flavonoids, quassinoids, steroid lactones and alkaloids. The most interesting were the diterpenes, lignans, quassinoids, and alkaloids. The tumor systems used included the regular screen at different times and also the slow-growing tumors, B16 melanoma and Lewis lung carcinoma. The interesting goal here was the structure-antitumor activity relationships, which had brought out the desirability for further investigation of certain types of compounds as possibilities for clinical studies.

Indicine-N-oxide from Heliotropium indicum was found to possess significant antitumor activity in acute leukemia while monocrotaline has been used against skin cancer in China.

A large number of natural and semi-synthetic derivatives of colchicines have been tested and several in clinical trials, e.g. demecolcine are being used in cancer treatment in some countries. Acronycine isolated from Achronychia baueri exhibited a very broad antitumor spectrum.

Pyridocarbazole alkaloids ellipticine and 9-methoxyellipticine from Ochrosia elliptica (Apocynaceae) and their derivatives, e.g. elliptinium acetate has produced a highly active material of value in some forms of breast cancer, and perhaps also in renal cell cancer. Nitidine, a benzophenanthridine alkaloid isolated from Zanthoxylum nitidum has been selected for development based on its exceptional antileukemic activity but was dropped owing to erratic toxicity while fagaronine, a closely related alkaloid, isolated from Z. xanthoxyloides, has been found to have greater antitumor activity than any of the natural benzophenanthridine structures, coupled with excellent stability, and has entered clinical trials in Japan.

The quassinoids or simaroubolides are a group of terpenoid-related compounds isolated from a variety of plants in the Simaroubaceae, e.g. bruceantin from Brucea antidysenterica showed high antileukemic activity at low dosages and over a wide dose range. It acts through inhibition of protein synthesis and has undergone clinical trials in man.

The diterpenes triptolide and tripdiolide isolated from Tripterygium wilfordi are potent antileukemic agents that contain a reactive triepoxide system.

The Central American tree Phyllanthus acuminatus contains in its roots a complex mixture of glycosides, two of which, phyllanthostatin 1 and phyllanthoside have demonstrated marked antitumor properties. Phyllanthoside is in early clinical trials.

FUTURE DEVELOPMENTS

The search for new and potent antitumor compounds in nature is by no means confined to plants, but also to microorganisms, marine habitats. Microorganisms, widely employed as sources of antibiotics, produced a considerable number of metabolites having antitumor activity.

The identification of epothilones from the bacterium Sorangium cellulosum has thus generated considerable interest since these agents mimic the effects of taxol, and some analogs are much more potent than taxol, especially towards multidrug-resistant cell lines.

A natural product of high interest is 4-ipomeanol, a toxin isolated from mould-infected sweet potatoes (Ipomoea batatus) is undergoing clinical trials against lung cancers.

Natural product extracts for testing programs are to be selected from plants, microorganisms and marine animals with emphasis on plants used locally as medicinals and on species and groups which have not been extensively studied in the past (Treese and Evans, 2006).

Turmeric, derived from the plant Curcuma longa, is a gold-colored spice commonly used in the Indian subcontinent, not only for health care but also for the preservation of food and as yellow dye for textiles. Curcumin, a diferuloylmethane was determined in 1910. Extensive research within the last half century has proven that most of the activities, once associated with turmeric, are due to curcumin. Curcumin has been shown to exhibit antioxidant, anti-inflammatory, antiviral, antibacterial, antifungal, and anticancer activities. Curcumin can thus be considered an ideal "spice of life" (Aggarwal et al., 2007). It has been extensively investigated for its cancer chemopreventive potential.

Plant species such as Panax ginseng and Allium sativum, antitumor activity has been evaluated in experimental studies using cultured cells and animal models, but the therapeutic potentials in patients remain to be determined. Antitumor activity derived from medicinal plants may produce results via a number of mechanisms, including effects on cytoskeletal proteins, which play a key role in mitosis (e.g., paclitaxel), inhibition of activity of topoisomerase enzymes I (camptothecin) or II (etoposide), stimulation of the immune system (Viscum album) (Mantle et al., 2000).

Medicinal plant derived antineoplastic agents may be used in single agent or in combinational therapies, and have been used in first-line or second-line (including anthracycline-refractory patients) treatment of localized or metastatic breast cancer. Adverse effects resulting from the use of these agents include neutropenia and peripheral neuropathies.

Plants are of relevance to dermatology for both their adverse and beneficial effects on skin and skin disorders respectively. Beneficial aspects of medicinal plants on skin include: healing of wounds and burns (especially Aloe vera); antifungal, antiviral, antibacterial and acaricidal activity against skin infections such as acne, herpes and scabies (especially tea tree, Melaleuca alternifolia oil); activity against inflammatory and immune disorders affecting skin (e.g., psoriasis); antitumor promoting activity against skin cancer (identified using chemically-induced two-stage carcinogenesis in mine, while some adverse effects include irritant contact dermatitis, phytophotodermatitis, etc. (Mantle et al., 2001).

Soybeans are unique among the legumes because they are a concentrated source of isoflavones. Soyfoods and isoflavones have received considerable attention for their potential role in preventing and treating cancer and osteoporosis. The low breast cancer mortality rates in Asian countries and the putative antiestrogenic effects of isoflavones have fueled speculation that soyfood intake reduces breast cancer risk (Messina, 1999).

In brief, ascorbic acid, soybean lecithin, capsaicin, biochanin A, Ganoderma lucidum, caffeine, and a novel synthetic 2-(allylthio)pyrazine decrease the incidence of mouse lung tumors, whereas fresh ginseng (4 years old), carrot, spinach, Sesamum indicum, beta-carotene, and 13-cis-retanoic acid do not. Subsequently, (-)-epigallocatechin gallate, crytoporic acid E, and sarcophytol A from natural products, and synthetic acyclic retinoid and canventol were shown to be anticarcinogenic or chemopreventive in human subjects (Yun, 1999).

Extracts produced from Viscum album L. (mistletoe) as well as certain isolated components are able to stimulate different functions of the immune system. The natural killer cells have been suggested as one of the candidates for direct tumor cell destruction. It is interesting that mistletoe extracts are able to stimulate natural killer cell-mediated cytotoxicity in vitro directly as well as indirectly in a cytokine-like manner, with the active components being carbohydrates rather than lectins (Schink, 1997).

Dietary factors are regarded as exerting major influences on cancer development in various organ sites and in Asia there is particular interest in the potential preventive effects of foodstuffs such as soy products and ginseng. The so-called phytoestrogens, like genistein and daidzein in soy, can bind to estrogen receptors and therefore interfere with the action of estrogen itself, a well-established risk factor for breast, ovarian and endometrial cancers (Kim, 2008).

Ukrain is an anticancer drug base on the plant Chelidonium majus L. Numerous preclinical and clinical investigations seem to suggest that ukrain is pharmacologically active, having curative effects on a range of cancer (Ernest and Schmidt, 2005).

Epidemiologic case-control studies in China and Italy on gastric carcinoma in relation do diet suggest that consuming garlic may reduce the risk of gastric cancer. Chemical constituents of garlic have been tested for their inhibiting effect on carcinogenesis, using in vitro and in vivo models. In most experiments inhibiting tumor growth was accomplished using fresh garlic extract, garlic compounds or synthetically prepared analogs. The available evidence however, warrants further research into the possible role of garlic in the prevention of cancer in humans (Dorant et al., 1993).

Botanicals have been used for the treatment of various human diseases throughout history. They also play a role in disease prevention. For example, epidemiologic studies have suggested that a reduce risk of cancer is associated with high consumption of vegetables and fruits. Thus, the cancer chemopreventive potential of naturally occurring phytochemicals is a great interest. Some examples are cruciferous vegetables such as cabbage and broccoli, Allium vegetables such as garlic and onion, green tea, citrus fruits, tomatoes, berries, ginger and ginseng, as well as some medicinal plants (Peterson et al., 1995) Several lead compounds, such as brassinin from Chinese cabbage, sulforaphane (from broccoli) and its analog sulforamate, withanolides (from tomatillos), and resveratrol (from grapes and peanuts among other foods), had been subjected to preclinical or clinical trials for cancer chemoprevention. Phytochemicals of these types therefore have great potential in the fight against human cancer (Park and Pezzuto, 2002).

The number of novel natural products isolated from microbial origins is continuing to increase and is doubling every 10 years. The used Hsp90 inhibitors, geldanamycin, herbimycin A and radicicol were isolated from Streptomyces and fungi originally for their antiprotozoal, herbicidal and antifungal activities respectively. In the mid 1980s it was found that the benzoquinone ansamycin antibiotics (herbimycin A, geldanamycin, and macbecin) reversed v-Src transformed cells to normal phenotypes and Bcr-abl was subsequently suggested to be the molecular target for the treatment of chronic myelogenous leukemia through a study using herbimycin A for its selective antioncogenic activity. In 1994, these ansamycins were found to bind to Hsp90 and to cause the degradation of client proteins including Src kinases; further efforts to develop anticancer drugs were made using geldanamycin analogs and 17AAG was chosen as the best candidate for clinical trials (Uehara, 2003).

As cancer is the second leading cause of death worldwide, natural products have played a significant role in drug discovery and development especially for agents against cancer and infectious disease. An analysis of new and approved drugs for cancer by the US FDA over the period 1981-2002 showed that 62% of these cancer drugs were of natural origin. A number of native Andean and Amazonian medicine of plant origin for example are used as traditional medicine in Peru to treat different diseases. Of particular interest are three plant materials endemic to Peru with the common names of cat's claw (Uncaria tomentosa), Maca (Lepidium meyenii), and dragon's blood (Croton lechleri) each having been scientifically investigated for a wide range of therapeutic uses including as specific anticancer agents through an evidence-based analysis of the chemistry, biological properties, and antitumor activities (Gonzales and Valerio, 2006).

Cancer chemoprevention has traditionally been defined as a dietary or therapeutic approach for the prevention, delay, or reversal of carcinogenesis. Using biologic response as a guide for fractionation, over 200 active compounds have been identified. Some of the most interesting include brassinin and 4'-bromoflavone as inducers of quinine reductase, deguelin as an inhibitor of ornithine decarboxylase, resveratrol as an inhibitor of cyclooxygenase, and brusatol as an inducer of cellular differentiation. These agents have demonstrated effectiveness in experimental models of carcinogenesis. Chemoprevention therefore offers great hope in reducing the morbidity and mortality associated with cancer (Mehta and Pezzuto, 2002).

Historically, herbs and spices have enjoyed a rich tradition of use for their flavor enhancement characteristics and for their medicinal properties. The rising prevalence of chronic diseases worldwide and the corresponding rise in health care costs is propelling interest among researchers and the public for multiple health benefits related to herbs and spices, including a reduction in cancer risk and modification of tumor behavior. A growing body of epidemiological and preclinical evidence points to culinary herbs and spices as minor dietary constituents with multiple anticancer characteristics such as their ability to influence carcinogen bioactivation and antioxidant activity (Kaefer and Milner, 2008).

Capsaicin (trans-8-methyl-N-vanillyl-6-nonenamide), a pungent ingredient of hot chili pepper, protects against experimentally induced mutagenesis and tumorigenesis. It also induces apoptosis in various immortalized or malignant cell lines. Zingiber officinale Roscoe, contains such pungent ingredients as [6]-gingerol and [6]-paradol, which also have antitumor promotional and antiproliferative effects. Curcumin, a yellow ingredient from turmeric (Curcuma longa L., Zingiberaceae), has been extensively investigated for its cancer chemopreventive potential.

Yakuchinone A [1-(4′-hydroxy-3′-methoxyphenyl)-7-phenyl-3-heptanone] and yakuchinone B [1-(4′-hydroxy-3′-methoxyphenyl)-7-phenyl-3-hept-1-en-3-one] present in Alpinia oxyphylla Miquel (Zingiberaceae) have inhibitory effects on phorbol ester-induced inflammation and skin carcinogenesis in mice, and oxidative stress in vitro. These diarylheptanoids suppress phorbol ester-induced activation of ornithine decarboxylase and production of tumor necrosis factor-alpha or interleukin-1 alpha and their mRNA expression. They also nullified the phorbol ester-stimulated induction of activator protein 1(AP-1) in culture human promyelocytic leukemia (HL-60) cells. In addition, both yakuchinone A and B induced apoptotic death in HL-60 cells.

Resveratrol (3, 5, 4′-trihydroxy-trans-stilbene) a phytoalexin found in grapes and other dietary and medicinal plants, and (–)-epigallocatechin gallate, a major antioxidative green tea polyphenols exert striking inhibitory effects on diverse cellular events associated with multi-stage carcinogenesis. In addition, these compounds have ability to suppress proliferation of human cancer cells via induction of apoptosis (Surh, 1999).

There has been the discovery of several plant isolates and derivatives with activities in in vivo models of cancer chemoprevention, including deguelin, resveratrol, bruceatin, brassinin, 4′-bromoflavone, and oxomate. Using a panel of in vitro bioassays to monitor chromatographic fractionation, a diverse group of plant secondary metabolites has been identified as potential cancer chemopreventive agents from mainly edible plants. Nearly 50 new compounds have been isolated as bioactive principles in one or more in vitro bioassays. These active compounds are alkaloids, flavonoids, stilbenoids, and withanolides, as well as a novel stilbenolignan and the first representatives of the norwithanolides, which have a 27-carbon atom skeleton.

Several of these compounds were found to be active when evaluated in a mouse mammary organ culture assay, when used as a secondary discriminator.

The compounds (2S)-abyssinone II, (2S)-2′,4′-dihydroxy-2″-(1-hydroxy-1-methylethyl)-dihydrofuro-[2,3-h]-flavanone,3′-[gamma-hydroxymethyl-(E)-gamma-methylallyl]-2,4,2′,4′-tetrahydroxychalcone-11′-O-coumarate, isolicoflavonol, isoliquiritigenin, and ixocarpalactone A are regarded as promising leads as potential cancer chemopreventive agents (Kinghorn et al., 2004).

ANTI-HIV/AIDS

The identification of the human immunodeficiency virus (HIV) as the causative agent of AIDS has stimulated the search for novel antiviral agents. Large screening program for anti-HIV drugs are underway across the globe especially at the US National Institute of Health and leading Pharmaceutical companies. Two plant derived compounds have emerged from these screenings: castanospermine and hypericin. The tetrahydroxyindolizidine alkaloid castanospermine occurs in the toxic chesnut-like seeds of the evergreen Australian tree Castanospermum australe A. Cunn et Fras. (Leguminosae). The compound is a potent inhibitor of β-glucosidase, β-glucocerebrosinase and lysosomal a- and β-glucosidases. It is recently found to inhibit replication of HIV. Several O-acyl derivative of castanospermine are as much as 20 times more active than the present compound in inhibiting HIV-virus replication. Another interesting lead is the aromatic polycyclicdione hypericin. This anthraquinone derivative occurs in certain species of Hypericum (Guttiferae), such as H. perforatum L (St. John's wort) with antiretroviral activity. It inhibits the propagation of

Friend (leukemia virus (FLV) and radiation leukemia virus both in vitro and in vivo. A single dose of hypericin can prolong survival of FLV-induced mice. Hypericin is being developed for clinical trials. Anti HIV/AIDS -Despite continuous advances made in antiretroviral therapy, AIDS has become the leading cause of death in Africa and fourth worldwide; the number of people with HIV is increasing at an alarming rate in India and Southeast Asia. The number of compounds exhibiting anti-HIV activity and isolated from natural sources is increasing steadily. Examples are Calanolide A, a coumarin isolated from Callophyllum lanigerum, and two other natural product-derived molecules, DSB and 3-hydroxymethyl-4-methyl DCK are phase II clinical candidates, with potential to come up as drugs for treatment of HIV infection (Singh et al., 2005).

A phorbol derivative, prostratin, was discovered as possessing good anti-HIV activity, following the lead of a plant, Samoan plant Homalanthus nutans used locally for yellow fever.

Acquired immunodeficiency syndrome (AIDS), caused by the human immunodeficiency virus (HIV), is an immunosuppressive disease that results in life-threatening opportunistic infections and malignancies. Despite continuous advances made in antiretroviral therapy, AIDS has become the leading cause of death in Africa and fourth worldwide; the number of people with HIV is increasing at an alarming rate in India and Southeast Asia. Biodiversity of the plant kingdom has always provided a source of new drug candidates for almost all disease areas. Therefore, the number of compounds exhibiting anti-HIV activity and isolated from plant sources is increasing steadily (Singh et al., 2005).

Natural products anti-AIDS studies discovered many potent anti-HIV agents, which inhibit viral replication in H9 lymphocytes. Two lead compounds showed remarkable activities in this assay: DSB, a synthetic analog of the natural triterpenoid betulinic acid and DCK, a coumarin based analog of the natural product suksdorfin (Yu et al., 2007). Both classes of compounds were patented and licensed to Panacos Pharmaceuticals (Gaithersburg, MD) for development into clinical trials candidates. DSB was renamed PA-457 and then Bevirimat and is in fast-track drug development status. Bevirimat is the first in a new class of HIV drugs called maturation inhibitors, and its novel mechanism of action makes it promising for use alone or together with current anti-AIDS agents (Yu et al., 2005).

Notable HIV inhibitory natural products that were discovered since 1990 include prostratin (Gustafson et al., 1992), michellamine B (Boyd et al., 1994), and catanolide A (Kashmah et al., 1992). Calanolide A, a coumarin isolated from Callophyllum lanigerum was licensed to Sarawak Medichem, and it progressed into Phase II clinical trials against HIV. A summary of natural products that were active at various stages of HIV's life cycle has thus been adopted: absorption and penetration (polysaccharides, glycyrrhizin, phenolic compounds, pseudomonas exotoxin, lectins, 'sugar alkaloids' such as castanospermine); reverse transcription and integration (tannins, flavonoids, sesquiterpenes, coumarins and liganolides); transcription and translation, post-translational modification (didemnaketal A); viral assembly and release (hypericin); and other undetermined steps (gossypol, michellamine B, prostratin, trichosanthin); and finally immunomodulators (pine cone extracts and acemannan); (Wright, 1995).

The life forms from which the bioactive compounds have been isolated are equally as diverse as the compounds and comprise terrestrial and marine plants, microorganisms and marine animals. Again, notable amongst them is the calanolide A, a reverse transcriptase inhibitor (Matthew et al., 1999).

Therefore as an approach, traditional medicines from different places of the world were evaluated with a panel of in vitro bioassays (designed to monitor inhibition of HIV-1-induced cytopathic effect (CPE), and HIV essential enzymes; reverse transcriptase (RT), protease (PR), and integrase (IN), and active leads were then isolated and identified. Structurally diverse compounds that have potent anti-HIV activity were classified to CPE inhibitors (phorbol diterpenes), RT inhibitors (derivatives of caffeic acid and polyphenols), PR-inhibitors (derivatives of oleanane, ursane, and lupane type triterpenes), and the IN inhibitors (Meselhy et al., 2005).

The anti-HIV agents have been also classified according to their chemical classes rather than their target in the HIV replicative cycle, which is the most frequently encountered approach. They are thus, the flavonoids, coumarins, terpenoids, alkaloids, polyphenols, polysaccharides or proteins. It is the general conviction that the results and experiences with many of the anti-HIV natural products has inspired and motivate even more researchers to look for new leads from plants and other natural sources (Kaleab Asres et al., 2005).

Sumbul root (Ferula sumbul, Umbelliferae), a drug formerly used for its stimulant and anti-spasmodic properties, contains at least 27 coumarins and possesses anti-HIV activity (Zhou et al., 2000).

Sometimes anti-AIDS agents of more than one chemical class occur in the same plant, e.g. coumarins, flavonoids, and pentacyclic triterpenoids in liquorice. Also salaspermic acid, a pentacyclic triterpene, from the roots of Tripterygium wilfordii (Celastraceae) shows inhibition of HIV reverse transcriptase and HIV replication in HG lymphocyte cells. Also active, from the same plant, is tripterifordin, a kaurene-type diterpene lactone.

Many polysaccharides, e.g. sulphated polysaccharides with in vitro inhibitory activity against HIV have been isolated from Viola yedoensis (Violaceae), Prunella vulgaris (Labiatae), Alternanthera philoxeroides (Amaranthaceae) (Trease and Evans, 2006).

For approximately 24 years the AIDS pandemic has claimed approximately 30 million lives, causing approximately 14,000 new HIV-1 infections daily worldwide in 2003. About 80% of infections occur by heterosexual transmission. In the absence of vaccines, topical microbiocides, expected to block virus transmission, offer hope for controlling the pandemic. Antiretroviral chemotherapeutics have decreased AIDS mortality in industrialized countries. To prevent an analogous dichotomy, affordable, and accelerative in transition from development to marketing. Many fruit juices have been screened for inhibitory activity against HIV-1 IIIB using CD4 and CXCR4 as cell receptors. It was found that HIV-1 entry inhibitors from pomegranate juice absorb onto corn starch. The resulting complex blocks virus binding to CD4 and CXCR4/CCR5 and inhibits infection by primary virus clades A to G and group O, which suggest the possibility of producing an anti-HIV-1 microbiocide from inexpensive, widely available sources, whose safety has been established throughout centuries (Neurath et al., 2005).

The biochemical characteristics and biological activities of eight Cucurbitaceae plant proteins designated trichosanthin (isolated from tubers of Trichosanthes kirilowii), beta-trichosanthin (from tubers of Trichosanthes cucumeroides), alpha and beta-momorcharins (from seeds of Momordica charantia), momorchochin (from tubers of Momordica cochinchinensis), luffaculin (from seeds of Luffa acutangula) and luffin-a and luffin-b (from seeds of Luffa cylindrica) have been established. Most of the proteins are immunologically distinct and exhibit abortifacient, antitumor, ribosome inactivating and immunomodulatory activities while trichosanthin (the only non-glycoprotein) manifests anti-human immunodeficiency virus activity (Ng et al., 1992).

The target of action of several anti-HIV compounds including alkaloids (O-demethyl-buchenavianine, papaverine), polysaccharides (acemannan), lignans (intheriotherins, schisantherin), phenolics (gossypol, lignins, catechol dimers such as peltatols, napthoquinones such as conocurvone) and saponins (celasdin B, Gleditsia and Gymnocladus saponins), has not been elucidated.

Only a very few of these plant-derived anti-HIV products have been used in a limited number of patients suffering from AIDS viz-glycyrrhizin, papaverine, trichosanthin, castanospermine, N-butyl-1-deoxynojirimicin and acemannan (Vlietinck et al., 1998).

There is a continuous need for new drugs effective against otherwise drug-resistant HIV strains. Chemical compounds from natural sources provide a large variety of potential anti-HIV compounds. The most promising natural products are highlighted by Hupfeld and Efferth, 2009. In 2007, an estimated 33.2 million people globally were infected with AIDS. The virus represents a major threat in developing countries, where over 95% of all infected people worldwide are living. In Africa, AIDS remains the main cause of death. Sub-Saharan Africa is most vigorously affected, with over two-thirds of the population infected with HIV. Even though there is still no cure for AIDS, advances in HIV treatment have improved patients' quality of life and prolong their lives. In this regard, medicinal plants and their chemical constituents with activity against HIV have come into focus of virus research.

Currently 24 drugs for HIV treatment are approved by the US Food and Drug Administration (FDA). They are classified into four different groups based on their virus life cycle target: fusion or entry inhibitors (FI), reverse transcriptase inhibitors, integrase inhibitors (IN), and protease inhibitors (PI). All current anti-HIV treatments eventually lead to drug resistant mutants, which is one of the main reasons for therapy failure. There is therefore a continuing interest in finding new agents, which are not only well tolerated, convenient and less expensive, but which are also active against resistant virus strains and do not show cross resistance to other drugs.

Some of these natural products have already entered clinical trials. An example is betulinic acid, a triterpene isolated from Syzygium claviflorum and many other plants. It has been shown to inhibit HIV replication in vitro with an EC_{50} of 1.4 µM. Modifications of betulinic acid lead to even more potent derivatives, such as the 3-O-(3',3'-dimethyl-succinyl)-betulinic acid (DSB, bevirimat, PA-457) exhibits remarkable anti-HIV activity with an EC_{50} of 0.35 µM, with promising reduction of viral load and a promising safety profile in several clinical studies.

Various calanolides, isolated from Calophyllum langerium reveal anti-HIV activity, the most promising being calanolide A. It is an NNRTI with EC_{50} values between 0.02 and 0.5 µM. The compound is active against a broad range of HIV-1 strains, including otherwise drug-resistant variants. Phase Ia clinical trials have shown the compound to be safe and well tolerated at oral doses between 200 and 800 mg. A Phase Ib study showed a significant mean viral load reduction with oral dosage of 600 mg, while Phase II studies are ongoing.

(–)Epigallocatechin gallate (EGCG), a flavonoid isolated from the green tea plant Camellia sinensis. It inhibits several steps in the HIV life cycle such as post-adsorption entry and protease kinetics. Its IC_{50} value is 0.01-0.02 µg/ml for inhibition of the viral RT. Besides antiviral activities, EGCG also has antitumor promoting, anti-inflammatory and antioxidant activities.

Glycyrrhizin (GL), a terpenoid from the roots of Glycyrrhiza glabra, improved the CD4+ T-cell count In AIDS patients. In in vitro, GL had an IC_{50} of 0.15 mM, it inhibits virus binding to the host cell and inhibition of protein kinase C (PKC). It also has affinity to HIV surface proteins.

Andrographolide is a diterpene lactone isolated from Andrographis paniculata. In a Phase I clinical trial, it caused significant rise in CD4+ T-cells from 405 cells/ml to 501 cells/ml in HIV positive patients at a dosage of 10 mg/kg. Andrographolide probably acts through inhibition of the dysregulation of the cell cycle in HIV infected cells.

Polycitone A, an aromatic alkaloid isolated from marine Polycitor sp., inhibits RT of wild-type and some resistant HIV-1 strains as well as of HIV-2 strains. It has a low IC_{50} of 245 nM for RNA-directed DNA polymerase function of RT. Inhibition of the RT-DNA complex formation is an anti-HIV mechanism not used by any currently approved drug. Therefore, polycitone A is an interesting model compound for drug development.

Geranin, isolated from Phyllanthus amarus, inhibits HIV-1 replication in MT-4 cells and its $IC_{50} = 0.22$ μM. It acts through two different mechanisms, as a competitive RT inhibitor and also inhibits viral uptake, which makes it interesting for therapeutic use.

3′R,4′R-di-O-(-)camphanoyl-(+)-cis-khellactone (DCK), a derivative of suksdorfin, a pyranocoumarin isolated from Lomatium suksdorfii, demonstrated promising anti-HIV activity in vitro (EC_{50} of 0.049 μM). Several modifications of DCK were performed to further increase potency and bioavailability, while the mechanism of action is similar to other RT inhibitors.

Dietary and plant-derived compounds have advantages over synthetic drugs, exhibiting minimum side effects and are available in cost effective manner. Studies exploring the effects of dietary and plant-derived compounds targeting lipid rafts could be an evolving strategy to control the progression of AIDS; with the attendant composition or structure and conditions for the formation of lipid rafts in plasma membranes, interaction of HIV-1 with lipid rafts and introduce a novel concept that dietary and plant-derived compounds, which can target lipid rafts, could have potential preventive or therapeutic values against the progression of AIDS.

The important roles of omega-3-fatty acids and plant-derived various triterpenes, especially euphane types extracted from neem tree (Azadirachta indica), have been established as a target of lipid rafts and its major component cholesterol (Verma, 2009).

A long-term screening of plant extracts, particularly anti-infective or immunomodulative Chinese herbal medicines has focused on lead identification followed by the structural optimization of biologically active natural product leads, then a major approach for new lead generation through bioactivity-directed fractionation and isolation (BDFI). This has led to the generation of an abundance of structurally novel compounds displaying in vitro anti-HIV activity from natural resources, such as the 3′3′-dimethylsuccinyl-betulinic acid (DSB, PA-457, bevirimat), derived from a triterpene, is currently in Phase II clinical trial as an HIV-1 maturation inhibitor (MI).

A 3-hydroxy methyl-4-methyl-3′R,4′R-di-O-(-)-camphanoyl-(+)-cis-khellactone (HMDCK) was modified from suksdorfin, a khellactone coumarin, and exhibited extremely high potency in H9 lymphocytes. It is in preclinical testing. Other natural products and their derivatives include alkaloids, hexahydroxybiphenyls, flavonoids, and other compound classes (Yu et al., 2007).

Hundreds of terpenes have been isolated and assayed for their antiretroviral potency. Two new kaurane-type diterpene lactones isolated from the ethanolic extract of Tripterygium wilfordii (Celastraceae) exhibited potent anti-HIV activity in H9 lymphocytes. Neotripterifordin was the most potent diterpene from this plant with an EC_{50} value of 0.025 μM and therapeutic index (TI = IC_{50}/EC_{50}) of 125.

Another kaurane diterpene 16-β-17-dihydroxy-ent-kauran-19-oic acid was isolated from Annona squamosa (Amonaceae). This compound also showed anti-HIV activity ($EC_{50} = 2.4$ μM, TI >5).

Two know anti-HIV triterpenoid saponins, Gleditsia saponin C and Gymnocladus saponin G, were isolated from the fruit extracts of the two leguminosae plants, Gleditsia japonia and Gymnocladus chinensis, respectively. These two compounds prevented 50% of HIV IIIB replication in H9 lymphocytes at 1.1 μM (TI = 8.9) and 2.7 microM (TI = 5.2), respectively.

A new C-31 lanostane-type tetracyclic triterpene, suberosol, isolated from Polyalthia suberosa, was found to show anti-HIV replication activity in H9 lymphocyte cells with an EC_{50} of 6.78 μM.

Four cucurbitacins isolated from the methanolic extract of the leaves of Cowania mexicana (Rosaceae) also exhibited anti-HIV activity. 15-oxo-cucurbitacin F demonstrated potent anti-HIV activity and much lower cytotoxicity (IC_{50} = 9.6 microM, EC_{50} = 0.56 μM, and TI = 17).

The terpenoid saponin actein was identified as the anti-HIV principle of the methanol extract of the rhizome of Cimicifuga racemosa, commonly known as black cohosh. It exhibited promising antiviral activity with an EC_{50} of 0.55 μM and TI of 144.

Salaspermic acid, a friedelane pentacyclic triterpenoid from the roots of Tripterygiun wilfordii inhibited HIV replication in H9 lymphocytes with an EC_{50} value of 10 μM and also showed moderate inhibitory activity against recombinant RT as a template primer.

Several triterpenes from oleananes, ursanes, lupanes groups were reported to inhibit HIV replication in H9 lymphocytes. Oleanolic acid inhibited HIV-replication in H9 lymphocytes with an EC_{50} of 3.7 μM and TI of 12.8. Morolic acid, which has a double bond at C-18 rather than C-12, exhibited similar activity with EC_{50} of 5.9 μM and TI of 8.2. The 3-oxo analog morolic acid was reported to be more active and less toxic (EC_{50} <0.22 μM, TI >186).

Two lupane triterpenes, betulinic acid and platonic acid, from Rosa woodsii (Rosaceae) were reported to suppress HIV-1IIIB replication in vitro with EC_{50} of 1.4 and 6.5 μM, respectively. Dihydrobetulinic acid, which lacks the delta 29-20 double bond in betulinic acid, exhibited slightly better anti-HIV activity with an in vitro EC_{50} of 0.9 μM and TI of 14.

Three new triterpene lactone were isolated from the stems and roots of Kadsura lancilimba. Both A and B rings are seven membered, and ring A is a lactone, for example, lancilactone A. The active compound lancilactone C has an open A-ring, and inhibited HIV replication with an EC_{50} of 3.0μM and TI >71.4. Another example of an anti-HIV seco-ring A triterpene is nigranoic acid, isolated from Schisandra sphaerandra (Schisandraceae). This compound exhibited moderate activity against HIV-1 RT. and was found to inhibit DNA-dependent DNA polymerase activity.

Shinjulactone C, a degraded triterpene known as a quassinoid, which was originally purified from Allanthus altissima, was the most active quassinoid (EC_{50} = 10.6μM, TI >25) among a series of 18 quassinoid glycosides and 9 quassinoids.

An anti-HIV coumarin, suksdorfin, from Lomatium suksdorfii had been reported to suppress viral replication in 11 separate acute HIV-1IIIB infections of H9 lymphocyte cells with an average EC_{50} of 2.6 ± 2.1 μM. It is worthy of note that its structural modification confirmed that the 3′ and 4′ positions should be R-configured, as the stereoisomer 3′R,4′R-di-O-(-)-camphanoyl-(+)-cis-khellactone (DCK) showed over 100-fold improved activity (EC_{50} = 0.049 μM, TI >328).

Anti-HIV (-)-Calanolide B or costatolide from Calophyllum lanigerum, demonstrated comparable in vitro anti-HIV activity to calanolide A, and also demonstrates in vitro activity towards Mycobacterium tuberculosis and human cytomegalovirus (HCMV).

Oxocalanolide, a semi-synthetic calanolide analog, possesses activity against both HCMV and HIV. These dual therapeutic properties make it potentially suitable for immuno-compromised patients who are co-infected with both viruses. It is therefore, currently undergoing pre-clinical studies.

Various alkaloids have shown viral inhibition in HIV-infected cells. The well-known benzyl-isoquinoline alkaloid papaverine from Papaver somniferum, which is prescribed as a vasodilator, exhibited moderate inhibitory effects on HIV replication in the H9 cell line and in peripheral blood mononuclear cell (PBMC) culture.

A group of naphthylisoquinoline alkaloid dimers, including michellamine B, which were isolated from Ancistrocladus korupensis found in the Korup rainforest of Cameroon, were active against a panel of biologically diverse laboratory and clinical strains of HIV-1 and HIV-2.

Also known is the isolation of (+)-1(R)-coclaurine and (-)-1(S)-norcoclaurine from the leaves of Nelumbo nucifera (Nymphaceae) and their potent anti-HIV activity to be EC_{50} = 2.8 and <2.9 μM, TI >125 and >25, respectively.

Nuciferine, an aporphine alkaloid, had a potent EC_{50} of 2.6 μM and TI of 36. (±)-6-Acetonyldihydrochelerythine, a benzo[c]phenanthridine alkaloid isolated from the chloroform fraction of Argemone mexicana, exhibited significant anti-HIV-1 activity in H9 lymphocytes with an EC_{50} of 4.37 μM and TI of 14.6.

Some interesting positional effects were found with certain beta-carboline alkaloids, therefore the 1-methoxycanthinone, a beta-carboline alkaloid isolated from Leitneria floridana, exhibited an anti-HIV effect in H9 lymphocytes with an EC_{50} of 1.04 βM and TI of 39. The related drymaritin, a μ-carboline from Drymaria diandra with a 4-carbonyl and 5-methoxy, was also active with EC_{50} = 2.80 μM, TI = 20.6.

Harman, another beta-carboline alkaloid isolated from Symplocos setchuensis (Symphocaceae), exhibited moderate anti-HIV activity with an EC_{50} of 10.7 μM and TI of 10.4.

Sesquiterpene alkaloids are another series of alkaloids showing potent anti-HIV activity. More than 20 sesquiterpene alkaloids were isolated from plants of Tripterygium spp. and nine of them had TI values over 100. Triptonine B, hypoglaunine B, hyponine B, and wilfortrine are among the most potent sesquiterpene alkaloids with EC_{50} of 0.11-0.12 μM and TI values over 1000.

The tannin (polyphenols) classes screened for anti-HIV activity have included gallotannins, ellagitannins, condensed tannins, complex tannins, and other related compounds. Among 56 tannins isolated from plant materials, some gallotannins and ellagitannins showed anti-HIV activity and are structurally unique RT inhibitors.

It has further been shown that ellagitannins like punicalin, punicalagin, and punicacortein-C are the most potent inhibitors of HIV replication. Punicalin and punicacortein-C were the most potent RT inhibitors with IC_{50} of 8 and 5 μM respectively.

The polyphenols that inhibit upon preincubation may bind tightly to virions, causing their inactivation and preventing infection. Of 38 tea polyphenols isolated from various teas, 8-C-ascorbyl-(-)-epigallocatechin and theasinensin D were the most potent inhibitors of HIV replication with EC_{50} of 8.3 and 8.8 μM, and TI values of 9.5 and 5, respectively.

In the search for potent anti-HIV lignans, podophyllotoxin and dibenzylbutyrolactone lignans have received considerable interest in recent decades because of their wide-ranging biological activities. Several members of this family and their analogs have been shown to possess potent antiviral properties. For example, the clinically useful anti-cancer drug etoposide has in vitro anti-HIV activity with an EC_{50} of 0.03 μM and TI of 42.7, while the parent compound podophyllotoxin was toxic at all tested concentrations.

Several dibenzylbutyrolactones found in Symplocos setchuensis also exhibited anti-HIV activity. The subsequent BDFI of the chloroform fraction of this plant led to the isolation of an anti-HIV dibenzylbutyrolactone, matairesinol, as one of the major components. This compound and its diacetate exhibited moderate in vitro anti-HIV activity in H9 lymphocytes, with EC_{50} of 2.0 and 6.9 microM and TI of 11.0 and 7.1, respectively.

Arctiin (109), the β-D-glucoside of (-)-arctigenin, was reported to inhibit HIV replication in H9 cells with EC_{50} and TI values of 1.59 μM and >118, respectively, while (-)-arctigenin produced slightly better anti-HIV activity (EC_{50} = 0.43 μM) but higher cytotoxicity (TI = 5).

An ethanolic extract of the stems of Kadsura interior showed significant activity. The BDFI led to the isolation of 12 dibenzocyclooctadiene lignans. Among them, gomisin G showed the most potent anti-HIV activity, with EC_{50} and TI values of 0.011 μM and 300, respectively.

In the past two decades, the discovery and development of flavonoids and their analogs as anti-HIV agents have been widely investigated, and significant progress has been achieved. Acacetin-7-O-β-D-galactopyranoside, isolated from the methanol extract of the flower heads of Chrysanthemum morifolium, exhibited potent anti-HIV activity. It was found the most active flavonoid with EC_{50} = 4.2 μM, TI > 55.6. The BDFI of the active flavonoid fraction from Kummerowia striata led to the isolation and characterization of an anti-HIV principle, apigenin-7-O-β-D-glucopyranoside.

Lawina, a flavonoid from Desmos spp, demonstrated anti-HIV activity (EC_{50} = 7.72 μM, TI = 45). However, the most potent flavonoid-related compound was the chalcone 2-methoxy-3-methyl-4,6-dihydrox-5-(3′-hydroxy) cinnamoylbenzaldehyde (EC_{50} = 0.067 μM, TI = 489). This compound has provided an excellent lead compound for further anti-HIV drug development (Yu et al., 2007).

CONCLUSION

Notable among the active anti-cancer compounds isolated from numerous plants are taxol, one of the most outstanding agents, has been found beneficial in treatment of refractory ovarian, breast and other cancers. Another prominent molecule is podophyllotoxin, a synthetic modification of this molecule led to the development of etoposide, known to be effective for small cell cancers of the lung and testes. Camptothecin isolated from Camptotheca acuminate. Other important molecules include vincristine, vinblastine, colchicines, ellipticine and lepachol along with flavopiridol, a semi-synthetic analogue of the chromone-alkaloid rohitukine from India a pyridoindole alkaloid from the leaves of Ochrosia species (Mukherjee, 2001).

By applying BDFI, potential anti-HIV drugs derived from natural product leads are continuously discovered – encompassing a wide range of structural classes and mechanisms of action. Modern medicinal chemistry-based molecular modification has led to numerous compounds with more potent anti-HIV activity while as expected, a few have shown less potency or completely loose activity. This in effect will play an important role in developing the new leads into useful drugs (Yu et al., 2007).

Natural products and their derivatives provide an excellent sources for new anti-HIV drugs. Since many natural products are present in medicinal plants, which can be abundantly found in developing countries, a straightforward idea might be to propose administration of natural anti-HIV products in forms of tea or by direct consumption of the plant by patients in these countries. However, there are several limitations to this kind of application, such as concentration in a tea extract, bioavailability.

It has been documented that some of the most promising compounds are derivative of natural products, hence chemical modifications are sometimes necessary for improved antiviral activity.

A few of them have already been investigated in clinical trials. The vast majority of natural compounds have, however, only been analyzed in vitro leaving the treasure of potential novel HIV drugs from natural origin to be unearthed in the future (Hupfeld and Efferth, 2009).

Recently, there has been a renewed interest in natural product research due to the failure of alternative drug discovery methods to deliver many lead compounds in key therapeutic areas such as immunosupprerssion, cancer, anti-infectives, and metabolic diseases.

As a result of what is already in literature, it is very obvious that scientists, phytochemists and/or natural products chemists, pharmacognosists and pharmacologists must continue to screen our endowed medicinal plants for biological activities with the use of advanced bioactivity directed isolation and characterization of active compounds.

One key challenge to natural products chemistry research in the very near future is the loss of presently cheap and ready availability of our medicinal plants to the present rate of destruction of vegetation to make way for human development and economic exploitation.

It is quite encouraging that natural (plant) derived or originated compounds still play a major role as drugs, and as lead structures for the development of synthetic molecules. About 50% of the drugs introduced to the market during the last 20 years are derived directly or indirectly from natural products.

Hence, in conclusion, a multidisciplinary approach to drug discovery involving the generation of truly novel molecular diversity from natural product sources, combine with total and combinatorial synthetic methodologies provides the best solution to increase the productivity in drug discovery and development (Vuorelaa et al., 2004; Peterson et al., 2005).

REFERENCES

Aggarwal BB, Sundaram C, Malani N, Ichikawa H. Curcumin: the Indian solid gold. *Advances in Experimental Medicine and Biology*, 595, 1-75, (2007).

Beutler JA, Robert H. Shoemaker, Tanya Johnson, Michael R. Boyd. Cytotoxic Geranyl Stilbenes from *Macaranga schweinfurthii*. *J. Nat. Prod.*, 61, 1509-1512, (1998).

Boyd MR, Hallock YF, Cardellina JH, Manfredi KP, Blunt JW, McMahon JB, Buckheit Jr. RW, Bringmann G, Schaffer M, Cragg GM, Thomas DW, Jato JG. Anti-HIV michellamines from *Ancistrocladus korupensis*. *J.Med.Chem.*37, 1740-1745, (1994).

Cassady JM, Chan KK, Foss HG, Leistner E. Recent developments in the maytansinoid antitumor agents.*Chem. Pharm. Bull.*, 52, 1-26, (2004).

Cragg GM, Beutler JA, Jones WP. The American Society of Pharmacognosy 50 years of Progress in Natural Products Research 1959-2009. Omnipress, Madison, Wisconsin, U.S.A. pp. 197-199, (2009).

Cragg GM, Kingston DGI, Newman DJ. (eds), Antitumor Agents from Natural Products. Taylor and Francis, New York, pp. 71-87; 123-135; 321-337 (2005).

Crews P, Gerwick W, Schmitz F, France D, Bair K, Wright A, Hallock Y. Molecular approaches to discover marine natural product anticancer leads – An update from a drug discovery group collaboration. *Pharm. Biol.*, 41, 39-52, (2004).

Dorant E, van den Brandt PA, Goldbohm RA, Hermus RJ, Sturmans F. Garlic and its significance for the prevention of cancer in humans: a critical view. *British J. Cancer*, 67(3), 424-429, (1993).

Doskotch RW, Wilton JH, Fathallam MH, FAIRCHILD EH, Huang CT, El-FERALY FS. Six additional sesquiterpene lactones from *Liriodendron tulipifera*. *J. Nat. Prod.*, 46, 923-929, (1983).

El-Naggar SR, El-Feraly FS, Foos JS, Doskotch RW. Flavonoids from the leaves of *Kalmia latifolia*. *J. Nat. Prod.*, 43, 739-751, (1980).

Ernest E, Schmidt K. Ukrain - a new cancer cure? A systematic review of randomised clinical trials. *BMC Cancer*, 5, 69, (2005).

Evans WC. Pharmacognosy. Saunders, New Delhi, India, pp 394, 432, (2006).

Furia MD. de Paclitaxel (Taxol reg.): a new natural product with major anticancer activity. *Phytomedicine* 4 (3), 273-282, (1997).

Gonzales GF, Valerio LG Jr. Medicinal plants from Peru: a review of plants as potential agents against cancer. *Current Medicinal Chemistry–Anti-Cancer_Agents*, 6(5), 429-444, (2006).

Guenard D, Gueritte-Voegelein F, Potier P. Taxol and taxotere: Discovery, chemistry, and structure-activity relationships. *Accounts Chemical Res.*, 26, 160-167, (1993).

Gustafson KR, Cardellina II JH, McMahon JB, Gulakowaki RJ, Ishitoya J, Szallasi Z. Lewin NE, Blumberg PM, Weislow OS, Beutler JA, Buckheit Jr. RW, Cragg GM, Cox PA, Bader JP, Boyd MR. A nonpromoting phorbol from the Samoan medicinal plant *Homalanthus nutans* inhibits cell killing by HIV-1. *J. Med. Chem.*, 35, 1978-1986, (1992).

Hartwell JL. Types of anticancer agents isolated from plants. *Cancer Treatment Reports*, 60(8), 1031-1067, (1976).

Hartwell JL, Shear MJ. Chemotherapy of cancer. Classes of compounds under investigation and active components or podophilin. *Cancer Res.*, 7, 716-717, (1947).

Holmes FA, Walters RS, Theriault RL, Forman AD, Newton LK, Raber MN, Buzdar AU, Frye DK, Hortobagyi GN. Phase II trial of taxol, an active drug in the treatment of metastatic breast cancer. *J. Nat. Cancer Inst.*, 83, 1797-1805, (1991).

Hupfeld J, Efferth T. Drug resistance of human immunodeficiency virus and overcoming it by natural products. *In Vivo*, 23, 1-6, (2009).

Ireland CM, Aalbersberg W, Andersen R, Ayral-Kaloustian S, Berlinck R, Berman V, Carter G, Churchill A, Clardy J, Concepcion G, De Silva D, Discafani C, Fojo T, Frost P, Gibson D, Greenberger L, Greenstein M, Harper MK, Mallon R, Loganzo F. Anticancer agents from unique natural products sources. *Pharm. Biol.*, 41 Supplement, 15-38, (2003).

Jodi Laakso Chris M. Ireland, Leanne Murray, Robert J. Capon,? Michael R. Boyd..The lobatamides, novel cytotoxic macrolides from Southwestern Pacific Tunicates. *J. Org. Chem.*, 63, 7805-7810, (1998).

Johnson SA, Harpar P, Hortobagyi GN, Pouill P. Vinorelbine: An overview. *Cancer Treat. Rev.*, 22, 127-142, (1996).

Joshi SP. Plant products as anti-HIV agents. *J. Medicinal and Aromatic Plant*, 24(4), 1006-1023, (2002).

Kaefer CM, Milner JA. The role of herbs and spices in cancer prevention. *J. Nutritional Biochemistry*, 19(6), 347-361, (2008).

Kaleab Asres, Ameha Seyoum, Ciddi Veeresham, Bucar F, Gibbons S. Naturally derived anti HIV agents. *Phytotherapy Research*, 19(7), 557-581, (2005).

Kantarjian HM, Talpaz M, Santini V, Murgo A, Cheson B, O'Brien SM. Homoharringtonine: History, current research, and future directions. ***Cancer***, 92, 1591-1605, (2001).

Kaplan IW. et al., *New Orleans Med. Surg. J.*, 94, 388, (1942).

Kashman Y, Gustafson KR, Fuller RW, Cardellina, II JH, McMahon JB, Currens MJ, Buckheit, Jr. RW, Hughes SH, Cragg GM, Boyd MR. The calanolides, a novel HIV-inhibitory class of coumarin derivatives from the tropical rainforest tree, *Calophyllum lanigerum*. *J. Med. Chem.*, 35, 2735-2743, (1992).

Kim J. Protective effects of Asian dietary items on cancers- soy and ginseng. *Asian Pacific J. Cancer Prevention*, 9(4), 543-548, (2008).

Kinghorn AD, Su BN, Jang DS, Chang LC, Lee D, Gu JQ , Carcache-Blanco EJ, Pawlus AD, Lee SK, Park EJ, Cuendet M, Gills JJ, Bhat, K, Park HS, Mata-Greenwood E, Song LL, Jang M, Pezzuto JM. Natural inhibitors of carcinogenesis. <u>Planta Medica</u>, 70(8), 691-705, (2004).

Kinghorn AD, Farnsworth N, Soejarto D, Cordell G, Swanson S, Pezzuto J, Wani M, Wall M, Oberlies N, Kroll D, Kramer R, Rose W, Vite G, Fairchild C, Peterson R, Wild R. Novel strategies for the discovery of plant-derived anticancer agents. *Pharm. Biol.*, 41 Supplement, 53-67, (2003).

Kinghorn AD, Farnsworth NR, Soejarto DD, Cordell GA, Pezzuto JM, Udeani GO, Wani MC, Wall ME, Navarro HA, Kramer RA, Menendez AT, Fairchild CR, Lane KE, Forenza S, Vyas DM, Lam KS, Shu YZ. Novel strategies for the discovery of plant-derived anticancer agents. *Pure Appl. Chem.*, 71, 1611-1618, (1999).

Kupchan SM, Sigel CW, Guttman LJ, Restivo RJ, Bryan RF. Datiscoside, a novel antileukemic cucurbitacin glycoside from Datisca glomerata. *J. Am. Chem. Soc.*, 94, 1354-1356, (1972).

Lin L, Shi Q, Nyarko AK, Bastow KF, Wu CC, Su CY, Shih CCY, Lee KH. Antitumor agents. 250. Design and synthesis of new curcumin analogues as potential anti-prostate cancer agents. *J. Med. Chem.* 49, 3963-3972, (2006).

Mantle D, Gok MA, Lennard TW. Adverse and beneficial effects of plant extracts on skin and skin disorders. *Adverse Drug Reactions and Toxicological_Reviews,* 20(2), 89-103, (2001).

Mantle D, Lennard TW, Pickering AT. Therapeutic applications of medicinal plants in the treatment of breast cancer: a review of their pharmacology, efficacy and tolerability. *Adverse Drug Reactions and Toxicological Reviews*, 19(3), 223-240, (2000).

Marin D, Kaeda JS, Andreasson C, Saunders SM, Bua M, Olavarria E, Goldman JM, Apperley JF. Phase I/II trial of adding semisynthetic homoharringtonine in chronic myeloid leukemia patients who have achieved partial or complete cytogenetic response on imatinib. *Cancer*, 103, 1850-1855, (2005).

Matthee G, Wright AD, Konig GM. HIV reverse transcriptase inhibitors of natural origin. *Planta Medica*, 65 (6), 493-506, (1999).

McGuire WP, Rowinsky EK, ; Neil B. Rosenshein, NB, Grumbine FC, Ettinger DS, Armstrong DK, Ross C. Donehower RC. Taxol: A unique antineoplastic agent with significant activity in advanced ovarian epithelial neoplasms. *Ann. Intern. Med.*, 111, 273-279, (1989).

Mehta RG, Pezzuto JM. Discovery of cancer preventive agents from natural products: from plants to prevention. *Current Oncology Reports,* 4(6), 478-486, (2002).

Meselhy MR, El-Mekkawy S, Ma ChaoMei, Nakamura N, Tewtrakul S, Hattori M. Developing of anti-HIV agents from natural resources. *J. Traditional_Medicines*, 22 Suppl.1, 116-128, (2005).

Messina MJ. Legumes and soybeans: overview of their nutritional profiles and health effects. *American J. Clinical Nutrition,* 70(3 suppl.), 439S-450S, (1999).

Mukherjee AK, Sourav Basu, Nabanita Sarkar, Ghosh AC. Advances in cancer therapy with plant based natural products. *Current Medicinal Chemistry*, 8(12), 1467-1486, (2001).

Neurath AR, Strick N, Li YY, Debnath AK. Punica granatum (pomegranate) juice provides an HIV-1 entry inhibitor and candidate topical microbicide. *Annals of the New York Academy of Sciences*, 1056, 311-327, (2005).

Ng TB, Chan WY, Yeung HW. Proteins with abortifacient, ribosome inactivating, immunomodulatory, antitumor and anti-AIDS activities from Cucurbitaceae plants. *General Pharmacology*, 23(4), 579-590, (1992).

O'Brien SM, Kantarjian H. Keating M, Beran M, Koller C, Robertson LE, Hester J, Rios MB, Andreeff M, Talpaz M. Homoharringtonine therapy induces responses in patients with chronic myelogenous leukemia in late chronic phase. *Blood*, 86, 3322-3326, (1995).

Oberlies NH, Kroll DJ. Camptothecin and taxol: historic achievements in natural products research? *J. Nat. Prod.*, 67, 129-135, (2004).

Park EJ, Pezzuto JM. Botanicals in cancer chemoprevention. *Cancer and Metastasis Reviews*, 21 (3-4), 231-255, (2002).

Peterson J, Dwyer J, Bhagwat S, Haytowitz D, Holden J, Eldridge AL, Beecher G. and Aladesanmi, J. Major flavonoids in dry tea, *J. Food Composition and Anal.* 18, 487-501, (2005).

Pettit GR, Cichacz ZA, Gao F, Boyd MR, Schmidt, J.M. Isolation and structure of dictyostatin. *J. Chem. Soc. Chem. Commun.* 11-1112, (1994).

Pettit GR, Lippert JW, III. Tubulin binding liganols and corresponding prodrug constructs. Anti-Cancer Drug Design, 15, 203-216, (2000).

Pettit GR, Melody N, Herald DL, Knight JC, Chapuis JC. Antineoplastic agents 550. Synthesis of 10b (S)-epipancratistatin from (+)-Narciclasine. *J. Nat. Prod.*, 70, 417, (2007).

Pettit GR, Rhodes M. Antineoplastic agents 389. New syntheses of the combretastatin. *Anti-Cancer Drug Design*, 13, 189-191, (1998).

Pettit GR, Tan R, Pettit RK, Smith TH, Feng S, Doubek DL, Richert L, Hamblin J, Weber C, Chapuis JC. Antineoplastic agents 560. Isolation and structure of kitastatin 1 from an Alaskan Kitasatospora sp. *J. Nat. Prod.*, 70, 1069-1072, (2007).

Potier P, *Seminars in Oncology*, 16, 2-4, (1989).

Powell RG, Weisleder D, Smith CR. Antitumor alkaloids from *Cephalotaxus harringtonia*: Structure and activity. *J. Pharm. Sci.*, 61, 1227-1230, (1972).

Powell RG, Weisleder D, Smith Jr, CR, Rohwedder TK. Structures of Harringtonine, isoharringtonine, and homoharringtonine. *Tetrahedron Lett.* 11, 815-818, (1970).

Schiff PB. et al., *Nature*, 277, 665-667, (1979).

Schink M. Mistletoe therapy for human cancer: the role of natural killer cells. *Anti- Cancer Drugs*, 8 suppl 1, S47-51, (1997).

Shohat B. et al., *Cancer Chemotherapy Reports*, 51, 271-276, (1967).

Singh IP, Bharate SB, Bhutani KK. Anti-HIV natural products. *Current Science*, 89(2), 269-290, (2005).

Stahelin H F, Wartburg A. The chemical and biological route from podophyllotoxin glucoside to etoposide: Ninth Cain Memorial Award Lecture. *Cancer Res.*, 51, 5-15, (1991).

Sullivan BJ, Wechsler HI. The cytological effects of Podophyllin. *Science*, 105, 433, (1947).

Sun NJ, Woo SH, Cassady JM, Snapka RM. DNA polymerase and Topoisomerase II inhibitors from *Psoraea corylifolia. J. Nat. Prod.*, 61, 362-366, (1998).

Surh Y. Molecular mechanisms of chemopreventive effects of selected dietary and medicinal phenolic substances. *Mutation Research*, 428(1-2), 305-327, (1999).

Svoboda GH. et al., *J. Amer. Pharm. Ass. Sci. Ed.*, 48 (11), 659-666, (1959).

Svoboda GH. Alkaloids of *Vinca rosea*. IX. Extraction and characterization of leurosidine and leurocristine. *Lloydia*, 24(4), 173-178, (1961).

Tilleqyin F. *Phytochemical Reviews* 6, 65-79, (2007).

Uehara Y. Natural product origins of Hsp 90 inhibitors. *Current Cancer Drug_Targets*, 3(5), 325-330, (2003).

Verma SP. HIV: A raft-targeting approach for prevention and therapy using plant-derived compounds (Review). *Current Drug Targets*, 10(1), 51-59, (2009).

Vlietinck AJ, De Bruyne T, Apers S, Pieters LA. Plant-derived leading compounds for chemotherapy of human immunodeficiency virus (HIV) infection. *Planta Medica*, 64(2), 97-109, (1998).

Vuorelaa P, Leinonenb M, Saikkuc P, Tammelaa P, Rauhad JP, Wennberge T and Vuorelaa H. Natural products in the process of finding new drug candidates. *Current Medicinal Chemistry,* 11 (11), 1375-1389, (2004).

Wall ME, Wani MC, Cook CE, Palmer, K.H., McPhail, A.T., Sim, G.A. Plant antitumor agents. I. the isolation and structure of camptothecin, a novel alkaloidal leukemia and tumor inhibitor from Camptotheca acuminate. *J. Am. Chem. Soc.*, 88, 3888-3890, (1966).

Wambebe CON. The place of natural products in health care delivery system, a key note address to the Nigeria Society of Pharmacognosy Annual Conference, Jos, 1995, pp.1-12.

Wani MC, Taylor HL, Wall ME, Coggon P, McPhall AT. Plant antitumor agents. VI. The isolation and strurcture of taxol, a novel antileukemic and antitumor agent from *Taxus brevifolia. J. Am. Chem. Soc.*, 93, 2325-2327, (1971).

Wright CW. Natural products in the fight against AIDS. *Pharmaceutical Journal*, 254(6838), 583-587, (1995).

Xue H, Aziz RM, Sun N, Cassady JM, Kamendulis LM, Xu Y, Stonerr GD, Klaunig, J.E. Inhibition of cellular transformation by berry extracts. *Carcinogenesis*, 22, 351-356, (2001).

Yu D, Morris-Natschke SL, Lee KH. New developments in natural products-based anti-AIDS research. *Med. Res. Rev.* 27(1), 108-132, (2007).

Yu D, Wild CT, Martin DE, Morris-Natschke SL, Chen CH, Allaway GP, Lee KH. The discovery of a class of novel HIV-1 maturation inhibitors and their potential in the therapy of HIV. *Expert Opin. Invest. Drugs*, 14, 681-693, (2005).

Yun TK. Update from Asia. Asian studies on cancer chemoprevention. *Annals of the New York Academy of Sciences*, 889, 157-192, (1999).

Zhang YL, Lee KH. Recent progress in the development of novel antitumour etoposide analogues. *Chin. Pharm. J.*, 46, 319-369, (1994).

Zhou P, Takaishi Y, Duan H, Chen B, Honda G, Itoh M, Takeda Y, Kodzhimatov OK, Lee KH. Coumarins and bicoumarin from Felula sumbul: anti-HIV and inhibition of cytokine release. *Phytochemistry*, 53, 689-697, (2000).

chapter 12

Natural Therapies for Ocular Disorders

V. Kalaiselvan

INTRODUCTION

Eye is the most vulnerable part of the human body; it expresses the inner feelings, ailments of body, mind and beauty of the face. Eyes being one of the most important organs in Ayurveda, all five elements play a role in maintaining eye health. Earth (Prithivi) governs the muscular part of the eye, fire (Tejas) controls the blood vessels, air (Vayu) maintains the color, water (Apu) dominates the white area, and space (Akasha) controls the tear ducts and channels. According to Ayurvedic knowledge, eye diseases and disorders are caused by imbalance of the three doshas namely vata, pitta or kapha, doshas. The eye is organ of vision; it plays a very important role not only in life but also the human body, which gives us the sense of sight, allowing us to learn more about the surroundings than we do with any of the other four senses. The eye allows us to see and interpret the shapes, colors, and dimensions of object in the world by processing the light they reflect or emit. Eye acts as a camera. A camera needs a lens and a film to produce an image. In the same way, the eyeball needs a lens (cornea, crystalline lens, vitreous) to refract, or focus the light and a film (retina) on which to focus the rays (Figure 12.1). If any one or more of these components is not functioning correctly, the result is a poor picture. The care of eye is always a preventive stage towards the good health of eye. Eyes need to be protected from various environmental factors such as UV, sunlight etc., and from ocular diseases.

Based on projected increases in the prevalence of diabétes, the number of people with diabetes-related ocular diseases such as cataract, glaucoma, age macular degeneration, diabetic retinopathy etc., are the major problems. According to the Vision Council ocular diseases are the second most prevalent health issues in US. A recent report estimates the total economic burden of eye diseases in the U.S. at $51.4 billion annually (http://www.preventblindness.org/). These diseases cause 80% of blindness in Hong Kong. In India, cataract is responsible for almost 80% of blindness (Gupta et al., 1999). As per WHO report 2005, cataract causes 50% blindness globally; glaucoma and age macular degeneration is the second leading is the other leading factor for blindness.

Surgical and medication facilities are available for the treatment and management of ocular diseases. However cost of the surgical procedure and adverse effects of synthetic medicines, unable to reduce the avoidable blindness worldwide. Therefore researchers focused the pharmacological intervention for the treatment of ocular diseases. Herbal Medicine is the oldest form of medicine known to mankind and herbs have played an important part in our development. More than 2,000 years ago, Hippocrates wrote extensively about herbal medicine and healing. Herbal and nutritional supplements have gained considerable attention over the past few years, with many people hoping to maintain or improve their eyesight. Also Ayurvedic system of medicine described the usage of herbal extracts to treat various eye diseases. In recent times scientifically and clinically validated that herbal drugs are more effective in the management and prevention of ocular diseases.

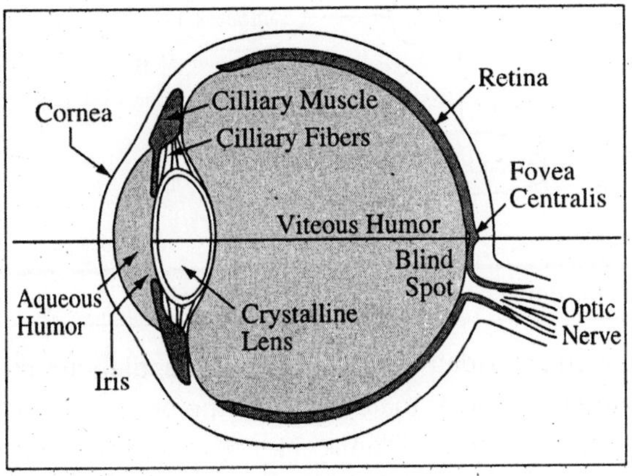

Fig. 12.1: Human Eye Section view

Cataract

The term 'Cataract'is used to describe an opacification of the lens substance. It may be localized to certain lens parts or may affect the whole lens. According to its localization, the opacity may cause a more or less pronounced disturbance of light transmission. Several risk factors have been identified in the pathogenesis of senile cataract. Apart from ageing, diabetes, smoking, gender, steroids and nitric oxide are responsible for the development of cataract. There are complex metabolic functions are responsible for cataract. The main three mechanisms are involved in the progress of cataractogenesis as follows:

a. Nonenzymatic glycation

b. Oxidative stress

c. Polyol pathway

It is widely accepted that oxidative stress is the major factor in the progression of cataractogenesis (Truscott, 2005). Oxidative stress is associated with increased reactive oxygen and known to accelerate cataract formation since superoxide is converted to toxic substance namely hydrogen peroxide. This reaction can be prevented by antioxidant enzymes. Hence antioxidants and herbal drugs contain antioxidant potential could play a significant role in the prevention of cataract. In recent years great emphasis had been laid on exploring the possibility of using our natural resources to delay the onset and progression of cataract. A large number of natural drugs and their formulations have been studied for the potential in the prevention of cataract.

Glaucoma

Glaucoma is the second leading cause of blindness. Globally, it is estimated that about 66.8 million people have visual impairment from glaucoma, with 6.7 million suffering from blindness. The prevalence of glaucoma increases with age. Two per cent of the population older than 40 years of age and five to nine per cent of those older than 65 years have glaucoma. It is estimated that there will be 60.5 million people with OAG (open angle glaucoma) and ACG (angle closure glaucoma) in 2010, which will increase to 79.6 million by 2020. Of these, 74% will have OAG. From 2010 to 2020, the most detectable change in glaucoma worldwide will be an increase of the incidence of glaucoma in India. As the proportion of those over age 40 increases, the proportional increase in glaucoma will challenge our resources and ingenuity (Gupta et al., 2008). Glaucoma is a disorder in eye that develops when too much fluid pressure builds up inside the eye. The increased internal pressure can damage the optic nerve, which transmits images to the brain. If this pressure and damage continues, vision will worsen and leads to blindness. Intraocular pressure is only one of the major risk factors for glaucoma, lowering it via various pharmaceuticals and/or surgical techniques are currently the mainstay of glaucoma treatment. Intraocular pressure can be lowered with medication, usually eye drops. There are several different classes of medications to treat glaucoma with several different medications in each class. Each of these medicines may have local and systemic side effects. Figure 12.2 shows the major risk factors responsible for the progression of cataract and development of glaucoma.

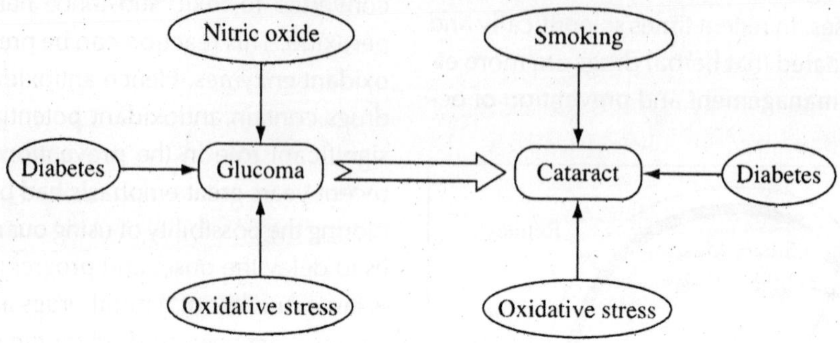

Fig. 12.2: Major risk factors and mechanisms associated with the development of cataract and glaucoma

How natural medicines can be a potential anticataract and antiglaucoma agents?

Cataract and glaucoma are the diseases characterized by opacification in the eye lens and increase in intraocular pressure respectively. There is large number of complex metabolic disorders such as oxidative stress, nitric oxide, diabetes etc are involved as major factor in the progression of cataract and glaucoma. Hence the herbal drugs possesses potential antioxidant, nitric oxide scavenging, antidiabetic and neuroprotection would be a novel and effective therapeutic agent for the prevention of ocular diseases especially cataract and glaucoma. (Figure 12.3).

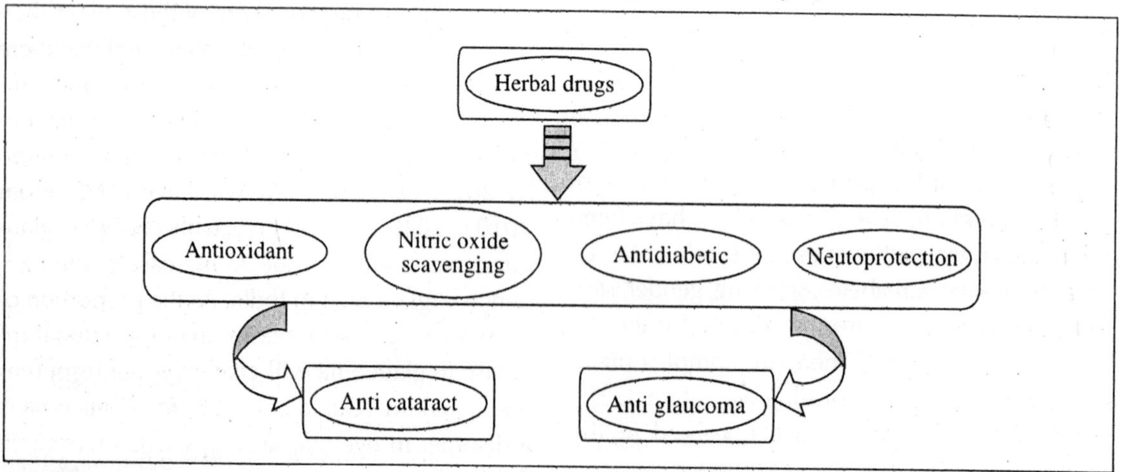

Fig. 12.3: Anti cataract and anti glaucoma property of herbal drugs due to various mechanisms

Emblica officinalis

Commonly known as amla, is extensively used in many preparations of Ayurveda and also against many chronic ailments including diabetes it contains rich source of ascorbic acid and tannins (Satyavati et al., 1976, Thakur, 1985, Sabu and Kuttan, 2002). In the recent experimental studies demonstrated *E. officinalis* inhibited the activity of enzyme aldose reductase (which is the responsible for the conversion of glucose to sorbitol via polyol pathway) *in vitro* cultured rat lens. Also showed significant inhibition against purified recombinant human aldose reductase at the concentration of 10 µg/ml respectively. The inhibition of aldose reductase by *E. officinalis* tannoids is 100 times higher than its aqueous extract and comparable to or better than quercetin (Suryanarayana et al., 2004).

Camellia sinensis

It is commonly known as green tea. The protection offered by various antioxidants in cataract development is well established. Polyphenolic compounds present in green tea are reported to possess antioxidant property in various pathological conditions. The anti cataract potential of green tea extract was established now. Green tea leaf extracts positively modulated antioxidant enzymes such as superoxide dismutase (SOD), catalase (CAT) and glutathione peroxidase (GPX). These antioxidant enzymes protecting the eye lens from various type of oxidative stress. Also it was found to reduce the incidence of selenite induced cataract *in vivo* (Gupta et al., 2002). The antioxidant effect of green tea also preventing glaucoma and age related macular degeneration (Shixian et al., 2006).

Glycine max

It is commonly referred as Soya bean, (Fam: Leguminosae) playing important role in traditional diets of many regions throughout the world. Soya bean contains isoflavones namely genistein, daidzein and glycetein and extensive research has been done on these compounds and showed potential antioxidant property (Corinna et al., 2006). The anticataract potential of soya bean was investigated in our laboratory. *In vitro* the aqueous extract of soya bean showed a concentration dependent protection against oxidative and osmotic stress; 200 µg/ml showed significant protection. *In vivo* 10% soya bean diet significantly delayed the onset and progression of 30% galactose induced cataract in rats (Agrawal et al., 2008).

Ocimum sanctum

It is generally referred as Tulsi. Aqueous extract of Tulsi possesses potential anticataract activity against selenite-induced experimental cataractogenesis. It showed different degrees of positive modulation in selenite-induced morphological as well as biochemical changes. At the concentration of 140 µg/ml significantly modulated glutathione and thiobarbituric acid reacting substances and also increased the activity of antioxidant enzyme levels with preservation of normal lens protein profile. *In vivo*, 5 and 10 mg/kg of reduced the incidence of selenite cataract by 20% and 60%, respectively, and prevented protein insolubilization as well (Gupta et al., 2005).

Allium cepa

Flavonoids are a group of substances that are widely distributed in various herbals and natural products and possess strong antioxidant activity. The potential of dietary flavonoids in the prevention of cataract has been investigated in some experimental studies (Durukan et al., 2006). In the recent study reported that topical administration of onion juice into the rat eyes effectively prevented selenite-induced cataract formation. This effect was associated with increased total antioxidant level, SOD and GPX activities in the lens (Javadzadeh et al., 2009).

Trigonella foenum-graecum

Trigonella foenum-graecum is known as Fenugreek is a plant in the family Fabaceae. The seeds of this plant are widely used in Indian cuisine. Fenugreek seeds are a rich source of the polysaccharide galactomannan. They are also a source of saponins such as diosgenin, yamogenin, gitogenin, tigogenin, and neotigogens. Other bioactive constituents of fenugreek include mucilage, volatile oils, and alkaloids such as choline and trigonelline. Experimental studies on alcoholic extract of Fenugreek at the dose of 2g/kg exerted significant effect in alloxan induced diabetic rats by showing the decreased opacity index (Vats et al., 2004).

Ginkgo biloba

It is also known as the Maidenhair Tree found in China; the leaves contain flavonoid, glycosides and terpenoids (ginkgolides, bilobalides) and have been used pharmaceutically. *Ginkgo biloba* has been extensively studied for its cognitive effects in patients with dementia (DeKosky et al., 2008). The extract have been found to possess potential therapeutic effect in radiation-induced cataract (Ertekin et al., 2004). The extract is used for the treatment of glaucoma; the mechanism of the activity is due to the improvement of central and peripheral blood flow, reduction of vasospasm, reduction of serum viscosity, antioxidant activity, platelet activating factor inhibitory activity, inhibition of apoptosis, and inhibition of excitotoxicity (Ritch, 2000).

Pilocarpus jaborandi

It is commonly known as jaborandi, Pilocarpus and Indian hemp. (Fam: Rutaceae). *P. jaborandi* is small shrub 120-150 cm in height, but in some species can the height of a medium-sized tree. Various species of Jaborandi are native South America, occurring most densely in Brazil, and to a much lesser extent in Central America. An herbal jaborandi leaf tea has a long history of use in Brazilian traditional folk medicine; the indigenous peoples of Amazonia used the herbal tea in treating many different problems including diuretic. The majority of pilocarpine drugs are derived from the natural alkaloid extracted from jaborandi leaves produced in Brazil. After extensive research, the alkaloid pilocarpine was identified in the plant. It is about 200 year's old medicine for the treatment of glaucoma. Pilocarpine eye drops are still sold as a prescription drug worldwide for the treatment of glaucoma and as an agent to cause constriction of the pupil of the eye (useful in some eye surgeries and procedures). This substance has the ability to lower pressure within the eye of a person with glaucoma. As a result of that finding, pilocarpine is used in modern ophthalmology in the treatment of glaucoma.

Coleus forskohlii

The plant is also called coleus (Family: Lamiaceae); an aromatic perennial plant about two feet tall when fully mature. Coleus possesses tuber like roots and a straight and erect stem with colorful leaves. The coleus has an aromatic fragrance resembling the scent of the camphor plant. Forskolin (7 beta-acetoxy-8, 13-epoxy-1 alpha, 6 beta, 9 alpha-trihydroxy-labd-14-ene-11-one) is the main active ingredient in the Ayurvedic herb *Coleus forskohlii*. Coleus is a member of the mint family and grows in subtropical areas in India, Burma, and Thialand. Forskolin has been extensively evaluated in the field of pharmaceutical sciences for use in the treatment of allergies, respiratory problems, cardiovascular diseases and glaucoma. Clinical studies have shown that topical application of one per cent forskolin eye drops resulted in significant decreases in intraocular pressure for up to five hours. Limited clinical experience suggests that oral forskolin appears to offer significant potential for sufferers of glaucoma. Indian pharmaceutical companies are currently engaged in clinical trials of a forskolin eye drop product in the treatment of glaucoma.

Grape Seed Extract

Grape Seed Extract which is high in Oligomeric Proanthocyanidins (OPC's or PCO's) is powerful antioxidant which can reduce the damage done by free radicals, strengthen and repair connective tissue, and promote enzyme activity. OPC's can also help moderate allergic and inflammatory responses by reducing histamine production. Proanthocyanidin is one of the names used to describe a powerful bioflavonoid complex known as Procyanidolic Oligomers. Clinical studies have shown that antioxidants can halt cataract progression. PCO has a strong affinity for the portion of the retina that is responsible for visual acuity. It prevents free radical damage and reinforces the collagen structures of the retina. In clinical trials of patients with various types of retinal disease, including macular degeneration, all patients given PCO showed significant improvement following therapy. Health professionals monitoring the effects of PCO have reported that it also has helped in the prevention and treatment of glaucoma. Grape seed extract considerably decreased the development of cataract in rats (Durukan et al., 2006).

Dregea volubilis

Dregea volubilis is a woody climbing plant commonly found in the hotter parts of India. The leaves are edible and used as a green vegetable, while the plant extract has been used traditionally to treat several diseases including eye ailments. Research studies have evaluated the potential anticataract effect and it has also been found that the effect is due to drevogenin D, a triterpenoid aglycone (Biju et al., 2007).

Vaccinium myritillus

It is commonly known as Bilberry; is a small, wild, perennial shrub that grows throughout Europe and is now cultivated from the Far East to the United States. The shrub yields large amounts of small, darkish blue berries. Besides their medicinal use, they are often eaten fresh or made into jams. It has a long history of use for various eye conditions in a clinical study report of 50 patients with senile cataracts, a combination of bilberry and vitamin E stopped the progression of cataracts up to 96% (Bravetti et al., 1989). Bilberry flavonoids can increase certain enzymes and substances in the eyes that are crucial to good vision and eye function. Furthermore, anthocyanosides can increase circulation in the blood vessels in the eyes, and help these blood vessels repair and protect themselves. Specifically, research has shown that anthocyanosides help stabilize and protect a protein called collagen, which is a basic building block of veins, arteries, capillaries, and connective tissue. Particularly, anthocyanosides seem to work favorably in the tissues found in the retina, the back of the eye where major functions of vision take place (Pizzorno and Murray, 1996). The recent study also established that the combination of a standardized extract of bilberry and French maritime pine bark reduces the risk of glaucoma (Steigerwalt et al., 2008).

Salvia miltiorrhiza

It is commonly known as Red sage, Chinese sage, Tan shen, is a perennial flowering plant in the genus Salvia, roots are widely used in traditional Chinese medicine. Experiments on rabbits found it protected the optic nerve from the damaging effects of increased Intra ocular pressure (IOP), with better results when used in conjunction with a medication to IOP pressure (Zhu and Cai, 1993). The effect of *Salvia miltiorrhiza* on human glaucoma is well established. In a clinical study, Intra muscular injection (2 g/mL) of *Salvia miltiorrhiza* and in combination with other Chinese herbs significantly controlled the IOP in 121 glaucoma patients. After 30 days visual acuity had improved in 43.8 per cent of the eyes and visual field improvement was noted in 49.7 per cent of eyes. There were no significant differences among the four herbal preparations; but the effect was a statistically significant (Wu et al., 1983).

Emilia sonchifolia

It is known as lilac tassel flower genus of Emilia. The juice of the leaves is used in treating eye inflammations and night blindness. Flavonoids from *Emilia sonchifolia* modulate the lens opacification and oxidative stress in selenite-induced cataract (Lija et al., 2006).

Antioxidants

Carotenoids: Beta-carotene-a naturally occurring antioxidant found in fruits and vegetables. They are natural lipid soluble antioxidants. It is reported that high intake of carotene reduce the risk of incidence of cataract (Cumming et al., 2000).

Lycopene: It is present in many fruits and vegetables. It is a red, fat-soluble pigment found in certain plants and microorganisms, where it serves as an accessory light-gathering pigment and protects these organisms against the toxic effects of oxygen and light. Tomato products, including ketchup, tomato juice, and pizza sauce, are the richest sources of lycopene. In addition to tomatoes (*Lycopersicon esculentum*) and tomato-based products, lycopene is also found in watermelon, papaya, pink grapefruit, and pink guava. Experimental studies have been reported the incorporation of lycopene on diet retard the onset and progression of cataract (Pollack et al., 1999). Similarly the role of lycopene in human cataract also has been established. Lycopene 5, 10 and 20 mM significantly increased the activities of glutathione and antioxidant enzymes where as the lipid peroxidation product namely malondialdehyde level was reduced in human lens epithelial cells culture *in vitro* (Mohanty et al., 2002). *In vivo* experimental study showed that 200 mg/kg significantly delayed the onset and progression of 30% galactose induced cataract on rats; the protective effect is to due to the antioxidant potential (Gupta et al., 2003).

Curcumin: Curcumin (1,7-bis (4-hydroxy-3-methoxyphenyl)-1,6. heptadiene-3,5-dione), is the major active compound of turmeric, has been shown to have significant antioxidant activity, both *in vitro* and *in vivo* (Joe et al., 2004). Curcumin 0.002% and 0.01% in the diet are effective against the development of streptozotocin induced diabetic cataract in rats (Suryanarayana et al., 2005). It is also effective against 30% galactose induced cataract in rats (Suryanarayana et al., 2003). Recent study demonstrated that topical application of aqueous extract of *Curcuma longa* showed potent anti-inflammatory activity against endotoxin induced uveitis in rabbits eye (Gupta et al., 2008).

Lutein: It is one of over 600 known naturally occurring carotenoids. Found in green leafy vegetables such as spinach and kale. Lutein is present in the plant as fatty-acid ester, with one or two fatty acids bound to the two hydroxyl-groups. It is a natural antioxidant; experimental studies reported that combination of lutein and insulin retard the progression of cataract (Arnal et al., 2009). Lutein was found to be concentrated in the macula, a small area of the retina responsible for central vision. The hypothesis for the natural concentration is that lutein helps protect from oxidative stress and high-energy light. Various research studies have shown that a direct relationship exists between lutein intake and pigmentation in the eye.

Vitamin E: As a fat-soluble antioxidant, the beneficial role in the prevention and delay of cataract in experimental and epidemiological studies has well documented (Ross et al., 1990). Recently 10 years of observational study concluded that intake of Vitamin E along with other antioxidants in middle age women significantly reduced the development of cataract (Christen, 2008).

MISCELLANEOUS

Omega 3 fatty acids include DHA-docosahexaenoic acid is important to eye health and brain functioning. EPA-eicosapentaenoic acid and Alpha-linolenic acid are also Omega 3 fatty acids and together are believed to support good health. Omega 6 fatty acids are composed of Linoleic and Arachadonic acid. Epidemiological and animal studies point to a possible protective effect of omega-3 fatty acids in glaucoma. Both topical administration of prostaglandin E3 and D3 (end products of omega 3 fatty acid metabolisms) and Intra muscular injections of cod liver oil (which is high in omega-3 fatty acids) led to decreased IOP in rabbits (Kulkarni and Srinivasan, 1983; Mancino et al., 1992). Specific studies have not been done to test the viability of using Omega 3 fatty acids in the treatment of Glaucoma. They have been known to have benefits in other eye problems such as retinal issues and Macular Degeneration. It would be interesting if the future studies are focusing on Omega 3 fatty acid in the treatments ocular diseases.

HERBAL FORMULATIONS

The herbal formulation namely Diabecon (used for diabetics, contains 25 herbal drugs) inhibited the sugar-induced lens opacity in organ culture and also demonstrated that the effect is mainly due to *Gymnema sylvestre*, which is one of its constituents (Moghaddam et al., 2005). A study by our laboratory on polyherbal preparation, Chyavanprash (containing about 35 natural herbs including amla), found it to be protective against steroid-induced opacities in lens of chick embryo (Velpandian et al., 1998). *Triphala* is a traditional Ayurvedic system of medicine comprised of mixture of equal parts of *Emblica officinalis, Terminallia chebula, Terminallia belarica*. In folk medicine and ancient literature it has been mentioned as one of the best formulation for the treatment of eye diseases. In the recent *in vivo* and *in vitro* experimental study, it has been validated that *Triphala* has potential role in the prevention of cataract (Kalaiselvan, 2008).

Table 12.1 Summarizes potential antioxidants and herbal drugs for the prevention and treatment of cataract.

Supplement	Mechanism of action
Vitamin C	Preserves glutathione levels; protects the Na^+/K^+ pump
Vitamin E	Precursor to FAD, a coenzyme for glutathione reductase which recycles glutathione
Glutathione	Deficiency noted in cataractous lenses; important component of the innate antioxidant system in the lens
Carotenes	Antioxidant; higher levels associated with decreased risk for cataract
Lycopene	Major carotenoid; possesses potential antioxidative property; reduces the risk associated with osmotic stress
Curcumin	Antioxidant; reduces apoptosis in sugar cataract; inhibits the enzyme Aldose Reductase in polyol pathway
Ocimum sanctum	Restores the antioxidant defense system; inhibits lens protein degradation
Emblica officinalis	Potent inhibitors of AR; reduces the osmotic stress

Contd. to next page.

Emilia sonchifolia	Acts as a antioxidant and inhibits the lipid peroxidation reaction
Dregea volubilis	Preserve the antioxidant mechanisms and lower the level of lipid peroxidation
Vaccinium myritillus	Potent antioxidant
Ginkgo biloba	Antioxidant that protects the lens from various oxidative damage
Camellia sinensis	Inhibits oxidative stress by balancing the antioxidant defense mechanisms
Trigonella foenum-graceum	Prevents diabetic cataract by reduces the risk associated with osmotic stress
Grape seed	Increases glutathione level; reduces the lipid peroxidation
Coleus forskohlii	Increases cyclic adenosine monophosphate, inhibits glucose transport in erythrocytes

Table 12.1: Antioxidants and herbal drugs for the prevention and treatment of cataract and glaucoma.

CONCLUSION

Extensive research has been done to explore the natural sources especially herbal drugs for the prevention and treatment of ocular diseases. Even with the use of conventional medications, and surgical procedure are maintaining IOP and preventing cataract in patients can be challenging. There are several nutrients, vitamins and botanicals that hold anticataract and antiglaucoma potential. However, most studies are merely preliminary larger and prospective clinical studies on the use of nutrients and herbal drugs for the treatment of cataract and glaucoma are needed. Also ocular toxicity of the natural therapies claiming for ocular diseases is warranted.

REFERENCES

Agrawal SS, Gupta SK, Kalaiselvan V, Srivastava S, Saxena R. Potential of traditional food supplement soya bean as a novel amticataract agent. IJIB, 3, 1-9, (2008).

Arnal E, Miranda M, Almansa, Muriach M, Jorge M, Francisco BJ, Romero, Manuel, Diaz-Llopis M, Bosch-Morell F. Lutein prevents cataract development and progression in diabetic rats. Graefe's Archive for Clinical and Experimental Ophthalmology, 247, 115-120, (2009).

Biju PG, Devi VG, Lija Y, Abraham A. Protection against selenite cataract in rat lens by drevogenin D: A triterpenoid aglycone from Dregea volubilis. J Med Food, 10, 308-315, (2007).

Bravetti G. Preventive medical treatment of senile cataract with vitamin E and anthocyanosides: Clinical evaluation. Ann Ottalmol Clin Ocul, 115, 109, (1989).

Christen W. Dietary Carotenoids, Vitamins C and E, and Risk of Cataract in Women. Archives of Ophthalmology, 126, 102-109, (2008).

Corinna E, Rufer E, Sabine E, Kulling. Antioxidant activity of isoflavones and their major metabolites using different in vitro assays. J Agric Food Chem 54, 2926-2931, (2006).

Cumming RG, Mitchell P, Smith W. Diet and cataract: The Blue Mountains eye studies. Ophthalmol, 107, 450-456, (2000) damage in chronic glaucomatous rabbit. Chin Med J, 106, 922-927, (1993).

DeKosky ST, Williamson JD, Fitzpatrick AL. Ginkgo biloba for prevention of dementia: a randomized controlled trial. JAMA, 300, 2253-2262, (2008).

Durukan AH, Evereklioglu C, Hurmeric V, Kerimoglu H, Erdurman C, Bayraktar MZ. Ingestion of IH636 grape seed proanthocyanidin extract to prevent selenite-induced oxidative stress in experimental cataract. J Cataract Refract Surg, 32, 1041-1055 (2006).

Ertekin MV, Kocccer I, Karslioglu I, Taysi S, Gepdiremen A, Sezen O. Effects of oral Ginkgo biloba supplementation on cataract formation and oxidative stress occurring in lenses of rats exposed to total cranium radiotherapy. Jpn J Opthalmol, 48, 499-502, (2004).

Gupta SK, Galpalli ND, Agrawal SS, Srivastava S, Saxena R. Recent advances in pharmacotherapy of glaucoma. Indian J Pharmacol, 40, 197-208, (2008).

Gupta SK, Halder N, Srivastavaa S, Trivedi D, Joshi S, Varma SD. Green Tea (Camellia sinensis) Protects against Selenite-Induced Oxidative Stress in Experimental Cataractogenesis. Ophthalmic Res, 34, 258-263, (2002).

Gupta SK, Joshi S, Vajpayee RB, Saxena R. Epidemiology cataract in India: Combating plans and strategies. Ophthalmic, 31, 86-92, (1999).

Gupta SK., Srivastava S, Agrawal P, Agrawal SS, Saxena R, Galpalli N. The anti inflammatory effects of Curcuma longa and Berberis aristata in Endotoxin induced Uveitis in rabbits. Invest Ophthalmol & Visual Sci, 49, 4036-4040, (2008).

Gupta SK, Srivastava S, Trivedi D, Joshi S, Halder N. Ocimum sanctum modulates selenite-induced cataractogenic changes and prevents rat lens opacification. Curr Eye Res, 30, 583-591, (2005).

Gupta SK, Trivedi D, Srivastava S, Joshi S, Halder N, Verma SD. Lycopene attenuates oxidative stress induced experimental cataract development: an in vitro and in vivo study. Nutrition, 19, 794-799, (2003).

Javadzadeh A, Ghorbanihaghjo A, Bonyadi S, Rashidi MR, Mesgari M, Rashtchizadeh N, Argani H. Preventive effect of onion juice on selenite-induced experimental cataract. Indian J Ophthalmol, 57, 185-189, (2009).

Joe B, Vijaykumar M, Lokesh BR. Biological properties of curcumin-cellular and molecular mechanisms of action. Crit Rev Food Sci Nutr, 44, 97-111, (2004).

Johnson EJ, Hammond BR, Yeum KJ, Qin J, Wang ZD, Castaneda C, Snodderly DM, Russell RM. Relation among serum and tissue concentrations of lutein and zeaxanthin and macular pigment density. Am J Clin Nutr. 2000 Jun; 71(6): 1555-62.

Kalaiselvan V. Prevention of cataract development by herbal ophthalmic formulation: *In vitro, In vivo* and ocular toxicity studies. Dissertation, University of Delhi (2008).

Kulkarni PS, Srinivasan BD. Prostaglandins E3 and D3 lower intraocular pressure. Invest Lija Y, Biju PG, Reeni A, Cibin TR, Sahasranamam V, Abraham A. Modulation of selenite cataract by the flavonoid fraction of Emilia sonchifolia in experimental animal models. Phytother Res, 20, 1092-1095, (2006).

Mancino M, Ohia E, Kulkarni P. A comparative study between cod liver oil and liquid lard intake on intraocular pressure on rabbits. Prostaglandins Leukot Essent Fatty Acids, 45, 239-43, (1992).

Moghaddam MS, Kumar PA, Reddy GB, Ghole VS. Effect of Diabecon on sugar-induced lens opacity in organ culture: Mechanism of action. J Ethnopharmacol, 97, 397-403, (2005).

Mohanty I, Joshi S, Trivedi D, Srivastava S, Gupta SK. Lycopene prevents sugar-induced morphological changes and modulates antioxidant status of human lens epithelial cells. Br J Nutr, 88, 347-354, (2002).

Ophthalmol Vis Sci, 26, 1178-1182, (1985).

Pizzorno J, Murray M. A Textbook of Natural Medicine: Vaccinium Myrtillus. Bothell, WA: Bastyr University Publications, Vol. 1, (1996).

Pollack A, Oren P, Stark AH, Eisner Z, Nyska, Madar Z. Cataract development in sand and galactosemic rats fed a natural tomato extract. Journal of Agriculture Food Chemistry, 47, 5122-5126, (1999).

Ritch R. Potential role for Ginkgo biloba extract in the treatment of glaucoma. Medical Hypotheses, 54, 221-235, (2000).

Ross WM, Creighton MO. Trevithick JR. Radiation cataractogenesis induced by neutron or gamma irradiation in the rat lens is reduced by vitamin E. Scannin Microsc, 4, 641-649, (1990).

Sabu MC, Kuttan R. Anti-diabetic activity of medicinal plants and its relationship with their antioxidant property. J Ethnopharmacol, 81,155-160, (2002).

Satyavati GV, Raina MK, Sharma M. Medicinal plants of India. New Delhi: Indian Council of Medical Research; (1976).

Shixian Q, VanCrey B, Shi J, Kakuda Y, Jiang Y. Green tea extract thermogenesis-induced weight loss by epigallocatechin gallate inhibition of catechol-O-methyltransferase. J Med Food, 9, 451-458, (2006).

Steigerwalt R, Gianni B, Paolo M, Bombardell E, Burki C, Schönlau F. Effects of Mirtogenol on ocular blood flow and intraocular hypertension in asymptomatic subjects. Mol Vis, 14, 1288-1292, (2008).

Suryanarayana P, Anil Kumar P, Saraswat M, Mark P, Reddy GB. Inhibition of aldose reductase by tannoid principles of Emblica officinalis: implications for the prevention of sugar cataract. Mol Vis, 10, 148-154, (2004).

Suryanarayana P, Krishnaswamy K, Reddy GB. Effect of curcumin on galactose-induced cataractogenesis in rats. Mol Vis, 9, 223-230 (2003).

Suryanarayana P, Saraswat M, Mrudula TT, Krishna TP, Krishnaswamy K, Reddy GB. Investigative Ophthalmology and Visual Science, 46, 2092-2099, (2005).

Thakur CP. Emblica officinalis reduces serum, aortic and hepatic cholesterol in rabbits. Experientia, 41, 423-424, (1985).

Truscott RJ. Age related nuclear cataract-oxidation is the key. Exp Eye Res, 80, 709-725. (2005).

Vats V, Yadav SP, Biswas NR, Grover JK. Anti-cataract activity of Pterocarpus marsupium bark and Trigonella foenum-graecum seeds extract in alloxan diabetic rats. J Ethnopharmacol, 2004, 93, 289-294.

Velpandian T, Mathur P, Sengupta S, Gupta SK. Preventive effect of Chyavanprash against steroid induced cataract in the developing chick embryo. Phytother Res, 12, 320-323. (1998).

Wu ZZ, Jiang YQ, Yi SM, Xia MT. Radix salviae miltiorrhizae in middle and late stage glaucoma. Chin Med J, 96, 445-447, (1983).

Zhu MD, Cai FY. Evidence of compromised circulation in the pathogenesis of optic nerve.

chapter 13

Chemical Entities from Traditional Medicine

R. Venkidesh, Hauzel Lalhlenmawia, Rajarajan Amirthalingam Thandavarayan and Subhash C Mandal

INTRODUCTION

The knowledge of medicinal plants has been accumulated across many centuries based on different medicinal systems such as Ayurveda, Unani and Siddha. Plants have been used in traditional medicine for cure of various ailments since thousands of years (Abu-Rabia, 2005). Medicinal and aromatic plants are local heritage of global importance (Purohit and Vyas, 2004). Total 60% of the population of world and 80% of the population in developing countries rely on traditional medicine, mostly plant drugs, for their primary health care needs (Shrestha and Dhillion, 2003). An account of 70% of the population of India (Gadgil and Rao, 1998), 80% of Pakistan (Ahmad and Ghafoor, 2002) and 80% of Nepal are dependent on traditional plant based medicines. According to the World Health Organization (WHO), nearly 80% of the world's people depend on traditional medicine for their primary healthcare needs.

There are considerable economic benefits in the development of indigenous medicines and in the use of medicinal plants for the treatment of various diseases (Azaizeh et al., 2003). The term "Complementary and Alternative Medicine" (CAM) includes various system of traditional medicinal practices like, Siddha, Unani, Ayurveda, Homoeopathy, Chinese Traditional Medicine. The commercial market estimated for the CAM is over 60 billion US $. (Samir et al., 2006).

ETHNOBIOLOGY

During the last few decades there has been an increasing interest in the study of medicinal plants and their traditional use in different parts of the world (Gazzaneo et al., 2005). Documenting the indigenous knowledge through ethnobotanical studies is important for the conservation and utilization of biological resources. Local communities still possess invaluable knowledge of plants and their uses. Large numbers of people are engaged in collection of medicinal and aromatic plants.

Ethnobiology deals in studying the traditional values of plants and animals.

Ethnomedicinal data can be collected through general conversations with the informants. Questionnaires can be framed and used to obtain information on medicinal plants with their local names, parts used treatment for, mode of preparation and administration, subsequently, the plants can be located with the help of the local informants, and herbarium copies can be prepared and can be identified for their genus and species. The information collected can be checked for any available reference in any traditional books like books on Ayurveda, Siddha, Chinese Traditional

Medicine or any books or recordings indigenous to the place of practice. Such recordings can be the good start for successful Research Projects with an appreciable commercial hit. A great number of these natural products have come to us from the scientific study of remedies traditionally employed by various cultures, most of them being plant-derived (Farnsworth and Bingel, 1997). It is cited that (Farnsworth, 1990), 74% of the chemical compounds used as drugs have the same or related use of nearly hundred plants from which they were derived.

Clinical trials in complementary and alternative medicine systems

Clinical trials are done to estimate the safety, efficacy and dosage level or dosage adjustments any needed for the new drug under investigation. Clinical trials are the main requisite for the approval of the drug in any country for the western medicine. However the need for clinical trials is foreseen for the Alternative Medicines also.

Clinical trials normally involves phase I, II and III. The objective of Phase I trial is to identify the dosage level for the newly identified chemical entity and subsequently identify the side effects in humans. For this study healthy volunteers are preferred and monitoring of untoward effects, toxicity will be on the priority. Normally a group of six to eight participants are utilised for this study and the initial doses for the participants are arrived at from the animal studies conducted earlier.

Phase II is conducted to identify the usefulness of the drug by giving to few hundreds of patients at the safe dose derived in the earlier Phase I. When there is significant safety and efficacy the drug goes for the Phase III trials.

Phase III is to confirm the drugs efficacy at different target population of different age groups. Normally this study is conducted on different ethnic groups across the globe to evaluate the safety and efficacy of the drug. The data collected from this study is used for the dose adjustments in various population and disease conditions.

The above process normally involves a span of 12-15 years and a whooping cost of US $ 900-1500 millions.

Subjecting the CAM to such phased clinical studies is not in strict practice. However few drugs like St.John's Wort, Ginko biloba have been subjected to such clinical trials. The common problem faced when doing clinical studies with CAM is that the problem with placebo preparation where in a drug like sample without effect resembling the drug to be tested has to be prepared. As there is no adequate data about the toxicity of the drug, monitoring the particular organs for toxic effects are also difficult. Also as the CAM mostly involves the dissemination of knowledge from one person to the other person without any standard scientific communication, the required clarity and openness with respect to their data for the drug utilisation normally is not available. The non availability of analytical methods in-vitro and in-vivo makes it difficult to monitor the drug in the patients at parts per billion levels. The difficulty in procuring or extracting the relatively low levels of Marker compounds present in the extracted preparation adds to tediousness in the process.

At present many reports from the British and other European Journals about the higher levels of heavy metals in the CAM cautions for the free usage of these formulations. Strict standardization of the drug if used in as such formulation in terms of the clinical utility and the analytical qualification for the active ingredients and the heavy metals becomes mandatory for bringing the CAM on par with the western medicine to the entire world.

Discovering potential therapeutic molecules

In spite of the minor setbacks with respect to utilisation of the formulations identified in the CAM at par with the western medicines, identifying potential therapeutic molecules from such formulations or the knowledge is a viable alternative.

Several works have been published in terms of integrating the Traditional Knowledge into a fruitful drug discovery Platforms. Do and Bernard has recently introduced a new phrase called "Reverse Pharmacognosy". In Reverse Pharmacognosy, the compounds are selected based on their chance to be a lead compound from any available software or by their mere functional or structural group .The chosen compounds are checked for their activity by means of Biological assays or Tests. Finally the compounds are checked for their source from the plant data base.

This Startup knowledge backed with scientific aids helps a scientist in identifying a viable Lead Molecule Discovery. The ethnobotanical knowledge once gained with a rare variety of plant with no documented evidence on any modern communication system has a relatively good project Potential to start with and can guide through a prospective Compound without any Patent Infringement. The advent of high-throughput, mechanism-based in vitro bioassays coupled with candidate plants derived from ethno biological research has resulted in the discovery of new pharmaceuticals such as "Prostratin", a drug candidate for treatment of human immunodeficiency virus.

The initial Morphological and Taxonomical screening of the identified species may further predispose a researcher to investigate on the phytochemical component present in the species of interest. The harvested plant species can be suitably extracted with the solvents and can be subjected to chromatographic separation.

In course of the extraction a suitable crystallisation technique to identify a pure or relatively pure crystal can be of considerable importance and is a requirement for Molecular Characterisation. An ideal crystallisation technique involves recrystallisation with varying ratios of polar and non polar solvents. The successful separation and identification of the Phytochemical analytes using the present day analytical techniques and instruments like HPTLC, NMR, X-Ray Crystallograph, can yield a quantum leap in one's idea of the molecule or group of the isolated compound. The structure of the compound can be extrapolated or mapped with any renowned Structure activity relationship software.

Say, the Ethnomedical data of the species of interest is of a particular antiemetic, and then the receptor mapping can be narrowed for any sub class of the 5 Hydroxytryptamine Receptors or of their related class. The positive correlation from the software can be a good project to implement for allied field of study.

The molecule can now be attempted for scale up using the preparative column chromatography for which the required plant material can be obtained either from the field or can be harnessed using tissue culture techniques.

Initially to test the activity of the Investigational Compound, Ligand Binding Assay techniques can be employed to identify the interaction or the affinity of the said compound with any protein or nucleic Acids or in specific with any enzyme moiety. Particular plant extracts exhibited selective action to a single receptor. Suitable Bio-analytical methods have to be developed at this stage to validate the outcome against the activity of the Investigational Compound. In a research work to identify the active molecules for alleviating mental disorder, approaches were made to correlate the extracts with Bioassays. The total crude extracts of selected plants were identified to have potent selectivity to various receptors, like gamma-Amino Butyric Acid (GABA), N-Methyl-D-Aspartic Acid (NMDA), and Mono Amino Oxidase (MAO), Cholecystokinin (CCK), Benzodiazepines receptors, which are associated to be involved in mental disorders. The extracts showing the highest displacement of such receptors were perceived to have potent receptor specific activity. Bioassay aided fractionation of the most active extracts resulted in pure compounds which retained the original activity of the crude extract validating the Ethnobotanical use. A bioactivity-guided fractionation of *Terminalia bellerica* fruit extract led to the isolation of several pure compounds which retained the original activity of the crude extract for CCK, and GABA receptors (Misra, 2007).

To site an another example of a bioanalytical method, specifically receptor binding study, utilised for validating the ethnobotanical knowledge of selected citing from the medicinal and scientific literature of China, South America, Asia and West Africa, the crude Extracts of the plants, *Ageratum conyzoides, Barringtonia edulis, Croton tiglium, Ipomea pescaprae, Panax ginseng, Physostigma venenosum, Sinomenium acutum, Solidago virgaurea, Symplocos leptophylla* and *Typhonium giganteum* were worked on. The extracts were prepared and tested in vitro receptor radioligand binding assays to determine whether there was an indication of biological activity, in particular their selectivity to a single receptor implicated in the mediation of pain. The three neuropeptide receptors chosen were Bradykinin (BK II), expressed in Chinese hamster ovary cells (CHO), neurokinin 1 (NK 1) expressed in astrocytoma cells, and calcitonin gene related peptide (CGRP) which were all implicated in the mediation of acute pain in the mammalian central nervous system. The results showed that there was a strong indication of biological activity for the above studied plants which are used ethnomedicinally to treat pain (Sampson et al., 2000).

The results of the particular tests if overwhelming or if the statistical treatment of the Bio-analytical technique correlates with that of the preliminary animal assay, then this can be a prospective compound for filling for Investigational New Drug (IND) Molecule. The second phase of the investigational activity involves the animal study. Toxicity and Phase I animal studies of the Investigational New Drug. The subsequent phases of clinical studies will be carried out with every positive outcome from each stage as sited in the earlier part of this chapter. The Phase IV of the clinical studies involves post-marketing surveillance to identify any untoward toxicity in the utilised patients.

To review few examples of drug developed from the natural source gained from traditional knowledge, Ziconotide, (Miljanich, 1997) a prospective research compound derived from cone snails has thousand folds higher analgesic potency than that of Morphine however the compound is devoid of all the tolerance, addiction or the related side effects associated with morphine. In another work, the skin secretions of "dendrobatid" frogs from Ecuador, and of other "poison dart" frog species in Central and South America. This work has led to the identification of a number of alkaloid toxins that bind to multiple receptors in the membranes of nerve and muscle cells. The above study leads to the discovery of a molecule by Abbot Laboratories which resulted in a prospective Morphine like compound having activity about hundred folds higher than morphine (Chivian, 2002).

Other than the traditionally valued medicines from plant origin, marine source of plants and animals are rich with traditionally valued medicinal compounds. An example for this is the sponge *Luffariella variabilis* which produces relatively large amounts of a chemical with anti-inflammatory activity known as Monoalide. It was found that monoalide inhibits the action of an enzyme called phospholipase A_2 (Carte, 1996).

Utilisation of Ethnobiology Knowledge From China

Traditional Chinese Medicine remains largely obscure to the Scientific Community. There are large Chinese Traditional Formulations for basic to higher level diseases, which involves the formulation of various crude extracts concocted to the type of ailments. The Chinese use the method of combining the drugs based on the characteristic of the drug to increase or decrease the body heat, those for the general maintenance of the body and the like.

In spite of the less knowledge of the outside world to the Chinese Medicine, the modern utilisation of "Ginseng" at present in various Pharmaceutical Formulations is an indication of the value of ethnomedical advances the country has gained. The utilisation of chemotaxonomic principles to related species of those plants used in traditional Chinese medicine has yielded an approach which can be used for the development of new drug moieties. Each herbal drug contains diverse families of chemical compounds, where each family comprises structurally related members that act with low affinity at multiple molecular targets (Nikolaus, 2006). The multicomponent, multitarget approach of traditional Chinese medicine has yielded promising drug moieties. To cite, the identification of compounds like "irisquinone" from *Iris lactea pallasii* and Zhuling polysaccharide from *Polyporus umbellate and indirubicin* (Dang et al., 1988) and their prospective utilisation in the antineoplastic therapy is overwhelming. Also further studies are in the process in the antineoplastic therapeutic segment on plants like *Cephalotaxus hainanesis* and *Camptotheca accuminata*.

In the line for identification of drugs for the ischemic heart disease, plants like *Fructus Forsythiae* and *Caulis Polygoni multiflori* has yielded active principles "Lianqiao" and "Shouwuteng" which can block the activity of the initiator caspase-8 as well as the effector caspase-3 and caspase-7 in a dose-dependent manner. In particular, activation of caspases is a critical step in neuronal apoptosis which lead to the activation of cell death programs during the ischemic stroke. Utilisation of Nuclear magnetic resonance and fluorescence assays, to identify the active principles from the aqueous extracts have been carried out (Fattorusso et al., 2006).

"Gossypol", a male contraceptive, has shown an antifertility effect in 99% of 8000 cases studied; however, hypokalemia and irreversibility of spermatogenesis were reported in some cases. Plants like *Radix Trichosanthis* and *lilac daphne terpine* are used as traditional abortifacients.

Another Chinese traditionally used plant "Muching" which has been highly effective in treating chronic bronchitis. *Salvia miltiorrhiza*, used in ancient times to activate blood circulation, is used to treat coronary artery diseases and has proved effective in 87% of angina pectoris cases are reported in literature.

Utilisation of ethnobiology knowledge from india

The utilisation of Ethnobiology knowledge in India can be evidenced by the modern Medicinal use of "Vasicine" from *Adothoda vasaica* utilized as cough suppressant and mucokinetic.The use of glycosides from the plant senna namely Sennoside groups are widely used as laxatives. Further the utility of the plants like tulsi, neem, turmeric, Sarasparilla, species of Solanum like *S.trilobatum, S.xanthocarpum* are reported traditionally. Further many terrestrial herbs like *oldenlandia, mimosa*, Shrubs and trees like *datura, ficus, terminalia, pavatta, smilex* are the few of the abundant resources sited in the traditional medicinal use. The traditional practice in India like Siddha, Ayurveda, Unani, system of medicine endorse the utilisation of the plant, mineral and animal sources for various ailments. The herbal practices are closely associated with the cultural integrity of the individual place in India. Say the Holy Basil, turmeric is culturally a sanctified species utilized in important cultural and religious practice. Plants like *Plumbago zeylanica, Hemidesmus indicus, Acorus calamus, Camellia sinensis, Terminalia chebula, Terminalia bellerica, Hollorheana antidysente-*

rica, *Lawsonia inermis*, *Mangifera indica*, *Punica granatum*, *Cichorium intybus*, *Delonix regia* traditionally merits activity.

List of Plants practiced and cited in Traditional Books

The below are the list of plants indicated in the traditional books like Guna Padam,Vaithia Thirattu, which are published several centuries back and are practiced by the local practitioners in southern India. The Botanical sources their respective indications and the constituents/Colloquial names mentioned in the below table are adopted from the book by Loganathan, N, Poorvigam Thoguppu Nool Kalangiam (Tamil), Printex Printing Imaginations, Chennai, (2007). The constituents hither to with reference indicate the source not referred in the mentioned book.

Botanical Source	Indication	Colloquial name/Constituents
Drosera burmannii *Drosera indica* *Drosera peltata*	Tuberculosis, General dibility, bronchial sputam, Asthma	Flavanoids like, Quercetin, Hyperoside
Codariocalyx motorius *(desmodium gyrans)*	Antidote for Snake poison, Skin ailments	(sun worship plant) Aminoacids,Peptides–Canavantine, Hypaphorine, Alkaloids–Bufotenine, Choline, Phenylethylamine
Spermacoce hispida *Spermacoce ocymoides* *Spermacoce decandollei* *Spermacoce pusilla*	Severe sinus, Diarrhoea, Dysentry	Ursolic Acid, beta cytosterols, D-Mannittol, calcium, Phosphorous, Iodine, Flavanoids, Isoramnidine
Anisomeles indica *Anisomeles malabarica*	Diaphoretic, Antipyretic, Skin ailments, Partial Paralysis	(Malabar catmint) Ovatodiolide, Iso-ovatodiolide
Corallocarpus epigaeus	Bloody Dysentry, Allergy, Ulcerative skin diseases	Bryonin, Glycoside
Imperata cylindrical	Tularemia, Micturition with irritation, Dysmennorohoea, Breast cancer, microlithiasis	Cylindrin, araundin, farnenol, isoarborinol, semiarenol
Tinospora sinensis, *Tinospora malabarica,* *Tinospora tomentosa,* *Tinospora cordifolia*	Antileprotic,Tuleremia, Immunomodulator, Digetive, splenomegaly, Eye ailments, Oligospermia, Tachicardia, Jaundice, Liver problems	(Moon creeper)Phenolic glycoside-Tinosinen (Yonemitsu et al., 1993)
Thespesia lampas, *Thespesia macrophylla*	Leucorrhoea, Dysmenorrhoea, Blood purifier, Syphlis, Gonorohoea, Nerve disorders, Skin ailments, Eye power enhanced & said can be used for star gazing in day light.	Quercetin, Protocatechuic acid, Gossipol
Ephedra gerardiana	Asthma, General well being, Sinusitis, Cardiac problems, For longevity of life (Ambrosia).	Ephedrine, Pseudo ephedrine

Contd. to next page.

Habenaria petalodes *Habenaria roxburghii* *Habenaria platyphylla,* *Habenaria sprengel*	Nerve tonic, Oligospermia, Aphrodisiac,	Loroglossin, Militarin, Isoquercitin, Isorhamnetin derivatives. (Betania et al., 2008)
Pouzolzia auriculata, *Pouzolzia wightii*	Urinary calculi, obstructive jaundice, boils	Ellagic acid, Betulinic acid, Quercetin, beta-cytosterol
Pleurospermum alatum	Epilepsy, paralysis	
Elephantopus scaber	Tuleremia, Urinery disorders, Neoplastic diseases	Lupeol, Stigmosterol, isodeoxylephantopin, and other terpenes
Utricularia minutissima *Utricularia bifida* *Utricularia aurea*	Wound healing, Tuleremia, Urinery diseases, treatment of boils	(common bladderwort) Tannins, Volatile oils
Diplocyclos palmatus	Constipation, Uterine problems, Leucorrohoea, Female infertility,	Punicic acid, Lecithin (Grubben, 2004)
Aristolochia tagala *Celastrus paniculatus*	Psoriasis, Epilepsy, Malarial fever Brain tonic, Leprosy, Cardiac ailment, Gastric ailments	Phenolic constituents. Alkoloids-Celestine, Paniculatin
Baliospermum montanum	Constipation, Urinery stone, Skin disorders, Asthma	Flavonoids, Tanins and steroids. (Prajakta et al., 2008)
Ampelocissus araneosa	General body coolant	Lawson
Cycas circinalis	Male infertility, oligospermia, Inflammation, Antinauseant, irritable micturition, Nerve stimulant	Glycoside-Cycasin;Methylazoxy–methanol. (Cycasin, Safety data sheet, 2008)
Artocarpus hirsutus	Acne, Inflammation, Somatocoel, Gastric Problems	Wild jack fruit
Aphanamixis polystachya	Hepato-Splenomegaly, Inflammation	LLignan-Polystachol, Lyoniside, Nudiposide. (Samir, 2006)
Coscinium fenestratum	Boils,Infection, Diabetes, Snake bite, Skin disease, Jaundice	Alkaloid-Berberine
Caralluma umbellata	Diabetes, Jaundice	Pregnane, Flavone, megastigmine, Saponin and flavonoids
Cocculus hirsutus	Diabetes, Jaundice	Beta Sitosterol, Glycoside, Sterols, Alkoloids-Shaheenine, Cohirsine (Viqaruddin, 1991)
Hybanthus enneaspermus	Leucorrhoea, Nervous dibility, Uterine problem	Triterpenes,Steroids. Alkaloids, Flavonoids. (Saxena, 1975; Majumdader et al.,1979)
Hygrophila auriculata	Diabetes, Jaundice	Mucilagenous substances, Phytosterol,Alkaloids and fixed oils
Clistanthus collinus	Antineoplastic	Clistanthin
Tribulus terrestris	Aphrodisiac, Liver enlargement	Saponin

Table: 1

List of plants practiced in traditional Indian medicine for Skin Diseases (Loganathan, 2007)

Gloriosa superba, Urgenia indica, Cuscuta reflexa, Calamus rotang, Smilax chinensis, Azadirachta indica, Pongamia glabra, Madhuca longifolia, Ricinus communis, Allium sativum.

List of plants practiced in traditional Indian medicine for Leucoderma (Loganathan, 2007)

Centella asiatica, Aegle marmelos, Andrographis paniculata, Wrightia tinctoria, Lawsonia inermis.

List of plants practiced in traditional Indian medicine for urinal stone (Loganathan , 2007)

Pavonia odorata, Zingiber officinale, Crateva manga, Tribulus terrestris, Aerva lanata, Hygrophila auriculata, Musa paradisiaca.

List of plants practiced in traditional Indian medicine for Piles (Loganathan, 2007)

Solanum trilobatum, Hygrophila auriculata, Cynodon dactylum, Marsilea quadrifolia, Vitis quadrangularis, Amorphophallus campanulatus, Sansevieria roxburghiana, Draconitum polyphyllum.

List of plants practiced in traditional Indian medicine for Bile stones (Loganathan, 2007)

Boerhaavia diffusa, Achyranthes aspera, Ocimum sanctum, Aloe barbadensis, Crataeva magna, Premna tomentosa, Wedelia chinensis.

CONCLUSION

Traditional medicine as such is being brought to the scrutiny of Modern methods of Instrumental analysis. Considerable views on the presence of heavy metals in the traditional preparation are taken up by regulatory authorities. Many compounds and preparation of traditional medicine are finding their entry into modern pharmacopoeias after a strict regulatory scrutiny.

Ethnopharmacological information can be used as a general indicator of non-specific bioactivity suitable for screening and high-resolution bioassays other than the discovery of a New Chemical Entity. Indigenous ethnomedical traditions are rapidly disappearing. To preserve indigenous discoveries and make them accessible and useful to Western medicine, collaboration is required between linguistically sophisticated Ethnobotanists, Pharmacognosists, Synthetic Chemist, Molecular Modeling Personnel and Pharmacologists. Preserving the cultural tradition and values of native people facilitates the discovery of new compounds and information to the modern medicine.

REFERENCES

Abu-Rabia A. Urinary diseases and ethnobotany among pastoral nomads in the Middle East. *J Ethnobiol Ethnomed.* 1, 4, (2005).

Ahmad Z, Ghafoor A. Resource Base and Conservation Strategies of MAPs in Pakistan. In *Sharing Local and National Experience in Conservation of Medicinal and Aromatic Plants in South Asia* Edited by: Bhattarai N, Karki M. HMGN, IDRC and MAPPA, 105-109, (2002).

Azaizeh H, Fulder S, Khalil K, Said O. Ethnomedicinal knowledge of local Arab practitioners in the Middle East Region. *Fitoterapia,* 74, 98-108, (2003).

Betania BC, Alvicler M; Adrino MCP Ezequinas PS, Tana MAA, Carlos LZ, Chemical Constituents of Habenaria petalodes Lindl, J Braz. Chem. Soc. vol.19 no. 6Sao Paulo 2008.

Carte BK. Biomedical potential of marine natural products. *BioScience,* 46, 271-286, (1996).

Chivian E. *Biodiversity: Its Importance to Human Health:* Center for Health and the Global Environment. Harvard Medical School, (2002).

Cycasin safety Data Sheet, Div. of OHS, NIH; http://dohs.ors.od.nih.gov/pdf/cycasin.

Dang Gui LHW, Jui H. Traditional Chinese medicine and the search for new antineoplastic drugs. *J Ethnopharmacol,* 24, 1-17, (1988).

Farnsworth NR. The role of ethnopharmacology in drug development. In *Bioactive Compounds from Plants*. Edited by: Anonymous. Ciba Foundation Symposium 154. Wiley Interscience, New York, 2-1, (1990).

Farnsworth NR, Bingel AS. Problems and prospects of discovering new drugs from higher plants by pharmacological screening. In *New Natural Products and Plant Drugs with Pharmacological, Biological or Therapeutic Activity.* Edited by: Wagner H Wolff P. Berlin: Springer, 1-22, (1997).

Fattorusso S, Frutos X, Sun NJ, Sucher M. Traditional Chinese medicines with caspase-inhibitory activity. *Phytomedicine*, 13, 16-22, (2006).

Gadgil M, Rao PRS. Nurturing Biodiversity: An Indian Agenda. Center for Environment Education, Ahamadabad, India, (1998).

Gazzaneo LR, Paiva de Lucena RF, Paulino de Albuquerque U. Knowledge and use of medicinal plants by local specialists in an region of Atlantic Forest in the state of Pernambuco (Northeastern Brazil). *J Ethnobiol Ethnomed* 1, 9, (2005).

Grubben GJH, Plant Resources of Tropical Africa, Backhuys Publishers, (2004).

Loganathan N, Poorvigam Thoguppu Nool Kalangiam (Tamil), Printex Printing Imaginations, Chennai, (2007).

Majumder PL, Basu A, Mal D. Chemical constituents of Hybanthus enneaspermus F. Muell (Violaceae). Indian Journal of Chemistry Section B 17, 297-298, (1979).

Miljanich GP. Venom peptides as human pharmaceuticals. *Sci Med*, 4, 6-15, (1997).

Misra R. Modern drug development from traditional medicinal plants using radioligand receptor-binding assays. Methods Find Exp Clin Pharmacol, 29, 79-92, (2007).

Nikolaus. Insights from molecular investigations of traditional Chinese herbal stroke medicines: Implications for neuroprotective epilepsy therapy. *J. Sucher. Epilepsy & Behavior,* 8, 350-362, (2006).

Prajakta VD, Raju RW, Girish HK, Kalpana SP, Free radical Scavanging activity of aqueous Extract of Roots of *Baliospermum montanum* Muell-Arg, *IJGP*, Vol. 2, 31-33, (2008).

Purohit SS, Vyas SP. Medicinal Plant Cultivation: A Scientific Approach. Agrobois, India. 624, (2004).

Samir M, Nusrat S, Promila P, Clinical Research,Ind-Swift, Chandigarh (2006).

Samir KS, Panadda P, ShahabuddinM, Takashi O, Masami I, A new lignin from *Aphanamixis polystachya, J of Natural Medicines*, 60, pp. 258-260, (2006).

Sampson JH, Phillipson JD, Bowery NG, Neill MJ, Houston JG, Lewis JA. Ethnomedicinally selected plants as sources of potential analgesic compounds: indication of in vitro biological activity in receptor binding assays. *Phytother Res,* 14, 9-24, (2000).

Saxena HO. A survey of the plants of Orissa (India) for tannins, saponins, flavonoids and alkaloids, Lioydia 38, 346-374, (1975).

Shrestha PM, Dhillion SS: Medicinal Plant Diversity and Use in the Highlands of Dolakha District, Nepal. *J Ethnopharm* 2003, 86:81-96, (2003).

Viquaruddin A, Tahir R, Shaista I, Coohirsine an alkaloid from cocculus hirsutus, Phytochemistry 62, 8-157, (1991).

chapter 14

Role of Garlic on Cardio-vascular Disorders: A New Look of an Old Healing Herb

Sanjay K. Banerjee

INTRODUCTION

In recent years, there has been growing interest in garlic for cardiovascular health. Garlic acquired a reputation in the folklore of many cultures over centuries as a formidable prophylactic and therapeutic medicinal agent. Garlic has attracted particular attention of modern medicine because of its widespread health use around the world, and the cherished belief that it helps in maintaining good health warding off illnesses and providing more vigor. In USA, one study used the 2002 National Health Interview Survey and analyzed data on complementary and alternative medicine (CAM) use in 10,572 respondents with cardiovascular disease (Gloria et al., 2006). Among those with cardiovascular disease, 36% had used CAM (excluding prayer) in the previous 12 months. The most commonly used therapies were herbal products (18%) and among herbs, garlic was most commonly used. To date, many favorable experimental and clinical effects of garlic preparations, including garlic extract, have been reported. These biological responses have been largely attributed to i) reduction of risk factors for cardiovascular diseases and cancer, ii) stimulation of immune function, iii) enhanced detoxification of foreign compound, iv) hepatoprotection, v) antimicrobial effect and vi) antioxidant effect. This chapter has been made indicating an overall view of the efficacy of garlic in cardiovascular disease conditions both in human and animals. Cardiovascular disease is associated with multiple factors such as raised serum total cholesterol, raised LDL and an increase in LDL oxidation, Inhibition of fibrinolytic activity, increased platelet aggregation, hypertension, arrhythmia and decrease myocardial endogenous antioxidants or increased oxidative stress. The role of garlic in reducing each risk factor is described here.

HISTORICAL PERSPECTIVE OF GARLIC

It is fascinating to observe how cultures that never came into contact with one another came to the same conclusions about the role of garlic in health and disease. If folk wisdom is not ignored, it may teach us valuable lessons. Some of the earliest references to this medicinal and culinary plant are found on Sumerian clay tablets dating from 2600–2100 BC. Garlic was an important medicine to the ancient Egyptians listed in the medical text *Codex Ebers* (ca. 1550 BC) specially for the working class involved in heavy labor (Lawson, 1998). There is evidence that during the earliest Olympics in Greece, garlic was fed to the athletes for increasing stamina (Lawson, 1998). The leading Indian ancient medical text, *Charaka-Samhita* recommends garlic for the treatment of heart disease and arthritis for over many centuries. In modern era scientists have been trying to validate many of these properties of garlic, specially in terms of the identity of the active components, their mechanisms of action and exploring the potential benefits as food supplements.

ATHEROSCLEROSIS AND LIPID METABOLISM

Atherosclerosis is a complex disease, characterized by an excessive inflammatory, fibro-fatty, proliferative response to damage of the artery wall involving several cell types, particularly smooth muscle cells, monocyte-derived macrophages, T-lymphocyte and platelets (Schwartz et al., 1993). Hyperlipidemia constitutes a major etiopathological factor for atherosclerosis. The medicinal value of garlic is best known for its lipid lowering and antiatherogenic effects.

Animal Studies

Several groups of investigators studied the effects of long term (2–9 months) feeding of garlic and garlic preparations (2% garlic powder in diet) on experimental atherosclerosis induced by a high-cholesterol diet in rabbits (Banerjee and Maulik, 2002). Most of these studies reported a statistically significant reduction in atheromatous lesions, particularly in the aorta, that averaged about 50%. The chronic effects of garlic on lipid metabolism in rats were also encouraging. The duration of these studies was at least 4 weeks. Garlic (1–4% in diet) and garlic protein administration in hypercholesterolemic rats induced by a high-cholesterol diet, significantly reduced serum cholesterol, triglyceride and LDL cholesterol (Banerjee and Maulik, 2002) but there was no effect on serum HDL. Total lipid content and cholesterol levels in liver were also decreased in rat after chronic garlic consumption. Abramoviz et al. (1999) investigated the effect of allicin as an active component of garlic on the formation of fatty streaks in aorta and lipid profile in mice (Abramovitz et al., 1999). While no significant differences were observed between blood lipid profiles, the microscopic evaluation of formation of fatty streaks in the aortic sinus showed that values for mice in the allicin treated groups were significantly lower by nearly 50%. Aged garlic extract 'Kyolic' also significantly inhibited the development of thickened, lipid-filled lesions in the preformed neointimas produced by balloon-catheter injury of the right carotid artery in cholesterol-fed rabbits (Efendy et al., 1997; Campbell et al., 2001).

Human Studies

Since 1975 there have been more than 46 (from medline search) human studies on lipid-lowering effects of garlic and garlic preparations. These studies, were mostly randomized, double blind, placebo-controlled using garlic powder rather than raw gàrlic of 4–16 weeks, in hyperlipidemic patients. Most of these studies showed significant decrease in serum cholesterol and serum triglyceride. Only about one-third of these studies measured lipoproteins, where significant favorable changes in LDL-cholesterol level (11–26% decrease) were consistently observed. A few studies using garlic powder (having low allicin yields) failed to show any lipid lowering effects. During the last one decade (1993–2002), 18 clinical studies have been published regarding the hypolipedemic effect of garlic. Nine studies showed negative results and garlic powder was used in seven of these studies (Banerjee and Maulik, 2002). The different composition and quantity of sulfur components of different garlic preparations used in various studies could account for the inconsistent findings. It highlights the need for standardization of different garlic preparations and to arrive at a valid conclusion. Other factors might include the subject recruitment, duration of study, dietary control, lifestyle and methods of lipid analyses (Silagy and Neil; 1994; Warshafsky et al., 1993). Four meta-analysis of randomized, placebo-controlled human studies on hypocholesterolemic effects of garlic are available. The analyses further detected that the extent of cholesterol-lowering properties of garlic differed markedly from one study to another. Warshafsky and his colleagues deduced from five randomized clinical trials that hypercholesterolemic patients treated with garlic had a mean plasma cholesterol concentration, that was 9% lower than that of patients treated with placebo (Warshafsky et al., 1993). Silagy and Neil (1994) analyzed sixteen trials, with data from 952 subjects in the meta-analysis (Silagy and Neil, 1994). Garlic, in powder and non-powder form, significantly lowered serum lipid levels over a 1–3 month period. Serum cholesterol fell by 8% with dried powder preparations and 15% with non-powder preparations. Serum triglyceride level also dropped significantly, while HDL-cholesterol was essentially unchanged. Amongst the garlic powder preparations these effects appeared to be similar across the daily dose range of 600–900 mg. Another meta-analysis (Neil et al., 1996) revealed that there was no significant difference in the mean concentrations of serum lipids, lipoproteins or apo A1 or B amongst the groups receiving garlic (900 mg/day of dried garlic powder standardized to 1.3% allicin) and placebo. In this meta-analysis, garlic was less effective in reducing total cholesterol than suggested by previous meta-analyses. However, in a more recent meta-analysis of thirteen trials (Stevinson et al., 2000), garlic reduced total cholesterol level from baseline significantly more than placebo, while six dietcontrolled trials with the highest scores for methodological quality revealed a nonsignificant difference between garlic and placebo groups. The available data suggests that garlic is superior to placebo in reducing total cholesterol levels. However, the size of the effect is modest, and the robustness of the effect is debatable. Therefore, the hypocholesterolemic effect of garlic remains to be firmly established. In contrast, cardiovascular calcification (CAC), a marker of atherosclerosis, is inhibited by garlic. A recent small pilot study showed that, compared with placebo, AGE may inhibit the rate of progression of CAC in the general population (Budoff et al., 2004).

Possible Mechanism/s

Protective effect of garlic on atherosclerosis has been attributed to its capacity to reduce lipid content in arterial wall. Garlic causes direct antiatherogenic (preventive) and antiatherosclerotic (causing regression) effects at the level of artery wall (Orekhov and Grunwald, 1997). Garlic depressed the hepatic activities of lipogenic and cholesterogenic enzymes such as malic enzyme, fatty acid synthase, glucose-6 phosphate dehydrogenase and 3-hydroxy-3-methyl-glutaryl-CoA (HMG CoA) reductase (Yu-Yan and Liu, 2001). Garlic also increased the excretion of cholesterol, as manifested by enhanced excretion of acidic and neutral steroids after garlic feeding (Banerjee and Maulik, 2002). LDL isolated from human subjects given AGE and aqueous garlic extract (Lewin and Popov, 1994) was found to be significantly more resistant to oxidation. These data indicate that suppressed LDL oxidation may be one of the powerful mechanisms accounted for the benefits of garlic in atherosclerosis. Allicin was identified as the active compound responsible for antiatherosclerotic effect. Allicin affect atherosclerosis not only by acting as an antioxidant, but also by other mechanisms, such as lipoprotein modification and inhibition of LDL uptake and degradation by macrophages (Cohen et al., 2005). Other *in vitro* studies revealed that water-soluble organosulfur compounds, especially S-allyl cysteine (SAC), present in aged garlic extract and diallyl-di-sulfide (DADS), present in garlic oil are also potent inhibitors of cholesterol synthesis (Yu-Yan and Liu, 2001; Gebhardt R, Beck, 1996). Inhibition of blood vessel calcification might be another promising mechanism of anti-atherosclerotic effect of garlic (Budoff et al., 2004).

Fibrinolytic Activity

Inhibition of fibrinolytic activity (FA) or deficiency of the factors involved might upset the hemostatic balance and allow excessive fibrin deposition. In diabetes, hypertension and hypercholesterolemia, it is possible that disturbance in the coagulation-fibrinolytic system may be an important factor leading to the development of thrombosis and ischemia. Accordingly, the greater the FA, the more favorable is the antithrombic effect. FA is generally determined by euglobulin lysis time. The patients who died with acute or old myocardial infarction showed the highest values of plasma fibrinogen, euglobulin lysis time and antiplasmin. This suggests that prognosis in myocardial infarction is partly influenced by the degree to which plasma fibrinolysis is impaired (Rodger et al., 1972).

Animals Studies

Marked rise in blood coagulability of rabbits that followed 3 months of cholesterol feeding (0.2 g/kg/day) was significantly reduced by the essential oils of garlic. Fibrinolytic activity was actually increased even above the normal control levels. The essential oils of garlic (equivalent to 1 g/kg/day of raw bulbs) proved effective in mediating fibrinolytic activity (Bordia et al., 1975). Experimental study also revealed that garlic juice (raw garlic; 250 mg/day) had significant effect in enhancing the fibrinolytic activity in rabbit after receiving a cholesterol rich diet for 13 weeks (Sainani et al., 1979). The plasma fibrinolytic activity in rabbit, which was decreased on cholesterol feeding, was considerably increased when this diet was supplemented with garlic (Mirhadi et al., 1991).

Human Studies

Almost all human studies on fibrinolytic activity of garlic have been found to have positive effect. Acute as well as chronic intake of garlic oil and raw garlic increased fibrinolytic activity (FA). In 1975, Bordia first demonstrated that garlic oil increased FA after 3 hours of administration. Bordia also reported that chronic (3 weeks to 3 months) administration of garlic oil (dose: equivalent to 1 gm/kg of fresh garlic) increased FA significantly ranging from 36% to 130% in healthy as well as acute myocardial infarction patients (Banerjee and Maulik, 2002). Dried garlic powder has been also tested for its fribinolytic activity. While two studies (Lutomski, 1984; Luley et al., 1986) showed no difference in FA, one study (Legnani et al., 1993) showed increased FA as well as tissue plasminogen activator activity after acute and chronic garlic powder intake. Chutani and Bordia (1981) designed one study to show that both raw and fried garlic significantly enhance FA (Sainani et al., 1979). Frying removes the strong acrid smell of garlic, but preserves it useful effects on FA. The rise in FA has been observed within 6 hours of garlic administration, which showed that garlic has a rapid onset of action and the effect is well maintained as long as garlic is being taken. Recently Bordia (1998) found that intake (3 months) of ethyl acetate extract of crushed raw garlic also increased FA (Bordia et al., 1998).

Platelet Aggregation

Platelet aggregation superimposed on an atherosclerosis vessel is an antecedent event causing total blockage of blood flow leading to myocardial infarction and thromboembolic diseases. Platelets adhere to the exposed collagen, laminin and von Willebrand factor in the injured vessel wall. This process is called platelet activation. Activation can also be produced by ADP and thrombin. The activated platelets change shape, put out pseudopodia, discharge their granules, and stick to other platelets, initiating the process of platelet aggregation. Aggregation is also fostered by platelet activating factor (PAF), a cytokine secreted by neutrophil and monocytes as well as platelets (Harfenist et al., 2000). Studies have shown that garlic has great potential in inhibiting platelet aggregation.

Animal Studies

Pretreatment of rabbits with an aqueous extract of garlic (500 mg/kg) significantly inhibited thromboxane-B2 (TXB2) synthesis (a potent platelet aggregator) and protected against thrombocy-topenia induced by collagen or arachidonate infusion. These observations indicate that garlic may be beneficial in the prevention of thrombosis (Ali et al., 1990). Aqueous extract of garlic was found to inhibit platelet aggregation induced by ADP, epinephrine, collagen and arachidonate in a dose-dependent manner *in vitro* and inhibited biosynthesis of prostacyclin in rat aorta (Srivastava, 1984). A dose-dependent inhibition of cyclooxygenase activity and collagen-induced platelet aggregation was observed in rabbit platelets treated with raw garlic *in vitro*. The concentration required for 50% inhibition of the platelet aggregation for garlic was calculated to be approximately 6.6 mg/ml plasma. But boiled garlic was found to be of little effect. This finding indicates that garlic may be beneficial in the prevention of thrombosis if ingested raw rather in a cooked form (Ali, 1995). Garlic extract containing diallyl disulfide and diallyl trisulfide, prevented acute platelet thrombus formation in stenosed canine coronary arteries (Laurence and John, 1989). Fresh garlic extract is effective in reducing thromboxane formation by platelets both *in vivo* and *in vitro* animal models of thrombosis. It was observed that garlic inhibits thrombin-induced platelet synthesis of TXB2 in a dose-and time-dependent manner in rabbits. Maximum inhibition of TXB2 occurred between 0.5 h and 6 h at 25 and 100 mg/kg garlic. The rapid recovery of platelet cyclooxygenase activity after infusion of a single dose of garlic suggests that garlic should be taken more frequently in order to achieve beneficial effects in the prevention of thrombosis (Thomson et al., 2000). Garlic was also capable of delaying hyperthermia-induced platelet aggregation in mouse pial arterioles, *in vivo*, which was comparable to acetyl salicylic acid (el-Sabban and Radwan, 1997). Ajoene, a constituent of essential oil of garlic, has been shown to inhibit *in vitro* platelet aggregation in different species of animals i.e. cow, dog, guinea-pig, horse, monkey, pig, rabbit and rat (Apitz-Castro et al., 1986). Under *in vivo* flow conditions and in the presence of physiological calcium levels, ajoene prevented thrombus formation induced by severe vascular damage, mainly in arterial sites with local low shear stress (Apitz-Castro et al., 1994). Makheja and Bailey (1990) identified three main antiplatelet constituents, namely adenosine, allicin and polysulfides in garlic. Adenosine and allicin both inhibited platelet aggregation without affecting cyclooxygenase and lipoxygenase metabolites of arachidonic acid. The polysulfides inhibited platelet aggregation as well as thromboxane synthesis. The observed *in vivo* antiplatelet effects of ingesting garlic are attributable more to adenosine than to allicin and polysulfide constituents.

Human Studies

In human studies a positive response to garlic has been observed. Like enhancement of fibrinolysis, garlic also has a beneficial effect on platelet adhesion or aggregation in human. Bordia (1978) first showed the dosedependent inhibition of platelet aggregation by garlic. Raw garlic, garlic oil and other extract of garlic have been shown to inhibit platelet aggregation in *in vitro* induced by ADP, collagen, arachidonate, epinephrine and calcium ionophore (Banerjee and Maulik, 2002). Single dose as well as chronic intake of garlic powder and garlic oil also inhibits platelet aggregation (Banerjee and Maulik, 2002).

Possible Mechanism/s

The antiplatelet mechanism of garlic is much more established than its any other biological effects. Aqueous extract of garlic inhibited platelet aggregation induced by ADP, collagen, arachidonate, epinephrine and calcium ionophore A23187 in a dose-dependent manner (Srivastava, 1986). It was found that garlic reduced the formation of thromboxane, inhibited the phospholipase activity and lipoxygenase products formed in platelets. These effects may explain, in part, inhibition of platelet aggregation. Further, since garlic was also effective in inhibiting aggregation induced by calcium ionophore A23187 it may be suggested that the antiaggregation effect may be related to intraplatelet mobilization of calcium. Inhibition of epinephrine-induced aggregation by garlic extract may suggest that it may be inhibiting uptake of calcium into platelets thereby lowering cytosolic calcium concentrations (Srivastava, 1986).

In regard to a specific mechanism of ajoene's antiplatelet action, several suggestions have been made. Ajoene strongly inhibits the metabolism of arachidonic acid by both cyclooxygenase and lipoxygenase pathways (Srivastava and Tyagi, 1993), thus inhibiting the synthesis of thromboxane A2 and 12-HETE. Antiaggregatory effect of ajoene may also be causally related to its direct interaction with the putative fibrinogen receptor (GPIIb/IIa) (Apitz-Castro et al., 1986). The studies of Jamaluddin et al. (1988) demonstrated that ajoene interacts with a purified hemoprotein implicated in platelet activation. Ajoene modifies the binding of the hemoprotein with ligands deemed to be physiologically relevant as effectors. Allicin inhibits human platelet aggregation in vitro without affecting cyclooxygenase or thromboxane synthase activity or cyclic adenosine monophosphate (AMP) levels. Allicin also inhibits platelet aggregation but does not alter the activity of vascular prostacyclin synthase. However, it inhibits ionophore A23187-stimulated human neutrophil lysosomal enzyme release. Thus garlic appears to be in possession of components which might exert their effects at various stages involved in the process of platelet aggregation.

Blood pressure lowering effect

A general definition of hypertension is a systolic blood pressure (SBP) of 140 mm Hg or higher or a diastolic blood pressure (DBP) of 90 mm Hg or higher or both. Prevention and proper management of hypertension decreases the incidence of related morbidity and mortality. A downward shift of 3 mm Hg in SBP decreases the mortality from stroke by 8% and from ischemic heart disease by 5% (Joint National Committee, 1993). Life style modification are definitive therapy for some and adjunctive therapy for all persons with hypertension (Joint National Committee, 1997). Diets that are high in fruits, vegetables and low-fat dairy products; have been shown to reduce hypertension. Increased consumption of garlic is associated with lower incidence of hypertension in population. Based on current information, garlic powder preparations are considered for recommendation as adjuncts in the treatment of hypertensive patients (Schulz et al., 2001).

Animal Studies

In experimental animals, intravenous injection of garlic extracts produced slight reductions in both systolic and diastolic pressures (Rashid and Khan, 1985). Oral administration of garlic reduced experimentally induced hypertension, bringing blood pressure back to the normal range. For example 2.5 to 25 mg per kg of alcoholic garlic extract reduced blood pressure by 10 to 50 mm Hg (Chanderkar and Jain, 1993). Blood pressure in dogs has been significantly reduced for several hours following intragastric administration of a small dose of garlic powder (as low as 2.5 mg/kg b.wt) (Pantoja et al., 1991). Other animal experiments on rats and dogs also indicate a 'normalizing' effect of garlic on elevated blood pressure (Banerjee and Maulik, 2002). The antihypertensive effect of garlic in these studies has been repeatedly confirmed.

Allicin, a major constituent of garlic, was also evaluated for its antihypertensive effects. Chronic oral administration of allicin lowered blood pressure in hypertensive rats (Ali et al., 2000). Allicin also caused pulmonary vasodilatation in isolated lung of rat (Kaye et al., 2000). Single as well as multiple doses of aqueous garlic extract reduced thromboxane B2 and prostaglandin E2 level and thereby reduced hypertension in '2 kidney 1-clip' model of hypertension in rat (Al-Qattan et al., 2001). Garlic also inhibited endothelin-1 induced contraction in a dose-dependent manner in isolated rat pulmonary arteries (Kim-Park and Ku, 2000).

Garlic (100 mg/kg) administration for 5 days resulted in a complete inhibition of acute hypoxic pulmonary vasoconstriction in rat (Fallon et al., 1998). There was a marked decrease in systolic blood pressure in spontaneously hypertensive rats after oral administration of single dose of garlic (Foushee et al., 1982). Prolongation of life span was also found in hypertensive rats by dietary supplementation with garlic (Brandle et al., 1997).

Human Studies

Leoper and DeBray recognized the hypotensive effect of garlic in 1921 (Leoper and DeBray, 1921). Damrau (1941) has reviewed the earlier literature, including his own investigations on 26 patients. Blood pressure reduction was observed in 85% of the patients, the average decline being 12.3 mm Hg systolic (SBP) and 6.5 mm Hg diastolic (DBP) blood pressure, over one-quarter of the subjects experienced a decline in SBP of 20 mm Hg or more. Piotrowski (1948) has reviewed some of the early clinical studies in which garlic was administered under controlled conditions to hypertensive patients. Two-fifths of 100 patients exhibited a 20 mm Hg or greater decline in SBP generally within 1 week after initiation of treatment with 0.6 to 1.2 g daily of dialyzed, alcoholic garlic extract.

Studies with a dried garlic powder (Kwai tablets) showed an average decrease in blood pressure of about 9% with 0.6 g garlic powder per day (Konig and Scineider, 1986) and in a randomized double blind trial, a beneficial effect of garlic on blood pressure and blood lipids in mildly hypertensive subjects was demonstrated (Auer et al., 1989). Those reports point in the same direction, that garlic can be useful in the control of mild hypertension in many if not all cases. Pektov (1979) has also cited several studies, mostly from the Soviet Union and Bulgaria, which indicate that garlic and its extracts exhibit antihypertensive activity. Besides subjective improvement, the results of these studies indicated a moderate hypotensive effect involving a drop in SBP of 20–30 mm Hg and in DBP of 10–20 mm Hg. Another study in China (1986) on 70 hypertensive patients who were given garlic oil equivalent to 50 gm of raw garlic/day, 47 patients showed moderate to marked reduction in blood pressure (Zheziang Institute of Traditional Chinese Medicine, 1986). There is only one meta-analysis done by Silagy and Neil (1994). Eight trials were identified all using the same dried garlic powder preparation (Kwai). Data from 415 subjects were included in the analysis. Only three trials were specifically conducted in hypertensive subjects. Of the seven trials that compared the effect of garlic with that of placebo, three showed a significant reduction in systolic blood pressure (SBP) and four in diastolic blood pressure (DBP). The overall pooled mean difference in the absolute change (from baseline to final measurement) of SBP was greater in the subjects who were treated with garlic than in those treated with placebo. For DBP the corresponding reduction in the garlic-treated subjects was slightly smaller. This meta-analysis suggest that this "garlic powder preparation may be of some clinical use in subjects with mild hypertension". However, there is still insufficient evidence to recommend it as a routine clinical therapy for the treatment of hypertensive subjects. More rigorously designed and analyzed trials are needed for firm conclusion.

Possible Mechanism/s

Rashid and Khan (1985) have postulated that mechanism of antihypertensive action of garlic is due to its prostaglandin like effects, which decreases peripheral vascular resistance. The gamma-glutamylcysteines are the compounds in garlic that may lower blood pressure, as indicated by their ability to inhibit angiotensin-converting enzyme in *in vitro* (Sendl et al., 1992). Garlic modulates the production and function of both endothelium derived relaxing and constricting factors and this may contribute to its protective effect against hypoxic pulmonary vasoconstriction (Kim-Park and Ku, 2000). Garlic elicits nitric-oxide-dependent relaxation in pulmonary arteries. This hypothesis was explained by the fact that NG-nitro-L-arginine methyl ester (L-NAME, a NOS inhibitor) abolished the vasodilatory effect of garlic (Fallon et al., 1998; Kim-Park and Ku, 2000). But another study reported that pulmonary vasodilatory effect of allicin are independent of the synthesis of NO, ATP-sensitive (K+) channel, activation of cyclooxygenase enzyme (Kaye et al., 2000).

Diabetes Mellitus

Diabetes mellitus is a group of diseases characterized by high blood glucose levels resulting from defects in insulin secretion, insulin action, or both. Abnormalities in the metabolism of carbohydrate, protein, and fat are also present (Granner et al., 2000). Nutrition plays a primary role to control blood glucose level and further complication.

Animal Studies

Garlic was effective in reducing blood glucose in streptozotocin-induced as well as alloxan-induced diabetes mellitus in rats and mice. Most of the studies showed that garlic can reduce blood glucose level in diabetic mice, rats, and rabbit (Banerjee and Maulik, 2002). Augusti & Sheela consistently showed that S-allyl cysteine sulfoxide (alliin), a sulfur containing amino acid in garlic (200 mg/kg b.wt.) has a potential to reduce diabetic condition in rat almost to the same extent as did glibenclamide and insulin (Augusti and Sheela, 1996). Treatment of diabetic rats with garlic oil decreased serum acid and alkaline phosphatase, serum alanine and asparate transferases, as well as serum amylase in diabetic rats (Ohaeri, 2001). Aged garlic extract is also effective to prevent adrenal hypertrophy, hyperglycemia and elevation of corticosterone in hyperglycemic mice induced by immobilization stress (Kasuga et al., 1999). Garlic intake (6.25% by weight in diet) for 12 days reduced hyperphagia and polydipsia but did not alter hyperglycemia and hypoinsulinaemia in streptozotocin-induced diabetic mice (Swanston-Flatt et al., 1990). Ingestion of garlic juice resulted in better utilization of glucose in glucose tolerance test performed in rabbits (Mathew and Augusti, 1973). The ethyl alcohol, petroleum ether and ethyl ether extracts of garlic produced a significant fall in blood sugar levels in rabbits (Jain and Vyas, 1975). Allicin at a dose of 250 mg/kg is 60% as effective as tolbutamide in alloxan-induced diabetic rabbit (Mathew and Augusti, 1973).

Human Studies

Hypoglycemic effect of garlic in human is not well studied. Chronic feeding of garlic oil and garlic powder showed significant decrease in blood glucose level whereas some other studies (Bordia et al., 1998; Kiesewetter et al., 1991; Banerjee and Maulik, 2002) showed no change of blood glucose level. All human studies, except one or two, showing effect of garlic on blood glucose level on normal healthy individuals but not in diabetic patients. Thus the role of garlic in diabetic condition is yet to be confirmed.

Possible Mechanism/s

Though the exact mechanism/s of garlic as antidiabetic agent is still not clear but *invivo* (Patumraj et al., 2000; Mathew and Augusti, 1973) as well as *invitro* (Augusti and Sheela, 1996) studies showed that garlic acts as an insulin secretagogue in diabetic rats. Augusti & Sheela also proposed that antioxidant effect of S-allyl cysteine sulfoxide (isolated product from garlic) may also contribute for its beneficial effect in diabetes (Augusti and Sheela, 1996). Another proposed mechanism is due to spare insulin from sulphydryl group. Inactivation of insulin by sulphydryl group is a common phenomenon. Garlic (allicin) can effectively combine with compounds like cysteine and enhance serum insulin (Mathew and Augusti, 1973). Jain & Vyas proposed that garlic can act as an antidiabetic agent by increasing either the pancreatic secretion of insulin from the beta cells or its release from bound insulin (Jain and Vyas, 1975).

Antioxidant Effects

Oxidative stress plays a pathological role in the development of heart failure. Oxidative stress caused specific morphological changes of mitochondria, excess formation of superoxide (O_2^-), reduction of ATP, and transcriptional alterations of genes associated with heart failure in respect to cardiac contractility. Administration of antioxidants or agents which mimic cardiac endogenous antioxidants may reduce the progression of heart failure (Hill and Singal, 1996). The beneficial effect of garlic in heart might be partly through its antioxidant activity.

Animal Studies

Garlic extracts and its component have direct free radical scavenging activity as shown by different invitro studies (Banerjee et al., 2003). LDL isolated from allicin-treated (one component of raw garlic extract) groups was more resistant to $CuSO_4$ induced oxidation than LDL isolated from control mice (Gonen et al., 2005). Incubation of mouse plasma with (3)H-labeled allicin showed binding of allicin to lipoproteins. Raw garlic homogenate augmented endogenous antioxidants along with reduction of basal lipid peroxidation in rat heart, liver and kidney in a dose dependent manner (Banerjee et al., 2002; Banerjee et al., 2001). Aged garlic extract (AGE) also exerted its antioxidant action by scavenging reactive oxygen species (Imai, 1994) and enhancing the cellular antioxidants, like reduced glutathione, superoxide dismutase, catalase and glutathione peroxidase of vascular endothelial cells (Wei and Lau, 1998). Augmented endogenous antioxidants on heart and endothelial cells have important direct cytoprotective effects, especially in the event of oxidant stress induced injury.

Recently, in our laboratory, we found that chronic oral administration of garlic homogenate protected rat heart from *in vitro* ischemic reperfusion injury (Banerjee et al., 2002a) and oxidative stress induced by single dose of adriamycin (Mukherjee et al., 2003) and isoproterenol (Banerjee et al., 2003b). AGE has been shown to offer protection against the cardiotoxic effects of doxorubicin, an antineoplastic agent used in cancer therapy (Kojima et al., 1994). Feeding of garlic powder in rats for 11 days had a protective effect on isoproterenol-induced myocardial damage (Ciplea and Richter, 1988). Aqueous garlic extract was also found to be effective in reducing Cu (+)-initiated oxidation of low density lipoprotein (LDL) as measured by photochemiluminescence method (Lewin and Popov, 1994). AGE also protected vascular endothelial cells from H_2O_2-induced oxidant injury (Yamasaki and Lau, 1997).

Human Studies

One human study show that ingestion of garlic leads to significantly lowered plasma and erythrocyte MDA (a byproduct of lipid peroxidation) levels and to increased activities of some antioxidant enzymes, which indicates that consumption of garlic decreases oxidation reactions (Avci et al., 2008). Another human study suggests that garlic preparation may be tentatively used as an adjunct agent in treatment of arterial hypertension because of its hypolipemic and antioxidant properties (Duda et al., 2008). It is quite possible that increased endogenous antioxidants and reduced peroxidation processes due to garlic consumption may play a part in some of the beneficial effects of garlic in elderly subjects and might be true for all other organ as suggested in experimental studies (Banerjee et al., 2003). One case study from Nepal reported that garlic (9 months treatment) prevented heart failure of a 50 year old breast cancer patient from adriamycin treatment (Das et al., 2006). As the mechanism of adverse effects is due to oxidative stress, improvement of heart failure suggests the antioxidant effect of garlic. In contrast to above reports, one human study with 2 weeks treatment of Aged Garlic extract in coronary artery disease did not change the markers of oxidant stress (plasma oxidized low density lipoprotein and peroxides) and systemic inflammation (plasma C-reactive protein ad interleukin-6) (Williams et al., 2005).

Possible Mechanism/s

Direct free radical scavenging activity of garlic extracts and its component was responsible for antioxidant activity of garlic. Augmentation of endogenous antioxidant enzymes might be another possible mechanism for cardioprotective effect of garlic against oxidative stress (Banerjee et al., 2003).

Arrhythmia and others cardiovascular effects

Animal Studies

Garlic has a significant antiarrhythmic effect in both ventricular and supraventricular arrhythmias. Garlic powder (1% added to a standard chow for an 8 week period) significantly reduced ischemia reperfusion-induced ventricular fibrillation (VF) in isolated perfused rat heart (Rietz et al., 1995). Size of the ischemic zone was significantly reduced and the onset of arrhythmia after occlusion of the descending branch of the left coronary artery was significantly prolonged in rats fed with a standard chow enriched with 1% garlic powder for 10 weeks (Isensee et al., 1993). Garlic dialysate suppressed premature ventricular contractions and ventricular tachycardia in ouabain-intoxicated dogs as well as ectopic rhythms induced by isoprenaline and aconitine on electrically driven left rat atria (Martin et al., 1994). Garlic dialysate decreased the positive inotropic and chronotropic effects of isoproterenol in a concentration dependent manner. β-receptor blocking action of garlic was also suggested by Martin et al. The positive inotropism and chronotorpism induced by isoproterenol were partially antagonized by preincubation of the rat atria with the garlic dialysate. The ECG showed a regular sinus bradycardic rhythm in garlic dialysate fed anaesthetized rat (Martin et al., 1994). Direct relaxant effect of cardiac muscles was reported by Aqel et al., (1991). Garlic juice inhibited norepinephrine-induced contractions of rabbit and guinea pig aortic rings. It also inhibited the force of contraction of isolated rabbit heart in a concentration-dependent manner (Aqel et al., 1991). In contrast, one study showed that aqueous garlic extract increased the amplitudes of atrial complex 'p' wave and the ventricular complex 'QRS' of the rat ECG. This is suggestive of increase in voltage output of the atria and ventricles probably in accordance with positive inotropism (Tongia, 1984).

Human Studies

Aortic stiffening is as much an important risk factor in cardiovascular morbidity and mortality, as it serves as reliable surrogate marker for clinical endpoints like myocardial and cerebrovascular incidents. Elevated aortic stiffness induces high systolic blood pressure, augmented pulse pressure with increased ventricular afterload, reduced subendocardial blood flow and augmented pulsatile stress in the peripheral arteries (Breithaupt-Grogler and Belz, 1999). In population, consuming garlic for long period, attenuation of age-related increase in aortic stiffness has been observed. This suggests a protective effect on the elastic properties of the aorta related to aging in human. This study also showed that regular long term garlic powder intake protected endothelial cell from oxidative injury (Breithaupt-Grogler et al., 1997). Twelve week therapy with garlic powder (800 mg/day) was effective in patients with peripheral arterial occlusive disease Stage II. A significant decrease of plasma viscosity was observed. It is also quite interesting that the garlic-specific increase in walking distance did not appear to occur until the 5th week of treatment (Kiesewetter et al., 1993). Microcirculation of skin increased by 48% after administration of 800 mg/day garlic powder over a period of four weeks. Plasma viscosity was decreased by 3.2% (Kiesewetter et al., 1991). Kiesewetter also reported that garlic improved blood fluidity and increased capillary perfusion (Kiesewetter et al., 1990). Decreased plasma viscosity and increased (55%) capillary skin perfusion were observed even after 5 hours of garlic powder administration (Jung et al., 1991).

Toxicity Study

Considering the fact that garlic has been an integral part of our diet for centuries, it is taken for granted that garlic is safe in a wide range of doses. But a few isolated reports highlight some of the adverse and toxic effects of garlic.

Animal Studies

Higher concentrations of garlic extract have been shown to be clastogenic (Das et al., 1996) in mice, which was appreciably reduced at lower concentrations. Prolong feeding of high levels of raw garlic in rats has resulted in anemia, weight loss and failure to grow due to lysis of red blood cells (Augusti, 1996). Raw garlic juice at a high dose has resulted in death of rats due to stomach injury (Nakagawa et al., 1980). Surviving rats exhibited swelling of the liver, hypertrophy of the spleen and adrenal glands, and the decrease of erythrocyte count with various morphological changes after 3 and 8 days. Aqueous garlic extract (200 gm/l drinking water) for 10 days exhibited significantly higher levels of aspartate aminotransferase (AST) due to liver injury. Histopathological examination of liver showed focal nonspecific injury with inflammatory cell infiltration in hepatocytes (Joseph et al., 1989). Chen *et al.*, (1999) have reported that treatment of rats with fresh garlic homogenate for 7 days caused a significant decrease in liver catalase activity in doses of 2 and 4 gm/kg. The ultrastructural study carried out in our laboratory revealed significant loss of normal cellular architecture of heart, liver and kidneys after 30 days feeding of raw garlic homogenate at 1000 mg/kg/day dose (Banerjee et al., 2001; Banerjee et al., 2002). Feeding of allicin (100 mg/kg/day) for 15 days in rats increased the activity of liver lipase and alpha glucal phosphorylase and decreased glucose-6-phosphatase activity (Augusti and Mathew, 1975). The exact mechanism of such garlic induced alteration in cell structure and function is not clear. There is also some reported toxicity with garlic powder. Chronic administration of garlic powder (50 mg/day) resulted in inhibition of spermatogenesis in rats. Reduced concentration of sialic acid in the testes, epididymis and seminal vesicles together with decreased leydig cell function reflects antiandrogenic effect of garlic (Dixit and Joshi, 1982). Higher concentration of garlic powder (200 mg/ml) or allicin isolated from garlic caused considerable cell injuries in the porta hepatis zone in isolated perfused rat liver (Egen-Schwind et al., 1992), which was not observed at a lower concentration. Another *in vitro* study showed that diallyl sulfide (oxidized product of allicin) at 5 mM significantly decreased cell viability in liver (Sheen et al., 1996).

Garlic oil fed at a dose of 100 mg/kg after 24 hour fasting has also been found to be lethal. The cause of death appears to be acute pulmonary edema with severe congestion (Joseph et al., 1989). Garlic oil and Diallyl-disulfide (200 mg/kg b.w.) significantly reduced body weight gain of rats (Sheen et al., 1999). Ajoene, a garlic derived natural compound, present in other types of garlic oil, is an inhibitor as well as a substrate of human glutathione reductase and expected to increase the oxidative stress of the respective cell (Gallwitz et al., 1999). All the above mentioned toxicity reports can not be explained to its fullest extent but the sulphoxides present in the garlic extract can undergo exchange reaction with the titratable SH-groups of enzymes and other proteins in the body spontaneously at physiological pH and temperature, inhibiting their activity. Garlic has been demonstrated to inhibit the alkaline phosphatase (Joseph et al., 1989), papain, and alcohol dehydrogenase (Rabinkov et al., 2000). These enzyme interactions with garlic components may be a reason for its toxicity.

Human Studies

Relatively few side effects were reported in clinical studies using garlic and its preparations. Most of the reported side effects were non-specific. Gastrointestinal discomfort and nausea were the most frequent complaint (Beck and Grunwald, 1993). A survey by Koch et al., (1995) showed that allergic reactions to garlic were reported in a total of 39 publications between 1938 and 1994. Most of these cases involved an allergic contact dermatitis, sometimes severe (Eming et al., 1999), which has been reported in people with occupational exposure to garlic. There have also been sporadic reports of allergic conjunctivitis, rhinitis, or bronchospasms occurring in response to garlic inhalation or ingestion (Papageogiou et al., 1983). Other reported side effects included bloating, headache, dizziness, and profuse sweating (Beck and Grunwald, 1993). Ingestion of fresh garlic and garlic powder may have additive effects with anticoagulants or platelet aggregation inhibitors, leading in one case to a life-threatening hemorrhage (Burnham, 1995, Banerjee and Maulik, 2002).

CONCLUSIONS

Epidemiologic studies show an inverse correlation between garlic consumption and progression of cardiovascular disease (Kendler, 1987; Keys, 1980). The wealth of scientific literature supports the proposal that garlic consumption have significant cardioprotective effect, which includes both animal and human studies. But certain issues regarding the proper use of garlic, i.e. use of different preparations available, dose, duration and interaction with generic drugs should be optimized. Compounds in garlic work synergistically to produce various effects, but, because of garlic's chemical complexity, the efficacy and safety of different garlic preparations differ widely. Further research should also be carried out to identify specific compounds from garlic or garlic products that are responsible for most of its biological effects. It is a great challenge for scientists all over the world to make a proper use of garlic and enjoy its maximum beneficial effect as it is the cheapest way to prevent cardiovascular disease.

REFERENCES

Abramovitz D, Gavri S, Harats D, Levkovitz H, Mirelman D, Miron T, Eilat-Adar S, Rabinkov A, Wilchek M, Eldar M, Vered Z. Allicin-induced decrease in formation of fatty streaks (atherosclerosis) in mice fed a cholesterol-rich diet. *Coron Artery Dis*, 10, 515-519, (1999).

Ali M. Mechanism by which garlic (Allium sativum) inhibits cyclooxygenase activity. Effect of raw versus boiled garlic extract on the synthesis of prostanoids. *Prostaglandins Leukot Essent Fatty Acids*, 53:397-400, (1995).

Ali M, Al-Qattan KK, Al-Enezi F, Khanafer RM, Mustafa T. Effect of allicin from garlic powder on serum lipids and blood pressure in rats fed with a high cholesterol diet. *Prostaglandins Leukot Essent Fatty Acids*, 62, 253-259, (2000).

Ali M, Thomson M, Alnaqeeb MA, al-Hassan JM, Khater SH, Gomes A. Antithrombotic activity of garlic: its inhibition of the synthesis of thromboxane-B2 during infusion of arachidonic acid and collagen in rabbits. *Prostaglandins Leukot Essent Fatty Acids*, 41, 95-99, (1990).

Al-Qattan KK, Khan I, Alnaqeeb MA, Ali M. Thromboxane-B2, prostaglandin-E2 and hypertension in the rat 2-kidney 1-clip model: a possible mechanism of the garlic induced hypotension. *Prostaglandins Leukot Essent Fatty Acids*, 64, 5-10, (2001).

Apitz-Castro R, Badimon JJ, Badimon LA. garlic derivative, ajoene, inhibits platelet deposition on severely damaged vessel wall in an in vivo porcine experimental model. *Thromb Res*, 75, 243-249, (1994).

Apitz-Castro R, Escalante J, Vargas R, Jain MK. Ajoene, the antiplatelet principle of garlic, synergistically potentiates the antiaggregatory action of prostacyclin, forskolin, indomethacin and dypiridamole on human platelets. *Thromb Res*, 42, 303-311, (1986).

Apitz-Castro R, Ledezma E, Escalante J, Jain MK. The molecular basis of the antiplatelet action of ajoene: direct interaction with the fibrinogen receptor. *Biochem Biophys Res Commun.*, 141, 145-150, (1986).

Aqel MB, Gharaibah MN, Salhab AS. Direct relaxant effects of garlic juice on smooth and cardiac muscles. *J Ethnopharmacol*, 33, 13-19, (1991).

Auer W, Eiber A, Hertkom E, Kohrle U, Lenz A, Mader F, Merx W, Otto G, Schmid-Oto B, benheim H. Hypertonie and Hyperlipidamie: In leichterenauch Knoblauch. *Der Allgemeinarzi.*, 3, 205-208 (1989).

Augusti KT. Therapeutic values of onion (Allium cepa L) and garlic (Allium sativum L). *Ind J Exp Biol.* 34, 634-640, (1996).

Augusti KT, Mathew PT. Effect of allicin on certain enzymes of liver after a short term feeding to normal rats. *Experentia.* 31, 148-149, (1975).

Augusti KT, Sheela CG. Antiperoxide effect of S-allyl cysteine sulfoxide, a insulin secretagogue, in diabetic rats. Experientia, 52, 115-120, (1996).

Avci A, Atli T, Ergüder IB, Varli M, Devrim E, Aras S, Durak I. Effects of garlic consumption on plasma and erythrocyte antioxidant parameters in elderly subjects. *Gerontology*, 54(3):173-176 (2008).

Banerjee SK, Maulik SK. Effect of garlic on cardiovascular disorders: a review. *Nutr J*, 1, 4, (2002).

Banerjee SK, Maulik M, Manchanda SC, Dinda AK, Das TK, Maulik SK. Garlic-induced alteration in rat liver and kidney morphology and associated changes in endogenous antioxidant status. *Food Chem Toxicol*, 39, 793-797 (2001).

Banerjee SK, Dinda AK, Manchanda SC, Maulik SK. Chronic garlic administration protects rat heart against oxidative stress induced by ischemic reperfusion injury. *BMC Pharmacology*, 2, 16 (2002a).

Banerjee SK, Maulik M, Mancahanda SC, Dinda AK, Gupta SK, Maulik SK. Dose-dependent induction of endogenous antioxidants in rat heart by chronic administration of garlic. *Life Sciences*, 70, 1509-1518, (2002).

Banerjee SK, Sood S, Dinda AK, Das TK, Maulik SK. Chronic oral administration of raw garlic protects against isoproterenol-induced myocardial necrosis in rat. *Comp Biochem Physiol C Toxicol Pharmacol*, 136(4), 377-386, (2003b).

Banerjee SK, Mukherjee PK, Maulik SK. Garlic as an antioxidant: the good, the bad and the ugly. *Phytother Res*, 17(2), 97-106, (2003).

Beck E, Grunwald J. Allium sativum in der Stufentherapie der Hyperlipidamie. *Med Welt*, 44, 516-520, (1993).

Bordia A. Effect of garlic on human platelet aggregation in vitro. *Atherosclerosis*, 30, 355-360, (1978).

Bordia A, Arora SK, Kothari LK, Jain KC, Rathore BS, Rathore AS, Dube MK, Bhu N. The protective action of essential oils of onion and garlic in cholesterol-fed rabbits. *Atherosclerosis*, 22, 103-109, (1975).

Bordia A, Verma SK, Srivastava KC. Effect of garlic (Allium sativum) on blood lipids, blood sugar, fibrinogen and fibrinolytic activity in patients with coronary artery disease. *Prostaglandins Leukot Essent Fatty Acids*, 58, 257–263, (1998).

Bordia AK, Joshi HK. Garlic on fibrinolytic activity in cases of acute myocardial infarction. *J Assoc Physiol In*, 26, 323-326, (1978).

Brandle M, al Makdessi S, Weber RK, Dietz K, Jacob R. Prolongation of life span in hypertensive rats by dietary interventions. Effects of garlic and linseed oil. *Basic Res Cardiol*, 92, 223-232, (1997).

Breithaupt-Grogler K, Belz GG. Epidemiology of the arterial stiffness. *Pathol Biol (Paris)*, 47, 604-613, (1999).

Breithaupt-Grogler K, Ling M, Boudoulas H, Belz GG. Protective effect of chronic garlic intake on elastic properties of aorta in the elderly. *Circulation*, 96, 2649-2655, (1997).

Budoff MJ, Takasu J, Flores FR, Niihara Y, Lu B, Lau BH, Rosen RT, Amagase H: Inhibiting progression of coronary calcification using aged garlic extract in patients receiving statin therapy: A preliminary study. *Prev Med*, 39, 985-991, (2004).

Burnham BE. Garlic as a possible risk for postoperative bleeding. *Plast Recon Surg*, 95, 213, (1995).

Campbell JH, Efendy JL, Smith NJ, Campbell GR. Molecular basis by which garlic suppresses atherosclerosis. *J Nutr*, 131, 1006S-1009S, (2001).

Chanderkar AG, Jain PK. Analysis of hypotensive action of Allium sativum (garlic). *Ind J Physiol Pharmacol*, 17, 132–133, (1973).

Chen L, Hong JY, So E, Hussain AH, Cheng WF. Decrease of hepatic catalase level by treatment with diallyl sulfide and garlic homogenates in rats and mice. *J Biochem Mol Toxicol*, 13, 127-133 (1999).

Ciplea AG, Richter KD. The protective effect of Allium sativum and crataegus on isoprenaline-induced tissue necrosis in rats. *Arzneim-Forsch / Drug Res*, 38, 1583-1592, (1988).

Damru F. The use of garlic concentrate in vascular hypertension. *Med Rec*, 153, 249-251, (1941).

Das RN, Poudel N. Could garlic be an useful adjuvant therapy in adriamycin heart failure? *Kathmandu Univ Med J (KUMJ)*, 4(3), 337-339, (2006).

Das T, Roychoudhury A, Sharma A, Talukder G. Effects of crude garlic extract on mouse chromosomes in vivo. *Food and Chemical Toxicology*, 34, 43-47, (1996).

Dixit VP, Joshi S. Effects of chronic administration of garlic (Allium sativum Linn) on testicular function. *Ind J Exp Biol*, 20, 534-536, (1982).

Duda G, Suliburska J, Pupek-Musialik D. Effects of short-term garlic supplementation on lipid metabolism and antioxidant status in hypertensive adults. *Pharmacol Rep*, 60(2), 163-170, (2008).

Efendy JL, Simmons DL, Campbell GR, Campbell JH. The effect of the aged garlic extract, 'Kyolic', on the development of experimental atherosclerosis. *Atherosclerosis*, 132, 37-42, (1997).

Egen-Schwind C, Eckard R, Kemper F. H. Metabolism of garlic constituents in the isolated perfused rat liver. *Planta Medica*, 58, 301-305, (1992).

El-Sabban F, Radwan GM. Influence of garlic compared to aspirin on induced photothrombosis in mouse pial microvessels, in vivo. *Thromb Res*, 88, 193-203, (1997).

Eming SA, Piontek JO, Hunzelmann N, Rasokat H, Scharffetter Kachanek K. Severe toxic contact dematitis caused by garlic. *Br J Dermatol*, 141, 391-392, (1999).

Fallon MB, Abrams GA, Abdel-Razek TT, Dai J, Chen SJ, Chen YF, Luo B, Oparil S, Ku DD. Garlic prevents hypoxic pulmonary hypertension in rats. *Am J Physiol*, 275, L283-L287, (1998).

Foushee DB, Ruffin J, Banerjee U. Garlic as a natural agent for the treatment of hypertension: A preliminary report. *Cytobios*, 34, 145-152, (1982).

Gallwitz H, Bonse S, Martinez-Cruz A, Schlichting I, Schumacher K, Krauth-Siege RL. Ajoene is an inhibitor and subversive substrate of human glutathione reductase and Trypanosoma cruzi trypanothione reductase: crystallographic, kinetic, and spectroscopic studies. *J Med Chem*, 42, 364-372, (1999).

Gebhardt R, Beck H. Differential inhibitory effects of garlic-derived organosulfur compounds on cholesterol biosynthesis in primary rat hepatocyte culture. *Lipids*, 31, 1269-1276, (1996).

Gonen A, Harats D, Rabinkov A, Miron T, Mirelman D, Wilchek M, Weiner L, Ulman E, Levkovitz H, Ben-Shushan D, Shaish A. The antiatherogenic effect of allicin: possible mode of action. *Pathobiology*, 72(6), 325-334, (2005).

Granner DK, Murry RK, Mayes PA, Grannen DK, Rodwell VW. Hormones of the pancreas and gastrontestinal tract. In: Barnes DA. (eds) Harper's Biochemistry. New York, A Lange Medical Book, pp. 610-626, (2000).

Harfenist WJ, Murry RK, Murry RK, Mayes PA, Grannen DK, Rodwell VW. Plasma proteins, immunoglobulin and clotting factors. In: Barnes DA (eds) Harper's Biochemistry. New York, A Lange Medical Book, pp. 737-762, (2000).

Hill MF, Singal PK. Antioxidant and oxidative stress changes during heart failure subsequent to myocardial infarction in rats. *Am J Pathology*, 148, 291-300, (1996).

Imai J, Ide N, Nagae S, Moriguchi T, Matsuura H, Itakura Y. Antioxidant and radical scavenging effects of aged garlic extract and its constituents. *Planta Med*, 60, 417-420, (1994).

Isensee H, Rietz B, Jacob R. Cardioprotective action of garlic (*Allium sativum*). *Arzneim Forsch / Drug Res*, 43, 94-98, (1993).

Jain RC, Vyas CR. Garlic in alloxan-induced diabetic rabbits. *Am J Clin Nutr*, 28, 684-685, (1975).

Jamaluddin MP, Krishnan LK, Thomas A. Ajoene inhibition of platelet aggregation: possible mediation by a hemoprotein. *Biochem Biophys Res Commun*, 153, 479-486, (1988).

Joseph PK, Rao KR, Sundaresh CS. Toxic effects of garlic extract and garlic oil in rats. *Ind J Exp Biol*, 27, 977-979, (1989).

Jung EM, Jung F, Mrowietz C, Kiesewetter H, Pindur G, Wenzel E. Influence of garlic powder on cutaneous microcirculation. A randomized placebo-controlled double-blind cross-over study in apparently healthy subjects. *Arzneimittelforschung*, 41, 626-630, (1991).

Kasuga S, Ushijima M, Morihara N, Itakura Y, Nakata Y. Effect of aged garlic extract (AGE) on hyperglycemia induced by immobilization stress in mice. *Nippon Yakurigaku Zassh*, 114, 191-197, (1999).

Kaye AD, De Witt BJ, Anwar M, Smith DE, Feng CJ, Kadowitz PJ, Nossaman BD. Analysis of responses of garlic derivatives in the pulmonary vascular bed of the rat. *J Appl Physiol*, 89, 353-358, (2000).

Kendler BS. Garlic (Allium sativum) and onion (Allium cepa): a review of their relationship to cardiovascular disease. *Prev Med*, 16, 670-685, (1987).

Keys A. Wine, garlic and CHD in seven countries. *Lancet*, 1, 145-146, (1980).

Kiesewetter H, Jung F, Mrowietz C, Pindur G, Heiden M, Wenzel E, Gu LD. Effects of garlic on blood fluidity and fibrinolytic activity: a randomised, placebo-controlled, double-blind study. *Br J Clin Pract*, 69, 24-29, (1990).

Kiesewetter H, Jung F, Pindur G, Jung EM, Mrowietz C, Wenzel E. Effect of garlic on thrombocyte aggregation, microcirculation, and other risk factors. *Int J Clin Pharmacol Ther Toxicol*, 29, 151-155, (1991).

Kiesewetter H, Jung F, Jung EM, Mroweitz C, Koscielny J, Wenzel E. Effect of garlic on platelet aggregation in patients with increased risk of juvenile ischaemic attack. *Eur J Clin Pharmacol*, 45, 333-336, (1993).

Kim-Park S, Ku DD. Garlic elicits a nitric oxide-dependent Exp Pharmacol relaxation and inhibits hypoxic pulmonary vasoconstriction in rats. *Clin Physiol*, 27, 780-786, (2000).

Koch HP, Hahn G, Lawşon L, Reuter HD, Siegers C P. Garlic-An introduction to the therapeutic application of Allium sativum L. Williams & Wilkins, Baltimore, im Druck. (1995).

Kojima R, Epstein CJ, Mizui T, Carlson E, Chaqn P H. Protective effects of aged garlic extracts on doxorubicin induced cardiotoxicity in the mouse. *Nutr Cancer*, 22, 163-173, (1994).

Konig FK, Scineider B. Knoblauch bessert Durchblutungstorungen Arztliche Praxis. pp. 44-35, (1986).

Laurence WVD, John DF. Garlic extract prevents acute platelet thrombus formation in stenosed canine coronary arteries. *Am Heart J*, 117, 973-975, (1989).

Lawson LD. Garlic: a review of its medicinal effects and indicated active compounds. In: Lawson LD, Bauer R (eds) Phytomedicines of Europe. Chemistry and Biological Activity. Series 691. American Chemical Society, Washington, DC, pp 176-209, (1998).

Legnani C, Frascaro M, Guazzaloca G, Ludovici S, Cesarano G, Coccheri S. Effects of a dried garlic preparation on fibrinolysis and platelet aggregation in healthy subjects. *Arzneimittelforschung*, 43, 119-122, (1993).

Leoper M, DeBray M. Hypotensive effect of tincture of garlic. *Prog Med*, 36, 391-392, (1921).

Lewin G, Popov I. Antioxidant effects of aqueous garlic extract. 2nd communication: Inhibition of the Cu(2+)-initiated oxidation of low density lipoproteins. *Arzneimittelforschung*, 44, 604-607, (1994).

Luley C, Lehmann-Leo W, Moller B, Martin T, Schwartzkopff W. Lack of efficacy of dried garlic in patients with hyperlipoproteinemia. *Arzneimittelforschung/Drug Res*, 36, 766-768, (1986).

Lutomski J. Klinische Untersuchungen Zur therapeutischen wirksamkeit von llya Rogiff knoblanchpillen mit Rutin. *Z Phytotherapia*, 5, 938-942, (1984).

Makheja AN, Bailey JM. Antiplatelet constituents of garlic and onion. *Agents Actions*, 29, 360-363, (1990).

Martin N, Bardisa L, Pantojaa C, Vargas M, Quezaada P, Valenzuela J. Antiarrhythmic profile of a gaarlic dialystate assaay ed in dogs and isolaated atrial preparations. *J Ethanophrmacol*, 43, 1-8, (1994).

Mathew PT, Augusti KT. Studies on the effect of allicin (diallyl disulphide-oxide) on alloxan diabetes. I. Hypoglycaemic action and enhancement of serum insulin effect and glycogen synthesis. *Indian J Biochem Biophys*, 10, 209-212, (1973).

Mirhadi SA, Singh S, Gupta PP. Effect of garlic supplementation to cholesterol-rich diet on development of atherosclerosis in rabbits. *Ind J Exp Biol*, 29, 162-168, (1991).

Mukherjee S, Banerjee SK, Maulik M, Dinda AK, Talwar KK, Maulik SK. Garlic protects against acute adriamycin induced cardiotoxicity: Role of endogenous antioxidants and inhibition of TNF—a expression. *BMC Pharmacology*, 3(1), 16, (2003).

Nakagawa S, Masamoto K, Sumiyoshi H, Kunihiro K, Fuwa T. Effect of raw and extracted aged garlic on growth of young rats and their organ after peroral administration. *J Toxicol Sci*, 5, 91-112, (1980).

Neil HA, Silagy CA, Lancaster T, Hodgeman J, Vos K, Moore JW, Jones L, Cahill J, Fowler GH. Garlic powder in the treatment of moderate hyperlipidaemia: a controlled trial and meta-analysis. *J R Coll Physicians Lond*, 30, 329-334, (1996).

Ohaeri OC. Effect of garlic oil on the levels of various enzyme in the serum and tissue of streptozotocin diabtic rats. *Biosci Rep*, 21, 19-24, (2001).

Orekhov AN, Grunwald J. Effects of garlic on atherosclerosis. *Nutrition*, 13, 656-663, (1997).

Pantoja CV, Chiang CL, Norris BC, Concha JB. Diuretic, natriuretic and hypotensive effects produced by Allium sativum (garlic) in anaesthetized dogs. *J Ethnopharmacol*, 31, 325-331, (1991).

Papageogiou D, Corbet JP, Menezes F, Pecegueiro M, Benezra C. Allergic: contact dermatitis to garlic (Allium sativum I) identification of the allergens: the role of mono-, di- and trisulfides present in garlic. *Arch Dermatol Res*, 275, 229-234, (1983).

Patumraj S, Tewit S, Amatyakul S, Jariyapongskul A, Maneesri S, Kasantikul V, Shepro D. Comparative effects of garlic and aspirin on diabetic cardiovascular complications. *Drug Deliv*, 7, 91-96, (2000).

Petkov V. Plants and hypotensive, antiatheromatous and coronarodilatating action: *Am J Chin Med*, 7, 197-236, (1979).

Piotrowski'ailen GL. therapeutique. *Praxis*, 26, 488-492, (1948).

Qidwai W, Qureshi R, Hasan SN, Azam SI. Effect of dietary garlic (Allium Sativum) on the blood pressure in humans – a pilot study. *J Pak Med Assoc*, 50, 204-207, (2000).

Rabinkov A, Miron T, Mirelman D, Wilchek M, Glozman S, Yavin E, Weiner L. S-Allylmercaptoglutathione: the reaction product of allicin with glutathione possesses SH-modifying and antioxidant properties. *Biochim Biophys Acta*, 1499, 144-153, (2000).

Rashid A, Khan HH. The mechanism of hypotensive effect of garlic extract. *J Pak Med Assoc*, 35, 357-362, (1985).

Rietz B, Belagyi J, Torok B, Jacob R. The radical scavenging ability of garlic examined in various models. *Bolletino Chimico Farmaceutico*, 134, 69-76, (1995).

Rodger B, Roberty B, Edward S. Fibrinolytic activity in acute myocardial infarction. *Am J Clin Pathol*, 57, 359-363, (1972).

Sainani GS, Desai DB, Natu MN, Katrodia KM, Valame VP, Sainani PG. Onion, garlic, and experimental atherosclerosis. *Jpn Heart J*, 20, 351-357, (1979).

Sainani GS, Desai DB, Gorha NH, Natu SM, Pise DV, Sainani PG. Effect of dietary garlic and onion on serum lipid profile in Jain Community. *Ind J of Med Res*, 69, 776-780, (1979).

Schulz V, Hansel R, Tyler VE. Rational Phytotherapy; physicians' guide to herbal medicine. Springer-verlag, Berlin, Cardiovascular system. pp. 107-168, (2001).

Schwartz CJ, Valente AJ, Sprague EA. A modern view of atherogenesis. *Am J Cardiol*, 71, 9b-14b, (1993).

Sendl A, Elbl G, Steinke B, Redl K, Breu W, Wagner H. Comparative pharmacological investigations of *Allium ursinum* and *Allium sativum*. *Planta Medica*, 58, 1-7, (1992).

Sheen LY, Chen HW, Kung YL, Liu CT, Li CK. Effects of garlic oil and its organosulfur compounds on the activities of hepatic drug-metabolizing and antioxidant enzymes in rats fed high- and low-fat diets. *Nutr Cancer*, 35, 160-166, (1999).

Sheen LY, Li CK, Sheu SF, Meng RHC, Tsai SJ. Effect of the active principle of garlic-diallyl sulfide- on cell viability, detoxification capability and the antioxidation system on primary rat hepatocytes. *Food Chem Toxicol*, 34, 971-978, (1996).

Silagy CA, Neil HA. A meta-analysis of the effect of garlic on blood pressure. *J Hyperten*, 12, 463-468, (1994).

Silagy C, Neil A. Garlic as a lipid lowering agent-a meta-analysis. *J R Coll Physician Lond*, 28, 39-45, (1994).

Srivastava KC. Effects of aqueous extracts of onion, garlic and ginger on platelet aggregation and metabolism of arachidonic acid in the blood vascular system: in vitro study. Prostaglandins *Leukot Med*, 13, 227-235, (1984).

Srivsatava KC. Evidence for the mechanism by which garlic inhibitors platelet aggregation. *Prostaglandin Leukot Med*, 22, 313-321, (1986).

Srivastava KC, Tyagi OD. Effects of a garlic-derived principle (ajoene) on aggregation and arachidonic acid metabolism in human blood platelets. *Prostaglandins Leukot Essent Fatty Acids*, 49, 587-595, (1993).

Stevinson C, Pittler MH, Ernst E. Garlic for treating hypercholesterolemia. A meta-analysis of randomized clinical trials. *Ann Intern Med*, 133, 420-429, (2000).

Swanston-Flatt SK, Day C, Bailey CJ, Flatt PR. Traditional plant treatments for diabetes. Studies in normal and streptozotocin diabetic mice. *Diabetologia*, 33, 462-464, (1990).

Thomson M, Mustafa M, Ali M. Thromboxane-B(2) levels in serum of rabbits receiving a single intravenous dose of aqueous extract of garlic and onion. Prostaglandins *Leukot Essent Fatty Acids*, 63, 217-221, (2000).

Tongia SK. Effects of intravenous garlic Juice Aallium sativum on rat Electrocardiogram. *Ind J Physiol Pharmacol*, 28, 250-252, (1984).

Vorberg G, Schneider B. Therapy with garlic: results of a placebo-controlled, double-blind study. Br J Clin Prac. 1990; 44:7-11.

Warshafsky S, Kamer RS, Sivak SL. Effect of garlic on total serum cholesterol, A meta-analysis. *Ann Intern Med*, 119, 599-605, (1993).

Wei Z, Lau BHA. Garlic inhibits free radical generation and augments antioxidant enzyme activity in vascular endothelial cells. *Nutr Res*, 18, 61-70, (1998).

Williams MJ, Sutherland WH, McCormick MP, Yeoman DJ, de Jong SA. Aged garlic extract improves endothelial function in men with coronary artery disease. *Phytother Res*, 19(4), 314-319, (2005).

Yamasaki T, Lau BH. Garlic compounds protect vascular endothelial cells from oxidant injury. *Nippon Yakurigaku Zasshi*, 110, 138P-141P, (1997).

Yu-Yan Y, Liu L. Cholesterol lowering effect of garlic extracts and organosulfur compounds: Human and animal studies. *J Nutr*, 131, 989S-993S, (2001).

Zheziang Institute of Traditional Chinese Medicine. The effect of essential oil of garlic on hyperlipemia and platelet aggregation – an analysis of 308 cases. Cooperative Group for Essential Oil of Garlic. *J Tradit Chin Med*, 6, 117-120, (1986).

chapter 15

HERBAL FORMULATIONS IN THE TREATMENT OF DIABETES AND ITS COMPLICATIONS

Nageswara Rao Thalapaneni, S. Mohanalakshmi, G. David Lin and Subhash C Mandal

INTRODUCTION

The role of herbal medicine in the treatment of diabetes mellitus has become well established over the past decade. Diabetes mellitus is a heterogeneous metabolic disorder characterized by altered carbohydrate, lipid and protein metabolism. The management of diabetes mellitus is considered a global problem and successful treatment yet to be discovered. The treatment of diabetes mellitus has been attempted with various indigenous plants and polyherbal formulations. In the traditional system of Indian medicine plant formulation and in several cases, combined extracts of plants are used as the drug of choice rather than individual. Many of these formulations have shown promising effects. In this review we have outlined the polyherbal formulations having scientific evidence for the treatment of diabetes and its complications. Plant drugs are frequently considered to be less toxic and more free from side effects than synthetic ones. All the polyherbal formulations were scientifically evaluated in alloxan and streptozotocin induced diabetes mellitus.

Diabetes mellitus is a major public health burden worldwide. In year 2000, there were about 171 million diabetes cases worldwide and the number is estimated to rise to 366 million by year 2030 (Wild et al., 2004). Type 2 diabetes (T2DM) results from the inability of the body to respond properly to the action of insulin produced by the pancreas. It is the most prevalent form of diabetes accounting for around 90% of all diabetes cases. Before the discovery of insulin and other drugs for diabetes control, herbal medicines were the major form of treatment for diabetes and its complications.

In the traditional system of Indian medicine plant formulation and in several cases, combined extracts of plants are used as the drug of choice rather than individual. Many of these have shown promising effects (Kumari and Devi, 1993). This paper reports a critical review of 23 herbal formulas in treating diabetes and its complications. Ovidmedline, pubmed and the Cochrane library were searched for pharmacological and clinical evidence of herbal formulas with antidiabetic activity. A systematic literature search was conducted to identify relevant trials of herbal formulations in the treatment of diabetes and its complications.

Cogent – db

The ingredients of cogent db are *Azardirachta indica, Phyllanthus emblica, Terminalia bellerica, Terminella chebula, Tribulus terrestris, Trigonella foenum graecum, Curcuma longa, Syzigium cumini and Rotula aquatica*. Cogent db, a compound herbal drug, was investigated for its possible antidiabetic effect in alloxan-induced diabetic rats. Oral administration of the aqueous solution of Cogent db for 40 days exhibited a significant reduction in blood glucose, glycosylated haemoglobin, increased plasma insulin and total haemoglobin along with antihyperlipidemic effects in diabetic rats. The effective dose was found to be 0.45 gm/kg body wt. It also prevents body weight loss in diabetic rats. An oral glucose tolerance test (OGTT) was also performed in experimental diabetic rats in which there was a significant improvement in glucose tolerance in rats treated with Cogent db. A comparison was made between the action of cogent db and a known antidiabetic drug-glibenclamide (600 μg/kg body wt). The antidiabetic effect of Cogent db was more effective than that observed with glibenclamide. The significant and consistent antidiabetic effect of cogent db, the decreased glucose level in alloxan diabetic rats may also be due to enhanced glucose utilisation by peripheral tissues. The body weight was decreased in alloxan diabetic rats (Al-Shamaony et al., 1994). Administration of Cogent db increases the body weight in alloxan diabetic rats. The ability of Cogent db to protect massive body weight loss seems to be due to its ability to reduce hyperglycaemia. Cogent db might enhance glucose utilization because it significantly decreased the blood glucose level in glucose loaded rats. It may be due to restoration of delayed insulin response or due to inhibition of intestinal absorption of glucose. In this context, other workers have reported that *Azardirachta indica* (Bajaj and Srinivasan, 1999; Khosla et al., 2000), *Syzigium cumini*, *Tribulus terrestris* and *Curcuma longa* (Mitra et al., 1996). Ingredients of Cogent db have significant antidiabetic and glucose tolerance effect in experimentally induced diabetic rats. In the alloxan-induced diabetes mellitus, the rise in blood glucose is accompanied by an increase in serum cholesterol and triglycerides. The levels of cholesterol and triglycerides were brought to near normal by the treatment of Cogent db in alloxan diabetic rats. The effect of Cogent db on diabetic hypertriglyceridemia could be through its control of hyperglycaemia. Hence, Cogent db proves to be a safer antidiabetic agent and might help in preventing diabetic complications.

Aavirai Kudineer

Aavirai Kudineer (AK), a herbal formulation cited in the Tamil Siddha medical text 'Gunapadam' is suggested as panacea for diabetes (Murugesa Mudaliar, 1980). AK is composed of seven herbs, viz. *Cassia auiriculata* (bark), *Cassia fistula* (bark), *Cyperus rotundus* (tubers), *Saussurrea lappa* (tubers), *Salacia prinoides* (roots), *Eugenia jambolina* (bark) and *Terminalia arjuna* (bark). Tablets prepared from root bark of *Salacia prinoides* have been clinically demonstrated to have significant hypoglycemic activity (Kowsalya et al., 1996). Leaves of *Cassia fistula* significantly reduced hyperglycemia in experimental diabetic mice (Esposito et al., 1991). Decoctions prepared from fruit pulp, kernel and seeds of *Eugenia jambolina* exhibit marked anti diabetic effect in humans (Espinas et al., 1993), rabbits (Randriamampandry and Ramarojoana 1972) and rats (Grover et al., 2000). Alcoholic extracts of roots of *Saussurrea lappa* elicited significant hypoglycemic response in normal albino rats (Chaturvedi et al., 1993). AK treatment has reversed the diabetic status. It increased hexokinase activity up to 82% as compared to *Eugenia jambolina* which increased hexokinase activity by 72.7% when used singly, replenished liver glycogen stores and suppressed the hepatic gluconeogenesis by reducing activities of fructose 1,6 – biphosphatase and glucose – 6 phosphatase significantly. It can be safely concluded that Aavirai kudineer is potently hypoglycemic. The antidiabetic activity of AK seems superior as compared to similar effect of the some of the individual plants used in this formulation. Hypoglycemic efficacy could be attributed to the synchronicity and the additive effects of the constituents, reducing the possibility of side effects. The mechanism by which hypoglycemia is achieved by this herbal formulation needs to be further investigated. Estimation of insulin level and insulin receptor may give more insight into its mechanism of action (Bhavapriya et al., 2001).

D-400

It is a crude drug formulation consisting of herbs and minerals derived from the traditional system of medicine in India. After D-400 treatment a significant reduction in blood sugar levels in alloxan induced diabetes was observed. The main ingredients of D-400 are *Eugenia jambulana, Pterocarpus marsupium, Ficus glomerulata* and *Ocimum sanctum* in addition to other herbs, which have blood sugar lowering effect. In one of the study D-400 a herbo mineral preparation has shown significant hypoglycemic action and proved to be effective on alloxan-induced nephrotoxicity. An oral glucose tolerance test (OGTT) showed a significant lowering of AUC in streptozotocin induced diabetes in rats. There was a rise in hepatic glycogen level closer to normal after D-400 treatment. In the pancreas of diabetic rats, D-400 therapy showed a significant increase in islet number and beta cell count and appeared to bring about blood glucose homeostasis by increasing insulin secretion through repair/regeneration of endocrine pancreas which may be responsible for the prevention of hepatic glycogenolysis. There was a significant reduction in pancreatic weight, number of islets, diameter of each islet and beta cell counts/ islet in Streptozotocin treated group. Treatment with D–400 resulted in restoration of near normal architecture of pancreatic islet. This suggests a possible regeneration or repair of the cells of the islets of langerhans in the Streptozotocin treated group. Unlike sulphonylureas D-400 did not have any hypoglycaemic effect in normal rats. It is here that D-400 assumes significance, because of its capacity to partially regenerate the damaged endocrine tissue so that the islet number increases with therapy. The elevation of depressed glycogen stores by D-400 in alloxan treated rats may be attributed to either an inhibition of hepatic glucose output by improvement in plasma insulin levels or by stimulating the enzyme glycogen synthetase responsible for the incorporation of glucose moieties into pre-existing glycogen chains. The findings of the present study lend credence to the use of D-400 as an anti-hyperglycaemic agent (Mitra et al., 1996).

Diakyur

Diakyur a polyherbal Antidiabetic formulation containing seven ingredients of herbal origin that is used in traditional medicine to treat type II diabetes contains both antidiabetic and antioxidant principles. It contains dried extracts of *Cassia auriculata, Gymnema sylvestre, Mucuna pruriens, Syzygium jambolanum, Terminalia arjuna, Salacia reticulata* and crude powder of *Cassia javanica*. The findings suggest that *Salacia reticulate, Gymnema sylvestre and Syzygium jambolanum* are proven antidiabetic drugs (Yashikawa et al., 1998). *Terminalia arjuna* is a proven cardiotonic (Karthikeyan et al., 2003) and antioxidant drug that protects the heart and blood vessels from the oxidative stress of free radicals (Chander et al., 2004). *Cassia auriculata* and *Cassia javanica*, which are rich in bioflavonoids, are hypocholesterolemic and hypolipidemic agents that maintain favourable High Density Lipoprotein (HDL): Low Density Lipoprotein (LDL) cholesterol ratio. *Mucuna pruriens* is a rejuvenator drug also found to have a neuroprotective action (Manyam et al., 2004) which may help to prevent the neuropathic complications of diabetes. Findings suggest that Diakyur is non toxic since no marked changes in hematological, biochemical and histopathological parameters were observed. Thus, at normal therapeutic doses, Diakyur is considered to be safe for long term treatment in diabetic conditions.

Dangnyosoko (DNSK)

Dangnyosoko, an herbal medicine, is an extract of a mixture of *Coptidis rhizoma (Coptis chinensis)* and *Trichosanthis radix (Trichosanthes kirilowii)*. It has been used in the treatment of diabetes in Korea in folk medicine. The preventive anti – diabetic effect of dangnyosoko (DNSK), a Chinese herbal medicine, was evaluated in STZ – induced diabetic rats. Continous treatment with DNSK for a period of 28 days produced significant decrease in the blood and urine glucose levels of STZ – diabetic rats, which inhibited the decrease in insulin producing cells in the pancreatic islets, and consequently inhibited the increase in glucagon - producing cells. In addition, DNSK significantly and dose dependently increased plasma insulin levels as compared to the diabetic control. It is concluded that DNSK has favourable effects in preventing changes in blood and urine glucose levels, body weight, and the histopathological changes in the pancreas in STZ – induced diabetes (Jong et al., 2007).

Diasulin

The ingredients of this formulation are *Cassia auriculata, Coccinia indica, Curcuma longa, Emblica officinalis, Gymnema sylvestre, Momordica charantia, Scoparia dulcis, Syzigium cumini, Tinospora cardifolia, Trigonella foenum graecum*. Diasulin decreases blood glucose in alloxan diabetic rats. The possible mechanism of action of extract could be correlated with the reminiscent effect of the hypoglycemic sulphonylureas that promote insulin secretion by closure of K^+- ATP channels, membrane depolarization and stimulation of Ca^{2+} influx, an initial key step in insulin secretion. Antidiabetic and antihyperlipidemic effect of Diasulin may be due to the effect of active constituents of different plants, viz, alkaloid and pectins from *Coccinia indica* (Hossain et al., 1992) alkaloids from *Tinospora cordifolia* (Prince et al., 2002), emlicanin A and B from *Emblica officinalis* (Aruna et al., 1999), trigonelline and scopoltin from *Trigonella foenum graecum* (Jachak, 2002), alkaloid-6-methoxybenzoxazolinone and terpenoids such as scoparic acids A,B,C and scopadulcic acid A and B from *Scoparia dulcis* (Pari and Latha, 2004), which may be responsible for scavenging free radicals liberated by alloxan in diabetic rats. Diasulin, a combination of ten herbal plants exert a significant antihyperlipidemic and antiperoxidative effect. This could be due to different types of active principles, each with a single or a diverse range of biological activities, which serves as a good adjuvant in the present armamentarium of antidiabetic drugs.

Diarunplus

Diarunplus is a polyherbal formulation containing seeds of *Eugenia jambolana, Trigonella foneun graceum, Momardica charantia*, leaves of *Gymnema sylvestre*, Fruits of *Emblica officinalis*, Rhizomes of *Curcuma longa* and roots of *Salacia reticulata*. All these ingredients have traditional claim for their beneficial effects for the management of diabetes mellitus (Sathyavathi et al., 1976; Chopra et al., 1956; Nadkarni, 1954). The herbal ingredients present in the formulation had been proved to exhibit hypoglycemic effect in many experimental diabetic models (Senthilvel et al, 2006). Ethanolic extract of *C. longa* rhizome lowered blood sugar in alloxan – induced diabetic rats by vitalization of pancreatic cells and stimulation of insulin production (Anonymous, 2001). Ethanolic extracts of *M.charantia* seeds lowered fasting blood glucose and improved glucose tolerance (Karunanayake et al., 1984). Fruits of *E. officinalis* are potent antioxidant, which are free radical scavengers and lipid peroxide inhibitors (Jose and Kuttan, 1995). Powdered seeds and aqueous extract of *E. jambolana* lowered blood glucose in diabetic rabbits and produced a marked symptomatic relief in diabetic patients (Kohli and Singh, 1993). Aqueous extract of *T. foenum-graceum* exhibited potent hypoglycemic effect in alloxan induced diabetic rats (Abdel Barry et al., 1997). The seed extract also induced hyperinsulinemia and hypercholesterolemia. The alcoholic extract of *Gymnema sylvestre* lowered blood glucose in diabetic animals and stimulates insulin secretion in rabbits. Salacino isolated from *S. reticulatta* is also been reported to be a potent inhibitory activity against several alpha glucosidases and found that more potent than acarbose, a commercial alpha glucosidase inhibitor (Yoshikawa et al., 2002). A combination of these herbs can be naturally expected to lower the blood glucose level and exert beneficial effects in diabetic patients.

DCBT 2345

DCBT 2345, an ayurvedic formulation, has three herbal ingredients *Gymnema sylvestre, Syzygium jambolinium* and *Cephalandra indica*. These herbal extracts have been claimed to have some antidiabetic action (Baskaran et al., 1990, Raj, 1995, Shanmugasundaram et al., 1990). Review of literature provides interesting information on the herbal composition of DCBT 2345. *Gymnema sylvestre*, which is also known as "sugar buster" has been shown to reduce blood sugar levels in diabetic patients. The hypoglycemic nature of this drug was documented 70 years earlier (Mhaskar and Caius, 1930). Later, extensive observational and experimental studies have shown that *Gymnema sylvestre* increases insulin production by regenerating islet cells and increasing cell permeability and it is also reported to decrease intestinal absorption of glucose (Persaud et al., 1999; Shimizu et al., 1997). Herbs that belong to the genera *Syzygium* have been shown to effectively reduce hyperglycemia. *Syzygium cumini* seed powder reduces the sugar in urine and ameliorates polydipsia (Raj, 1995). Extensive studies on experimental models have revealed that this herb promotes endogenous release of insulin. The glucoside jamboline has been shown to control polyuria and glycosuria equally well (Kedar and Chakrabarti, 1983). *Cephalandra indica* is also referred to as an "Indian substitute: for insulin" and has glucokenin, which has a property of reducing glucose in blood. The lowering of glycosylated hemoglobin and the maintenance of pancreatic beta cell function as assessed by plasma insulin and C-peptide estimations in the drug treated group, while there was a 30-37% deterioration in beta cell function in the placebo treated group. This might suggest that the drug helps to improve/maintain insulin secretion providing optimal stimulation of pancreatic beta cells. Alternatively, the drug may have improved insulin sensitivity thus resulting in less exhaustion of beta cells. Further studies are needed to assess the mechanism of action of DCBT 2345.

OB 200G

OB-200G is a polyherbal formulation containing aqueous extracts of *Garcinia cambogia, Zingiber officinale, Piper longum, Gymnema sylvestre* and resin of *Commiphora mukul*. The ingredients in the formulation have been reported to possess thermogenic, hypocholesterolemic, body weight lowering, antidiabetic and digestive stimulant properties. the antiobesity effect of OB- 200G was studied using the dietary (cafeteria and atherogenic diets) animal models of obesity as they have been reported to bear close resemblance to human obesity. The weight reducing effect of the formulation may be attributed to *Garcinia cambogia* (contains Hydroxy citric acid reported to inhibit lipogenesis13) and *Commiphora mukul* (Sanskrit name palkash, pal = flesh, kash = reduce, is reported as one of the best herbs for treatment of obesity (Seth et al., 1996). All the ingredients of the formulation possessed thermogenic property (Varier, 1996; Varier, 1995; Varier, 1997). Since obesity is associated with defective thermogenesis (Pasquali and Casimirri, 1993) OB-200G may offer enormous therapeutic potential for its treatment. *Commiphora mukul* (Satyavati et al., 1969; Singh et al., 1994) and *Zingiber officinale* (Bhandari et al., 1998, Guh et al., 1995) have been reported to exert hypolipidemic effect and lower cholesterol levels. Gymnemic acid isolated from the leaves of *Gymnema sylvestre* has been reported to inhibit the intestinal absorption of glucose and oleic acid (Waang et al., 1998) and reported to exert beneficial effect in diabetes (Baskaran et al., 1990) and obesity. *Piper longum* (pippali) has heat generating property and has been referred by Charak as the best digestive stimulant (Seth et al., 1996). The increases in rectal temperature and ambulatory activity by OB-200G may be attributed to the overall stimulant and thermogenic property of the ingredients of the formulation. The underlying mechanism by which OB-200G increases blood glucose levels as compared to controls could not be defined. Thus, in conclusion OB-200G exerted significant antiobesity effect in rats fed on cafeteria and atherogenic diets.

Antidiabetic foot ulcer formula

Before the discovery of insulin and other drugs for diabetes control, herbal medicines were the major form of treatment for diabetes and its complications. Formula 1, the 'Herbal drink to strengthen muscle and control swelling', is a Chinese herbal medicine formula used when local circulation needs to be improved. It has been shown to effectively promote the healing of diabetic foot ulcers. Formula 1 consists of six Chinese medicinal herbs, including *Radix Astragali, Radix Rehmanniae, Rhizoma Atractylodis Macrocephalae, Radix Polygoni Multiflori Preparata, Rhizoma Smilacis Chinensis and Radix Stephania Tetrandrae*. It is speculated that the limb salvage power of this formula may be associated with the normalization of glycaemic control in diabetes. To test the hypothesis that Formula 1 and its component herbs modify tissue glucose homeostasis and elicit anti-diabetic activities, *in vitro* and *in vivo* systems have been established to study the effects of the herbal extracts. The extracts of Formula 1 and its components were first tested for their effects on tissue glucose homeostasis *in vitro* including: (1) glucose absorption into intestinal brush border membrane vesicles (BBMV); (2) gluconeogenesis by H4IIE rat hepatoma cells; (3) glucose uptake by Hs68 human skin fibroblasts and 3T3-L_1 mouse adipocytes. The active herbal extracts in the *in vitro* systems were selected for further evaluation of their antidiabetic activities *in vivo* using streptozotocin (STZ)-induced diabetic rat model. Clinical studies have demonstrated prominent effects of formula 1 on healing diabetic foot ulcers (Wong et al., 2001). Antidiabetic foot ulcer formula 1 contains ingredients active in modifying tissue glucose homeostasis *in vitro,* it doesn't elicit *in vivo* anti diabetic effects in this study. Results support that mechanisms other than normalizing systemic glycemic control underlie the clinically observed diabetic foot ulcer healing effects of Formula 1 (Chan et al., 2007).

Diabegon

Polyherbal preparation diabegon, containing 18 plant extracts with hypoglycemic activity (i.e. *Momordica charantia, Swertia chirata, Gymnema sylvestre, Trigonella foenum-graecum, Plumbago zeylanica, Eugena jambolana, Aegle marmelos, Terminalia chebula, Terminalia balerica, Emblica officinalis, Curcuma longa, Pterocarpus marsupion, Berberis aristata, Citrullus culocynthis, Cyperus rotondous, Piper longum, Root of Piper longum, Zingiber officinale, Asfetum punjabinum*), was evaluated for its preventive effect during progression of type 2 diabetes in high-fructose-diet–fed rats. Oral administration of diabegon (100 mg/kg body weight) delayed development of glucose intolerance for 4 weeks in comparison with the diabetic control group, and the effect of diabegon was compared to that of the standard insulin sensitizer drug rosiglitazone. Diabegon treatment also ameliorated the elevation of glycosylated haemoglobin, liver glycogen content, plasma insulin, homeostasis model assessment, free fatty acids, triglycerides, total cholesterol, LDL-cholesterol, and VLDL-cholesterol, whereas it increased HDL-cholesterol after 56 days of treatment ($P<0.05$). The mechanism of action by which diabegon attenuates insulin resistance and dyslipidemia may be through induction of peroxisome proliferator-activated receptor-ã and lipoprotein lipase activity in peripheral tissues (muscles). Moreover, diabegon administration for 56 days also produced no alteration in liver and kidney function tests, which seems to indicate its non-toxicity during treatment. Our present results suggest that diabegon may be included in diabetes mellitus treatment regimens, as a drug with good antidiabetic actions but no toxic manifestations (Hariom et al., 2007).

ADD -199

ADD-199 is an herbal medicine that is prepared from *Maytenus senegalensis* (Lam.) Exell. (Celastraceae), *Annona senegalensis Per var senegalensis*, Robyns and Ghesquiere (Annonaceae), *Kigelia africana* (Lam.) Benth. (Bignoniaceae) and *Lannea welwitschii* (Hiein) Engl. (Anacardiaceae), is used by some Ghanaian diabetic patients to manage the disease. The antidiabetic and antioxidant effects of the herbal preparation ADD-199 were investigated in STZ-induced diabetic mice and results were compared with two allopathic hypoglycaemic drugs, glibenclamide and metformin. Plasma glucose, insulin and lipids as well as liver glycogen, lipids and lipid peroxidation were measured following treatment for 8 weeks. The results indicated that plasma insulin levels in normal controls at termination were about 76 µmol/L compared to trace levels in untreated diabetic mice. Glibenclamide and ADD-199 increased insulin levels in diabetic mice up to 70% of levels in untreated non-diabetic mice while metformin had no effect. Basal plasma glucose levels in diabetic controls (18.8 mM) were reduced to 14.0 mM by 100 mg/kg ADD-199 in <2 weeks compared to 4 and 6 weeks for glibenclamide and metformin, respectively. This hypoglycaemic effect of ADD-199 appeared to be associated with the alkaloidal content of the extract. Treatment with ADD-199 or the hypoglycaemic agents reversed the observed elevation in plasma lipids but increased hepatic glycogen, triacylglycerol and cholesterol levels. Treatment also increased glucose uptake by isolated diaphragms and attenuated hepatic lipid peroxidation. These antihyperglycaemic and antioxidant actions of ADD-199 at a dose of 100 mg/kg/day are comparable to those of the maximum daily therapeutic doses of glibenclamide (0.25 mg/kg) and metformin (50 mg/kg). These could explain the basis for use of this plant extract to manage diabetes mellitus (DM) (Okine et al., 2005). Findings suggest that ADD-199 had no overt organ specific toxicity and did not demonstrate a potential for drug interactions via CYP-mediated metabolism in the rat on subchronic administration (Nyarko, 2005).

Gosha-jinki-gan (GJG)

Recently, traditional Chinese medicine (called Kampo medicine in Japan) has been recognized for its efficacy and there has been a noticeable increase in its popularity around the world (Borchers et al., 2000) because of its supposedly less frequent side effects (Nishizawa et al., 1995). The two noteworthy findings of this formulation are, firstly, GJG with or without a small dose of exogenous insulin produced a significant improvement in the insulin sensitivity in STZ-diabetes and, secondly, the molecular effect of GJG probably occurred via correction of the abnormal early steps of the insulin signaling pathway. Thus, correction of the abnormal early step of insulin signaling in skeletal muscle of GJG-treated STZ-diabetic rats may play an important role in improving insulin sensitivity *in vivo*. In conclusion, the current study suggests that long-term GJG administration would ameliorate the insulin sensitivity, at least in part, by correcting the abnormal insulin signaling in STZ-diabetes. However, further investigation on other molecular details regarding GJG is needed (Bolin et al., 2004). The ingredients of this formulation is Rehmanniae Radix, Achyranthis Radix, Coprni Fructus, Dioscoreae Rhizoma, Plantaginis Semen, Alismatis Rhizoma.

Hachimi-jio-gan (Ba-Wei-Di-Huang-Wan)

The herbal prescription Hachimi-jio-gan (HJ) (Ba-Wei-Di- Huang-Wan) has been widely used for the treatment of patients with diabetes mellitus, hypertension, nephrotic syndromes, and glomerulonephritis since the late middle ages. HJ is used as a Kampo formula for diabetes and the package insert for HJ extract for medical use states that HJ suppresses experimentally induced diabetes, inhibits reduction in vascular elasticity due to high-cholesterol diets, hinders aldose reductase activity, and protects the renal tissue of rats that are genetically sensitive to salt.

The composition of HJ is as follows: Rehmanniae radix, Corni fructus, Dioscoreae rhizoma, Alismatis rhizoma, Hoelen, Moutan cortex, Cinnamomi cortex, and Aconiti tuber. Animal studies have shown that Rehmanniae radix, Corni fructus and Hoelen lower blood sugar, but HJ does not contain ginseng which is frequently used to treat diabetes in the clinical setting (Yoshihiko et al., 2007). This formulation is used in the treatment of diabetes for a long period of time. Although no clinical studies have found these herbal formulas to lower blood glucose levels, these agents have been given to diabetics. It has clinically been evaluated that although Chinese medicine doesn't improve hyperglycemia, it can alleviate diabetes related symptoms such as dry mouth, frequent thurst, frequent urination and fatigue. In STZ induced diabetic rats, HJ didn't increase the number of pancreatic β-cells which had been reduced by STZ, but it increased insulin production and release by residual pancreatic β-cells and significantly suppressed the expression of hepatic GLUT2 protein, which is involved in glucose uptake and release in the liver. HJ also increased the amylase secretion by the liver and had favourable effects on pancreatic secretion. Because HJ appears to be involved in hepatic glucose release as well as in suppressing hyperglycemia by increasing insulin secretion from residual pancreatic cells, long term administration to diabetics may aid therapy.

Dianex

Dianex, a polyherbal formulation consisting of the aqueous extracts of *Gymnema sylvestre, Eugenia jambolana, Momordica charantia Azadirachta indica, Cassia auriculata, Aegle marmelose, Withania somnifera and Curcuma longa* was screened for hypoglycemic activity in normal and streptozotocin induced diabetic mice. In oral glucose tolerance test, Dianex treated mice (both normal and diabetic) showed significant decrease in blood glucose levels, indicating increased glucose tolerance. *Momordica charantia, Cassia auriculata, Azadirachta indica and Aegle marmelose* have been reported to increase the glucose tolerance in laboratory animals (Pari et al., 2001). Dianex produced significant hypoglycemic activity in experimental animals besides reversing other diabetic complications. In other studie, Dianex was well tolerated in laboratory animals at higher doses (up to 10 g / kg in mice, acute toxicity up to 2.5 g/ kg in rats, subacute toxicity studies for 30 days). Without exhibiting any toxic manifestation (Mutalik et al., 2003). Hence, Dianex may be effectively used in the treatment of diabetes mellitus. Studies on diabetic patients are under progress to confirm its effectiveness in human volunteers.

Keishi-ka Shakuyaku-to (TJ-60)

The ingredients of this formulation is Peony root (*root of Peonylactiflora* Pall) (6.0 g), Cinnamon bark (*bark of Cinnamomum cassia* BL) (4.0 g). Jujube (fruit of *Zizyphus jujuba* MILL var inermis REHD) (4.0 g), Glycyrrhiza (root and stolon of *Glycyr-rhiza glaba* L,*Glycyrrhizauralensis* FISCH) (2.0 g) and Ginger (*rhizome of Zingiber officinale* ROSC) (1.0 g). The yield of extract was 22 %. The extract contained glycyrrhizin (1.22 %) and paeoniflorin (1.78 %). To examine the effects of kampo medicine, Keshi-ka-Shakuyaku-to (TJ-60) on the signal transduction in diabetic gastrointestinal dysfunction experimental diabetic animals were prepared using streptozotocin treated wistar rats. Diacylglycerol (DG) and DG kinase activities were quantified in isolated arotic smooth muscle tissue. Treatment with TJ-60 indicated resistant effects for the alteration of DG kinase activities in diabetic intestinal tissues. In order to reveal the mechanism of effects, total content of DG was measured. Dysfunction of gastrointestinal smoothmuscle in diabetes is mediated by an alteration of DG and DG kinase. TJ-60 influences the alteration and relief the dysfunction (Nobe et al., 2002).

Okchun-San

In traditional medicine in Asian countries, many herbal drugs are combined in the form of a multiherbal formula to enhance their functions. The composition of this formulation is Trichosanthis radix (*Trichosanthes kirilowii* Max., Cucurbitaceae), Puerariae radix (*Pueraria thunbergiana* Benth., Leguminosae), Rehmanniae radix (*Rehmannia glutinosa* Libosch., Scrophulariaceae), *Schizandrae fructus* (*Schizandra chinensis* Baill., Magnoliaceae), Glycyrrhizae radix (*Glycyrrhiza uralensis* Fisch., Leguminosae), *Coicis semen* (Coix lachryma-jobi L. var. mayuen Stapf., Poaceae), and Oryzae semen (*Oryza sativa* L., Gramineae) The effective control of blood glucose is the key to preventing or reversing diabetic complications. In this study, the effects of Okchun-San (OCS), a Korean herbal medicine formula, on the blood glucose levels in diabetic C57BL/KsJ *db/db* mice were studied. Herbal medicines were prepared from dried herbs by adding Coicis semen (OCS-C) or Oryzae semen (OCS-O). The experimental animals were divided into a control group and three sample groups; the sample groups received OCS-C (200 mg/kg), OCS-O (200 mg/kg), or acarbose (5 mg/kg) orally once a day for 12 days. On days 5 and 12, the fasting blood glucose levels of vehicle-treated *db/db* mice were significantly higher than day 0, while those of OCS-C, OCS-O, or acarbose-treated mice had not increased compared to the control group ($p < 0.01$). During intraperitoneal glucose tolerance test (IPGTT), OCS-C group showed improved glucose sensitivity compared to the control group. These results suggest that OCS-C can be useful as an anti-diabetic therapy for Type 2 diabetic patients by lowering the blood glucose level (Chang et al., 2006).

Seishin-renshi-in

Composition of Seishin-renshi-in (Qing-Xin-Lian-Zi-Yin) is Ophiopogonis tuber, Hoelen, Scutellariae radix, Plantaginis semen, Ginseng radix, Astragali radix, lycyrrhizae radix, Nehunbinis semen, Lycii radicis cortex. Although there is no concept of insulin resistance in traditional Kampo (Chinese) medicine and Indian medicine, there is hypothesis that some drug in a mixture of crude drugs which was believed to ameliorate diabetes mellitus may have had the effect of improving insulin resistance. To test this hypothesis, the effects of Seishin-renshi-in (Chinese medicine) and *Gymne-*

ma sylvestre (Indian medicine) on the insulin resistance of streptozotocin-induced diabetic rats was studied by the glucose clamp technique. Oral administration of Seishin-renshi-in (800 mg/kg/day) with injections of a minimum dose of Ultralente insulin decreased urine volume and urinary glucose excretion during a 7-day treatment period and improved the insulin stimulated glucose uptake in peripheral tissues, as well as improving the insulin suppressed hepatic glucose output during glucose clamp. However, *G. sylvestre* (120 mg/kg/day) treatment did not improve insulin resistance. The conclusion is Seishin-renshi-in, with a small dose of insulin, improved insulin resistance in streptozotocin-induced diabetic rats, but *Gymnema sylvestre* did not (Tominaga et al., 1995).

Keishi-bukuryo-gan

It consisted of equal amounts of the following five crude drugs: Cinnamomi Cortex (*Cinnamomum cassia* Blume), Poria (*Poria cocos*Wolf), Moutan Cortex (*Paeonia suffruticosa* Andrews), Persicae Semen (*Purnus persicae* Batasch), and Paeonia Radix (*Paeoniae lactiflora* Pall). Keishi-bukuryo-gan is a Chinese traditional herbal medicine, which is used clinically as a vascular system disorder-eliminating drug. The effects of Keishi-bukuryo-gan on the occurrence and progression of diabetic nephropathy, employed two kinds of experimental model animals, namely diabetic nephropathy rats induced by subtotal nephrectomy plus streptozotocin injection and spontaneously diabetic WBN/Kob rats. In both animal models, Keishi-bukuryo-gan treatment suppressed the increase of urinary protein excretion, which is a prognostically important clinical manifestation for renal functional deterioration in diabetic patients, and preserved renal morphological changes peculiar to diabetic glomerulosclerosis. On the other hand, disorders of the metabolic pathway mediated by persistent hyperglycaemia (the glycation reaction, excessive polyol pathway and oxidative stress) were observed. However, oral administration of Keishi-bukuryo-gan normalized the accumulation of advanced glycation endproducts (AGEs), determined by measuring fluorescence, and lipid peroxidation levels in the kidney. Furthermore, by comparison with aminoguanidine (an AGEs inhibitor), butylated hydroxytoluene (an antioxidant) and captopril (an angiotensin-converting enzyme inhibitor), so confirmed that Keishi-bukuryo-gan prevents diabetic kidney damage from developing and has inhibitory effects against AGEs accumulation and oxidative stress. From these results, we proposed the potential usefulness of Keishi-bukuryo-gan in the treatment of diabetic nephropathy (Nakagawa et al., 2004).

Hyponidd

Hyponidd is a herbomineral formulation composed of the extracts of ten medicinal plants (*Momordica charantia, Melia azadirachta, Pterocarpus marsupium, Tinospora cordifolia, Gymnema sylvestre, Enicostemma littorale, Emblica officinalis, Eugenia jambolana, Cassia auriculata and Curcuma longa*). Investigations on hyponidd for its possible antihyperglycaemic and antioxidant effect in diabetic rats. Rats were rendered diabetic by streptozotocin (STZ) (45 mg kg^{-1} body weight). Oral administration of hyponidd (100 mg kg^{-1} and 200 mg kg^{-1}) for 45 days resulted in significant lowered levels of blood glucose and significant increased levels of hepatic glycogen and total haemoglobin. An oral glucose tolerance test was also performed in experimental diabetic rats in which there was a significant improvement in blood glucose tolerance in the rats treated with hyponidd. Hyponidd administration also decreased levels of glycosylated haemoglobin, plasma thiobarbituric acid reactive substances, hydroperoxides, ceruloplasmin and á-tocopherol in diabetic rats. Plasma reduced glutathione and vitamin C were significantly elevated by oral administration of hyponidd. The effect of hyponidd at a dose of 200 mg kg^{-1} was more effective than glibenclamide (600 g kg^{-1}) in restoring the values to near normal. The results showed that Hyponidd exhibits antihyperglycaemic and antioxidant activity in STZ-induced diabetic rats (Babu et al., 2004).

Diamed

Diamed is a herbal formulation composed of the aqueous extracts of three medicinal plants (*Azardirachta indica, Cassia auriculata* and *Momordica charantia*). We have investigated Diamed for its possible antihyperglycaemic action in rats with alloxan-induced experimental diabetes. Oral administration of Diamed (1.39 (0.25g), 1.67 (0.30g) or 1.94 (0.35g) mL kg^{-1}) for 30 days resulted in a significant reduction in blood glucose, glycosylated haemoglobin, and an increase in plasma insulin and total haemoglobin. The effect was highly significant after administration of the 1.94mL (0.35g) g^{-1} body weight dose. Diamed also prevented a decrease in body weight. An oral glucose tolerance test was performed in experimental diabetic rats in which there was a significant improvement in glucose tolerance in the animals treated with Diamed. The effect was compared with 600ìg kg^{-1} glibenclamide. The results showed that Diamed had antihyperglycaemic action in experimental diabetes in rats (Pari et al., 2001).

KIOM-79

KIOM-79 is composed of four herbal medicines, which are parched *Puerariae radix*, gingered *Magnoliae cortex, Glycyrrhizae radix* and *Euphorbiae radix*. These herbal medicines are frequently used for the treatment of diabetes or diabetic complications in traditional medicine in Korea and other countries. Investigations on the effect of KIOM-79, 80% ethanolic extract of a new herbal prescription, on non-obese type 2 diabetic Goto-Kakizaki (GK) rats were carried out. The rats were treated orally with KIOM-79 (500 mg/kg body weight) once a day for 13 weeks to examine the long-term effects on hyperglycemia and glomerular histology as well as biochemical and functional abnormalities in kidney. The results found that KIOM-79 reduced hyperglycemia ($p < 0.01$), ameliorated insulin resistance ($p < 0.001$), urinary protein excretion ($p < 0.01$) and creatinine clearance (Ccr) ($p < 0.001$), and inhibited glomerular AGE formation ($p < 0.001$) in diabetic GK rats. KIOM-79 prevented the glomeruli enlargement, overexpression of type IV collagen ($p < 0.001$), PKC protein ($p < 0.01$), TGF-β mRNA ($p < 0.05$) and VEGF mRNA ($p < 0.05$). Thus, based on our finding, KIOM-79 could reduce the hyperglycemia, and prevent or retard the development of diabetic nephropathy (Kim et al., 2007).

Die-Huang-Wan

The composition of this formulation is *Rehmanniae Radix et Rhizoma, Corni Fructus, Dioscoreae Rhizoma, Moutan Radics Cortex, Alismatis Rhizoma, Hoelen*. Effects of insulin sensitivity of Die-Huang-Wan, the herbal mixture widely used to treat diabetic disorder in Chinese traditional medicine, were investigated *invivo*. Die- Huang-Wan in the modulation of insulin sensitivity using an animal model of obesity-associated insulin resistance, the obese Zucker rats, which accompanied by mild hyperglycemia, glucose intolerance and hyperinsulinemia (Kasiske et al., 1992). It has been documented that tolbutamide- induced hypoglycemia occurs through the stimulation of endogenous insulin release (Chi et al., 1998, Shennan et al., 1987, Chang et al., 1999). Whole body insulin sensitivity, as reflected in the plasma glucose lowering action of tolbutamide, was significantly enhanced in obese Zucker rats receiving the repeated administration of Die-Huang-Wan for 3 days. However, the plasma glucose concentrations in these insulin-resistant animals with same treatment did not change significantly. These results suggest that Die-Huang- Wan might enhance insulin sensitivity in the insulin-resistant animal. Die-Huang-Wan could delay the formation of insulin-resistance in association with an increase of insulin sensitivity. Thus, Die-Huang-Wan may be used as an adjuvant for the handling of the diabetic patients with clinically manifested insulin resistance (Chang et al., 2002).

REFERENCE

Abdel-Barry JA, Abdel-Hassan I, Al-Hakiem A. Hypoglycemic and antihyperglycemic effects of *Trigonella foenumgraecum* leaf in normal and alloxan induced diabetic rats. J. Ethnopharmacol, 58, 149-155, (1997).

Al-Shamaony SM, Al-Khazraji Twaiji HA. Hypoglycaemic effect of *Artemisia herba alba* II. Effect of a valuable extract on some blood parameters in diabetic animals. J. Ethnopharmacol, 43, 167-171, (1994).

Satyavati GV, Raina MK, Sharma M. Medicinal plants of India, Vol. 1, 147 (1976) Indian Council of Medical Research, New Delhi.

Anonymous. The wealth of India, Vol. 2, 264 (2001) National institute of Science communication, CSIR, New Delhi.

Aruna Bhattacharya, Chatterjee A, Hosal S, Sail K. Antioxidant activity of active tannoid principles of *Emblica officinalis* (amala). Indian J Exp Biol, 137, 676-680, (1999).

Babu PS, Prince PS. M. Antihyperglycaemic and antioxidant effect of hyponidd, an ayurvedic herbomineral formulation in streptozotocin-induced diabetic rats. J Pharm Pharmacol, 56, 1435-1442, (2004).

Bajaj, Srinivasan BP. Investigations into the anti-diabetic activity of *Azardirchta indica*. Ind. J Pharmacol, 31, 138-141, (1999).

Baskaran K, Kizar Ahamath, B, Radha Shanmugasundaram K, Shanmugasundaram ER. Antidiabetic effect of a leaf extract from *Gymnema sylvestre* in non-insulin-dependent diabetes mellitus patients. J. Ethnopharmacol, 30, 295-300, (1990).

Bhandari U, Sharma JN, Zafar R. The protective action of ethanolic ginger (*Zingiber officinale*) extract in cholesterol fed rabbits. J Ethno Pharmacol, 61, 167-71, (1998).

Bhavapriya V, Kalpana S, Govindasamy S, Apparanantham T. Biochemical studies on hypoglycemic effect of Aavirai kudineer : A herbal formulation in alloxan diabetic rats. Ind J Exp Biol, 39, 925-928, (2001).

Bolin Q, Masaru N, Ming R, Gustavo B, Yoshiharu O, Yuzo S. Gosha-jinki-gan (a Herbal Complex) Corrects Abnormal Insulin Signaling. eCAM, 1, 269-276, (2004).

Borchers A, Sakai S, Henderson G. Shosaiko-to and other Kampo (Japanese herbal) medicines: a review of their immunomodulatory activities. J Ethnopharmacol, 73, 1-13, (2000).

Chan CM, Chan YW, Lau CH, Lau TW, Lau KM, Lam FC, Che CT, Leung PC, Fung KP, Lau CBS, Ho YY. Influence of an anti-diabetic foot ulcer formula and its component herbs on tissue and systemic glucose homeostasis. J Ethno Pharmacol, 109, 10-20, (2007).

Chander R, Kavita S, Khanna AK, Kaul SM, Anju P, Rashmi S, Gitika B, Farha R, Rastogi AK. Antidyslipidemic and antioxidant activities of different fractions of *Terminalia arjuna* stem bark. Indian J. Clin. Biochem, 19, 141-148, (2004).

Chang SL, Lin JG, Chi TC, Liu IM, Cheng JT. An insulindependent hypoglycemia induced by electroacupuncture at the Zhongwan (CV12) acupoint in diabetic rats. Diabetologia, 42, 250-5, (1999).

Chang SM, Myung SO, Do RK, Kye JJ, Sunmin P, Soo BC, Byoung SK, Seong KP. Effects of Okchun-San, a herbal formulation, on blood glucose levels and body weight in a model of Type

2 diabetes. J Ethno Pharmacol, 103, 3, 491-495, (2006).

Chang WUY, Hao HSUJ, Min LIUI, Shii LIOUS, Chen SUH, Tang CJ. Increase of insulin sensitivity in diabetic rats received Die-Huang-Wan, a herbal mixture used in Chinese traditional medicine. Acta Pharmacol Sin, 23, 1181-1187,(2002).

Chaturvedi P, Tripathi P, Pandey S, Singh U, Tripathi VB. Effect of *Saussurrea lappa* on different endocrine glands in relation to glucose metabolism in the rat. Phytother Res, 7, 205, (1993).

Chi TC, Liu IM, Cheng JT. A simple and rapid model of insulin-resistance in Wistar rats. Chin Pharm J, 50, 113-21, (1998).

Chopra RN, Nayar SL, Chopra IC. The glossary of Indian medicinal plants, 127, Publications and Information Directorate, Council of Scientific and Industrial Research, New Delhi.

Eposito, Avella M, Diaz A, De GI, De TR, Gupta M. P. Evaluation of traditional medicine, Effect of *Cajanas cajan* L. and of *Cassia fistula* on carbohydrate metabolism in mice. Rev Med Panama, 16, 39, (1991) .

Espinas J, Salla RM, Bellvehi M. A re-evaluation of the programme of diabetes mellitus type 2. A proposal for quality indices. Aten Primaria, 11, 123, (1993).

Grover JK, Vats V, Raathi SS. Anti hyperglycemic effect of *Eugenia jambolina* and *Tinospora cordifolia* in experimental diabetes and their effects on key metabolic enzymes involved in carbohydrate metabolism. J Ethnopharmacol, 73, 461, (2000).

Guh JH, Ko FN, Jong TT, Teng CM. Antiplatelet effect of gingerol isolated from *Zingiber officinale*. J Pharm Pharmacol, 47, 329-32, (1995).

Hariom Y, Shalini J, Prasad GBKS, Mukesh Y. Preventive Effect of Diabegon, a Polyherbal Preparation, During Progression of Diabetes Induced by High-Fructose Feeding in Rats. J Pharmacol Sci, 105, 12-21, (2007).

Hossain MZ, Shibib BA, Rahman R. Hypoglycemic effect of *Coccinia indica* inhibition if key gluconeogenic enzyme, glugose- 6-phosphate. Indian J Biol, 30, 418-420, (1992).

Jachak SM. Herbal drugs as antidiabetics. An overview. CRIPS, 3, 2, (2002).

Jong DK, Seock MK, Mee YP, Tae YJ, Hae YC, Sae KK. Ameliorative anti – diabetic activity of *Dangnyosoko*, a Chinese herbal medicine, in diabetic rats. Biosci. Biotechnol. Biochem, 71, 1527-1534, (2007).

Jose JK, Kuttan R. Antioxidant activity of *Emblica officinalis*. J Clin Biochem Nut, 19, 63-70, (1995).

Karthikeyan K, Bai BR, Gauthaman K, Sathish KS, Devaraj SN. Cardioprotective effect of the alcoholic extract of *Terminalia arjuna* bark in an *in-vivo* model of myocardial ischemic reperfusion injury. Lif Sci, 73, 2727-2739, (2003).

Karunanayake EH, Welihinda J, Sirimanne SR, Sinnadorai G. Oral hypoglycemic activity of some medicinal plants of Srilanka. J Ethnopharmacol, 11, 223-231, (1984).

Kasiske BL, Donnell MP, Keane WF. The Zucker rat model of obesity, insulin resis tance, hyperlipidemia, and renal injury. Hypertension, 19, I110-5, (1992).

Kedar P, Chakrabarti CH. Effects of Jambolan seed treatment on blood sugar, lipids and urea on streptozotocin induced diabetes in rabbits. Ind J Physio Pharmac, 27, 135-40, (1983).

Khosla P, Bhanwra S, Singh J, Seth S, Srivastava RK. A study of hypoglycaemic effects of *Azardirachta indica* (neem) in normal and alloxan diabetic rabbits. Ind. J. Pharmacol, 44, 69-74, (2000).

Kim CS, Sohn EJ, Kim YS, Jung DH, Jang DS, Lee YM, Kim DH, Kim JS. Effects of KIOM-79 on hyperglycemia and diabetic nephropathy in type 2 diabetic Goto-Kakizaki rats. J Ethnopharmacol, 111, 240-247, (2007).

Kohli KR, Singh RH. A clinical trial of Jambu (*Eugenia jambolana*) in non insulin dependent diabetes mellitus. J. Res. Ayur.Sid, 14, 89-97, (1993).

Kowsalya S, Usha C, Sharmila JB. Development and evaluation of hypoglycemic tablets from selected herbs. Ind J Nutr Diet, 33, 240, (1996).

Kumari KS, Devi KS. Effect of indigenous drugs on glucuronoglycan metabolism in diabetic hypertensive rabbits. Ind. J. Exp. Biol, 31, 595-599, (1993).

Manyam BV, Dhanasekaran M, Hare TA. Neuroprotective effects of antiparkinson drug *Mucuna pruriens*. Phytother Res, 18, 706-712, (2004).

Mhaskar KS, Caius JF. A study of Indian medicinal plants II. Gymnema sylvestre R. Br. Indian Medical Research Memoirs, 16, 2-75, (1930).

Mitra SK, Gopumadhavan S, Muralidhar TS. Effect of D-400, an Ayurvedic Herbal Formulation on Experimentally-induced Diabetes Mellitus. Phytotherapy Res, 10, 433-435, (1996).

Mitra SK, Gopumadhavan S, Muralidhar TS, Anturlikar SD, Sujatha MB. Effect of a herbomineral preparation D-400 in streptozotocin-induced diabetic rats. J. Ethnopharmacol, 54, 41-46, (1996).

Murugesa Mudaliar CS. Gunapadam, Vegetable section, Vol. 1, 65 (1980) 3rd edition.

Mutalik S, Sulochana B, Chetana M. Preliminary studies on acute and subacute toxicity of an Antidiabetic herbal preparation, Dianex. Ind J Exp Biol, 4, 316-320, (2003).

Nadkarni KM, Indian Materia Medica, Vol. 1, (1954) Popular Book Depot, Bombay.

Nakagawa T. Therapeutic potential of Keishi-bukuryo-gan on diabetic nephropathy, J Trad Med, 21, 7-16, (2004).

Nishizawa M, Sutherland W, Nukada H. Gosha-jinki-gan (herbal medicine) in streptozocin-induced diabetic neuropathy. J Neurol Sci. 132, 177-81, (1995).

Nobe K, Momose K, Sakai Y. Effects of Kampo medicine, Keishi – Ka- Shakuyaku-to (TJ – 60) on alteration of diacyl glycerol metabolism in gastrointestinal smoothmuscle of diabetic rats. Acta Pharm. Sinica, 23, 1173-1180, (2002).

Nyarko AK, Okine LKN, Wedzi RK, Addo PA, Ofosuhene M. Subchronic toxicity studies of the antidiabetic herbal preparation ADD-199 in the rat: absence of organ toxicity and modulation of cytochrome P450. J Ethnopharmacol, 97, 2, 319-325, (2005).

Okine LKN, Nyarko AK, Osei-Kwabena N, Oppong, IV, Barnes F, Ofosuhene M. The antidiabetic activity of the herbal preparation ADD-199 in mice: a comparative study with two oral hypoglycaemic drugs. J Ethnopharmacol, 97, 1, 31-38, (2005).

Pari L, Latha L. Protective role of *scopari dulcis* plant extract on brain antioxidant status and lipid peroxidation in STZ diabetic male wistar rats. BMC Compliment Altern Med. 4, 16, (2004).

Pari L, Ramakrishnan R, Venkateswaran S. Antihyperglycaemic effect of Diamed, a herbal formulation, in experimental diabetes in rats. J Pharm Pharmacol, 53, 1139-1143, (2001).

Pasquali R, Casimirri F. Clinical aspects of ephedrine in the treatment of obesity. Int J Obes, 17, 65-8, (1993).

Persaud SJ, Ai-Majed H, Raman A, Jones PM. *Gymnema sylvestre* stimulates insulin release in vitro by increased membrane permeability. J. Endocrinol, 163, 207-12, (1999).

Prince PSM, Menon VP, Pari L. Antioxidant action of *Tinosfora cordifolia* root extract in alloxan diabetic rats. Phytother Res, 15, 213-218, (2002).

Raj MK. A review on some antidiabetic plants of India. Ancient Science of Life, XIV, 168-80, (1995).

Randriamampandry, Ramarojoana J. Hypoglycemic effects of Rotra (*Eugenia jambolina* Lamarck) on the rabbit with alloxan diabetes. C R Seances Soc Biol Fil, 166, 484, (1972).

Satyavati GV, Dwarakanath C, Tripathi SN. Experimental studies on the hypocholesterolemic effect of *Commiphora mukul* Engl. (Guggul). Indian J Med Res, 57, 1950-62, (1969).

Senthilvel G, Austin A, Thirugnanasambantham Mayiswaran E, Balasubramanian, Jagadeesan M. Effect of a polyherbal formulation (Diarunplus) on streptozotocin induced experimental diabetes. Int. J. Trop. Med, 1, 88-92, (2006).

Seth S. Guggul (Commiphora mukul). Herbs for health and beauty, 113, (1996) India Book House Publishers, Bombay.

Seth S. Pippali (Piper Longum). Herbs for health and beauty, 1996, 115-6, India Book House Publishers, Bombay.

Shanmugasundaram ER, Rajeswari G, Baskaran K. Use of *Gymnema sylvestre* leaf extract in the control of blood glucose in insulin-dependent diabetes mellitus. J. Ethnopharmacol, 30, 281-94, (1990).

Shennan NM, Godsland IF, Wynn V. Derivation of a quantitative measure of insulin sensitivity from the intravenous tolbutamide test using the minimal model of glucose dynamics. Diabetologia. 30, 314-22, (1987).

Shimizu K, Ozeki M, Tanaka K, Itoh K, Nakajyo S, Urakawa N, Atsuchi M. Suppression of glucose absorption by extracts from the leaves of *Gymnema inodorum*. J. Vet. Med. Sci, 59, 753-7, (1997).

Singh RB, Niaz MA, Ghosh S. Hypolipidemic and antioxidant effects of Commiphora mukul as an adjunct to dietary therapy in patients with hypercholesterolemia. Cardiovas. Drugs Ther, 8, 659-64, (1994).

Tominaga M, Kimura M, Sugiyama K. Abe T, Igarashi K, Igarashi M, Eguchi H, Sekikawa A, Ogawa A, Manaka H, Sasaki H. Effects of Seishin – renshi – in and *Gymnema sylvestre* on insulin resistance in streptozotocin induced diabetic rats. Diabetes Res and Clinical Practice, 29, 1, 11-17, (1995).

Varier NKV. Indian medicinal plants, a compendium of 500 species, Vol. 3, 107-9 (1996) Orient Longman Ltd, Madras.

Varier NKV. Indian medicinal plants, a compendium of 500 species, Vol. 4, 290-2 (1995) Orient Longman Ltd., Madras.

Varier NKV. Indian medicinal plants, a compendium of 500 species, Vol. 2, 164-72 (1997) Orient Longman Ltd., Madras.

Wang LF, Luo H, Miyoshi M, Imoteo T, Hiji Y, Sasaki T. Inhibitory effect of gymnemic acid on intestinal absorption of oleic acid in rats. Can J Physiol Pharmacol, 76, 1017-23, (1998).

Wild S, Roglic G, Green A, Sicree R, King H. Global prevalence of diabetes: estimates for the year 2000 and projections for 2030. Diabetes Care, 27, 1047-1053, (2004).

Wong MW, Leung PC, Wong WC. Limb salvage in extensive diabetic foot ulceration—a preliminary clinical study using simple debridement and herbal drinks. Hong Kong Medical Journal, 7, 403-407, (2001).

Yashikawa M, Murakami T, Yashiro K, Matsuda H: Kotalanol, a potent alpha glucosidase inhibitor with thio sugar sulfonium sulfate structure from anti diabetic ayurvedic medicine Salacia reticulate. Chem. Pharm. Bull, 46, 1339 -1340, (1998).

Yoshihiko H, Takuya I, Kaoru Y, Nobuo K. Effects of Hachimi-jio-gan (Ba-Wei-Di-Huang-Wan) on hyperglycemia in Streptozotocin-Induced Diabetic Rats. Biol.Pharm. Bull. 30, 1015-1020, (2007).

Yoshikawa M, Morikawa T, Matsuda H, Tanabe G, Muraoka O. Absolute stereostructure of potent alpha glucosidase inhibitor, salacinol, with unique thiosugar sulfonium sulfate inner salt structure from *Salacia reticulata*. Bioorb. Med. Chem, 10, 1514-1547, (2002).

chapter 16

HERBAL LEADS FOR LIVER DISORDERS

Nilanjan Ghosh, Vivekananda Mandal, Hauzel Lalhlenmawia and Subhash C Mandal

INTRODUCTION

Chronic liver diseases represent a major health burden worldwide, with liver cirrhosis being the ninth leading cause of death in Western countries (Kim et al., 2002). Chronic viral hepatitis B and C, alcoholic liver disease, non-alcoholic fatty liver disease and hepatocellular carcinoma are the major entities and many problems remain unresolved. Treatment options for common liver diseases such as cirrhosis, fatty liver and chronic hepatitis are often limited in efficacy, carry the risk of adverse effects and are often too costly, especially for the developing world. The effectiveness of treatments such as interferon, colchicine, penicillamine and corticosteroids are inconsistent and the incidence of side-effects profound. Physicians and patients are in need of effective therapeutic agents with a low incidence of side-effects. Herbal medicines potentially constitute such a group. In recent years many researchers have examined the effects of plants used traditionally by indigenous healers to support liver function and treat diseases of the liver. In most cases, research has confirmed traditional experience and wisdom by discovering the mechanisms and modes of action of these plants as well as reaffirming the therapeutic effectiveness of certain plants or plant extracts in clinical studies.

Causative factors for liver toxicity mainly are alcohol, viral and induced by drugs. Alcoholic liver damage is differentiated by three main histological stages, that is, steatosis, acute alcoholic hepatitis and cirrhosis. In alcoholic liver disease, oxidative stress is caused by pro-oxidant formation, inadequate intake of antioxidants, antioxidant depletion, and alcohol-mediated inhibition of glutathione synthesis. Alcohol-induced liver diseases are mediated by cytokines, which are secreted by liver and other parts of the body. The second is the viral hepatitis, mainly responsible for both acute and chronic liver diseases. So far hepatitis A, B, C, D, and E have been identified as causative in human. Drug induced hepatotoxicity is a dose limiting adverse effect for several drugs like paracetamol, isoniazid and rifampicin.

Therefore, treating liver diseases with plant-derived compounds which are accessible and do not require laborious pharmaceutical synthesis seems highly attractive. Furthermore, in spite of the advances in conventional medicine in the last decades, research professionals of developed countries are paying increasing attention to phytomedicine. Several recent surveys from Europe and the United States have demonstrated a sharp rise in the use of phytomedicine within a few years, and up to 65% of patients with liver disease take herbal preparations (Strader et al., 2002; De Smet, 2002). Many factors contribute to herbal medicine's appeal. It is claimed that herbal medicine may both treat and prevent diseases. This adds to a deep belief that these treatments are safe because they are "natural" and, therefore, harmless alternative to conventional medicine. In addition, herbal products are often exempt from rigorous regulations, such as in the U.S., and prescriptions are usually not required for these inexpensive products. The following review describes the current scientific evidence regarding herbal drugs and the liver, especially in regards to their presumed beneficial effect, and delineates the issues that need to be addressed to incorporate herbal medicine into the arsenal of therapies in the treatment of liver diseases.

Liver function tests

Liver has to perform different kinds of biochemical, synthetic and excretory functions, so no single biochemical test can detect the global functions of liver. Laboratories usually employ a battery of tests for initial detection and management of liver diseases and these tests are frequently termed "Liver function tests". Liver function tests (LFT) are a helpful screening tool, which are an effective modality to detect hepatic dysfunction. They also help to recognize the pattern of liver disease, to assess the severity of certain diseases.

Classification of Liver Function Tests

A. Tests of the liver's capacity to transport organic anions and to metabolize drugs- Serum bilirubin, urine bilirubin, urobilinogen *etc.*

B. Tests that detect injury to hepatocytes (serum enzyme tests)–Aminotransferases, alkaline phosphatase, γ-glutamyl transpeptidase, 5 nucleotidase, leucine aminopeptidase *etc.*

C. Tests of the Liver's biosynthetic capacity-Serum proteins, albumin, prealbumin, serum ceruloplasmin, procollagen III peptide, prothrombin time *etc.*

Diseases of the liver

Many diseases of the liver are accompanied by jaundice caused by increased levels of bilirubin in the system. The bilirubin results from the breakup of the hemoglobin of dead red blood cells. Normally, the liver removes bilirubin from the blood and excretes it through bile. The diseases of the liver are summarized below:

- Hepatitis, inflammation of the liver, is caused mainly by various viruses but also by some poisons, autoimmunity or hereditary conditions.
- Cirrhosis is the formation of fibrous tissue in the liver, replacing dead liver cells. The death of the liver cells can for example be caused by viral hepatitis, alcoholism or contact with other liver-toxic chemicals.
- Haemochromatosis is a hereditary disease causing the accumulation of iron in the body, eventually leading to liver damage.
- Cancer of the liver (primary hepatocellular carcinoma or cholangiocarcinoma and metastatic cancers, usually from other parts of the gastrointestinal tract).
- Wilson's disease is a hereditary disease which causes the body to retain copper.
- Primary sclerosing cholangitis, is an inflammatory disease of the bile duct, autoimmune in nature.
- Primary biliary cirrhosis is an autoimmune disease of small bile ducts.
- Budd-Chiari syndrome is the obstruction of the hepatic vein.
- Gilbert's syndrome is a genetic disorder of bilirubin metabolism, found in about 5% of the population.

- Glycogen storage disease type II, in which the build-up of glycogen causes progressive muscle weakness (myopathy) throughout the body and affects various body tissues, particularly in the heart, skeletal muscles, liver and nervous system.

Pathophysiology of Liver Injury

Irrespective of the underlying etiology, the process of liver damage shows a series of stereotyped features as the mechanisms of induction, the cells involved in overproduction of extra cellular matrix components, the tendency to progress into sclerosis, a proper degenerative evolution of the connective tissue, and, in a subgroup of patients, eventually to cirrhosis, the common endpoint of a variety of chronic liver diseases. Many if not all disease processes affecting hepatic tissue are accompanied by a certain degree of oxidative stress, i.e. an unbalanced increase of reactive oxygen species (ROS) with overall pro-oxidant activity exerted on the different molecules, potentially able to affect their structure and function. Reactive oxygen driven reactions are now increasingly recognized as taking place in both initiation and perpetuation of liver fibrosis. On this line, it seems feasible to believe that a moderate but sustained unbalance of redox cell equilibrium would represent a subtle but very efficient mechanism of progression of fibrotic lesion (Poli, 2000).

Following liver injury, wound repair mechanisms become activated that in turn lead to marked overproduction of the connective structure of the organ. Changes of extra cellular matrix are not merely quantitative but also involve marked qualitative modifications. The fibrotic process involves all cell types devoted to matrix synthesis, namely, stellate cells, sinusoidal endothelial cells and interstitial fibroblasts. Collagen type III is first increased after liver damage later on largely substituted by collagen type I. The amount of the latter type keeps increasing with the progression of the fibrotic process to sclerosis and cirrhosis.

Liver tissue injury, repair and fibrogenesis

Liver fibrosis occurs as a pathological sequel to chronic pro-inflammatory liver injury of many various etiologies (Bataller and Brenner, 2005; Friedman, 2004). The main causes of liver fibrosis in developed countries are chronic hepatitis virus infection, alcohol and non-alcoholic steatohepatitis (NASH) with other causes including autoimmune conditions and genetic disorders. The end stage of liver fibrosis, cirrhosis, is characterized by increased deposition and altered composition of the extracellular matrix (ECM) accompanied by hepatic failure and portal hypertension (Gines et al., 2004). Major complications of cirrhosis include ascites, variceal bleeding, renal failure and hepatic encephalopathy.

Fibrogenesis is currently viewed as a dynamic process strictly related to the extent and duration of parenchymal injury. This modern view implies that several fibrogenic disorders, once identified as "degenerative", are today considered as the result of events such as reiterative tissue damage and chronic inflammation (Schuppan et al., 1999). In general, the process leading to liver fibrosis, similar to the process of normal wound healing, includes three phases following tissue injury: acute inflammation, synthesis of collagenous and noncollagenous extracellular matrix (ECM) components, and tissue remodeling. Thus the persistence of the original insult causes the prolonged activation of the tissue repair mechanisms, thus leading to tissue fibrosis rather than to effective tissue repair (Brenner et al., 2000).

Fibrosis patterns in chronic liver diseases

Accumulation of fibrillar ECM is a common marker of chronic liver tissue damage and usually leads to the complex architectural changes typical of liver cirrhosis. Although nodular regeneration and septal fibrosis represent the common outcome of this process, several patterns of development can be distinguished according to different causes of liver damage and their typical temporal and pathophysiological features. In general, excessive amounts of fibrillar matrix are found in those areas of the liver lobule characterized by extensive hepatocellular necrosis and inflammatory infiltration. Accordingly, in chronic hepatitis due to chronic hepatitis B virus (HBV) or HCV infection, fibrosis initially develops at the edge of portal tracts where necrosis is present. This leads to the so-called *"portal tract enlargement"*. With the progression of the disease, fibrous septa develop from the enlarged portal tract and tend to proceed towards the centrilobular vein. This pattern, defined *"portal to central fibrosis"*, eventually results in the formation of cirrhotic nodules and is characterized by rapid metabolic and hemodynamic consequences, including the development of portal hypertension and its related complications in relatively early stages of the disease.

Liver fibrosis consequent to chronic alcohol abuse tends to follow a different pattern of development. In this clinical setting, accumulation of fibrillar ECM is first observed around the centrilobular vein *(pericentral fibrosis)* and particularly in the space of Disse, thus leading to capillarization of the sinusoids located in this area of the liver lobule. Only at later stages does fibrosis assume the typical features of septal fibrosis and nodular regeneration.

Cellular and molecular basis of liver fibrosis
Hepatic stellate cells: biology and role in hepatic fibrogenesis

Although different types of liver cells have the capacity to synthesize ECM components, hepatic stellate cells (HSC, also known as Ito cells/lipocytes/fat-storing cells) are currently considered the main connective tissue producing cells in fibrotic liver (Pinzani, 1995). HSC are located in the space of Disse in close contact with hepatocytes and sinusoidal endothelial cells. Their three-dimensional structure consists of the cell body and several long and branching cytoplasmic processes. Two main types of cytoplasmic process are recognized according to their spatial disposition: the intersinusoidal or interhepatocellular processes and the perisinusoidal or subendothelial processes. The interhepatocellular processes penetrate the hepatic cell plates and extend to nearby sinusoids (Friedman, 2000).

An intriguing aspect of stellate cell function is the capacity to express a dual phenotype. In healthy liver, the cells show the "quiescent phenotype", that is to say, they contain vitamin A-rich lipid droplets, under developed organelles and show a low proliferation rate. In the chronically diseased liver, the cells acquire the "activated phenotype" - they differentiate into myofibroblast-like cells with high proliferative capacity, thereby losing their vitamin A-containing fat droplets, and developing a prominent rough endoplasmic reticulum, extensive microtubules and bundles of actin filaments with local condensations (Freije et al., 1994). A variety of functions have been ascribed to the stellate cells and the myofibroblast-like cells derived from them: they take up, store, and release retinoids; they, particularly in their myofibroblast-like form, synthesize and secrete extracellular matrix proteins (collagens I, III, IV, V and VI, fibronectin, laminin, tenascin, undulin, hyaluronan and proteoglycans); stellate cells and derived myofibroblast like cells in particular synthesize and secrete extracellular matrix degrading metalloproteinases and tissue inhibitors of metalloproteinase-1; in both forms they synthesize and secrete cytokines and, especially, as myofibroblast-like cells they are able to contract in response to vasoactive substances and are thus potentially involved in the regulation of hepatic sinusoidal tone (Emonard and Emonard, 1990). The activated phenotype is characterised by a dramatically increased synthesis of collagen types I and III, that appears predominantly over the synthesis of collagen type IV (I>III>IV) and other ECM components. In conditions of chronic liver damage, HSC undergo a process of activation from the quiescent "storing" phenotype to the highly proliferative "myofibroblast-like" phenotype. This transition is gradual and occurs through an intermediate stage defined as "transitional cell" (Mak and Lieber, 1998; Burr et al., 1986). The phenotypic cascade of HSC activation involves both marked morphological changes and up-regulation of several functional components including ECM synthesis, expression of growth factor and cytokine receptors, contractile structures and metalloproteinases. Taken together these modifications lead to a cell type with remarkable proliferative, synthetic and contractile properties.

The presence of reiterated liver tissue damage leads to what has been defined as "perpetuation" of HSC activation. Activated HSC have been shown to increase the degradation of the normal subendothelial matrix as a result of an augmented secretion of type IV collagenase (gelatinase) and/or a reduced secretion of the tissue inhibitor of metalloproteinase (TIMP), a specific proteinase inhibitor (Arthur et al., 1989). Finally, recent experimental evidence suggests that following prolonged activation HSC undergo a down regulation of the gene encoding for matrix metalloproteinase (type I collagenase or fibroblast type interstitial collagenase) and an up-regulation of the gene encoding for the corresponding specific inhibitor (TIMP-1), thus leading to further accumulation of insoluble interstitial collagen (Iredale et al., 1992).

Growth factors, cytokines and other soluble mediators involved in HSC activation

Extensive HSC proliferation, migration and ECM synthesis occur in response to polypeptide growth factors and cytokines locally released as part of the inflammatory component of the tissue repair process (Pinzani, 1995). Among other polypeptide growth factors potentially involved in chronic liver tissue inflammation, platelet-derived growth factor (PDGF) has been shown to be the most potent mitogen for cultured HSC isolated from rat, mouse, or human liver (Pinzani et al., 1989). Of the three possible dimeric forms of PDGF (-AA, -AB, and -BB), PDGF-BB has been shown to be the most potent in stimulating HSC growth and the relative intracellular signaling, in agreement with a predominant expression of PDGF-receptor β (or type B) subunits compared to the expression of PDGF-receptor α (or type A) subunits in activated HSC. The PDGF receptors contain intrinsic tyrosine kinase activity and dimerize and become autophosphorylated on tyrosine residues upon binding to their ligand.

Another growth factor that has been recognized to play a definite pro-fibrogenic role is transforming growth factor-β (TGF-β). TGF-â is a multifunctional growth factor with stimulatory or inhibitory properties on cellular proliferation and/or differentiation. TGF-β has been shown to be clearly associated with hepatic fibrosis (Castilla et al., 1991). One of the most evident effects of TGF-β on fibroblasts, myofibroblasts and pericytes is the increased synthesis and deposition of ECM components (Raghow et al., 1987). In addition, TGF-β is capable of retarding the degradation of such products. For these reasons TGF-β is considered a key factor in the tissue repair process and in the development of fibrogenic disorders. TGF β stimulates procollagen I and III synthesis and release in rat as well as human cultured HSC (Weiner et al., 1990).

Fibrotic liver tissue: a new biological microenvironment

The abnormal matrix microenvironment characterizing the fibrogenic process may further contribute to perpetuation of HSC activation. Indeed, the progressive shift from a basal membrane-like ECM, rich in collagen type IV, to a fibrillar ECM in which type I collagen predominates, may be responsible for increasing the proliferative potential of HSC. Collagen type I, in addition directly to promoting HSC activation (Davis et al., 1987) may function as a reservoir of polypeptide mitogens released in active or inactive form by inflammatory cells or as a consequence of cell necrosis. For these reasons, the relationship occurring between HSC and the modified hepatic microenvironment typical of fibrotic liver, and particularly the interaction between HSC and ECM through integrin receptors, represents a relevant current issue. Indeed, this relationship may have, per se, profound implications in the acquisition of the proliferative/contractile phenotype typical of this stage of activation. Integrins are heterodimeric transmembrane proteins that consist of an α subunit and β subunit. The molecular masses of the various subunits range from 90 to 200 kDa. The α sub unit and β subunit are non-covalently bound, and this association is promoted by divalent cations. There are at least 8 β and 15 α subunits that can associate in various combinations to form 21 individual receptors. Activated HSC express several integrin β_1-associated α subunits. A particularly high expression has been demonstrated for $\alpha_1\beta_1$ and $\alpha_2\beta_1$. Integrin $\alpha_1\beta_1$ has been shown to be a dual receptor for collagen type IV, collagen type I, and laminin. Integrin $\alpha_2\beta_1$ is defined as a collagen receptor, but it can also interact with other ECM proteins such as laminin and fibronectin. However, $\alpha_2\beta_1$ binding affinity to laminin and collagen differs consistently, suggesting a cell type-dependent regulation. The signaling pathways activated by integrins have been identified through the analysis of biochemical events that are triggered by integrin engagement, and by the identification of proteins that associate with focal adhesion complexes. It is particularly relevant that many of the signaling proteins regulated by integrins are also involved in signal transduction pathways activated by growth factor receptors and agents inducing cell contraction (Carloni et al., 1987). Accordingly, synergistic interactions between growth factor and integrin signaling pathways are involved in the regulation of cell proliferation, adhesion and migration. For example, adherence to the ECM is critical for growth factor or serum dependent proliferation in most cell types or for cell contraction in response to vasoconstrictors.

In other words, a particular organization of the cytoskeleton deriving from integrin receptor engagement with different ECM components is likely to synergize with the signals deriving from multiple receptor systems to regulate biological phenomena such as cell proliferation, cell motility, ECM synthesis and cell contraction.

Agents which are used as hepatotoxins

1. Paracetamol at a dose of 250 mg/kg p.o. is known to cause liver damage in rats (Mitra et al., 1998).
2. CCl_4 a single dose of 2 ml/kg, i.p. is used for inducing hepatotoxicity in rats (Latha et al., 2006).
3. d-galactosamine at a dose of 400 mg/kg i.p. is used as a hepatotoxin (Latha et al., 2006).
4. LPS, a major cell wall molecule of Gram-negative bacteria and the principal initiator of septic shock, causes liver injury at doses from 1-10 mg/kg.
5. Diethylnitrosamine at a dose of 200 mg/kg iis used to indice hepatotoxicity.
6. Ethanol at dose of 5 g/kg/day for 21 days is used to induce liver injury.
7. Thioacetamide at a dose of 200 mg/kg is known to cause liver damage in rats.

Biomarkers used in detection of liver disease

Alanine transaminase

Alanine transaminase (ALT), also called Serum Glutamic Pyruvate Transaminase (SGPT) is an enzyme present in hepatocytes. When a cell is damaged, it leaks this enzyme into the blood, where it is measured. ALT rises dramatically in acute liver damage.

Principle of estimation

ALT catalyses the following reaction:

α-ketoglutarate + L- Alanine ! Pyruvate + L- Glutamate

Pyruvate reacts with 2,4 dinitrophenyl hydrazine (DNPH) to give pyruvate hydrazone, which gives brown color in alkaline condition and is measured colorimetrically at 505nm (Rietman and Frankel, 1957).

Aspartate transaminase

Aspartate transaminase (AST) also called Serum Glutamic Oxaloacetic Transaminase (SGOT) is similar to ALT in that it is another enzyme associated with liver parenchymal cells. It is raised in acute liver damage. The ratio of AST to ALT is sometimes useful in differentiating between causes of liver damage. Elevated AST levels are not specific for liver damage, and AST has also been used as a cardiac marker.

Principle of estimation

AST catalyses the following reaction:

α-ketoglutarate + L- Aspartate ↔ Oxaloacetate + L- Glutamate

Oxaloacetate so formed reacts with 2,4 dinitrophenyl hydrazine (DNPH) to give oxaloacetate hydrazone, which gives brown color in alkaline condition and is measured colorimetrically at 505nm (Rietman and Frankel, 1957).

Alkaline phosphatase

Alkaline phosphatase (ALP) is an enzyme in the cells lining the biliary ducts of the liver. ALP levels in plasma will rise with large bile duct obstruction, intrahepatic cholestasis or infiltrative diseases of the liver. ALP is also present in bone and placental tissue, so it is higher in growing children (as their bones are being remodelled) and elderly patients with Paget's disease.

Principle of estimation

Alkaline phosphatase from serum converts Phenyl phosphate to inorganic phosphate and phenol at pH 10. Phenol so formed reacts in alkaline medium with 4-aminoantipyrine in presence of oxidizing agent potassium ferricyanide and forms an orange red complex. This colored complex is estimated colorimetrically at 510nm (Kind and King, 1954).

$$\text{Phenyl phosphate} \xrightarrow[\text{pH 10}]{\text{ALP}} \text{Phenol} + \text{Phosphate}$$

$$\text{Phenol} + \text{4-aminoantipyrine} \xrightarrow[\text{OH}^-]{\text{Potassium ferricyanide}} \text{Orange red complex}$$

Bilirubin

Bilirubin is a breakdown product of heme. The liver is responsible for clearing bilirubin. It does this by the following mechanism: bilirubin is taken up into hepatocytes, conjugated (modified to make it water-soluble), and secreted into the bile, which is excreted into the intestine. Increased total bilirubin causes jaundice, and can signal a number of problems:

1. **Prehepatic:** Increased bilirubin production. This can be due to a number of causes, including hemolytic anemias and internal hemorrhage.
2. **Hepatic:** Problems with the liver, which are reflected as deficiencies in bilirubin metabolism (e.g. reduced hepatocyte uptake, impaired conjugation of bilirubin, and reduced hepatocyte secretion of bilirubin). Some examples would be cirrhosis and viral hepatitis.
3. **Posthepatic:** Obstruction of the bile ducts, reflected as deficiencies in bilirubin excretion. (Obstruction can be located either within the liver or in the bile duct.)

Principle of estimation

Direct or conjugated bilirubin couples with diazotized sulfanilic acid, forming azobilirubin, a red purple colored product in acidic medium, whereas unconjugated bilirubin is diazotized only in presence of methanol. The intensity of the red purple color so developed above is measured colorimetrically at 540nm (Malloy and Evelyn, 1937).

Gamma glutamyl transpeptidase

Gamma glutamyl transpeptidase (GGT) may be elevated with even minor, sub-clinical levels of liver dysfunction. It can also be helpful in identifying the cause of an isolated elevation in ALP. GGT is raised in alcohol toxicity (acute and chronic).

Histopathological examinations

Liver pieces are preserved in 10% formaldehyde solution for histopathological study. The pieces of liver were dehydrated with a sequence of ethanol solution and embedded in paraffin wax. Sections of about 4-6 μm thickness are cut. They are stained with hematoxylin and eosin and photographed using a photomicroscope. The haematoxylin and eosin stained section of paracetamol treated liver tissue with intense lymphocytic infiltration around central vein and centrilobular necrosis (zone 3 necrosis). Dilated sinusoids and hepatocytes with ballooning degeneration are also observed. Cellular boundary and normal architecture of hepatic lobule is also damaged. The haematoxylin and eosin stained section of CCl_4 shows distorted hepatic lobule with extensive fatty changes (steatosis i.e., accumulation of fat droplets), sinusoidal congestion, extensive lymphocytic infiltration around central vein and extensive vacuolization with loss of nuclei in hepatocytes and normal hepatic lobular architecture. The liver of d-galactosamine treated animals showed inflammation of lymphocytes and Kupffer cells and hyaline degeneration around the portal vein area.

Phytoconstituents with hepatoprotective potentials

Compounds with different structure but with the same therapeutic activity isolated from different plant species act as active moieties for the treatment of various diseases. Several phytomolecules including flavonoids, alkaloids, glycosides, and saponins obtained from various plant sources have been reported as potent hepatoprotective agents. Plant tissues contain a wide variety of compounds with antioxidant activity. Phenolic compounds (flavonoids and phenolic acids), nitrogen compounds (alkaloids, chlorophyll derivatives, amino acids and amines), carotenoids, lignans and terpenes were reported to possess antioxidative activity in suppressing the initiation or propagation of the chain reactions (Cuppett and Hall, 1997). Flavonoids and phenolic compounds are the main antioxidative compounds of herbal drugs.

The phenolic compounds exhibit considerable free radical scavenging activities, through their reactivity as hydrogen or electron-donating agents, and metal ion chelating properties (Rice-Evans et al., 1996). Flavonoids are polyphenolic compounds that occur ubiquitously in foods of plant origin. Over 4000 different flavonoids have been described. They may have beneficial health effects because of their antioxidant properties and their inhibitory role in various stages of tumor development. Some potent herbs with established hepatoprotective activity are described in the following section:

Silymarin (Family: Compositae)

Silymarin obtained from *Silybum marianum*, commonly known as 'milk thistle' is one of the oldest and thoroughly researched plants in the treatment of liver diseases (Luper, 1998). It is the gold standard of hepatoprotective agents and has been widely used as comparative standard for test drugs in preclinical studies. The pharmacological profile of silymarin has been well defined and hepatoprotective properties of silymarin were investigated both in vitro and in vivo. Experimental studies demonstrated antioxidant and free radical scavenging properties, improvement of the antioxidative defense by prevention of glutathione depletion, and antifibrotic activity. The active constituents of the plant are obtained from the dried seeds and consist of four flavonolignans which are collectively known as silymarin. Silymarin is extracted from the dried seeds of milk thistle plant, where it is present in higher concentrations than in other parts of the plant. Silymarin is a complex mixture of four flavonolignan isomers (Flora et al., 1998), namely silybin, isosilybin, silydianin and silychristin with an empirical formula $C_{25}H_{22}O_{10}$. The structural similarity of silymarin to steroid hormones is believed to be responsible for its protein synthesis facilitatory actions (Saller et al., 2001). Among the isomers silybin is the major and most active component and represents about 60-70%, followed by silychristin (20%), silydianin (10%), and isosilybin (5%).

The cytoprotective effects of silymarin are mainly attributable to its antioxidant and free radical scavenging properties (Miller, 1986). Silymarin can also interact directly with cell membrane components to prevent any abnormalities in the content of lipid fraction responsible for maintaining normal fluidity (Wiseman, 1996; Muriel and Mourelle, 1990). Silymarin also has anti-inflammatory actions due to inhibition of 5-lipoxygenase pathway which results in impaired leukotriene synthesis (Dehmlow et al., 1996). Liver fibrosis can result in remodeling of liver architecture leading to hepatic insufficiency, portal hypertension and hepatic encephalopathy. These processes involve complex interplay of cells and mediators. In the initial phase there will be proliferation of hepatic parenchymal cells. The conversion of hepatic stellate cells (HSC) into myofibroblast is considered as the central event in fibrogenesis. Silymarin inhibits NF-KB and also retards HSC activation. It also inhibits protein kinases and other kinases involved in signal transduction and may interact with intracellular signaling pathways (Saliou et al., 1998: Johnson et al., 2002). Stimulation of protein synthesis by Silymarin has important therapeutic implications in the repair of damaged hepatocytes and restoration of normal functions of liver (Sonnenbichler and Zetl, 1986).

Drugs in common use can cause toxic effects on the liver which can mimic almost every natural diseases of the liver. This is rarely due to the drug itself and a toxic metabolite is usually responsible. The drug metabolizing enzymes activate chemically stable drugs to produce electrophilic metabolites. These potent agents bind covalently to liver molecules such as proteins and fatty acids which are essential to the life of the hepatocyte and necrosis ensues. Free radicals are generated which results in lipid peroxidation and membrane damage. The end result is hepatocyte death related to failure to pump calcium from the cytosol and to depressed mitochondrial function. Drugs like paracetamol and halothane produce zone 3 (centrilobular) necrosis of liver (Sherlock and Dooley, 2002). Silymarin has a regulatory action on cellular and mitochondrial membrane permeability in association with an increase in membrane stability against xenobiotic injury. It can prevent the absorption of toxins into the hepatocytes by occupying the binding sites as well as inhibiting many transport proteins at the membrane. These actions along with antiperoxidative property make silymarin a suitable candidate for the treatment of iatrogenic and toxic liver diseases.

Glycyrrhizin (Family: Leguminosae)

Glycyrrhizin is an aqueous extract of the liquorice root (*Glycyrrhiza glabra*) and has been used in traditional medicine to alleviate bronchitis, gastritis and jaundice. The major constituents are glycyrrhetinic acid, flavonoids, hydroxycoumarins, and β-sitosterol, the latter with probable glucocorticoid and mineralocorticoid properties. Glycyrrhizin is capable of preventing various kinds of liver injury in animals. This drug possesses anti-inflammatory and antioxidant activities. Glycyrrhizin inhibits CD4+ T-cell and tumor necrosis factor (TNF)-mediated cytotoxicity (Yoshikawa et al., 1997). Glycyrrhizin has a membrane stabilizing effect (Shiki et al., 1992) and also stimulates endogenous production of interferon. In cell culture experiments, glycyrrhizin modifies glycosylation and blocks sialylation of hepatitis B surface antigen (HBsAg), leading to its retention in the Golgi apparatus. Glycyrrhizin counteracts several forms of experimental hepatic injury and partly inhibits the activity of 11-beta-hydroxysteroid dehydrogenase, prostaglandin E2 production by macrophages, and may have antioxidative properties through the induction of glutathione-S-transferases and catalase. Some evidence points to an antifibrotic effect in the rat CCl_4 model, possibly through inactivation of NFkB.

Phyllanthus niruri (Family: Euphorbiaceae)

Phyllanthus niruri is a small, erect, annual herb that grows 30-40 cm in height. It is indigenous to the rainforests of the Amazon and other tropical areas throughout the world, including the Bahamas, southern India, and China. The main plant chemicals include alkaloids, astragalin, brevifolin, carboxylic acids, corilagin, cymene, ellagic acid, ellagitannins, gallocatechins, geraniin, hypophyllanthin, lignans, lintetralins, lupeols, methyl salicylate, niranthin, nirtetralin, niruretin, nirurin, phyllanthin, phyllanthine, phyllanthenol, phyllochrysine, phyltetralin, repandusinic acids, quercetin, quercetol, quercitrin, rutin, saponins, triacontanal, and tricontanol.

Whole plant, fresh leaves and fruits are used to treat various ailments, particularly hepatitis. This herb has shown potent antioxidant activity and hepatoprotective activity (Harish and Shivanandappa, 2006). Methanolic and aqueous extract of leaves and fruits of *P. niruri* showed inhibition of membrane lipid peroxidation (LPO), scavenging of 1,1-diphenyl-2 picrylhydrazyl (DPPH) radical and inhibition of reactive oxygen species (ROS) *in vitro*. Antioxidant activities of the extracts were also demonstrable *in vivo* by the inhibition of the CCl_4 induced formation of lipid peroxides in the liver of rats by pretreatment with the extracts. CCl_4 induced hepatotoxicity in rats, as judged by the raised serum enzymes, glutamate oxaloacetate transaminase (GOT) and glutamate pyruvate transaminase (GPT) was prevented by pretreatment with the extracts, demonstrating the hepatoprotective action of *P. niruri*. Treatment with the protein isolates of *P. niruri* significantly increase SOD and catalase which were reduced due to CCl_4 administration (Bhattacharjee and Sil, 2007). Phyllanthin and hypophyllanthin have been established as the hepatoprotective agents.

Boerhaavia diffusa (Family: Nyctaginaceae)

Boerhaavia diffusa is a vigorous, low-growing, spreading vine with a long, tuberous tap root. It can be found in many tropical and warm-climate countries and is indigenous to Brazil. It is also found in abundance in warmer parts of India and called *punarnava*. It has a long history of use by indigenous and tribal people and in Ayurvedic herbal medicine systems. The roots of *Boerhaavia diffusa* are used by a large number of tribes in India for the treatment of various hepatic disorders.

The *Boerhaavia diffusa* plant contains a large number of such compounds as flavonoids, alkaloids, steroids, triterpenoids, lipids, lignins, carbohydrates, proteins, and glycoproteins. Punarnavine, punarnavoside and liirodendrin are the major active constituents. Punarnavoside and liirodendrin are thought to be responsible for the hepatopotective activity (Rawat et al., 1997). The hepatoprotective activity of roots of *Boerhaavia diffusa* was examined in thioacetamide intoxicated rats. The results showed that an aqueous extract (2 ml/kg) of roots exhibited marked protection of a majority of serum parameters, i.e. AST, ALT and ALP.

Eclipta alba (Family: Compositae)

It is widely used herbal medicine. Folklore suggests its hepatoprotective activity. It is widely distributed throughout India, China, Thailand, and Brazil. In Ayurvedic medicine, the leaf extract is considered a powerful liver tonic, rejuvenative, and especially good for the hair. Phytochemically, *Eclipta alba* is rich in coumestans i.e. wedelolactone (I) and demethylwedelolactone (II), polypeptides, β-amyrin, stigmasterol, luteolin-7-Glucoside, polyacetylenes, thiophene-derivatives, steroids, triterpenes and flavonoids. Wedelolactone possesses a wide range of biological activities and is used for the treatment of hepatitis and cirrhosis and for direct inhibition of IKK complex resulting in suppression of LPS-induced caspase-11 expression. The hepatoprotective activity has been experimentally established (Saxena et al., 1993). The hepatoprotective effect of the ethanol/water (1:1) extract of *Eclipta alba* has been studied in rats against CCl_4 induced hepatotoxicity. It significantly counteracted CCl_4 induced inhibition of the hepatic microsomal drug metabolising enzyme amidopyrine N-demethylase and membrane bound glucose 6-phosphatase, but failed to reverse the very high degree of inhibition of another drug metabolising enzyme aniline hydroxylase. The loss of hepatic lysosomal acid phosphatase and alkaline phosphatase by CCl_4 was significantly restored by extract of *Eclipta alba*. The study shows that hepatoprotective activity of extract of *Eclipta alba* is by regulating the levels of hepatic microsomal drug metabolising enzymes.

Berberis aristata (Family: Berberidaceae)

Berberis aristata is an erect, spinescent and glabrous shrub, ranging between 2 and 3 metres in height with lanceolate, simple spiny, toothed, leathery, sessile, acuminate leaves. The flowers are yellow coloured and are present in corymbose racemes. Fruits are in form of ovoid berries. It is an edible plant employed in the South Asian Traditional Medicine, particularly its fruits being used as a tonic remedy for liver and heart. It is rich in alkaloids like berberine, oxyberberine, berbamine, aromoline, karachine, and oxycanthine. Berberine is the major active constituent Berberine has experimentally established hepatoprotective activity (Gilani and Janbaz, 2000). In an investigation, berberine, a known compound from this plant, was studied for its possible anti-hepatotoxic action in rats. Pretreatment of animals with berberine (4 mg/kg; orally twice daily for 2 days) prevented the acetaminophen or CCl_4 induced rise in serum levels of alkaline phosphatase (ALP) and aminotransaminases (AST and ALT), suggestive of hepatoprotection. Post-treatment with three successive oral doses of berberine (4 mg/kg every 6 h) reduced the hepatic damage induced by acetaminophen, while CCl_4 induced hepatotoxicity was not modified, suggesting a selective curative effect against acetaminophen. Pretreatment of animals with a single oral dose of berberine (4 mg/kg) induced prolongation of the pentobarbital (60 mg/kg, i.p.) induced sleeping time as well as increased strychnine (0.3 mg/kg; i.p.) induced toxicity, suggestive of inhibitory effect on microsomal drug metabolizing enzymes; cytochrome P450s (CYPs).

Andrographis paniculata (Family: Acanthaceae)

Andrographis paniculata is a herbaceous plant in the family *Acanthaceae*, native to India and Sri Lanka. *Andrographis paniculata*, is an erect annual herb extremely bitter in taste in each and every part of the plant body. The stem is quadrangular with longitudinal furrows. The leaves are glabrous, dark green and arranged opposite decussate. Flowers are small and in terminal racemes. Mostly the leaves and roots were used for medicinal purposes. The principal constituents are 14-Deoxy-11-dehydroandrographolide, 14-Deoxy-11-oxoandrographolide, andrographolide, andrographine, neoandrographolide, panicoline, paniculide-A, paniculide-B and paniculide-C.

Andrographolide, chief constituent extracted from the leaves of the plant, is a bitter water-soluble lactone exhibiting protective effects in carbon tetrachloride induced hepatopathy in rats. It is very popular for its hepatoprotective activity. Andrographolide is the major active constituent and it has been established that it is responsible for the hepatoprotective activity of *Andrographis paniculata* (Visen et al., 1993). Andrographolide, the active constituent isolated from the plant *Andrographis paniculata*, showed a significant dose dependent (0.75–12 mg/kg p.o.× 7) protective activity against paracetamol-induced toxicity on *ex vivo* preparation of isolated rat hepatocytes. It significantly increased the percent viability of the hepatocytes as tested by trypan blue exclusion and oxygen uptake tests. It completely antagonized the toxic effects of paracetamol on certain enzymes (GOT, GPT and alkaline phosphatase) in serum as well as in isolated hepatic cells. Andrographolide was found to be more potent than silymarin, a standard hepatoprotective agent.

Picrorhiza kurroa (Family: Scrophulariaceae)

Picrorhiza kurroa is a well-known herb in the Ayurvedic system of medicine and has traditionally been used to treat disorders of the liver and upper respiratory tract, reduce fevers, and to treat dyspepsia, chronic diarrhea, and scorpion sting. It is a small perennial herb from the Scrophulariaceae family, found in the Himalayan region growing at elevations of 3,000-5,000 meters. The active constituents are obtained from the root and rhizomes.

Kutkin is the active principle of *Picrorhiza kurroa* and is comprised of kutkoside and the iridoid glycoside picrosides I, II, and III. Other identified active constituents are apocynin, drosin, and nine cucurbitacin glycosides. Picroliv is a standardized iridoid glycoside mixture isolated from the roots and rhizomes of the plant *Picrorhiza kurroa*. It contains at least 60% of a 1:1.5 mixture of picroside I and kutkoside; the remainder (40%)

is a mixture of iridoid as well as cucurbitacin glycosides and some still unidentified substances. This herb is one of the most important natural remedies for liver diseases. Picroliv has been found to possess potent hepatoprotective activity against different hepatotoxins (Dwivedi et al., 1993). The hepatoprotective activity of Picroliv, a standardized iridoid glycoside fraction of *Picrorhiza kurroa*, has been investigated by studying the protection of biochemical and histological changes induced in livers of rats given single oral doses (7 mg/kg) of aflatoxin B1. Administration of aflatoxin B1 resulted in a significant increase in 52-nucleotidase, γ-glutamyl transpeptidase, acid ribonuclease, total lipids, cholesterol and lipid peroxides in liver and transaminases, alkaline phosphatase and billrubin in serum. However, the activity of glucose 6-phosphatase and levels of cytochrome P450, cytochrome b5, DNA, RNA, proteins and glycogen in liver and total proteins in serum decreased. The liver histology showed ballooned hepatocytes, degeneration, microvesicular fat, focal necrosis, bile duct hyperplasia and proliferation of oval and spindle cells in portal tracts. When Picroliv (25 mg/kg × 7 days) was given to aflatoxin B1 toxicated rats, the majority of the biochemical and histological changes were significantly protected. The findings indicate a hepatoprotective activity of Picroliv against aflatoxin B1 toxicity in rats.

Cichorium intybus (Family: Compositae)

Cichorium intybus is a bushy perennial herb with a fleshy tap root and blue or lavender flowers. The leaves are broadly oblong, lanceolate, crowded at the base and arranged spirally on the stem. Principal chemical constituents are inulin (polysaccharide), cichoriin, lactucin and lactucopricin. The plant *Cichorium intybus* is used as liver tonic, cardiotonic, diuretic, stomachic, cholagogue, depurative, emmenagogue, hepatomegaly, cephalalgia, inflammations, anorexia, dyspepsia, flatulence, colic, jaundice, splenomegaly, amenorrhea dysmenorrhea, and asthma. It has been experimentally established as a potent hepatoprotective agent (Ahmed et al., 2003). The different fractions of alcoholic extract and one phenolic compound AB-IV of seeds of *Cichorium intybus* were screened for antihepatotoxic activity on carbon tetrachloride induced liver damage in albino rats. The degree of protection was measured using biochemical parameters like AST, ALT and ALP. The methanol fraction and compound AB-IV were found to possess a potent antihepatotoxic activity comparable to the standard drug Silymarin. The histopathological study of the liver was also carried out, wherein the methanolic fraction and compound AB-IV showed almost complete normalization of the tissues as neither fatty accumulation nor necrosis was observed.

Solanum nigrum (Family: Solanaceae)

Solanum nigrum has been widely used as hepatoprotective and anti-inflammation agent. The principal constituents are solamargine-A, solamargine-B, solasodine and solasodine. Its hepatoprotective and antioxidant activity has been established experimentally (Lin et al., 2008). In this study, the protective effects of aqueous extract of *Solanum nigrum* (SNE) against liver damage were evaluated in CCl_4 induced chronic hepatotoxicity in rats. *Solanum nigrum* extract was orally administered (0.2, 0.5 and 1.0 g/kg) along with administration of CCl_4 (20% CCl_4/corn oil; 0.5 mL/kg) for 6 weeks. The results showed that the treatment of SNE significantly lowered the CCl_4 induced serum levels of hepatic enzyme markers (GOT, GPT, ALP, and total bilirubin), superoxide and hydroxyl radical. The hepatic content of GSH, and activities and expressions of SOD, GST Al, and GST that were reduced by CCl_4 were normalized by the supplement of SNE. Liver histopathology confirmed hepatoprotection by SNE. The results of this study suggest that SNE could protect liver against the CCl_4 induced oxidative damage in rats, and this hepatoprotective effect might be contributed to its modulation on detoxification enzymes and its antioxidant and free radical scavenger effects.

Plumbago zeylanica (Family: Plumbaginaceae)

Plumbago zeylanica or White Leadwort is native to SE Asia. It is a highly branched, evergreen rambling subscandent shrub with white flowers that reaches about 6 feet (2 meters) in height. Leaves are Dark green, ovate and glabrous. *Plumbago zeylanica* is a very useful medicinal plant. The root of the plant and its constituents are credited with potential therapeutic properties including anti-atherogenic, cardiotonic, hepatoprotective and neuroprotective properties. The anti oxidant activity of this herb has been established. Plumbagin is the main active constituent responsible for antioxidant and hepatoprotective activity (Tilak et al., 2004).

Tinospora cordifolia (Family: Menispermaceae)

Tinospora cordifolia is a large, glabrous, deciduous climbing shrub belonging to the family Menispermaceae. It is distributed throughout tropical Indian subcontinent and China, ascending to an altitude of 300 m. In Hindi, the plant is commonly known as Giloya, which is a Hindu mythological term that refers to the heavenly elixir that have saved celestial beings from old age and kept them eternally young. Its principle chemical constituents are tinosporine, tinosporide, cordifol, cordifolide, heptacosanol, clerodane furano diterpene, columbin and β-sitosterol. It is widely used in Ayurvedic medicine in India as tonic, vitalizer and as a remedy for diabetes mellitus and metabolic disorders. It has been experimentally established that this herb also possess significant hepatoprotective and antioxidant activities (Beliga and Jagetia, 2004; Parabia et al., 2007).

Embelia ribes (Family: Myrsinaceae)

It is large scandent shrub with slender branches and elliptic-lanceolate and gland dotted leaves. The fruit is globular and wrinkled varying in color from dull red to black. The plant contains embelin, christembine, quercitol and resins. It is a widely used herb for its anthelmintic, analgesic, antifertility properties hepatoprotective and antitumour properties. Embelin is the major active constituent and is responsible for the antioxidant and hepatoprotective activity (Mukherjee et al., 2007).

Cassia occidentalis (Family: Caesalpiniaceae)

Cassia occidentalis commonly known as 'Kasondi', is used in Unani medicine for liver ailments and is an important ingredient of several polyherbal formulations marketed for liver diseases. The hepatoprotective effect of aqueous-ethanolic extract (50%, v/v) of leaves of *Cassia occidentalis* was studied on rat liver damage induced by paracetamol and ethyl alcohol by monitoring AST, ALT, ALP, serum cholesterol, serum total lipids and histopathological alterations. The extract of leaves of the plant produced significant hepatoprotection (Jafri et al., 1999).

Achillea millefolium (Family: Compositae)

The herb is used as antiseptic, antispasmodic, hepatoprotective, astringent, carminative, cholagogue, diaphoretic, digestive and stimulant. The crude extract of *Achillea millefolium* was studied for its possible hepatoprotective effect against d-galactosamine and lipopolysaccharide (LPS) induced hepatitis in mice to rationalize some of the folklore uses. Co-administration of d-galactosamine (700 mg/kg) and LPS (25 μ/kg) produced 100% mortality in mice. Pre-treatment of animals with *Achillea millefolium* extract (300 mg/kg) reduced the mortality to 40%. Co-administration of d-galactosamine (700 mg/kg) and LPS (1 μg/kg) significantly raised the plasma ALT and AST levels compared with values in the control group. Pre-treatment of mice with crude extract (150-600 mg/kg) significantly prevented the toxins induced rise in plasma ALT and AST. The hepatoprotective effect of *Achillea millefolium* extract was further verified by histopathology of the liver, which showed improved architecture, absence of parenchymal congestion, decreased cellular swelling and apoptotic cells, compared with the toxin group of animals (Yaeesh et al., 2006).

Vernonia amygdalina (Family: Compositae)

Vernonia amygdalina is widely used in tropical countries for treatment of fever, jaundice, stomach disorders and diabetes. The possible modulatory effect of methanolic extract of *Vernonia amygdalina*, on the toxicity of CCl_4, was investigated in rats. Oral administration of CCl_4 at a dose of 1.2 g/kg body weight 3 times a week for 3 weeks significantly induced marked hepatic injury as revealed by increased activity of the serum enzymes ALT, AST, SALP and γ-GT. Methanolic extract of *V. amygdalina* administered 5 times a week for 2 weeks before CCl_4 treatment at 250 and 500mg/kg doses of the extract ameliorated the increase in the activities of these enzymes. Likewise the methanolic extract of *V. amygdalina* reduced the CCl_4 induced increase in the concentrations of cholesterol, triglyceride and phospholipid by 37.8%, 30.6% and 8.5%, respectively, and a reduction in the cholesterol/phospholipids ratio. CCl_4 induced lipid peroxidation was likewise attenuated by 57.2% at 500mg/kg dose of the methanolic extract of *V. amygdalina*. Similarly, administration of the extract increased the activities of the antioxidant enzymes: SOD, glutathione S-transferase and reduced glutathione concentration significantly at 500mg/kg and catalase activity at 500-1000mg/kg doses. These results suggest that methanolic extract of *V. amygdalina* leaves possesses protective effect against CCl_4 induced hepatotoxicity by the antioxidant mechanism of action (Farombi and Adesanoye, 2009).

CONCLUSION

Popularity of herbal remedies is increasing and at least one quarter of patients with liver disease use botanicals. Unfortunately, well performed clinical trials on their therapeutic value in the treatment of certain liver diseases are infrequent and the possibilities in which herbal drugs can alleviate hepatotoxicity remain uncharted. Future efforts will have to implement extensive methodological improvements to separate the real therapeutic value of these agents from unsubstantiated hopes associated with them. Sound and controlled clinical studies with certain herbals and especially their active ingredients in chronic liver diseases are important, with regard to discover novel anti-fibrotic and anti-inflammatory activities. There is a huge demand for both experimental and clinical research to validate the potential of herbal drugs and rigorous scientific testing along the principles of evidence-based medicine will help herbal medicine to become a very justifiable scientific treatment regime.

REFERENCES

Ahmed B, Al-Howiriny TA, Siddiqui AB. Antihepatotoxic activity of *Cichorium intybus*. *J. Ethnopharmacol.*, 87, 237-40 (2003).

Arthur MJP, Friedman SL, Roll FJ, Bissell DM. Lipocytes from normal rat liver release a neutral metalloproteinase that degrades basement membrane (type IV) collagen. *J. Clin. Invest.*, 84, 1076-1085 (1989).

Bataller R, Brenner DA. Liver fibrosis. *J Clin Invest*, 115, 209-218 (2005).

Bhattacharjee R, Sil PC. Protein isolate from the herb, Phyllanthus niruri L. (Euphorbiaceae), plays hepatoprotective role against carbon tetrachloride induced liver damage via its antioxidant properties. *Food Chem Toxicol*, 45, 817-26 (2007).

Carloni V, Romanelli RG, Pinzani M, Latfi G, Gentilini P. Focal adhesion kinase and phospholipase Cγ involvement in adhesion and migration of human hepatic stellate cells. *Gastroenterol.*, 112, 522-531. (1997).

Castilla A, Prieto J, Fausto N. Transforming growth factor β1 and α in chronic liver disease. Effects of interferon α therapy. *N. Engl. J. Med.*, 324, 933-940 (1991).

Cuppett SL, Hall CA. Antioxidant activity of the Labiatae. *Adv Food Nutr Res*, 42, 245-71 (1998).

Davis BH, Pratt BM, Madri JA. Retinol and extracellular collagen matrices modulate hepatic Ito cell collagen phenotype and cellular retinol binding proteins levels. *J. Biol. Chem.*, 262, 10280-10286 (1987).

De Smet PA. Herbal remedies. *N Engl J Med*, 347, 2046–56 (2002).

Dehmlow C, Eahard J, Goot HD. Inhibition of Kupffer cells as an explanation for the hepatoprotective properties of silibinin. *Hepatology*, 23, 749-754 (1996).

Dwivedi Y, Rastogi R, Garg NK, Dhawan BN. Perfusion with picroliv reverses biochemical changes induced in livers of rats toxicated with galactosamine or thioacetamide. *Planta Med*, 59, 418-420 (1993).

Emonard H, Emonard JA. Matrix metalloproteinases. A review. *Cell. Mol. Biol.*, 36, 131-153 (1990).

Farombi EO, Adesanoye OA. Hepatoprotective effects of *Vernonia amygdalina* (astereaceae) in rats treated with carbon tetrachloride. *Exp Toxicol Pathol* (2009) article in press.

Flora K, Hahn M, Rosen H, Benner K. Milk thistle (*Silybum marianum*) for the therapy of liver disease. *J. Gastroenterol* 93, 139-143 (1998).

Freije JM, Balbin M, Sanchez LM, Blasco R, Tolivia J, Lopez-Otin C. Molecular cloning and expression of collagenase-3, a novel human matrix metalloproteinase produced by breast carcinomas. *J. Biol. Chem.*, 269, 16766-16773 (1994).

Friedman SL. Mechanisms of disease: Mechanisms of hepatic fibrosis and therapeutic implications. *Nat Clin Pract Gastroenterol Hepatol*,1, 98-105 (2004).

Friedman SL. Molecular regulation of hepatic fibrosis, an integrated cellular response to tissue injury. *J. Biol. Chem.*, 275, 2247-2250 (2000).

Gines P, Cardenas A, Arroyo V, Rodes J. Management of cirrhosis and ascites. *N Engl J Med*, 350, 1646-1654 (2004).

Harish, R., Shivanandappa, T. Antioxidant activity and hepatoprotective potential of *Phyllanthus niruri*. *Food Chem.* 95, 180-185 (2006).

Iredale JP, Murphy G, Hembry RM, Friedman SL, Arthur MJP. Human hepatic lipocytes synthesize tissue inhibitor of metalloproteinase-l: implication for regulation of matrix degradation in liver. *J. Clin. Invest.*, 90, 282-287 (1992).

Jafri MA, Jalis Subhani M, Javed K, Singh S. Hepatoprotective activity of leaves of Cassia occidentalis against paracetamol and ethyl alcohol intoxication in rats. *J Ethnopharmacol.* 66, 355-61 (1999).

Jagetia GC, Baliga MS. The evaluation of nitric oxide scavenging activity of certain Indian medicinal plants *in vitro*: a preliminary study. *J Med Food* 7, 343-348. (2004).

Janbaza KH, Gilanib AH. Studies on preventive and curative effects of berberine on chemical-induced hepatotoxicity in rodents. *Fitoterapia*, 71, 25-33 (2007).

Johnson VJ, Osuchowski MF, He Q, Sharma RP. Physiological responses to a natural antioxidant flavonoids mixture, silymarin, in BALB/c mice: II. Alterations on thymic differentiation correlate with changes in *c- myc* gene expression. *Planta Med.*, 68, 961-965 (2002).

Kim WR, Brown RS, Terrault NA, El-Serag H. Burden of liver disease in the United States: summary of a workshop. *Hepatology*, 36, 227-42 (2002).

Kind PRN, King EJ. Estimation of plasma phosphatase by determination of hydrolyzed phenol with anti-pyrine. *J. Clin. Path*, 7, 322-326 (1954).

Lin HM, Tseng HC, Wang CJ, Lin JJ, Lo CW, Chou FP. Hepatoprotective effects of *Solanum nigrum* Linn extract against CCl_4-induced oxidative damage in rats. *Chem. Biol. Interact.* 171, 283-293 (2008).

Luper S. A review of plants used in the treatment of liver diseases: Part 1. *Altern. Med. Rev*, 3 , 410-421 (1998).

Mak KM, Lieber CS. Lipocytes and transitional cells in alcoholic liver disease: a morphometric study. *Hepatology*, 8, 1027-1033 (1988).

Malloy HT, Evelyn KA. The determination of bilirubin with the photometric colorimeter. *J Biol Chem*, 119, 481-490 (1937).

Miller AL. Antioxidant flavonoids: Structure, function and clinical usage. *Altern. Med. Rev*, 1, 103-111 (1996).

Mitra SK, Venkataranganna MV, Sundaram K, Gopumadhavan S. Protective effect of HD-03, a herbal formulation against various hepatotoxic agents in rats. *J. Ethnopharmacol.*, 63, 181-186 (1998).

Mukherjee T, Joshi R, Kamat JP. Free radical scavenging reactions and antioxidant activity of embelin: Biochemical and pulse radiolytic studies. *Chem. Biol. Interact*, 167, 125-134 (2007).

Muriel P, Mourelle M. Prevention by silymarin of membrane alterations in acute CCl_4 liver damage. *J. Appl. Toxicol*, 10, 275-279 (1990).

Parabia MH, Adhvaryu MR, Reddy N. Effects of four Indian medicinal herbs on Isoniazid, Rifampicin and Pyrazinamide induced hepatic injury and immunosuppression in guinea pigs. *World J Gastroenterol*, 13, 3199-3205 (2007).

Pinzani M. Novel insight into the biology and physiology of the Ito cell. *Pharmacol. Ther.*, 66, 387-412 (1995).

Pinzani M, Gesualdo L, Sabbah GM, Abboud HE. Effects of platelet-derived growth factor and other polypeptide mitogens on DNA synthesis and growth of cultured rat liver fat-storing cells. *J. Clin. Invest.*, 84, 1786-1793 (1989).

Poli G. Pathogenesis of liver fibrosis: role of oxidative stress. *Mol Aspects Med*, 21, 49-98, (2000).

Raghow R, Postlethwaite AE, Keski-Oja J, Moses HL, Kang AH. Transforming growth factor-β increases the steady state levels of type I procollagen and fibronectin mRNAs post transcriptionally in cultured human dermal fibroblasts. *J. Clin. Invest.*, 79, 1285-1288 (1987).

Rawat AK, Mehrotra S, Tripathi SC, Shome U. Hepatoprotective activity of *Boerhaavia diffusa* roots-a popular Indian ethnomedicine. *J Ethnopharmacol*, 56, 61-66 (1997).

Reitman S, Frankel S. A colorimetric method for the determination of serum glutamate oxaloacetate & glutamate pyruvate transaminases. *Am. J. Clin. Pathol.*; 28: 56-63. (1957).

Rice-Evans CA, Miller NJ, Paganga G. Structure-antioxidant activity relationships of flavonoids and phenolic acids. *Free Radic Biol Med*, 20, 933-56 (1996).

Saller R, Meier R, Brignoli R. The use of silymarin in the treatment of liver diseases. *Drugs*, 61, 2035-2063 (2001).

Saxena AK, Singh B, Anand KK. Hepatoprotective effects of *Eclipta alba* on subcellular levels in rats. *J Ethnopharmacol*, 40, 155-161 (1993).

Schuppan D, Cho JJ, Jia JD, Hahn EG. Interplay of matrix and myofibroblasts during hepatic fibrogenesis. *Curr. Top. Pathol.*, 93, 205-218 (1999).

Shyamal S, Latha PG, Shine VJ, Suja SR, Rajasekharan S, Ganga Devi T. Hepatoprctective effects of Pittosporum neelgherrense Wight & Arn., a popular Indian ethnomedicine. *J Ethnopharmacol.* 107, 151-5 (2006).

Sonnenbichler J, Zetl I. Biochemical effects of the flavonolignan silibinin on RNA, protein, and DNA synthesis in rat liver. *Progr. Clin. Biol. Res*, 213, 319-31 (1986).

Strader DB, Bacon BR, Lindsay KL, La Breque DR, Morgan T, Wright EC, et al. Use of complementary and alternative medicine in patients with liver disease. *Am J Gastroenterol*, 97, 2391-7 (2002).

Tilak JC, Adhikari S, Devasagayam TP. Antioxidant properties of *plumbago zeylanica*, an Indian medicinal plant and its active ingredient plumbagin. *Redox Rep*, 9, 219-227 (2004).

Visen PKS, Shukia B, Patnaik GK, Dhawan BN. Andrographolide protects rat hepatocytes against paracetamol-induced damage. *J Ethnopharmacol* 40, 131-136. (1993).

Weiner FR, Giambrone MA, Czaja MJ, Shah A, Annoni G, Takahashi S, Eghbali M, Zern MA. Ito-cell gene expression and collagen regulation. *Hepatology*, 11, 111-117 (1990).

Wiseman H. Dietary influences on membrane function: Importance in protection against oxidative damage and disease. *J. Nutr. Biochem*, 7, 2-5 (1996).

Yaeesh S, Jamal Q, Khan AU, Gilani AH. Studies on hepatoprotective, antispasmodic and calcium antagonist activities of the aqueous-methanol extract of *Achillea millefolium. Phytother Res.*, 20, 546-51 (2006).

Yoshikawa M, Matsui Y, Kawamoto H, Umemoto N, Oku K, Koizumi M, Yamao J, Kuriyama S, Nakano H, Hozumi N, Ishizaka S, Fukui H. Effects of glycyrrhizin on immune-mediated cytotoxicity. *J Gastroenterol Hepatol.* 12, 243-8 (1997).

chapter 17

IN SEARCH OF PHYTOMEDICINE FOR ARTHRITIS

Rabish Chandra, Kamini Kumar, Jyoti Kumar and Subhash C Mandal

INTRODUCTION

By looking back the history of medicine, it can be traced that for most of the period, mankind had no other source of medicine than plants, either fresh or dried. In India the use of plants as a source of medicine is found in *Rigveda* and *Yajurveda* both around 2000 BC. No doubt, the synthetic medicines have found a good position in health care but its adverse effects cannot be neglected and also because of its high cost it is beyond the reach of common people. Considering the adverse effects of synthetic drugs almost whole part of the world is looking for natural remedies. It has become a very common data, found almost in all related articles that 80% of the world population is using natural products especially plants. The importance of medicinal plants is demonstrated by the fact that even in developed countries, about 35% of the prescribed drugs are from natural origin and 50% among these are of plant origin. During the last decade, consumption of medicinal plants has doubled in western Europe. Natural products, including plants, animals and minerals have been the basis of treatment of human disease. The basis of development of modern medicine or allopathy remains rooted in traditional medicines and therapies (Patwardhan et al., 2004; patwardhan and Hooper, 1992). Plants have been selected and used empirically as drugs for centuries, initially as traditional preparations then as pure active principles (Taylor and Staden, 2002). The medicines from plant origin are given different terms like phytomedicines, herbs, herbal materials, botanicals and botanical drugs. Phytomedicines are preparations consisting of complex mixture of one or more plant materials (Warude and Patwardhan, 2005). In these plant medicines anti arthritic medicinal plants are one of the important group and their therapeutic effects have been verified in numerous modern medical investigations, which are often complementary to those of western drugs.

Arthritis is a general term for approximately 100 named diseases. The term arthritis simply means joint inflammation. Among different types of arthritis, rheumatoid arthritis, osteo-arthritis and gout are the most frequent one. The last few years have witnessed tremendous advances in the treatment of rheumatoid arthritis (RA). New therapies include potentially safer (but not more effective in terms of pain control) cycloxygenase-2, specific nonsteroidal anti inflammatory drugs leflunomide and tumor necrosis factor (TNF) (Moreland, 2002), current treatments using therapeutic agents for RA such as anti rheumatic and anti-inflammatory drugs are inadequate in that they only partially control established RA. They also have side effects that limit their use their side effect and toxicity call for new and more effective natural drugs

(Dai Min et al., 2003). With the recent advancement analytical and bio-assay techniques (both *in vivo* and *in vitro*) effort has been made to discover phytodrugs for arthritis. Testing extracts prepared from widely utilized medicinal plants has become a rapidly growing and successful field in pharmacological science. This review discusses various botanicals, its bioassay method and other approaches related to scientific evaluation of anti arthritic phytomedicines.

Understanding Arthritis

Arthritis really means inflammation of a joint and nothing more specific than that. It is a general term for a group of more than 100 diseases. The most common among them are rheumatoid arthritis, osteo-arthritis and gout. In addition there are the collagen diseases. Rheumatoid arthritis is potentially the most serious of the three chief disease, which is the main focus of this review.

Osteoarthritis is a focal diarthroidial joint and is characterized by the degeneration of cartilage, thickening of subchrondal bone, formation of marginal osteophytes, sub articular bony cysts, eburnation and remodeling of the bone (Kalindi, 1988) it is the relatively mild and usually non crippling form of arthritis. The chance of getting it increases with age.

Gout is one of the first diseases ever described (by Hippocrates in 500 B.C). It is characterized by severe acute arthritis, generally affecting one or two joints only. The pain is extremely severe; heat, redness and tenderness in and about the joint are noted and a maximum intensity of pain is reached in only a few hours. Gout is related to a hereditary defect in the chemistry of the uric acid in the body. The clinical manifestations of this diseases are due to complex interactions between monosodium urate (MSU) crystals and various cell types including mast cells, endothelial cell, neutrophils, macrophages, and synovial fibroblasts. The inflammation may be characterized by initiatian of the acute attack, leucocyte recruitment, amplification and subsequent resolution (Dalbeth and Haskard, 2005).

Sir Alfred Baring Garrod first coined rheumatoid arthritis term in 1859. Rheumatoid arthritis (RA) is a chronic disorder having characteristic of inflammation of the lining of synovium of the joints. Insidious pain, stiffness and symmetrical swelling of small joints are some basic symptoms of the onset of RA. The 1987 American college of Rheumatology (ACR) has given seven criteria (viz. 1. morning stiffness 2. arthritis in three or more joint areas 4. symmetric arthritis 5. rheumatoid nodules 6. serum rheumatoid factor 7. radiographic changes) to diagnose RA clinically. Clinical evaluation, laboratory tests and radiological investigation are the 3 main categories for the diagnosis for RA. For clinical evaluation of RA; criterian of ACR and Health assessment questionnaire (HAQ) are used. Modified Indian version of HAQ in different language has been developed (Chopra et al., 1996). Laboratory tests in rheumatic disease include several biochemical and serological tests. It includes analysis of erythrocyte sedimentation (ESR), C-reactive protein (CRP), Rheumatoid factor (RF), Anti nuclear antibodies (ANA), leucocytes, thrombocytosis. Advanced laboratory testings include investigation of cytokines (IL 1, IL6, IL 18, etc. TNF) and HLA (human leukocyte antigen) typing. As far as the genetic aspects of rheumatoid arthritis is concerned, the most important genes that effect the susceptibility to the disease are located within the major histocompatibility complex (MHC). MHC is the most polymorphic genetic locus in mammals. In humans HLAs (the cell surface proteins) is encoded by MHC. Based on the structure of the cell – surface proteins they specify, the HLA molecules are divided into two major types, Class I and Class II. HLA-A, HLA-B, and HLA-C are the three types of class I antigens where as HLA-DR, HLA-DP, and HLA-DQ are the three antigens of class II (Rao and Firdaus F, 2004; Kondkor, 2004; Bhatia, 2004; Balakrishnan, 2004). Stastny was first to found that approximately 70% of white patients with classic rheumatoid arthritis, compared with 28% of patients with non rheumatoid arthritis expressed HLA-DR4 (Stastny, 1978).

Traditional Medicine and Arthritis

Traditional medicine is a comprehensive term used to refer both TM systems such as traditional Chinese medicine, Indian Ayurveda and Arabic Unani medicine and to various forms of indigenous medicine. Use of herbal medicines is a medication therapy of TM therapies. Herbal medicines include herbs, herbal materials, herbal preparations and finished herbal products that contain as active ingredients parts of plants or other materials or combination there of (WHO, Geneva, Traditional Medicine Strategy 2002-2005, Internet edition). The traditional systems of medicines are based on the experience in the use of plant products in amelioration of common disease. A vast majority of our population, particularly those living in villages depends largely on herbal remedies (Gupta, 1994), it has served as a source of alternative medicine, new pharmaceuticals and health care products.

Traditional Chinese medicine (TCM) is a system with its own rich tradition and sizeable collection of data from over 3,000 years of continuous use and refinement through observation, testing and critical thinking. It encompasses many practices classified as Complementary and Alternative medicine (CAM) that include herbal medicine, acupuncture and Tai Chi/Qi Gong in the US and Europe. However presently, only acupuncture and herbal drug therapies are practiced as major branches. TCM is widely used in China as a treatment of RA and is a major research interest of whole world in the field of CAM. Extract of *Tryptergym wilfordii* Hook. F has been presented for the treatment of RA since long centuries.

In India several medicinal plant having tremendous therapeutic effect have been used by Ayurvedic practitioners to cure all forms of arthritis (Chikitsasthana, 1994). A review of Ayurvedic Medicine have been published explaining the core concept, therapeutic principles with reference to rheumatism and arthritis (Chopra, 2000, 2001, 2002). The first recorded text available on Ayurveda is Charaka Samhita (900 B.C). The fundamental principle followed in Ayurvedic treatment is *Tridoshic* (tri- three; dosha- biologic humor) and is classified into *Vata, Pitta* and *Kapha*. They correspond primarily to the elements of air, fire and water. These are primary physiologic forces and are considered to govern the biomotor, metabolic and preservative activity. In Ayurvedic practice rheumatic disorders are often described as *Vat* and arthritis is *Sandhivat* (sandhi-joint). In Ayurvedic text it is mentioned that "if excess *vata* (one of the three *doshas,*or humours) is vitiated all over the body, there is quivering and breaking pain in limbs and joints as if cracking. If it is localized in the joints, it produces swelling that feels like an air filled bladder and produces pain on movement; this explanantion is more or less similar to that of inflammatory arthritis. The pathogenesis of arthritic disorders according to ayurvedic system has been explained by *ama* hypothesis which attributes to the affliction of the joints to the excess accumulation of viscous substances called ama. Some plant based ayurvedic therapies practiced since ancient times includes *Boswellia serrata, Zingiber officinale, Curcuma longa, Embellica officinalis, Tinospora cordifolia, Allium sativum, Withania sominifera, Terminalia chebula* etc.

The origin of Unani medicine in Greece and it was started by Hippocrates (460-377 BC). This system of medicine was introduced by the Arabs and Iranians, some times it is also termed as Graco-Arab medicine. The diagnosing methods is based *Nabz* (pulse), a rhythmic expansion of arteries which is felt by the fingers. *Baul* (urine), *Baraz* (stool) also include the diagnosis method in

Unani system of medicine. In Unani system of medicine Rheumatoid arthritis is known as Waja-Ul- Mafasil. Through the co-ordination of Central council for Research in Unani Medicine, New Delhi at different institutional network, a combination of oral drug UNIM-301 and an oil UNIM-304 has been clinically investigated for rheumatoid arthritis which shows complete relief in 76% of he cases. Regimental therapy namely *Hajamat* (cupping) is also a popular therapy in rheumatoid arthritis (Anonymous, 2002; Ali, 2003).

Ethnomedicine is the key system followed in the remote areas for treating various ailments, the literature of which is not available in any part of the world. Rather it is passing from generation to generation orally. People in the remote areas are said to suffer more from degenerative arthritis and they have their own prescriptions to treat it efficiently. They have their own classification and number of ethnomedicinal formulations to treat arthritis, which hardly match each other's (Mahato, 2002). Important is to document this precious knowledge. The gathering of information about the use of particular plants as medicine has been in progress for a least a century. Recently this documented information is made available in the Internet databases. One such database is http://herb.umd.umich.edu. By putting key words rheumatism it display 500 matches till date. Yet ethno-botanists continue to uncover additional medicinal plants and uses of the plants, however there is a great chance of redundancy and duplicity.

Preparation of herbal and mineral compounds is a distinct and exhaustive subject. Physicians are encouraged to make their own medicines.

Plants and Herbs for Arthritis

The use of herbal therapies for arthritis has been increasing among the patients. The simple reason is its availability in nature and is believed to be safer than synthetic or allopathic medicine. Furthermore, several herbs are being used from the dawn of civilization without any side effects in traditional medicine. Research communities, with the power of contemporary science and technology are exploring the active phytoconstituent responsible for the said ailments. The investigatory approaches are gradually being enhanced as a result of improved technology. The classical method of bio perspecting the botanicals relies on the phytochemical factors, serendipity and random screening approaches. Where as the modern method is following ethnopharmacological approach. The later is time and cost effective and could lead to better success than routine random screening. Traditional systems of medicine are becoming important bio-prospecting tools. (Patwardhan and Gautam, 2005). To explain the mechanism of action of botanicals effective in arthritis, the classical pharmacological parameters has been integrated with the molecular study. In a recent study, the plant extracts from *Utrica diocia* inhibit the pro-inflammatory transcription factor NF-Kβ. There is a long list of botanicals that have been studied for potential anti arthritic agents (Table 17.1). A few of them will be discussed briefly in subsequent sections that have been studied to a greater extent including its traditional uses, therapeutic value and mechanism of actions.

Curcuma Longa

Curcuma longa L. belongs to Zingiberaceae, commonly referred as turmeric is a perennial plant and being widely cultivated in Asiatic countries mainly in India and China. In Indian language it is commonly called as "Haldi". Some species including *Curcuma longa* can be distinguished and identified using single nucleotide polymorphism analysis of trnK gene (Sasaki et al., 2004). The rhizome of this plant is widely used in Indian traditional system of medicine. Other than medicine it is also used as food additive (spice), preservative and dye. Its biological activity, chemistry, medical applications etc. has been reviewed from time to time (Araujo & Leon 2001; Chainani, 2003, Chattopadhyay et al., 2004). Biologically active substances in turmeric rhizome include Curcumin (diferuloylmethane) and its derivatives. It has been studied since long time for its anti arthritic effect (Chandra and Gupta, 1972) and to understand its mechanism. Recently it has been reported that curcumin inhibits IL-1β induced PGE_2 formation by inhibiting the expression of m PGES-1 (Prostaglandin E synthase 1) that is mediated by suppression of EGR-1 expression as well as NF-κB and JNK ½ (Aggarwal & Shishodia, 2004, Yuseok Moon et al., 2005). Curcumin has also been studied for its effect on cytokine production by human peripheral blood monocytes and alveolar macrophages (Abe et al., 1999). In this studies it was found that curcumin inhibited the production of IL-8, MIP-1∝, MCP-1, IL-1β and TNF-∝ by 4β phorbor 12β- myristate-13 ∝ acetate (PMA) or lipopolysaccharide stimulated monocytes and alveolar macrophages.

Zingiber officinale

Zingiber officinale, the type genus of Zingiberaceae family, commonly reffered to as gingers, is one of the most common constituents of diets world wide. The rhizome of *Z.officinale* has been used in Indian ayurvedic medicine and traditional sino-japaneese medicine thousands of years to treat inflammatory and rheumatic disease. It has also been reported for its antioxidant, antiseptic, and carminative properties (Afzal et al., 2001; Langer et al., 1998). The chief constiuent of ginger includes volatile oils, oleoresins (gingerols), β-carotenecapsaicin, caffeic acid and curcumin (Schulick, 1996). The constituents of ginger hydroxy-alcoxy-phenyl compounds inhibits chondrocytes and synviocytes TNF-α expression, another constituent [6] –gingerol inhibited LPS –induced I NOS expression and production of NO and other RNS Species in macrophages and blocked peroxynitrite- induced oxidation and nitration reaction, both *invitro* (Frondoza et al., 2000; Ippooushi et al., 2003).

Boswellia Sps.

The genus Boswellia belonging to family Burseraceae, with its anti-arthritic properties and others are well documented in alternative medicine literature. Four species namely *Boswellia serrata* in India, *Boswellia carterii* in East Africa and China, *Boswellia frereana* in Somalia, and *Boswellia sacra* in Arabia are used to obtain the resins and gums because of its medicinal properties. The gum resins are collectively known as Guggals. In Ayurvedic medicine system of India, guggal has been successfully used for the treatment of inflammatory poly-arthritis and other forms of rheumatism (Martine et al., 1989). It has also been screened for immunostimulant activity and anti-inflammatory properties and the mechanism behind it (Ammon, 1996). Ethonalic extract of *Boswellia carterii* dissolved in sesame oil exerted a dose dependence inhibitory effect on *in vitro* IFN-γ and IL-2 production by splenocytes from B_6, DBA/2 and B_6 D2F1 hybrid mice. Human rheumatoid arthritis has a strong immune mediated component and is marked by increase activated levels of TH1 cells and their cytokines, IL-2 and IFN-γ (Chevrier Marc et al., 2005).

Uncaria sps.

Two species namely *Uncaria tomentosa* and *Uncaria guianensis* are well known for its antiarthritic properties. *U. tomentosa* is a Peruvian vine, also known as cats claw has been used by ethnic people to treat immunologic disorders. In Traditional medicine system, the decoctions of cat's claw bark are prescribed for the treatment of arthritis, bursitis, stomach disorders and chronic fatigue syndrome. The chemical composition of the aqueous extract of *U. tomentosa* vine includes oxindolealkaloids, tannins, quinolic acids, glycosides, flavonoids and steroids. The root contains pentacyclic oxindoles. (Sandoval et al, 1998, 2002).

Phytochemicals for arthritis and its separation strategies

The major compound types of anti rheumatism agents in herbs usually involve phenolic, stilbene and polyphenol compounds, flavonoids, terpenoids, alkaloids anthraquinones, lignans polysaccharides and peptides. Some chemical entities for Arthritis are presented in Table 17.2. These compounds may also be antibacterial. For the analysis of plant medicines, chromatographic techniques (TLC, GC, SFC, HPLC and HPTLC) are frequently used methods and act as standards for identification and quality control of the most herbal medicines as illustrated in pharmacopoeia of different countries. Structures of some antiarthritic leads are shown in Figure 17.1. In anti rheumatism plant medicines, terpenoids are the most typical kind of volatile active components.

Kutney et al (1992) isolated various metabolites of interest in rheumatoid arthritis from *Tripterigium wilfordii*. Triterpenoids, terpenoids etc. has also been isolated from this particular plant (Duan, 2000; Duan, 1997). Column Chromatographic fractionation of petroleum ether extract of *Strobilanthus* with petroleum ether and benzene (65: 35) yielded lupeol and 19á-H lupeol and was simultaneously evaluated for its antiarthritic effect (Agarwal and Rangari, 2003). Apocyanin, 1-(4-hydroxy-3-methoxy phenyl)-ethanone, is a plant derived drug discovered during activity-guided isolation of immunomodulatory constituents from *Picrorhiza kurroa*. Apocyanin is found to be inhibitory in inflammation mediated cartilage destruction and also decreases IL-1 and TNF-∝ production (Lafeber et al., 1999). Momordin Ic and its aglycone, oleanolic acid, isolated from *Kochia scoparia* fruits could be the active principles for rheumatoid arthritis. From the fraction of BuOh extract of *Kochia scoparia* in column chromatography, eluent $CHCl_3$–MeOH-H_2O (65:35:10), crystal of momordin Ic was obtained (Choi Jong-won et al., 2002). Isolation of acid hydrolysed from the same plant afforded oleanolic acid (Momordin Ib,3) and its 6′-0-methyl ester (2). Subramanian Sethi (1969) isolated withaferin A from withiana cougulans roots. The same was studied for anti-inflammatory and anti-arthritic activity (Sethi et al, 1970) in the same laboratory. It was concluded that Withaferin A, to be more potent than hydrocortisone, standard, in adjuvant induced arthritis in rats. The root of *Zizyphus vulgaris* is ethnomedicinallly used in gout and rheumatism (Nandkarni, 1985), Mukhtar et al, 2005 has isolated Ursane –Type triterpenes taking C_6H_6-$CHCl_3$ (3:1) as eluant. However this particular compound was not evaluated for the activity. *Myricaria paniculata* (Tamaricaceae) has been reported to cure arthritis in China. Li Shuai et al., 2004 isolated two new triterpenoids myricare A and B along with other previously reported phytochemicals from the stem. Alpha and beta boswellic acids (BA) and rerelated analogs were isolated from the ethanol extract of *Boswellia carterii*. 45 grams of etahnolic extract of *B. carterii* was chromotographed using 250 g silica gel column. The solvent consists a gradient solvent system consisting of n-hexane with increasing amounts of ethyl acetate. A total of 120 fractions (250 ml/ fraction) were collected. The fractions 33 through 68 and fractions 69-85 were sub purified by HPLC which yields acetyl-11- dien-beta-BA: acetyl-alpha-BA: acetyl1-Beta-BA and alpha-BA; beta-BA respectively. Fractions 86 through 98 and fractions 99 through 118 were recrystallized without subpurification. Acetyl-11-keto-beta-BA were obtained from fractions 86-98 and fractions 99-118 respectively (Chevrier et al., 2005).

Poly Herbal Formulations and Rheumatoid Arthritis

Due to the side effects of Non steroidal antinflammatory drugs, no doubt there is an increase of herbals for the treatment of arthritis. However the scientific study of these herbs is currently more focused on the identification, isolation and characterization of the active principle(s) from crude extracts. The fact that strong synergism of several constituent in the crude drug may prove more potent and effective than any single purified compound is being overlooked. Moreover this may help to nullify the toxic effects (if any) of individual constituents (Engel et al., 2002; Ahmed et al., 2005). A limited number of polyherbal formulations has been studied for antiarthritic activity (Table 17.3). Among them are various Kampo medicine (traditional Japanese herbal medicine). In a study total 8 Kampo medicines were evaluated and examined for their effects on collagen induced arthritis and PX transgenic mice (Ono Yuka et al., 2003). Among these Dia–bofu- to, Kanzo-bushi–to, and Makayo-yokkan-to significantly reduced the severity of arthritis in collagen induced arthritis mice.

Dai-bofu-to (DBT), includes 15 herbs in different proportion, was studied for clinical evaluation of PX transgenic mice, histological assessment, FACS analysis, RT-southern blot analysis. All these studies show positive results towards an alternative for the treatment of arthritis. Kanzo- Bushi-to (KBT), consists of four medical srude drugs: *Cinnamomi cortex, Glycyrrhizae radix, Atractylodis Lanceae* and *Aconitum* tuber, was studied to investigate the suppressive effect on collagen induced arthritis (CIA) along with the mechanism. It was found that KBT suppressed CIA development effectively and further protected focal bone erosion and bone destruction (Ono et al., 2004). PG201 that contains ethanolic extracts of 12 herbs was tested for the control of inflammatory proteins and cartilage degradation with adverse effects on collagen induced arthritis. Evidence showed that it suppressed the progression of CIA and erosion of cartilage was dramatically reduced (Shin et al., 2003). An Indian poly herbal drug Ease was evaluated for its anti arthritc and anti inflammatory effect and its mechanism of action (Chatterjee and Das, 1996), the results significant effect recommending for its clinical studies. The Himalaya Drug Company, Bangalore, India developed a poly herbal formulation Joint Care B, containing *Alpinia galanga* (rhizome), *Commiphora wightii* (oleo-gum-resin), *Boswellia serrata* (oleo-gum resin), *Foeniculum vulgare* (fruit), *Glycyrrhiza glabra* (root), *Vitex negundo* (seed), and *Anethum graveolens* (fruit). It was recommended that this formulation have anti inflammatory activity without any side effects (Venkatranganna et al., 2000).

CONCLUSION

It is well known that drugs used currently to treat arthritis have limitation in that they have many undesired effects, and there is therefore a need for improved treatments. The major concerns with glucocorticoids, NSAIDS and DMARDS are poor efficacy, delayed onset of action and toxic effects. Important is that, many arthritic patients despite the use of these agents, continued to show progression of irreversible joint destruction.

No doubt that the use of botanicals is becoming the first choice of the peoples to get cured in arthritis. For acute pain and inflammation more accurate methods for inhibiting cyclooxygenase and lipoxygenase pathways (the mechanism behind NSAIDs) is with herbal support such as ginger turmeric and boswellia and with bioflavonoids (Mark, 1999). The evidence based traditional system of medicine (alternative and complementary medicine) has been initiated. A large number of medicinal plants have been reported by the ethnobotanist that is used for the treatment of arthritis. The medicines prescribed by the traditional herbal practitioners are being continuously studied by the scientist for their evidence, safety and efficacy.

The reported botanicals either in single or in combination require standardization to prove its safety and efficacy. Standardization of botanicals does not mean just an analytical operation for identification and assay of active principles; rather, it comprises total information and controls to necessary guarantee consistent composition of botanicals. To integrate these traditional medicines of plant origin with national healthcare system, study and research must be continued focusing on isolating and characterizing the active principles of the crude extract, its pharmacological validation, standardization and formulation (Chandra et al., 2007). To meet the desired quality and consistency, pharmacoepial standards should be developed following Good manufacturing Practices (GMP) using the guidelines provided by World Health Organisation (WHO), European Agency for the evaluation of Medicinal products (EMEA) and AYUSH (Ayurveda Unani and Shidha) department of Indian Government (Simha and Laxminarayan, 2007).

The results and discussion of the several phytomedicines needs further studies to advocate strongly on their use for arthritic disease.

Table 17.1. Plant extracts summary showing anti arthritic activity

Sl.No.	Botanical Name	Family	Reference
1	*Chaenomeles speciosa*	Rosaceae	Zhang ling-ling et al., 2004; Min Dai et al., 2003
2	*Ageratum conyzoides*	Asteraceae	Moura et al., 2005
3	*Kochia scoparia*	Chenopodiaceae	Choi jongwon et al., 2005
4	*Crataeva nurvala*Buch.-Ham	Capparaceae	Ramjilal et al., 1972; Das et al., 1974
5	*Vanda roxburghii*	Orchidaceae	Prasad and Achari, 1996
6	*Balasamodendron mukul*	Burseraceae	Mishra and Singh, 1972
7	*Caralluma stalagmifera*	Asclepiadaceae	Reddy et al., 1996
8	*Costus speciosus*	Zingiberaceae	Debnath and Pandey, 1971
9	Achyranthes speciosa	Amaranthaceae	Gokhale et al., 2002
10	Achyranthes aspera	Amaranthaceae	Gokhale et al., 2002
11	*Vitex negundo*	Verbenaceae	Tamhankar and Saraf, 1993
12	*Ocimum scantum* L.	Lamiaceae	Singh and Majumdar, 1995
13	*Dalbergia lanceolaria*	Fabaceae	Singh and Chaturvedi, 1965
14	*Boswellia carterii*	Burseraceae	Chevrier et al., 2005
15	*Boswellia serrata*	Burseraceae	Ammon, 2002.
16	*Tripterygium wilfordii*	Celastraceae	Chen, 2001; Toa et al., 2002
17	*Sinomenium acutum*	Menispermaceae	Liu et al., 2003
18	*Yucca schidigera*	Liliaceae	Cheeke et al., 2006
19	*Camellia sinensis*	Theaceae	Haqqi et al., 2005
20	*Uncaria tomentosa*	Rubiaceae	Ahmeds et al., 2005
21	*Curcuma longa*	Zingiberaceae	Ahmed et al., 2005; Chandra and Gupta, 1972
22	*Zingiber officinale*	Zingiberaceae	Das, 1996; Afzal et al., 2001

Contd. to next page.

23	*Cyperus rotundus*	Cyperaceae	Chatterjee and Das, 1996
24	*Tinospora cordifolia*	Menispermiaceae	Chatterjee and Das, 1996
25	*Saussurea lappa*		Chatterjee and Das, 1996
26	*Picrorrhiza kurroa*	Scrophulariaceae	Laferber et al., 1999
27	*Cinnamomi cortex*	Lauraceae	ono yuka et. al., 2004
28	*Glyccyrhizae radix*	Leguminaceae	ono yuka et. al., 2004
29	*Atractylodis lanceae*	Apiaceae	ono yuka et. al., 2004
30	*Aconitum* sps.	Ranunculaceae	ono yuka et. al., 2004
31	*Dryobalanops aromatica*	Dipterocarpaceae	Kubo et al., 1996
32	*Capsicum frutescens*	Solanaceae	Han et al., 2001
33	*Cinnamomum cassia*	Lauraceae	Akira, 1987
34	*Panax notiginseng*	Araliaceae	Li and Chu, 1999
35	*Urtica dioica*	urticacea	Riehemann et al., 1999
36	*Strobilanthus callosus*	Acanthaceae	Agarwal and Rangari, 2003
37	*Strobilanthus ixiocephala*	Acanthaceae	Agarwal and Rangari, 2003
38	*Clematis mandshurica*	Ranunculaceae	Choi et al., 2002; Cutis et al., 2004
39	*Tricosanthes kirilowil*	Cucurbitaceae	Choi et al., 2002, Cutis et al., 2004
40	*Prunella vulgaris*	Lamiaceae	Choi et al., 2002, Cutis et al., 2004
41	*Kochia scoparia*	Chenopodiaceae	Choi Jangwon et al., 2002
42	*Witahania sominiferea*	Solanaceae	Sethi et al., 1970
43	*Tinospora smilacnia*	Menispermaceae	Cribb and Cribb, 1981, Li et al., 2004
44	*Boswellia carterii*	Bureraceae	Chevrier et al., 2005

Table 17.2. Some chemical entities for Arthritis

Compounds	*Plant Source*	*Chemical Class*	*References*
Curcumin	*Curcuma longa*	Phenol compound	Kohli et al., 2005
Gingerols	*Zingiber officinales*	Phenolic compound	Afzal et al., 2001
Boswellic acid	*Boswellia serrata*	Pentacyclic terpenoid	Mahajan et. al., 1995
Momordin Ic	*Kochia scoparia*	Triterpene saponin	Choi et al., 2002
Oleanolic acid	*Kochia scoparia*	Pentacyclic terpenoid	Choi et al., 2002
Withaferin A	*Withania somnifera*	Steroidal lactones	Sethi et al., 1970
Triptolide	*Tripterygium wilfordii*	Diterpenoid triepoxide	Chen, 2001
Apocyanin	*Picrorhiza kurroa*	Iridoid glycoside	Vanden et al., 2001
Sinomenine	*Sinomenium acutum*	Alkaloid	Liu et al., 2003
Caffeic malic acid	*Urtica dioica L.*	Phenol	Riehemann et al., 1998
Lupeol	*Strobilanthus callosus*	Triterpenoid	Agarwal and Rangari, 2003
19-α-H-lupeol	*Strobilanthus ixiocephala*	Triterpenoid	Agrawal and Rangari, 2003
Withanolides	*Witahnia sominifera*	Steroids	Sethi and Subramanium, 1972

Table 17.3. Ingredients of some poly herbal formulation

Name of Poly Herbal Formulation	Constituent Medicinal Plants	References
PG201	*Chaenomelis speciosa* Chaenomeles fructus Achyranthes bibentata Angelica sinensis Cnidium officinale Gastrodia elata Blume (Gastrodiae rhizoma) Achanthopanax Senticosus maxim Acanthopanacis cortyex) Carathamus tinctorius L. (Carthami Flos) Cinnamomum aromaticum Nees. (Cinnamomi cortex) *Gentiana macrophy*	Shin et al., 2003
Joint Care B	*Alpinia galanga* *Commiphora wightii* *Boswellia serrata* *Foeniculum vulgare* *Glycyrrhiza glabra* *Vitex negundo*	Venkataranganna et al., 2000
Ease@	*Cyperus rotundus* *Tinospora cordifolia* *Saussurea lappa* *Picrorrhiza kurroa* *Zingiber officinale*	Chatterjee and Das, 1996
Dai-bofu-to (Kampo Medicine	*Glycrrhizae radix* *Atractylodis* *Lancaea* *Zingiberis rhizoma* *Paconia radix* *Zizyphi fructus* *Aconiti* *Glchnia radix* *Angelicac radix* *Rchmannia* *Cnidii rhizoma*	Inoue et al., 2004
	Ginseng radix *Achyranthes radix* *Eucommiae cortex* *Notplerygii rhizoma* *Astragali radix*	
Qing-Luo_Yin	*Sophora flavescensAit.* *Phellodendron* *amurense Rupr.* *Discorea hypoglauca* *Palib.* *Sinomenium acutum*	Li et al., 2003
Articulin F	*Witahnia sominifera* *Boswellia serrata* *Curcuma longa*	Kulkarni et al., 1991
OK 205	*Codenopsis pilosula* *Nanaf.* *Angelica koreana* *Maxim.* *Acanthopanax* *Sessiliflorous Seem* *Chaenomeles sinensis* *Koehne.* *Eucommia ulmoides* *Oliv.* *Poria cocos Wolf* *Glycyrrhiza uralensis* *Fish.*	In-Young Choi et al., 2004
Cool – Cool (Cool-X-A)	*Rhemania glutinosa* *Achyranthes bidetata* *Acanthopanax* *sessiliflorus* *Perilla frutuscens L.* *Atractylodes macrocephala* *Glycyrrhiza uralensis*	Kim Mi Sun et al., 2003
Bouun–Myunyuk–Dm	I6 herbs	Jeong Hyun-Ja et al., 2004

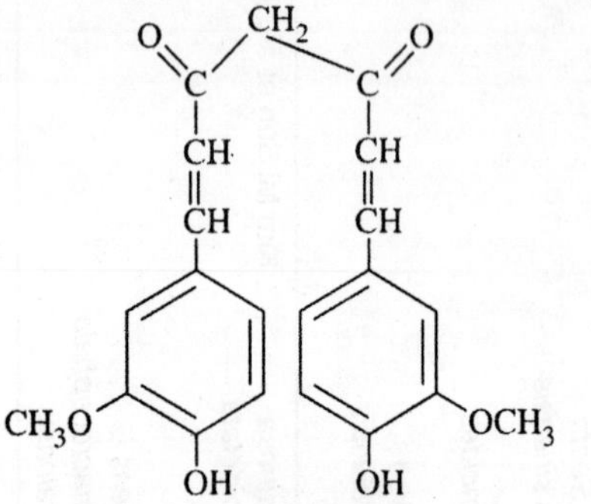

(A) Curcumin

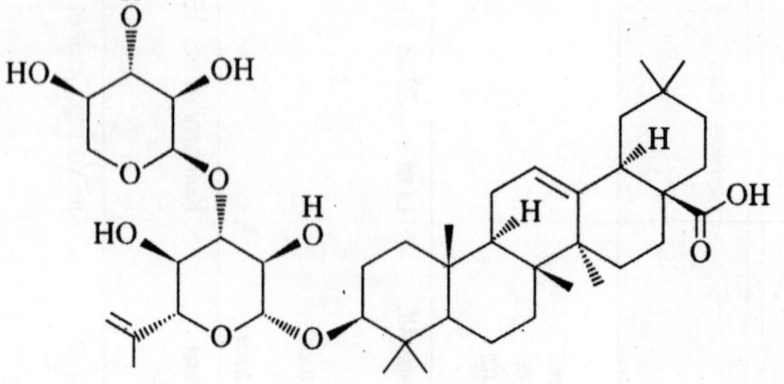

(B) Momordin Ic

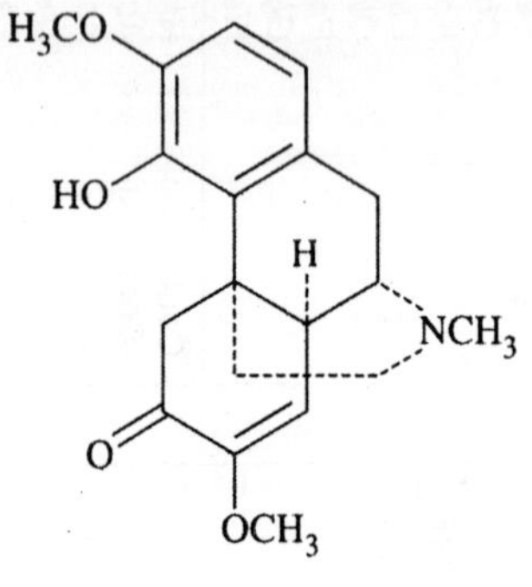

(C) Sinomenine

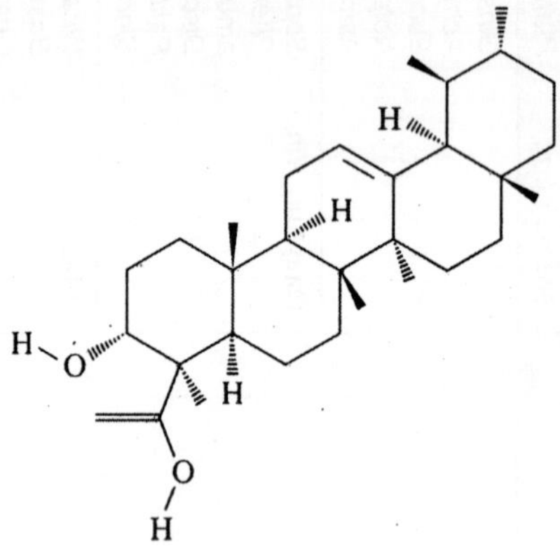

(D) Boswellic acid

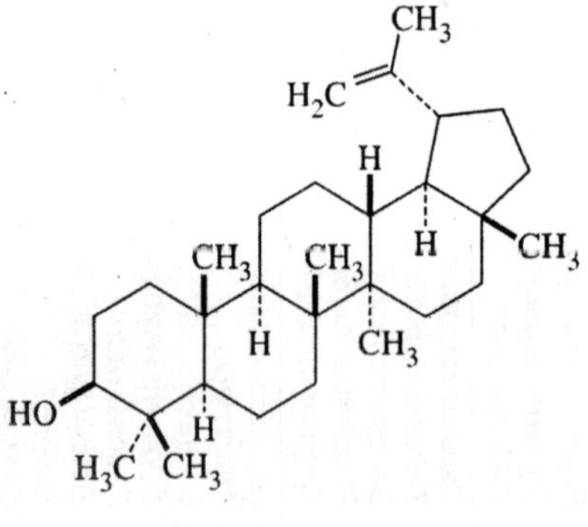

(E) Lupeol Acetae

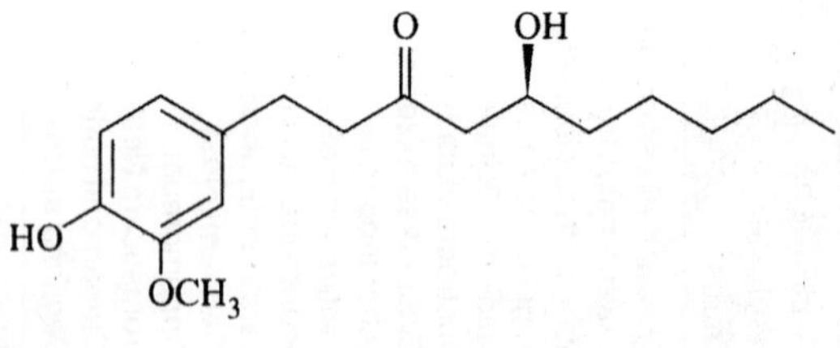

(F) Gingerols

Contd. to next page.

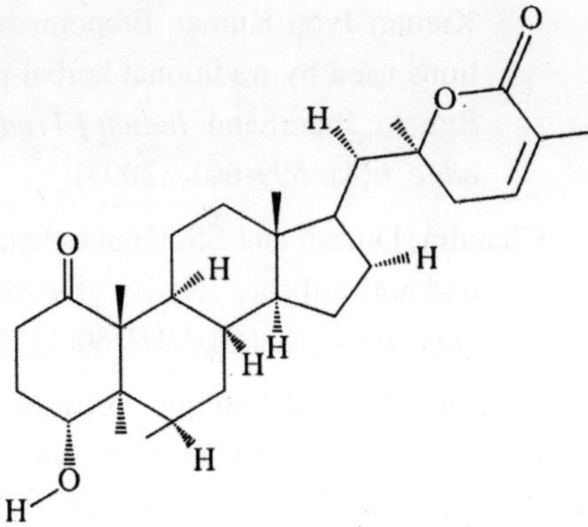

(G) Withaferin A

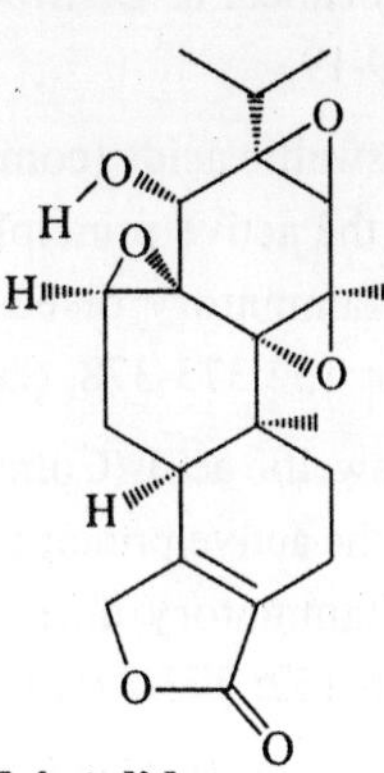

(H) Triptolide

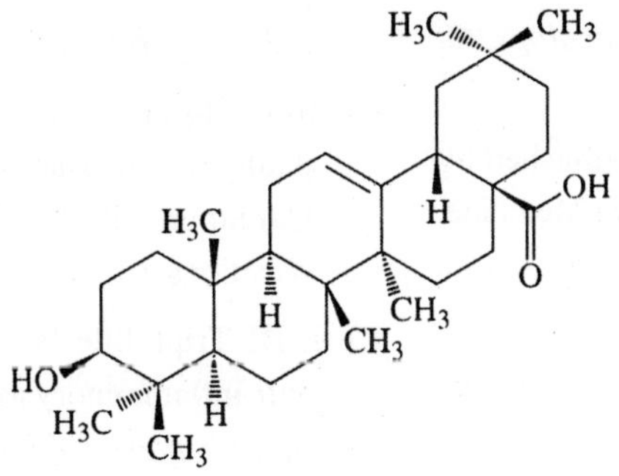

(I) Oleanolic acid

Fig. 17.1: Chemical structures of anti-arthritic leads from botanicals.

REFERENCES

Abe Y, Hashimoto S and Horie T Curcumin inhibition of inflammatory cytokine production by human peripheral blood monocytes and alveolar macrophages; *Pharmacol. Res.* 39: 41-47, (1999).

Afzal, Al- hadidi D, Menon M, Pesek J, Dhami M S. Ginger: an ethnomedicine, Chemical and pharmalogical Review. *Drug Metabol Drug Interact.*18: 159-90, (2001).

Agarwal R B and V D Rangari. Antiinflammatory and Antiarthritic activities of Lupeol and 19- alpha-H lupeol isolated from *Strobilanthus Callosus* and *Strobillanthus ixiocephala* roots. *Indian Journal of Pharmacology.* 35: 384-387, (2003).

Aggarwal BB, Shishodia S. Supression of the nuclear factor–KB activation pathway by spice derived phytochemicals :reasoning for seasoning. *Ann NY Acad Sci.* 1030: 434-441, (2004).

Ahmed S, Jeremy Anuntiyo, Charles J Malemud and Tariq M. Haqqi. 2005. Biological basis for the use of Botanicals in Osteo arthritis and Rheumatoid Arthritis: A Review. *eCAM* 2 (3): 301-308, (2005).

Akira T, The Pharmacological effects of *Cinnamomum* in ulcers. Foreign Medicine–Chinese Medicine Branch 9. 28, (1987).

Ali Mohammed. 2003. Text Book of Pharmacognosy. CBS Publishers & Distributors, New Delhi (India). Pp 9-19.

Ammon HP. Boswellic acids (components of frankincense) as the active principle in treatment of chronic inflammatory diseases. Wien. Med. Wochenschr. 152:373-378, (2002).

Amnon HP. Boswellic acids(Components of Frankincence) as the active principles in treatment of chronic inflammatory diseases. Wien. Med. Wochenschr. 152: 373-378, (2002).

Anita Jain SS. Katewa BL Chaudhary, Praveen Galav. Folk herbal medicines used in birth control and sexual disease by tribals of southern Rajasthan, India. *Journal of Ethnopharmacology*.90: 171-177, (2004).

Anonymous, Unani medicine in India, published by Central Council for Research in Unani Medicine, Govt. of India, New Delhi. Ed-Mehre-Alam Khan, (2002).

Araujo CAC, Leon LL, Biological activities of *Curcuma longa* L. Mem Inst Oswaldo Cruz Rio de Janeiro. 96 (5): 723-728, (2001).

Balakrishnan, Recent concepts in the therapy of Rheumatoid Arthritis based on advances in pathogenesis. *Clinical Labtechnology*, 14-17, (2004).

Bauer WW, Arthritis and Rheumatism. In: Todays Health Guide- A manual of health information & guidance for the American Family, eds. W.W. Bauer. Publisher-American Medical Association (USA) pp. 389-392, (1965).

Bhatia S. Laboratory investigations in Rheumatic Disease. Clinical Labtechnology : 9-13.

Chainani-Wu N. Safety and anti- inflammatory activity of curcumin a component of turmeric (*Curcuma longa) J Alternative Complementatry Medicine* 9: 161-168, (2004).

Chandra D. Analgesic effect of Aqueous and alcoholic extracts of Madhuka longifolia(Koeing). *Indian j Pharmacology*. 33: 108-111, (2001).

Chandra Rabish M. mahato, SC Mandal, Kamini Kumar, Jyoti Kumar. Ethnomedicinal formulations used by traditional herbal practitioners of Ranchi, Jharkhand. *Indian j Traditional Knowledge*. 6(4): 599-601, (2007).

Chandra, Dinesh and SS. Gupta. Anti-inflammatory and anti-arthritic activity of volatile oil of *Curcuma longa* (haldi), *IJMR* 60(1):138-142, (1972).

Chandra T and J Sadique. Anti-arthritic effect of *Cardiospermum halicacabum* in rats, *Indian Medicine* 1(2): 12-20, (1989).

Chatterjee S. and SN. Das Anti-arthritic and anti-inflammatory effect of a poly-herbal drug [Ease(R)]: its mechanism of action. *Indian Journal of Pharmacology* 28(2): 116-119, (1996).

Chattopadhyay Ishita, Bishwas kaushik, Bandopadhyay and Banerjee ranjit K Turmeric and Curcumin : Biological actions and medical applications. *Current science*.87 (1) : 44-53, (2004).

Chen BJ Triptolide, a novel immunosuressive and anti-inflammatory agent purified from a Chinese herb *Tripterygium wilfordii* Hook F. Leukemia and Lymphoma. 42: 253-265, (2001).

Chevrier MR, AE. Ryan DYW. Lee M Zhong Ze, Z wu-Yan, and C S Via. Boswellia carterii extracts inhibits TH1 Cytokines and promotes TH2 cytokines *in vitro*. *Clin. Diagn. Lab. Immunol.* 12(5): 575-580, (2005).

Chikitsasthana, Chapters XXVIII, XXIX. In Sharma PV,editor. Charaka Samhita (English Translation). Delhi: Chaukambha Orientalia.461, (1994).

Choi In-Young, Jung hyuk-sang, kim Hyung-Ryong, et al. OK205 regulates production of inflammatory cytokines in HMC-1 cells. *Biol.Pharm.Bull* 27 (11): 1871-1874, (2004).

Choi. J, Kyung-Tae Lee, et al. Anti-Rheumatoid Arthritis Effect of the *Kochia scoparia* fruits and activity comparision of Momordin Ic, it prosapogenin and Sapogenin. *Arch Pharm Res*.25(3): 336-342, (2002).

Chopra A et al., 2001. Exploring ancient Ayurveda for rheumatology: traditional therapy, Modern relevance and challenges. *APLAR J Rhematol.* 4: 190-199, (2002).

Chopra A, Gore A, Paranjape S, Edmonds J. Modified health assessment questionnaire (HAQ) : An Indian study for validity and relevance. Programme and Abstracts. 8th APLAR (Asia Pacific League Against Rheumatism) Congress, Melbourne, Australia, (1996).

Chopra A. Ayurvedic Medicine: Core Concept, therapeutic principles and Current Relavance. Med clin North Am.; 86: 75-89, (2002).

Chopra, A. 2000. Ayurvedic medicine and Arthritis. *Rheum Dis Clin North America* 26: 133-144.

Cribb AB, Cribb J w. 1981. Wild medicine in australia. William Collins: Sydney; 51, (2000).

Curtis clare L, John L: Harwood, Colin M. Dent and Bruce Caterson 2004, Bilogical basis for the benefit of nutraceutical supplementation in arthritis. *Drug Discovery Today.* 9(4): 165-172, (2004).

Dai Min, Wei W, Shen YX, Zheng Y Q. Glucosides of Chaenomeles speciosa remit rat adjuvant arthritis by inhibiting synoviocytes activites. *Acta pharmcol sin*; 24; 1161-6, (2003).

Dalbeth N and Haskard D.O, Mechanism of inflammation in Gout. *Rheumatology.* 44: 1090-1096, (2005).

Das PK, RS. Rathor, R Lal, RM Tripathi, AK Ram, and M Biswas. Anti-inflammatory and anti-arthritic activity of *Crataeva nurvala* Buch-Ham (varuna). *JRIM* 9(3) 9-16, (1974).

Debnath PK and VB. Pandey Investigation on the anti-inflammatory activities and anti-arthritic activities of saponin isolated from *Costus speciosus*. *JRIM.* 6:55, (1971).

Deodhar SD, Sethi R, Srimal R C. Preliminary studies on antirheumatic activity of Curcumin. *Indian J Med Res.* 71: 632-634, (1980).

Dinesh Chandra and SS. Gupta. Anti-inflammatory and anti-arthritic activity of volatile oil of *Curcuma longa* (haldi), *IJMR* 60(1):138-142, (1972).

Duan H, Yoshihisa Takaishi et al. Triterpenoids from *Tripterygium wilfordii. Phytochemistry.*53: 805-810, (2000).

Duan LK, Kawazoe K, and Takischi Y. Terpenoids from *Tripterygium wilfordii. Phytochemistry.*45:791-796, (1997).

Engel l W, Straus SE. Development of Therapeutics: opportunities within complementary and alternative medicine. *Nat. Rev.* 1:229-237, (2002).

Frondoza CG, Frazier C, Polotsky A, Lahiji K, Hungerford DS, Weinder MS. Inhibition of chondrocyte and synoviocyte TNF α expression by hydroxyl alcoxy–phenyl compound . *Trans ortho Res Soc.* 1038, (2000).

Gokhale AB, AS Damre KR Kulkarni MN. Saraf. Preliminary evaluation of anti-inflammatory and anti-arthritic activity of *S. lappa, A. speciosa* and *A. aspera. Phytomedicine.* 9(5):433-437, (2002).

Gupta SS. Prospects and perspectives of Natural Plant Products in Plants. *Indian J Pharmacology.*26: 1-12, (1994).

Han SS, Keum YS, Sco HJ, Chun KS, Lee SS, Suruh YJ. Capsaicin suppresses phorbol ester – induced activation of NF-kappa bbRel and AP- 1 transcription factors in mouse epidermis. *Cancer Letter.* 164: 119-126, (2001).

Haqqi TM, Antony DD, Gupta S, Ahmad N, Lee M-S, Kumar Gk et al. Prevention of collagen – induced arthritis in mice by a polyphenolic fraction from green tea. *Proc Natl Acad Sci* USA. 96: 4524- 4529, (1999).

Inoue m, Ono Y and Hajime Mizkami. Supressive effect of Dai-bofu-to on collagen induced arthritis. *Biol. Pharm Bull.* 27 (6): 857-862, (2004).

Ippoushi K, Azuma K, Ito H, Horie H, Higashio H. Gingerol inhibits nitric oxide synthesis inactivated J774.1 mouse macrophages and prevents peroxynitrate induced oxidation and nitration reactions. *Life Sciences.*73: 3427-37, (2003).

Jeong Hyun-Ja , Chung H S, An H J, Seo Sang wan, et al, 2004. The immune – enhancing Effect of the Herbal Combination Bouum-Myunyuk-Dan. *Biol. Pharm. Bull* 27 (1): 29-33, (2004).

Kim mi sun, Choi In-Young, Lee Si-Hyeong et al. The oriental medicine 'Cool-Cool (Cool-X-A)'inhibits inflammatorycytokine production and migration in mast cells. *Biol. Pharm. Bull* 27(1) 34-37, (2004).

Kohli K, MJ Ansari Z Ruheman. Curcumin: A natural anti-inflammatory agent. *Indian Journal Pharmacol.* 37(3): 141-147, (2005).

Kondkor A A. Genetic aspects of Rheumatoid arthritis. Clinical labtechnology. : 7-8.

Kubo M Ma, S Wu, J Matsuda H, 1996. Anti inflammatory activities of 70% methanolic extract from *Cinnamoni cortex. Biol. Pharm. Bull.* 19, 1041-1045, (2004).

Kulkarni RR, Patki PS, Jog VP, Gandage SG, Patwardhan B. Treatment of osteoarthritis with a herbomineral formulation: a double-blind, placebo-controlled, cross-over study. *J Ethnopharmacol.* 33(1-2): 91-5, (1991).

Kutney JP, Hewitt GM, Lee g, Piotrowskak, Roberto m& Retting SJ. Studies with tissue cultures of the Chinese herbal Plant *Tripterygium wilfordii.* Isolation of metabolites of interest in rheumatoid arthritis. Immunosupression and male contraceptive activity. *Canadian Journal of Chemistry.* 70. 1455-1480, (1992).

Lafeber, FPJG et al, Apocyanin, a plant derived, cartilage-saving drug might be useful in the treatment of rheumatoid arthritis. *Rheumatology.* 38: 1088-1093, (1998).

Langer E. Greifenberg S, Gruenwald J. Ginger: history and used. *Ad. Ther.*15: 25-44, (1998).

Li S, Lu Ai Ping, Wang Y Y, Li Y. Supressive effect of a Chinese herbal medicine Qing- Luo_Yin Extract on the angiogenesis of collagen induced arthritis in rats. *The American Journal of Chinese medicine.* 31(5): 713-720, (2003).

Li SH, Chu Y, Antiinflammatory effects of toatal saponins of *Panax notoginseng. Zhongguo Yao Li Xue Bao* 20: 551-554, (1999).

Liu M. et al Advance in the pharmacological research on matrine. *Zhongguo Zhong Yao Zay* 28: 801-804, (2003).

Mahajan B, SC. Taneja VK. Sethi and KL. Dhar. 1995. Two triterpenoids from *Boswellia serrata* gum resin. *Phytochemistry* 39: 453-455, (1995).

Mahato Malati, 2002. Investigations on ethnomedicinal plants for curing Rheumatism in Khunti Sub-Division of Ranchi District. PhD Thesis, (2002).

Martinez D, K Lohs, and J Janzen. Weihrauch als Arzneimittel. *In* D Martines (ed.), Weihrauch und myrrhe. Wisssenschaftliche Verlagsgesellschaft, Stuttgart, Germany. p. 125-140, (1989).

Mishra SS and HD Singh. Antiphlogistic action of some indigenous drugs, II. Anti-arthritic action of *Balsamodendron mukul. Indian Journal of Physiology and Allied Sciences* 16: 90, (1962).

Moreland L W. An Introduction to modern management of Rheumatoid arthritis. In: Moreland Larry E. editor, Rheumatoid Arthritis, epidemiology pathogenesis and treatment. 1st ed. New Delhi: Jaypee brothers Medical Publishers, (2002).

NK Dubey, Rajesh Kumar and Pramila Tripathi. Global Promotion of herbal medicine: India's opportunity. *Current Science* 86(1): 37-41, (2004).

Nandkarni AK. Indian Materia Medica, Vol. 6. Bombay, India, Popular Book Depot. p. 1317, (1985).

Ono Yuka, Makoti, Hajime Mizukumi and Yukio Ogihara. Suppressive effect of Kanzo – bushito, a kampo medicine, on collagen induced arthritis. *Biol. Pharm. Bull.* 27 (9): 1406-1413, (2004).

Ono Yuka, Yukio Ogihara, Shinobu Saijo, Yoichiro Iwakura, M Inoue. Evaluation of Kampo medicines used to treat rheumatoid arthritis in collagen- induced arthritic and pX transgenic mice. *Mod Rheumatol.* 13: 50-56, (2003).

OnoY, Yukio Ogihara, Shinobu Saijo, Evaluation of Kampo Medicines used to treat Rheumatoid Arthritis in Collagen induced arthritic and Px Transgenic mice. Mod. Rheumatoid.,13: 50-56, (2003).

P R Cheeke, S Piacente and W Oleszek, Anti inflammatory and anti –arthritic effects of Yucca Schidigern: A Review. *Journal of Inflammation* 3: 6, (2006).

Patwardhan B, Ashok DB. Vaidya and Mukund Chorghade. Ayurveda and natural products drug discovery. *Current Sience* 86(6): 789-799, (2004).

Patwardhan B & Manish Gautum. Botanical Immunodrugs: Scope and opportunities. *Drug Discovery Today.*10 (7): 495-502, (2005).

Patwardhan B and Hooper, M 1992. Ayurveda and future drug development. *Int. J. Alternative Complement. Med.*, 10: 9-11, (1992).

Phadke Kalindi. Review Article: In vivo and in vitro modelsfor arthritis. *Indian Drugs.* 25(9): 354-365, (1988).

Pillai NR and G Santhakumari a. Anti-arthritic and anti-inflammatory actions of nimbidin. Planta Medica. 43: 59-63, (1981).

Prasad DN and G Achari. Study of anti-arthritic action of *Vanda roxburghii* in albino rats, *Journal of The Indian Medical Association* 45(5): 234-237, (1966).

Rachel W Li David N, Leach, Stephen P. Myers, Gregorg J. Leach, G. David Lin, Donals J. brushetl and Peter G. Waterman. Anti inflammatory activity, cytotoxicity and active compounds of *Tinospora smilacina* Benth. *Phytother. Res* 18: 78-83, (2004).

Ramjilal, L. et al Preliminary studies on the anti-inflammatory and anti-arthritic activity of *Crataeva nurvala, Indian Journal of Pharmacology.* 4: 122, (1972).

Rao, URK., Firdaus F. Clinical Aspects of Rheumatoid Arthritis. *Clinical Labtechnology.* : 4-6, (2004).

Rathor SR. and HR. Goyal. Studies on the anti-inflammatory and anti-arthritic activity of an Indian medicinal plant, Cedrus deodara,. *Indian Journal of Pharmacology.* 5(2): 334-343, (1973).

Reddy BM, VV Byahatti AVN. Appa Rao and M. Ramesh. Anti-inflammatory activity of *Stapelia nobilis* and *Caralluma stalagmifera. Fitoterapia* 67(6): 545-547, (1996).

Riehemann K, Bert Behnke, Klaus schulze – O sthoff Plant extracts from stinging nettle (*Urtica dioica*), an antirheumatic remedy, inhibit the proinflammatory transcription factor NF-KB. *FEBS Letters.* 442: 89-94, (1999).

Sandoval M, Okuhama NN, Zhang XJ condezo LA, Angeles FM, Muash R M, et al. Anti inflammatory and antioxidant activities of cats claw (*Uncaria guianensis*) are independent of their alkaloid content. *Phytomedicine.*9: 325-337, (2002).

Sandoval-Chacon, M, Thompson JH, Zhang XJ, Mannick EE, Saowska- krowicka H, Charbonnet R M, et al. Anti inflammatory actions of cat's claw : the role of NF- KB. *Aliment Pharmacol Ther* 12: 1279-89, (1998).

Sasaki Y, Fushmi H and Komatsu k, Application of single nucleotide polymorphism analysis of the trnk Gene to the identification of *Curcuma* plants. *Biol pharm.bull.* 27 (1): 144-146, (2004).

Schulick P. Ginger: common spice and wonder drug. 3rd ed. Brattleboro (VT): Herbal Free Press Ltd.

Sethi PD, Thiabarajan and S Sankara Subramanian.1970. Studies on the anti inflammatory and antiarthritc activity of Withaferin A. *Ind J Pharmc.* 2(4): 165-72, (1996).

Sethi, P.D., A.R. Thiagarajan and S. Sankarasubramanian. Studies on the anti-inflammatory and anti-arthritic activity of Withaferin-A. *Indian Journal of Pharmacology* 2(4): 165-172, (1970).

Shim SS, M Jin et al. Supressive effects of PG 201, an ethanol extract from herbs on collagen induced arthritis in mice. *Rheumatology*.42:665-672, (2003).

Shin SS, M Jin, HJ Jung et al. Suppressive effects of PG 201, an etahnolic extract from herbs, on collagen induced arthritice in mice. *Rheumatology*. 42: 665-672, (2003).

Simha KR Gopala and V Laxminarayana. Standardsation of Ayurvedic Polyherbal formulation, Nyagrodhi Churna. *Indian J Traditional Knowledge*. 6 (4): 648-652, (2007).

Singh RH and GN Chaturvedi. Further studies on the anti-arthritic effect of an indigenous drug, *Dalbergia lanceolaria*. *IJMR* 54(4): 363-367, (1966).

Singh S and DK Majumdar. Anti-arthritic activity of Ocimum sanctum Linn. (tulsi). *Indian Journal of Pharmacology* 27(1): 50, (1995).

Srivastava KC, Mustafa T.Ginger (*Zingiber officinale*) in rheumatism and musculoskeletal disorders. Med Hypothesis. 39: 342-348, (1992).

Stastny P. Association of the B-Cell allo antigen DRW4 with rheumatoid arthritis. *N Engl J Med.* 298: 869-871, (1978).

Subramanian SS and Sethi PD. Withaferin A from *withania couglans* roots. *Curr. Sci.* (India), 38: 267, (1969).

Szabolcs Nyiredy. Separation Strategies of Plant Constituents – Current Status. *Journal of Chromatography B*, 81; 35-51, (2004).

Tamhankar CP, MN. Saraf Anti-arthritic activity of *Vitex negundo* Linn., *Indian Journal of Pharmaceutical Science* 56(4):158, (1993).

Tao X, Younger J, Fan Fz, Wang b, Lipsky P E. Benefit of an extract of *Tripterygium wilfordii* Hook F in Patients with Rheumatoid Arthritis. Arthritis Rheum 46: 1735-1743, (2002).

Taylor, J.L.S. & Van Staden, J. 2002. COX-1 and COX-2 inhibitory activity in extracts prepared from Eucomis species, with further reference to extracts from E. autumnalis autumnalis. *S. Afr. J. Bot.* 68: 80-85, (2002).

Venkatranganna MV, Gopumadhavan S Mitra Anturlikar SD. Anti-inflammatory activity of Joint Care B, a polyherbal formulation. *Indian Drugs* 37(11) 543-546, (2000).

Warude D, and Patwardhan B. Botanicals: Quality and regulatory issues. *Journal of Scientific & Industrial Research*.64:83-92, (2005).

Yuseok moon, Glasgow Wc, Eling ET. Curcumin suppresses interleukin 1B- mediated microsomal prostaglandin E synthase 1 by altering early growth response gene 1 and other signaling pathays. The *Journal of Pharmacology and Experimental Therapeutics* 315 (2): 788-795, (2005).

chapter 18

Fig Plants with Special Reference to Medicinal Values

Saikat Dewanjee and Subhash C Mandal

INTRODUCTION

Ficus is a genus of about under the family Moraceae, containing approximately 750 species of fig trees, 150 shrubs and vines native throughout the tropics with a few species extending into the warm temperate zone (Serrato *et al*, 2004). The genus includes one species, *Ficus carica* known as 'Common fig' that produces fruits commercially known as 'Fig'. A fig 'fruit' is derived from a specially adapted type of inflorescence (structural arrangement of flowers) is commonly called the 'fruit' is actually a specialized structure or accessory fruit called a syconium an involuted (nearly closed) receptacle with many small flowers arranged on the inner surface. Thus the actual flowers of the fig are unseen unless the fig is cut open.

The Taxonomical niche of Figs

Kingdom: Plantae

Subkingdom: *Tracheobionta*

Superdivision: *Spermatophyta*

Division: Magnoliophyta

Class: Magnoliopsida

Subclass: *Hamamelididae*

Order: Rosales

Family: Moraceae

Genus: Ficus

Species: more than 800 species available.

Among the more famous species are the Sacred Fig tree (*Ficus religiosa*) and the Banyan tree (*Ficus bengalensis*). Figs occupy a wide variety of ecological niche; from Common Fig (*Ficus carica*), a small temperate deciduous tree to Weeping Fig (*Ficus benjamina*) a hemi-epiphyte with thin tough leaves on pendulous stalks or to the Creeping Fig (*Ficus pumila*), a vine whose small, hard leaves form a dense carpet of foliage over rocks or garden walls. The figs with versatile plant habits have undergone adaptive radiation in different biogeographic regions. In the tropics, it is quite common to find that *Ficus* is the most species-rich plant genus in a particular forest. In Asia, as many as 70 or more species can co-exist. Although identification of many of the *Ficus* species can be difficult but figs as a group are relatively easy to recognize. The presence of aerial roots often gives the distinguished identity of figs. Figs clutch of vital importance throughout the tropics in cultural as well medicinal aspect.

Importance of Figs

Ficus is a relatively ancient genus being at least 60 million years old, and possibly as old as 80 million years. The fruits of most of Ficus species are edible and impart economic importance or eaten as bushfood. Figs are also of paramount cultural importance throughout the tropics, both as objects of worship and for their many medicinal uses (Watt and Breyer-Brandwijk, 1962). The fig trees have profoundly influenced culture through several religious traditions namely in Buddhism, Hinduism, Jainism and Islam. The medicinal values of different parts of different figs were demonstrated in different aboriginal literatures. Some of figs are cultivated ornamentals or as a source of rubber and paper (Ipulet, 2007) Fig tree's wood and the latex precludes were used for many purposes; it was for example used to make mummy caskets in Ancient Egypt. On the other hand, certain fig species mainly Ficus cotinifolia, Ficus glabrata and Ficus padifolia were traditionally used in Mesoamerica. Ficus natalensis bark was used to produce bark-cloth in Uganda (Ipulet, 2007). Weeping Fig (Ficus benjamina) and Indian Rubber Plant (Ficus elastica) are identified as powerful air-cleaning plants in the NASA Clean Air Study.

Medicinal values of figs

Since the evolution of mankind, man had no other source of medicine than plants and figs have served a successful history against an array of human as well animal ailments (Watt and Breyer-Brandwijk, 1962; Marimuthu and Subbarayalu, 1986). A number of medicinal values have been attributed by fig plants. Different traditional literatures are literal witness of it. Along with the progression of science, herbalists aimed to substantiate scientifically with the help of selected biological assays about the ethnomedicinal claims of figs. In this literature, it was attempted to give a view of medicinal uses of some of fig species.

Table 18.1. Some medicinally important fig species are mentioned hereunder

Biological source	Common name	Part used	Medicinal values
Ficus adenosperma Miq.	Ashuh	Leaf	Used for the treatment of cold and tuberculosis (Case, 2001); With coconut water possesses contraceptive action.
Ficus alba Reinw. Ex Blume. Syn. *Ficus grossularioes* Burm.	—	Leaf	Used for the treatment of Renosis.
Ficus amplissima Smith. Syn. *Ficus tsiela*	Bat tree, udumber	Aerial part	Possesses antitussive, antiasthmatic, anticancer and diuretic activity (Dhawan et al., 1980).
Ficus arbutifolia Link.	Pakur	Juice and milky secretion	Useful against poisoned wound, indolent ulcers and as a resolvent ((Nadkarni and Nadkarni, 1992).
Ficus arnottiana Miq. Syn *Urostigma arnottianum* Miq.	Crow fig (Ceylon), Paras papal,	Leaves	Useful as moderate sterilizer and to treat skin diseases (Asolkar et al., 1992; Chopra et al., 1992). In Ayurveda it is used to treat Blood diseases, apoplexy, vertigo and delirium (www.siu.edu/~ebl/leaflets/panca.htm).
Ficus asperrima Roxb. Syn. *Ficus exasperate* Vahl.	Kalumar	Bark	Useful against glandular enlargement of liver and spleen, cracks and fissures of palms, hands and soles of feet. (Dhawan et al., 1977). Bark is acrid and used as a tooth brush to remove tarter and cleansing teeth ((Nadkarni and Nadkarni, 1992).
Ficus bengalensis Linn. Syn. *Ficus indica*	Banyan tree, Sacred fig tree	Latex	Used to alleviate toothache.
		Young buds	Useful against diarrhoea, and dysentery.
		Root	Useful against arthritis (Daniel et al., 2003) obstinate vomiting (Asolkar et al., 1992) and immune-deficiency (Gabhe et al., 2006).
		Juice	Juice with sesame oil used externally in burn also found usefulness against diabetes and wound (Biswas and Mukherjee, 2003; Park and Chun, 2001).
		Bark and leaves	Bark with black pepper is useful against snake bite; decoction has strong antifertility activity in men and women. Useful to depress uterine and cardiac muscle also cholinergic blocking of smooth and skeletal muscles (Vohora et al., 1969).
		Milky latex	Used externally for pain, bruses, anodyne, rheumatism, lumbago, toothache (Chopra et al., 1992).
		Fruits	Useful against diabetes (Sharad et al., 2007).
Ficus benjamina Linn. Syn. *Ficus comosa,* and	Weeping fig, Java fig	Sap	Used for whitening of cornea, Useful against Liver disease (Miura et al., 1982).

Ficus retusa Auct.		Bark	Useful against rheumatoid arthritis and ulcer.
		Leaves	Juice of leaves along with ghrita is flatulent and colic, (Dhawan et al., 1977).
		Aerial part	Useful as poultice and possesses diuretic activity
Ficus callosa Willd. *Ficus basidentula*	—	Fruits and barks	Useful against leprosy, aphthous complaint and bladder complaint, (Nadkarni and Nadkarni, 1992; Chopra et al., 1992)
Ficus carica L. syn. *Ficus caprificus* Risso.	Caprifig, Wild Mediterranean fig	Leaves and Milky sap	Possesses anthelmintic (Wang et al., 2004), anti-HIV (Agabeili et al., 2005), antioxidant, antimutagenic (Agabeyli and Gasimova, 2005), antidiabetic (Pérez et al., 1998; Serraclara et al., 1998), antibacterial (Jang et al., 2004) activity.
Ficus citrifolia	Strangler Fig	Whole plant	Useful externally for the treatment of superficial infections. Possesses antispasmodic, antimicrobial and anticancer activity (Antoun et al., 2001; Simon et al., 2001).
Ficus Cunia Willd. Syn. *Ficus semicordata* Buch-Ham. Ex Smith., *Ficus conglomerata* Roxb.	Bhuin gular	Aerial part	Useful CNS depression activity (Dhawan et al., 1977).
		Latex	Useful to cure boils (reported from the Holy Bible) and fever (Rijal 1994).
		Fruits	Young fruit juice is applied in forehead to relieve headache (Manandhar 1998b). A bath made from the fruit is a cure for leprosy.
		Bark	Useful in ulcer and gastric (Manandhar 1993).
		Root	Root paste is taken to cure headache.
Ficus dalhausiae Miq.	—	Fruitsbark and leaves	Useful in cardiac problem.Possess hepatoprotective activity (Nadkarni and Nadkarni, 1992; Chopra et al., 1922).
Ficus elastica Roxb.	Indian rubber	Aerial partRoot bark	Possesses diuretic activity (Dhawan et al., 1980)Possesses anti-inflammatory activity (Madhavan and Benedict, 1986).
Ficus exasperate Vahl. Syn. *Ficus punctifera* Warb.	Kharapatra	Leaves	Useful in boils and ring worm. Possesses antibacterial (Macfoy and Cline, 1990), antitumor, antifungal (Okoli et al., 2007), antidiabetic (Nimenibo-Uadi, 2003) and gastro-protective (Akah et al., 1997) activity.
		Sap	The viscid non-milky sap is used for treating sores eye trouble and stomach pains (Burkill, 1997) arrest bleeding (Abbiw, 1990). It is also used by traditional birth attendants (TBAS) ease child-birth (Bouquet, 1969).

Ficus fistulosa Reinw. Ex Blume. ; syn. *Ficus harlandii* Benth., *Ficus rubrovenia* Merr.	Common yellow stem-fig	Aerial part	Used to treat malarial fever, headache and other symptoms. Possesses diuretic (Dhar et al., 1973) and antimalarial (Zhang et al., 2002) activity.
Ficus gibbosa Blume. syn. *Ficus tinctoria* G. Forst.	Udumber	Root bark	Useful against indigestion and loss of appetite (Nadkarni and Nadkarni, 1992).
Ficus glabrata Kunth. syn. *Ficus krugiana* Warb.	Red fig	Latex	Useful to treat intestinal flakes. Possess significant anthelmintic activity (Hansson, 1986).
Ficus heterophylla Linn. f.	—	Rootleaves	Used in asthma, cough and as gargle in salivation. Useful in chronic dysentery.
Ficus hirta Vahl. syn. *Ficus dumosa* King.	—	Root	Used as antidote: when eaten causes diarrhoea and vomiting which cleans out the poison from the affected person.
		Stem latex	Used for wounds (Manandhar 1990).
		Stem bark	Stem bark is boiled and its gel is used in fever (Manandhar 1998a).
Ficus hispida L. f. syn. *Ficus compressa* S. S. Chang	Rough-leaved fig	Leaf	Possesses antidiarrhoeal activity (Mandal et al., 2002). hepatoprotective (Mandal et al., 2000), antidiabetic (Ghosh et al., 2004).
Ficus infectoria Roxb. Syn.	Spotted fig, pakar	Bark	Useful against ulcer and an infection in leucorrhoea.
Ficus viren Aiton.,	Oje fig	Latex	Used to treat anemia, diarrhoeal, and abdominal distension.
Ficus insipida syn			(in pediatric cases) Possesses significant anthelmintic activity (Hansson, 1986).
Ficus lacor	Ashvatti	Stem bark	Used to in gastric and ulcer (Bajracharya et al., 1978; Pandey, 2001; Rai et al., 2004).
		Milky latex Buds Seeds	Blood diseases, apoplexy, vertigo and delirium. Used in typhoid and heavy fever, dysentery (Oli 2001) and boils.Decoction of buds is considered for ulcer and leucorrhoea (Chopra et al., 1956; HMG 1970), gargle in salivation (Malla 1994), boils (Manandhar 1985), pimples and blisters. Dried buds are used to treat harsa (Nakarmi 2001). Dried buds are used to treat harsa (Nakarmi 2001).Uses tonic and treatment of stomach disorder (Bhatt 1977).
Ficus megapoda Bak.	-	Leaf and bark	Possesses antimalarial activity (Randrianarivelojosia et al., 2003).
Ficus microcarpa L. syn. *Ficus rubra* Roth.	Laurel fig	Latexleaves	Possesses antifingal and cytotoxic activity (Taira et al., 2005). Possesses antioxidant activity (Li, 2003).
Ficus nemoralis Wall. syn.	—	Aerial part	Used as antispasmodic and anticancer agent.

Ficus neriifolia Sm.		Stem bark	Stem bark juice is given in conjunctivitis and boils (Manandhar 2001; Manandhar, 2002).
Ficus opposite Wild.	—	Bark Fruits and seeds	Used as antiperiodic, tonic and emetic. Used as emetic.
Ficus ovata Vahl. syn.	—	Bark, root	Possesses anti-viral (Hudson et al., 2000), anti-titenus, anti-
Ficus megaphylla Warb			convulsant activity (Ananil et al., 2000).
Ficus palmate Forsk	—	Latex of young twingsfruits	Stem latex is applied to extract spines deeply lodged in the flesh (Manandhar 1995; Manandhar, 2002). It is also applied to draw out prickles or other foreign matter in body Used to treat dysentery, vomiting (Devkota and Karmacharya 2003; Pant and Pant 2004) and the diseases of lung and bladder Possesses demulcent and laxative action.
Ficus platyphylla Delile.	—	Stem bark	Possesses anti-inflammatory, analgesic (Amos et al., 2002) and CNS depressant activity (Wakeel et al., 2004).
Ficus polita Vahl. syn. *Ficus repens* Hort.	Climbing fig, Creeping fig	Leaves	Possesses anti-inflammatory and analgesic activity (Recio et al., 1995; Gbeassor et al., 1990).
Ficus racemosa L. syn. *Ficus glomerata* Roxb., *Ficus goolereea* Roxb.	Cluster fig, Gular fig, Redwood fig, Dumur	Fruits Bark Leaf	Useful chemomodulatory and antifilarial agent (Mishra et al., 2005). Possesses wound healing activity (Biswas and Mukherjee, 2003). Use for the treatment of diabetes (Rao et al., 2002), liver diseases (Mandal et al., 1999) and diarrhoea (Mukherjee et al., 1998) Possesses anti-inflammatory (Li et al., 2004), antitussive (Rao et al., 2003), antipyretic (Rao et al., 2003), antidiabetic (Rao et al., 2002), and antibacterial (Mandal et al., 2000). Wound healing (Biswas and Mukherjee, 2003).
Ficus religiosa Linn.	Sacred fig, Bodhi tree, Pippal.	Bark Leaves and young shoot	useful in gonorrhoea, skin diseases and scabies; dried bark with milk aphrodisiac; bark infusion useful against ulcer and skin diseases Stem bark possesses antibacterial, antiprotozoal antiviral (Dhar et al., 1968) and cholinergic activity (Vinutha et al., 2006); root bark possesses hypoglycemic activity (Wadood et al., 2003). Young leaves with wet wheat flour effective against skin eruption and swelling. Used as purgative and produce estrogenic action.
Ficus retusa Linn. syn. *Ficus retusiformis* H. Léveillé	Indian laurel fig, Malay banyan	Bark Leaves	Possesses hepatoprotective and antirheumatic activity. Possesses wound healing and antirheumatic activity.

Ficus rumphii Blume. syn. *Ficus cordifolia*	Mock Bodh fig, Gaiaswat	Barks	Useful for the treatment of asthma, snake bite, ulcer of mouth and foot (Manandhar, 1992; Manandhar, 2002) and also employed to kill warms.
Ficus sarmentosa Buch. syn. *Ficus foveolata, Ficus luducca*	—	Stem bark	Bark powder is taken to cure boils and secrete more milk during delivery.
	—	Root	Used in malaria (Dangol and Gurung, 2000).
Ficus subincica Buch-Ham. Ex Smith. Syn. *Ficus clavata* Miq.	—	Aerial part	Useful spasmogenic agent.
Ficus sycomorus syn. *Ficus gnaphalocarpa* Miq.	—	Leaf	Possesses antibacterial and anti-diarrheal activity (Ahmadu et al., 2007).
Ficus thonningii Blume. *Ficus burkei* Miq.	Common wild fig.	Whole plant	Possesses amoebicidal activity (Moundipa et al., 2005).
Ficus tisela Roxb.	Pipat	Whole plant	Possesses antibacterial activity (Nair and Chanda, 2007).
Ficus vallis-choudae Del.	—	Whole plant	Possesses anthelmintic activity (Hudson et al., 2000).

Discussion

Observing the medicinal uses, *Ficus* may be described as the genus as a medicine cabinet. The medicinal values of only few of Ficus plants were discussed in this article. Fig trees have also been considered promising fodder trees for livestock. Beside the medicinal uses the *Ficus* plants impart significant socio-cultural impact in different countries namely in India, China, Japan, Fiji, Mexico, Uganda, USA and Mozambique. Thus *Ficus* is an important genus of interest for herbalist as well medicinal plant researchers.

REFERENCES

Abbiw T. Study of Tropical shrubs and plant. *J Bio*, 23, 591-602, (1990).

Agabeili RA, Kasimova TEV, Khan NU, Singhal KC. Potential antifilarial activity of fruit extracts of *Ficus racemosa* Linn. against Setaria cervi in vitro. *Ind J Exp Bio*, 43(4), 346-350, (2005).

Agabeyli RA, Gasimova TE. Antimutagenic activity of *Armoracia rusticana*, *Zea mays* and *Ficus carica* plant extracts and their mixture. *Cyto and Gen*, 39(3), 75-79, (2005).

Ahmadu AA, Agunu A, Enhimidu JO, Magiatis P, Skaltsounis AL. Antibacterial, anti-diarrheal activity of *Daniellia oliveri* and *Ficus sycomorus* and their constituents. *Plant Med*, 73, 878, (2007).

Akah PA, Gamaniel KS, Wambebe CN, Shittu A, Kapu SD, Kunle OO. Studies on the gastrointestinal properties of *Ficus exasperate*. *Fitotherapia*, 68(1), 17-20, (1997).

Amos S, Chindo B, Edmond I, Akah P, Wambebe C, Gamaniel K. Anti-inflammatory and anti-nociceptive effects of *Ficus platyphylla* extract in mice and rats. *J Herb Spic Med Plan*, 9(1), 47-53, (2002).

Ananil K, Hudson JB, Lee MX, De Souzâ K, Arnason JT, Gbeassor M. Anthelmintic activity of medicinal plants used in Northern Côte d'Ivoire Against Intestinal Helminthiasis. *Pharma Bio*, 43(1), 72-78, (2005).

Asolkar LV, Kakkar KK, Chakre OJ. Second supplement to Glossary of Indian Medicinal Plants with Active Principles. CSIR (PID), New Delhi Part-I (A-K), pp 312-313, (1992).

Bajracharya D, Rana SJB, Shrestha AK. A general survey and biochemical analysis of fodder plants found in Nagarjun hill forest of Kathmandu valley. *J Natur His Muse*, 2, 105-116, (1978).

Biswas TK, Mukherjee B. Plant Medicines of Indian Origin for Wound Healing Activity. *Inter J Low Extr Woun*, 2(1), 25-39, (2003).

Bouquet AJ. Natural products as an alternative remedy. Vol. 2, 4th edition, Royal Botanic Gardens Kew, pp. 166-179, (1969).

Burkill HM. The useful plants of tropical West Africa. Vol. 4, 3rd edition, Royal Botanic Gardens Kew, pp. 166-179, (1997).

Case RJ. Integrative pharmacognostic evaluation of anti-tb ethnobotanicals from Manus. In: Thesis, Illinois, Chicago, 32, (2001).

Chopra RN, Nayar SL, Chopra IC. Glossary of Indian Medicinal Plants, 3rd reprint, CSIR, New Delhi, pp. 118-119, (1992).

Dangol DR, Gurung, S.B., Ethnobotanical study of Darai tribe in Chitwan district, Nepal. In: Proceeding of III National Conference on Science and Technology, Royal Nepal Academy of Science and Technology, Nepal, pp 1194-1213, (2000).

Daniel RS, Devi KS, Augusti KT, Sudhakaran Nair, C.R. Mechanism of action of antiatherogenic and related effects of *Ficus bengalensis* Linn. flavonoids in experimental animals. *Ind J Exper Bio*, 41(4), 296-303, (2003).

Devkota R, Karmacharya SB. Documentation of indigenous knowledge of Meidicinal plants in Gwalek, Baitadi, Nepal. *Botanica Orientalis* 3, pp 135-143, (2003).

Dhar ML, Dhar, MM, Dhawan BN, Mehrotra BN, Ray C. Screening of Indian plants for biological activity: I. *Ind J Exper Bio,* 6(4), 232-247, (1968).

Dhar ML, Dhar MM, Dhawan BN, Mehrotra BN, Srimal RC, Tandon JS. Screening of Indian plants for biological activity. IV. *Ind J Exper Bio,*11(1), 43-54, (1973).

Dhawan BN, Dubey MP, Mehrotra BN, Rastogi RP, Tandon JS. Screening of Indian plants for biological activity: Part IX. *Ind J Exper Bio,* 18(6), 594-606, (1980).

Dhawan BN, Patnaik GK, Rastogi RP, Singh KK, Tandon JS. Screening of Indian plants for biological activity: part VI. *Ind J Exper Bio,*15(3), 208-219, (1977).

Gabhe SY, Tatke PA, Khan TA. Evaluation of the immunomodulatory activity of the methanol extract of *Ficus bengalensis* roots in rats. *Ind J Pharmacol,* 38(4), 271-275, (2006).

Gbeassor M, Kedjagni AY, Koumaglo K, De Souza C, Agbo Aklikokou K, Amegbo KA. *In vitro* antimalarial activity of six medicinal plants. *Phytother Res,* 4(3), 115-117, (1990).

Ghosh R, Sharatchandra KH, Rita S, Thokchom IS. Hypoglycemic activity of *Ficus hispida* (bark) in normal and diabetic albino rats. *Ind J Pharmaco,* 136(4), 222-225, (2004).

Hansson A. Preclinical and clinical studies with latex from *Ficus glabrata* HBK, a traditional intestinal antihelminthic in the Amazon area. *J. Ethnopharmacol.* 17, 105-138, (1986).

HMGN, Medicinal Plants of Nepal. Bulletin of the department of medicinal plants No. 3. MoFSC, Kathmandu, Nepal. pp 153, (1982).

Hudson JB, Anani K, Lee MK, Desouza C. Further investigations on the antiviral activities of medicinal plants of Togo. *Pharma Bio,* 38(l), 46-50, (2000).

Hudson JB, Ananil K, Lee MX, De Souzâ K, Arnason JT, Gbeassor M. Investigation of medicinal plants of Togo for antiviral and antimicrobial activities. *Pharma Bio,* 38(l), 40-45, (2000).

Ipulet P. Uses of genus Ficus (Moraceae) in Buganda region, central Uganda. *Afric. J. Eco.* 45 (3), 44-47, (2007).

Jang H, Kim S, Park Y, Kim T, Ahn SY, Heo B. Dyeability and antibacterial activity of the fabrics with *Ficus carica* extracts. *Korea J Horti Sci & amp Tech,* 22(1), 130-134, (2004).

Kortekangas-Savolainen O, Kalimo K, Savolainen J. Allergens of *Ficus benjamina* (weeping fig): unique allergens in sap. *Allergy,* 61(3), 393-394, (2006).

Li RW, Leach DN, Myers SP, Lin GD, Leach GJ, Waterman PG. A new anti-inflammatory glucoside from *Ficus racemosa* L. *Planta Med.* 70(5), 421-426, (2004).

Li MH. Peroxidase and superoxide dismutase activities in fig leaves in response to ambient air pollution in a subtropical city. *Archi. Enviro. Conta. & toxicol.* 45(2),168-176, (2003).

Macfoy CA, Cline EI. In-vitro antibacterial activities of three plants used in traditional medicine in Sierra Leone. *J Ethnopharmacol,* 28(3), 323-327, (1990).

Madhavan S, Benedict CR. The anti-inflammatory effect of a crude aqueous extract of the root bark of *Ficus elastica* in the rat. *Archi Inter de Pharmacody et de Thera,* 281(1), 169-176, (1986).

Malla SB. Medicinal herbs in the Bagmati zone, ADPI-Paper series 8. ICIMOD, Kathmandu, 85, (1994).

Manandhar NP. A survey of medicinal plants of Jajarkot district, Nepal. *J Ethnopharmacol* 48, 1-6, (1995).

Manandhar NP. Ethnobotanical note on folk lore remedies of Baglung district Nepal. *Contri Nepale Studi,* 20(2), 183-196, (1993).

Manandhar NP, Ethnobotanical notes on certain medicinal plants used by Tharus of Dang Deokhuri district, Nepal. *Inter J Cru Dr Res* 23(4), 153-159, (1985).

Manandhar NP. Folklore medicine of Dhading district, Nepal. *Fitotera,* 63(2), 163-177, (1992).

Manandhar NP. Herbal veterinary practices in Nepal. *Nep J Sci & Tech* 3, 65-68, (2001).

Manandhar NP. Plants and People of Nepal, Timbre Press, Oregon, USA, pp 599, (2002).

Manandhar NP. Native phytotherapy among the Raute tribe of Dadeldhura district, Nepal. *J Ethnopharmacol,* 60, 199-206, (1998a).

Manandhar NP. Native phytotherapy among the Raute tribe of Dadeldhura district, Nepal. *J Ethnopharmacol,* 60, 199-206, (1998b).

Manandhar NP. Traditional phytotherapy of Danuwar tribe of Kamlakhong in Sindhuli district, Nepal. *Fitotera,* 61(4), 325-332, (1990).

Mandal SC, Ashokkumar CK. Studies on anti-diarrhoeal activity of *Ficus hispida* leaf extract in rats. *Fitotera,* 73(7-8), 663-667, (2002).

Mandal SC, Maity TK, Das J, Pal M, Saha BP. Hepatoprotective activity of *Ficus racemosa* leaf extract on liver damage caused by carbon tetrachloride in rats. *Phytothera Res,* 13(5), 430-432, (1999).

Mandal SC, Saha BP, Pal M. Studies on antibacterial activity of Ficus racemosa Linn. leaf extract. *Phytothera Res,* 14(4), 278-280, (2000).

Mandal SC, Saraswathi B, Kumar CK, Mohana Lakshmi S, Maiti BC. Protective effect of leaf extract of *Ficus hispida* Linn. against paracetamol-induced hepatotoxicity in rats. *Phytothera Res,* 14(6), 457-459, (2000).

Marimuthu N, Subbarayalu M. Promising fodder trees for livestock feeding in the tropics. *Livesto Advis,* 663, 11-15, (1986).

Miura GA, Broomfield CA, Lawson MA, Worthley EG. Widespread occurrence of cholinesterase activity in plant leaves. *Physio Plan,* 56, 28-32, (1982).

Moundipa PF, Melanie Flore KG, Bilong Bilong CF, Bruchhaus I. *In vitro* amoebicidal activity of some medicinal plants of the Bamun region (Cameroon). *Africa J Trad Comple Alter Med,* 2(2), 113-121, (2005).

Mukherjee PK, Saha K, Murugesan T, Mandal SC, Pal M, Saha BP. Screening of anti-diarrhoeal profile of some plant extracts of a specific region of West Bengal. *India J Ethnopharmacol,* 60(1), 85-89, (1998).

Nair R, Chanda SV. Antibacterial Activities of Some Medicinal Plants of the Western Region of India. *Turki J Bio,* 31, 231-236, (2007).

Nadkarni KM, Nadkarni AK. Indian Materia Medica. Vol-I, 3rd edition, Popular Prakashan Pvt. Ltd., Mumbai, pp 542, 543, 547, (1992).

Nakarmi M. Medicinal plant used by Lama community of Ichhangu village in Kathmandu, Central Nepal,Central Department of Botany, Tribhuvan University, Nepal, 72, (2001).

Nimenibo-Uadi R. *Ficus exasperata*: effects on diabetes mellitus in an experimental rat model. *Glob J Pur & Appl Sci,* 9(4), 529-532, (2003).

Okoli RI, Aigbe O, Ohaju-Obodo JO, Mensah JK. Medicinal Herbs Used for Managing Some Common Ailments among Esan People of Edo State, Nigeria. *Pak J Nutri,* 6 (5), 490-496, (2007).

Oli BR. Local knowledge on plant utilization among the major ethnic communities in the eastern Churiya Nepal, Central Department of Botany, Tribhuvan University, Kathmandu, Nepal, M.Sc. Thesis, 137, (2001).

Pandey B. Environmental impacts of Kaligandaki A hydroelectric project on vegetation resource in the dam and reservoir area, Central Department of Botany, Tribhuvan University, Kathmandu, Nepal, 85, (2001).

Pant SR, Pant IR. Indigenous knowledge on medicinal plants in Bhagawati village, Darchula, Nepal. *Botani Orient,* 4, 79-83, (2004).

Park EH, Chun MJ. Wound healing activity of Opuntia *Ficus indica. Fitotera,* 72(2), 165-167, (2001).

Pérez C, Domínguez E., Ramiro, J.M., Romero, A., Campillo, J.E., Torres, M.D. A study on the glycaemic balance in streptozotocin-diabetic rats treated with an aqueous extract of *Ficus carica* (fig tree) leaves, *Phytothera Res*, 10(1), 82-83, (1998).

Rai SK, Subedi S, Mishra S. Utilization pattern of medicinal plants in Thumpakhar, Sindhupalchok, Nepal. *Botani Orient*, 4, 75-78, (2004).

Randrianarivelojosia M, Rasidimanana VT, Rabarison H, Cheplogoi PK, Ratsimbason M, Mulholland D, Mauclère A. Plants traditionally prescribed to treat *tazo* (malaria) in the eastern region of Madagascar. *Malari J*, 2, 25, (2003).

Rao BR, Murugesan T, Pal M, Saha BP, Mandal SC. Antitussive potential of methanol extract of stem bark of *Ficus racemosa* Linn. *Phytothera Res*, 17(9), 1117-1118, (2003).

Rao BR, Murugesan T, Sinha S, Saha BP, Pal M, Mandal SC. Glucose lowering efficacy of *Ficus racemosa* bark extract in normal and alloxan diabetic rats. *Phytothera Res*, 16(6), 590-592, (2002).

Rao RB, Anupama K, Swaroop KR, Murugesan, T., Pal, M., Mandal, S.C. Evaluation of anti-pyretic potential of Ficus racemosa bark. *Phytomed*, 9(8), 731-733, (2003).

Recio MC, Giner RM, Mánez S, Rios JL, Marston A, Hostettmann K. Screening of tropical medicinal plants for antiinflammatory activity. *Phytothera Res*, 9(8), 571-574, (1995).

Rijal A. Ethnobotany of Padampur: an analysis of dependency and conflict, Ph.D. Thesis, Agricultural University of Norway, Norway (1994).

Serraclara A, Hawkins F, Perez C, Dominguez E, Campillo JE, Torres MD. Hypoglycemic action of an oral fig-leaf decoction in type-I diabetic patients. *Diabet Res & Clin Prac*, 39(1), 19-22, (1998).

Serrato A, Ibarra-ManriqueZ G, Oyama K. Biogeography and conservation of the genus Ficus (Moraceae). *Mex J Biogeo*, 31, 475-485, (2004).

Sharma S, Chaturvedi M, Edwin E, Shukla S, Sagrawat H. Evaluation of the phytochemicals and antidiabetic activity of *Ficus bengalensis. Inter J Diabet Develop count*, 27(2), 56-59, (2007).

Taira T, Ohdomari A, Nakama N, Shimoji M, Ishihara M. Characterization and antifungal activity of gazyumaru (*Ficus microcarpa*) latex chitinases: both the chitin-binding and the antifungal activities of class I chitinase are reinforced with increasing ionoc strength. *Biosci Biotechnol Biochem*, 69(4), 811-818, (2005).

Vinutha B, Prashanth D, Salma K, Sreeja SL, Pratiti D, Padmaja R, Radhika S, Amit A, Venkateshwarlu, K., Deepak, M. Screening of selected Indian medicinal plants for acetylcholinesterase inhibitory activity. *J Ethnopharmacol*, 109(2), 359-363, (2007).

Vohora SB, Parasar, GC. Phytochemical and pharmacological studies on *Ficus bengalensis*, Linn. (Preliminary report). *Ind J Physio Pharmacol*, 13(3), 143-45, (1969).

Wadood N, Wadood A, Nisar M. Effect of *ficus relegiosa* on blood glucose and total lipid levels of normal and alloxan diabetic rabbits. *J Ayub Med Col Abbott*, 15(4), 40-42, (2003).

Wakeel OK, Aziba1 PI, Ashorobi RB, Umukoro S, Aderibigbe A, Awe EO. Neuropharmacological activities of *Ficus platyphylla* stem bark in mice. *Afric J Biomed Res*, 7, 75-78, (2004).

Wang G, Wang H, Song Y, Jia C, Wang Z, Xu H. Studies on anti-HSV effect of *Ficus carica* leaves. *Zhong Yao Cai*, 27(10), 754-756, (2004).

Watt JM, and Breyer-Brandwijk MG. The medicinal and poisonous plants of Southern Africa. 2nd edn. E. & S Livingstone Ltd, Edinburgh (1962).

Zhang HJ, Tamez PA, Aydogmus Z, Tan GT, Saikawa Y, Hashimoto K, Nakata M, Hung NV, Xuan Le T, Cuong NM, Soejarto DD, Pezzuto JM, Fong HH. Antimalarial agents from plants. III. Trichothecenes from *Ficus fistulosa* and *Rhaphidophora decursiva*. *Plant Med*, 68(12), 1088-1091, (2002).

chapter 19

Ethnomedicines of Kolli Hills at Namakkal District in Tamil Nadu and its Significance in Indian System of Medicines

G. Arunachalam and Subhash C Mandal

INTRODUCTION

The history of Kolli Hills is closely linked with ancient Tamil literature. It is believed that in the Ramayana, these hills are called madhuvanam (forest of honey), the abode of the monkey king Sugreva. In the ancient Tamil epics Silapadikaram and Manimekalai, there is an interesting reference to Kollipavai, the deity in the sacred grove, who is also considered the guardian of the forests here. There are many such legends and interesting myths associated with these hills, which make it all the more interesting and worth visiting. The drive up the 70-hairpin bend ghat road is truly an enjoyable experience. Contrary to ones expectations, the ghat road here is quite wide and well-laid, thanks to the tribal welfare funds allotted by the government.

They constitute about 95% of the total population of these sparsely populated hills. Researchers feel that these were not the people who lived here during King Oris time. The early natives were primarily hunters-gatherers, while the present tribes could have migrated from the plains, bringing farming and agriculture with them. About 4 miles from Solakkadu, an undulating track leads to the Christian settlements at Valavandhinadu established here by Mr.J.W.Brand, a Christian missionary who lived on the hills between 1913 and 1929. His work was carried on by his wife for many more years, in spite of the poor response from the tribals. But these missionaries were solely responsible for spreading literacy in this area, by establishing many elementary schools. A wide variety of medicinal plants and herbs used in Ayurvedic, Siddha and Unani medicine are nurtured, cultivated, gathered and sent from here. Even the most common medicinal plants, acquire a special value when grown here, as the medicinal plants from Kolli Hills are generally considered to be more potent and effective. For example, the Chitharathai (*galanga the lesser*), an effective remedy for cold, grown here is sold at Rs.400 per kg. Athimaduram (*Jamaica liquorice*), Karpooravalli (*Coleus aromaticus*), Thoothuvalai (*Trilobatum*), Tulasi (*Ocimum sanctum*), Kizhanelli (*Phyllanthus amarus*) and a host of other herbs, besides a variety of spices are also cultivated here.

Since ancient times, Kolli Hills has always been famous for its medicinal plants. It is believed that the Sithars (ancient medicine men) lived, researched and meditated here in the caves inside the sacred groves. Many such sacred groves are believed to be found in the forests here (near the Agasagangai falls) even today, and the adventurous go on trekking expeditions, to the caves where the Sithars lived. Stories abound of people chancing upon the stone mortars used by the Sithars to prepare their medicines and concoctions. The moss covering the inner walls of the Sithar caves is believed to have unique healing properties. The sacred groves are guarded by the local temple deities, and the felling of trees is prohibited here. There is also a popular belief among the locals here that a person could lose his mind while entering certain areas of the dense forest where the Sithars lived. No one knows where exactly these areas are, but these pockets, known as Mathikettan Solai are believed to completely wipe out a persons memory, for a period of time. A common explanation to this phenomenon is that it could be due to the effect of the concentration of so many highly potent medicinal plants in one place.

Kolli Hills is thus a naturalists haven-a treasure trove of medicinal plants, and the native home of traditional hill country and people. But like ecosystems elsewhere, these hills too have been invaded by modern farming practices and invasive methods. Tapioca, cassava and hybrid varieties of rice, which were introduced in this region recently, have overtaken the traditional paddy varieties, minor millets, pulses and fruit farms in terms of profitability. The M S Swaminathan Research Foundation has taken efforts to arrest this genetic erosion and rescue the traditional crop varieties. The local practice of burning the land after each yield has proven to be detrimental to the soil. The wiping out of traditional farmlands and orchards, has contributed to the near extinction of the mountain bees that produced the superior quality honey that Kolli Hills was once so famous for.

Ethno medicines

Plants have been used in traditional medicine for several thousand years (Abu-Rabia, 2005). The knowledge of medicinal plants has been accumulated in the course of many centuries based on different medicinal systems such as Ayurveda, Unani and Siddha. In India, it is reported that traditional healers use 2500 plant species and 100 species of plants serve as regular sources of medicine (Pei, 2001). During the last few decades there has been an increasing interest in the study of medicinal plants and their traditional use in different parts of the world (Lev, 2006, Gazzaneo *et al.*, 2005, Al-Qura'n, 2005, Hanazaki, *et al.*, 2000 and Rossato, *et al.*, 1999). Documenting the indigenous knowledge through ethnobotanical studies is important for the conservation and utilization of biological resources. Today according to the World Health Organization (WHO), as many as 80% of the world's people depend on traditional medicine for their primary healthcare needs. There are considerable economic benefits in the development of indigenous medicines and in the use of medicinal plants for the treatment of various diseases (Azaizeh, et al., 2003). Due to less communication means, poverty, ignorance and unavailability of modern health facilities, most people especially rural people are still forced to practice traditional medicines for their common day ailments. Most of these people form the poorest link in the trade of medicinal plants (Khan, 2002). A vast knowledge of how to use the plants against different illnesses may be expected to have accumulated in areas where the use of plants is still of great importance (Diallo, *et al.*, 1999).

In the developed countries, 25 per cent of the medical drugs are based on plants and their derivatives (Principe, 1991). A group of World Health Organization (WHO) experts, who met in Congo Brazzaville in 1976, sought to define traditional African medicine as 'the sum total of practices, measures, ingredients and procedures of all kinds whether material or not, which from time immemorial has enabled the African to guard against diseases, to alleviate his/her suffering and to cure him/herself' (Busia, 2005). Traditional medical knowledge of medicinal plants and their use by indigenous cultures are not only useful for conservation of cultural traditions and biodiversity but also for community healthcare and drug development in the present and future (Pei, 2001).

Ethno botany is not new to India because of its rich ethnic diversity. Jain (Jain, 1991) printed out that there are over 400 different tribal and other ethnic groups in India. The tribals constitute about 7.5 per cent of India's population. During the last few decades there has been an increasing interest in the study of medicinal plants and their traditional use in different parts of India and there are many reports on the use of plants in traditional healing by either tribal people or indigenous communities of India (Saikia, *et al.*,2006, Chhetri, *et al.*, 2005, Harsha, *et al.*, 2002, Natarajan and Paulsen, 2000, Maruthi, *et al.*, 2000, Samvatsar and Diwanji, 2000, Kala, 2005 and Hebbar, *et al.*, 2004). Apart from the tribal groups, many other forest dwellers and rural people also posses' unique knowledge about plants (Jain, 1991).

There has been a resurgence in the consumption and demand for medicinal plants. These plants are finding use as pharmaceuticals, neutraceuticals, cosmetics and food supplements. Even as traditional source of medicines and they continue to play pivotal rule. Modern pharmacopoeia contains at least 25% drugs derived from plants. Many other are synthetic analogues built on prototype compounds isolated from plants. Demand for medicinal plant is increasing in both developing and developed countries due to growing recognition of natural products, being non-toxic, having no side-effects, easily available at affordable prices. Medicinal plant sector has traditionally occupied an important position in the socio cultural, spiritual and medicinal arena of rural and tribal lives of Tamil Nadu. Millions of rural households use medicinal plants in a self-help mode. Over 20,000 practitioners of the Indian System of Medicine in the oral and codified streams use medicinal plants in preventive, promotive and curative applications in Tamil Nadu. There are estimated to be about 1000 manufacturing units in Tamil Nadu. In recent years, the growing demand for herbal product has led to a quantum jump in volume of plant materials traded within and across the countries. An estimate of the EXIM Bank puts the international market of medicinal plants related trade at US$ 60 billion per year growing at the rate of 7% only. Though India has a rich biodiversity, the growing demand is putting a heavy strain on the existing resources. While the demand for medicinal plants is growing, some of them are increasingly being threatened in their natural habitat. For meeting the future needs cultivation of medicinal plant has to be encouraged. According to an all India ethno biological survey carried out by the Ministry of Environment and Forests, Government of India, there are over 8000 species of plants being used by the people of India. Analysis of habits of medicinal plants indicates that they are distributed across various habitats. One third is trees and an equal portion shrub and the remaining one-third herbs, grasses and climbers. A very small proportion of the medicinal plants are lower plants like lichens, ferns algae, etc. Majority of the medicinal plant are higher flowering plants. The State of Tamil Nadu is endowed with a very rich flora. Due to the various physiographic features and physiognomic factors, different types of vegetation exists in the state–1. Coastal vegetation; 2. Island vegetation; 3. Vegetation of hills and mountains comprising of:

1) Dry deciduous forests
2) Moist deciduous forests
3) Semi-evergreen forests
4) Wet evergreen forests
5) Sholas (Southern montane wet temperate forests)

The altitude varies from sea level to 2637 m including the well known mountain ranges—the Nilgiri, the Anamalais and the Cardamom hills which harbours different types of ecological niches, ecosystem and innumerable medicinal plants. A few ethnic tribes like the Irular, Kaanikkara, Karumpar, Palliyan, Paniyar, Sholagar, Thodar and others dwell in these ecosystems and still depend on naturally occurring or cultivated from the state (N.C. Nair & A.N Henry, Flora of Tamil Nadu, India, Analysis–Vol. I, 1983, B.S.I., Coimbatore). Out of this, it is found that 1474 are medicinal plants. A total number are found to be used in Siddha system of medicine which is commonly practiced throughout the state.

Tampcol has two medicinal farms, one in Chennai city at Arumbakkam and at Valavandinadu, Kolli hills, Namakkal district. In Chennai farm six varieties of medicinal plants are cultivated in five acres to meet the fresh herb requirements for the production of herbal hair tonic, other medicated oils and also supplied to pharmacy at Arignar Anna Govt. Hospital for Indian medicine and Homoeopathy, Chennai. Another 150 varieties of medicinal plants are maintained in the parts as reference material. The farm is also visited by the students of all systems of Indian Medicine. Leading practitioners of Indian Medicine also make use of this farm as their reference for medicinal plants. This farm is very popular and has contributed for herbal awareness in Chennai city. The farm participates in the exhibitions conducted by Educational Institutions, Trade fairs and seminars/conferences in the city. The public are also encouraged to buy the medicinal plants at low prices to enhance the importance and awareness of herbal medicines. The Kolli Hills medicinal farm is situated in Valavandinadu at the altitude of 3600 ft. The land is undulating with rocky slopes. Out of 105 acres year-marked, the corporation has developed 55 acres and cultivating a dozen species of medicinal plants on large scale and another 50 varieties which includes trees, climbers and perennials are cultivated on bunds, hedges, fence line etc. as per suitability of the species. Further, the farm has a large nursery in which seedlings/saplings/cuttings/graftings are raised for own cultivation and to supply to the government institutions concerned and also to progressive farmers in the state and out side.

Siddha System of Medicine

The science of medicine is of fundamental importance to man's well being and his survival, and so it must have originated with man and developed as civilization advanced. It is therefore rather pointless to try to determine the exact point of time when any system of medicine was evolved and codified. A system of medicine is not a discovery but a gradual evolution during successive periods of history. It owes its progress to great men, who have not only enriched the science, but also society and civilization as a whole.

There are two ancient systems of medicine in India, the Siddha that flourished in the South and the Ayurveda prevalent in the North. Instead of giving the name of any one individual as the founder of either system, our ancients wisely attributed their origin to the Creator. According to tradition, it was Shiva who unfolded the knowledge of Siddha system of medicine to his consort, Parvati, who handed it down to Nandideva and he, to Siddhars. Therefore it is called 'Saiva Sampradayam' (tradition of Shive), or 'Siddha Sampradayam'. In the case of Ayurveda it was Brahma, the Creator of the Universe, who taught the science to Prajapati, he to Aswini Devatas and they, in their turn, to Atreya etc. So this tradition is called the Brahma or Arsha Sampradaya (the tradition of Rishis). The inference to be drawn from these traditions is that, there is no exact point of time to which the beginning of these systems could be traced. They are eternal, without a beginning or end; they began with man.The Tamils have a distinct civilization, which is not disputed by historians. The recorded history of the Tamils is thousands of years old. Apart from the literature of the first, the middle and the last Sangam periods which bears ample testimony to the extent of Tamil civilization and its eminence, mention is made even in contemporary Sanskrit literature about Cholas,

Pandiyas and Cheras and their kingdoms. A civilized society must naturally have had a system of medicine which catered to the health needs of its people. This was the Siddha system. The term 'Siddhi' means 'achievement' and the Siddhars were men who achieved certain results in medicine, as well as in yoga or tapas. The results in medicine were achieved by the Siddhars through their mental powers, they bequeathed to their 'Chilas' or pupils, who preserved and propagated the science.

Eighteen siddhas seem to have existed. They should have lived at different periods and bequeathed their experiences in medicine and yoga to posterity. The names of these eighteen Siddhas differ from one source to another. It is not necessary to dogmatise which of these enumerations is correct. Some of the Siddhas, for example, Kapila and Kakabujanda have written treatises both in Tamil and in Sanskrit. It is possible that the originals were written in Tamil and that they were translated into Sanskrit later. The following is the list of eighteen Siddhas according to one recension: 1. Nandi 2. Agasthiyar 3. Thirumular 4. Punnakkeesar 5. Pulasthiyar 6. Poonaikannar 7. Idaikadar 8. Bogar 9. Pulikai Isar 10. Karuvurar 11. Konkanavar 12. Kalangi 13. Sattainathar 14. Azhuganni 15. Agappai 16. Pambatti 17. Theraiyar and 18. Kudhambai.

Names like Bogar, Idaikadar and Theraiyar are of recent origin and these Siddhars lived probably in the middle ages. There are also authors of Siddha treatises like Sattaimuni, Yugimuni, Macha Muni, Kakabusundar etc. whose works are available in parts at the present day and are being used.

Siddha System is one of the ancient traditional systems of medicine in India. Siddhars the spiritual scientists of Tamil land are the founding fathers of this scientific system. According to Siddha System the human body is the replica of the universe so are the food and drugs irrespective of their origin. Siddha system believes that all objects in the universe including human body are composed of five basic primordial elements, namely earth, water, fire, air and space. The human body is a conglomeration of three humors and seven physical components. The Food is considered to be basic building material of human body, which gets processed into humors, tissues and wastes. The equilibrium of humors, body tissues and waste products is considered as health and its disturbance or imbalance leads to disease or pathologic state (Kurup, 1983).

This system also deals with the concept of immortality and salvation in this life. The exponents of this system consider that achievement of this state is possible by regulated diet, medicine and processing of mind by yogic or spiritual exercises like meditation and yoga. Siddhars described 96 principles as the constituents of Human Being. They include Physical, Physiological, Mental and Intellectual components of a person. They are nothing but the manifestations of the "Five Basic Elements ".

Disease

Disease is a condition in which there is imbalance in the "Five Elements, which alters the "Three Humours" which is also reflected in the seven physical constituents. The change disturbs the equilibrium and cause disease. The basic concept of Siddha system of medicine is

"Food is Medicine—Medicine is Food"

Saint Thiruvalluvar says

" Miginum Kuraiyinum Noi Seyyum Noolor
Vali Mudhala Enniya Moondru "
"Wind, bile and phlegm three cause disease
so Doctors deem it more or less"

Diagnosis

" Noi Naadi Noi Mudhal Naadi Athu thanikkum
Vaai Naadi Vayppa Seyal."
"Test disease, its causes and cure
and apply remedy that is sure"

—*Thiruvalluvar.*

It is always essential to identify the cause for any disease to be accepted as a "Scientific method" The Diagnostic methodology in Siddha Treatment is unique as it is made purely on the basis of the "Clinical Acumen" of the Physician. He examines the Tongue, complexion, speech, eyes, palpation in a patient and he also examines the urine and stools. The diagnosis is then confirmed by the "Pulse Diagnosis ". The above approach is collectively known as "Eight types of examinations". However, the Siddha Physician now also accepts the modern diagnostic methods for the purpose of diagonosis.

Treatment

The following line of treatment have been in practice in Siddha medicine.

- Using medicines like Choornam, Kudineer, Vadagam etc. made of herbs.
- Surgical methods like incision, excision, heat application, blood letting and leech application etc.
- Physiotherapy—Thokkanam and Varma, the Siddha way of Touch therapy, Medicated Oil application, Fomentation, herbal steam bath etc.
- Using medicines like Parpam, Chenduram, Chuxnam etc. made of minerals especially of metals.

Significance

The Siddha System is capable of treating all types of chronic diseases especially arthritis, skin problems urinary tract disorders, infertility, degenerative disorders like osteo arthritis, senile dementia, disease of the liver, medicinally treatable spinal disorders, general debility, diarrhoea and intractable allergic disorders. Aringnar Anna Govt Hospital of Indian Medicine, Arumbakkam, being the premier institute in Tamil Nadu for Indian Medicine and Homoeopathy treats both outpatient and inpatient.

Ayurveda System of Medicine

Ayurveda is an ancient system of medicine, which originated in northern India antiquity of which dates back to the period of vedas and this is said to be born from Atharva Veda. This knowledge has been gathered due to constant observation of nature for long years by men since the advent of civilization and cannot be attributed to any individual or a group of individuals by any stretch of imagination. Ayurveda is basically based on the predominance of three humours namely Vatha, Pittha and Kapha in the human body. Balanced state of these doshas denotes health and their imbalance produces disease.

Preceptors like Charaka, Susrutha have been benevolent enough to compile these invaluable treasure troves of knowledge to be passed on to posterity. The fact that Ayurveda has stood the test of time bears ample testimony to its efficacy till date. It comprises of eight branches namely.

1. Kaya Chikitsa (General Medicine)
2. Kaumara Bhruthya (Paediatrics)
3. Bhutha Vidhya (Psychiatry)
4. Salakya (ENT and Ophthalmology and dentistry)
5. Shalya (Surgery)
6. Agada Tantra (Toxicology)
7. Rasayana (Rejuvenation Therapy)
8. Vājeekarana (Aphrodisiac therapy)

Pancha karma one of the areas of specialization, which has earned public acclaim in recent times, is also a part of the above branches. It enjoys popularity because of its being hands on therapy and is very relaxing to the fatigued body and tired mind (Kurup, 1983).

Unani system of Medicine

Unani system of Medicine has originated in Greece. It was further enriched and developed by Arabs and Persians. Hippocrates explained that the disease was a normal process and its symptoms were the reaction of the body to the disease. The chief function of the physician was to aid the natural forces of the body. He held that there exists in the body four humours that keep up the balance of it. He also laid emphasis on diet, drugs of plants, animal and mineral origin for curing the disease.

The Unani system of Medicine is based on the Humoural theory. Humoural pathology which presupposes the presence of four humours namely - Blood (Dam), Phlegm (Balgham), Yellow bile (Safra) and Black bile (Sauda) in the body. The temperament of persons is expressed accordingly by the words Sanguine, Phlegmatic, Choleric and Melancholic according to the preponderance of them in the body. Everybody has got unique humoural constitution which represents the healthy state of humoural balance of the body. The Unani medicine plays a vital role when the individual experiences the humoural imbalance. The correct diet and digestion can bring back the humoural balance. Its main emphasis is on diagnosis of a disease through Nabz (Pulse), Baul (Urine), Baraz (stool) etc. It has laid down six essential prerequisites for the prevention of disease. They are known as 'Asbab-e-sitte Zarooriya' viz. air, drinks and foods; bodily movement and repose; psychic movement and repose; sleep and wakefulness; excretion and retention (Said, 1983).

The modes of treatment are as follows:

(i) Ilaj bid-Tadbeer (Regimental therapy)

(ii) Ilaj bid Ghiza (Dieto Therapy)

(iii) Ilaj bid Dawa (Pharmaco Therapy)

(iv) Jarahat (Surgery)

The regimental therapy includes venesection, cupping, sweating, diuresis, bath (Hammam), massage, cauterization, purging, vomiting, exercise and leeching etc. Dieto therapy aims at treating certain ailments by administration of specific diets, whereas pharmaco therapy deals with use of naturally occuring drugs, mostly herbals though drugs of animals and mineral origin are also used.

Diagnosis and Treatment

The unani system of diagnosis of diseases and treatment restoring health revolves round the concept of temperament or 'Mizaj'. The humours also have specific temperament. Changes in temperament are related to changes in the balance of humours. Any change in temperament brings about a change in the health of the individual. Thus imbalance of the harmony of humours and temperament along with failure of one or more parts of the body to eliminate pathogentic waste causes disease.The Government recognized the merit of Unani system and attempts were made to develop it as a viable system of medicine for National Health care. The Unani drugs are cost effective, safe and widely accepted by the people of India. Therefore, the Tamil Nadu Government have established a Unani Medical College and Unani dispensaries.

Homoeopathy System of Medicine

Homoeopathy is a system of treatment of the diseased by drugs usually prescribed in minute doses that in a healthy person would produce symptoms like those of disease. The Homoeopathy way of healing was devised by the Great German physician Dr.Christian Frederick Samuel Hahnemann in the late eighteenth century. He came across an old idea of the efficacy of 'Cinchona bark' in treating intermittent fever due to its toxic effect on the stomach and conducted experiments upon himself in order to get the truth. He deduced from the experiment that Cinchona was used as a remedy for intermittent fever and it could produce symptoms similar to those of intermittent fever in healthy people, if taken for a specific period of time. The law of 'Similia Similibus Curentur' or 'let likes be treated by the likes' thus forms the basis of treatment under the Homoeopathic method of drug therapy employed to cure the natural sufferings of person by the administration of drugs which have been experimentally proved to possess the power of producing similar artificial sufferings or symptoms of diseases in healthy human being (Vithoulkas, 1983).

In Homoeopathy, the main emphasis is on the remedial agents in illness and in health. It is a low cost system using only the non-toxic drugs. It has established a reputation for successful treatment of acute and chronic illness and in certain disease for which there is no or less treatment in other systems. Dr.Samuel Hanemann, who was the founder of this system, enunciated the basic concepts and its principles in "Organon the Art of Healing" in the year 1810. Due to various reasons like cost-effectiveness and non-toxic nature of its drugs, no side effects of easy in take. Homoeopathy is getting a very high recognition and acceptance from the people. Having its origin in the moden scientific age, it has the benefit of basing its theory and concept on demonstrable scientific principles and procedures.

It is based on the following cardinal principles

1. The law of Similars
2. The law of Single Remedy
3. The law of Minimum Dose
4. Doctrine of Drug proving
5. Doctrine of dynamisation
6. Doctrine of vital force
7. Doctrine of Chronic disease

Among this, the most fundamental is the 'law of Similars'. This law states that the symptoms experienced by the sick person are reactions of the body which it mobilizes in order to counteract a morbid influence, be it a specific stress such as bacteria or viruses, or a non-specific stress such as climatic changes, environmental pollution, mental and emotional disturbances etc. Among the seven, first three are having more therapeutic importance and value.

Health and Disease

This system assumes that any disease symptoms, syndrome is the reaction of the defence mechanism of human body against the disease-causing agent. The symptoms are the means through which the body tries to regain its lost balance. According to it, the symptoms syndrome in a disease is not the disease per se but the reaction of the defense mechanism mobilized by the body in order to counteract a morbific influence existing in the body and causing the loss of balance of the healthy body. Thus the disequilibrium in the normal functioning of the organs of body implies sickness.

Diagnosis and Treatment

In Homoeopathy patients are diagnosed (their individual symptoms) but not their disease. As there is specific medicine for specific disease, unless the diseases are diagnosed, they cannot be treated, in other systems of medicine, where as in Homoeopathy, medicine are proved in healthy individuals are their symptoms are recorded. In order to treat the diseased individual their symptoms are to be matched with the patients' symptoms. Therefore, importance is given to the symptomatology than the diagnosis. By treating in this way, the natural defence mechanism (Immunity) of the individual is strengthened and recurrence of the disease is curtailed.

In deciding the treatment, the Homoeopathic practitioner follows the well-known principles of 'Similia Similibus Curentur'. In simple terms it means let the similar substance which can produce specific symptoms in a healthy individual cure those similar symptoms in a sick individual, although the symptoms have arisen from another cause i.e. Bacteria, Virus etc., The cure is based on the assumption that the patient is extremely sensitive to that particular remedy and only to that remedy which can produce his/her symptomatology. Homoeopathy has a definite and effective treatment for some disease such as Diabetes, Arthritis, Bronchial Asthma, Epilepsy, Skin Eruption, Allergic conditions and Mental or Emotional disorders. Even, some surgical disease gets cured in Homoeopathy with out undergoing surgery. Thus the sick person after taking treatment not only gets cured of his disease, but simultaneously regains a perfect state of health.

Naturopathy & Yoga System of Medicine

Naturopathy is not just a system of medicine but a way of life. It is often referred as drugless therapy. It is based mainly on the ancient practice of the application of the simple laws of nature. There are two schools of thought regarding the approach of Naturopathy. One group believes in the ancient Indian methods. The advocacy of Naturopathy pay particular attention to eating and living habits, adoption of purificatory measures, use of hydrotherapy, cold packs, mud packs, massage and a variety of measure based on their innovative talent.

A carefully supervised total fast or partial fast is advocated to clear the system of toxic accumulation. Water or dilute fruit juices are permitted. The Naturopathy has to keep a strict supervision lest the patient may develop physical and emotional untoward effects. The system believes that, if the way of life is properly organised, one can get the bounties of energy, health and happiness from the benevolent nature. What one has to do for prevention of disease, promotion of health and to get therapeutic advantages is to adopt natural means to living. Naturopathy is based on various treatments like magneto therapy, massage therapy, physiotherapy, phychotherapy, reflexology, chromotherapy, accupuncture, accupressure, yoga therapy and diet therapy (Sachidananda, 1978 and Bloomfield, 1983).

REFERENCES

Abu-Rabia A: Urinary diseases and ethnobotany among pastoral nomads in the Middle East. J. Ethnobio and Ethnomed. 1:4, (2005).

Al-Qura'n S: Ethnobotanical survey of folk toxic plants in southern part of Jordan. Toxicon. 46:119-126, (2005).

Azaizeh H, Fulder S, Khalil K, Said O: Ethnomedicinal knowledge of local Arab practitioners in the Middle East Region. Fitoterapia. 74:98-108, (2003).

Bloomfield RJ. Traditional Medicine and Health Care Coverage. World Health Organization Geneva. 116-122, (1983).

Busia K: Medical provision in Africa – Past and present. Phytother Res. 19:919-923, (2005).

Chhetri DR, Parajuli P, Subba GC: Antidiabetic plants used by Sikkim and Darjeeling Himalayan tribes, India. J Ethnopharmacol. 99:199-202(2005).

Diallo D, Hveem B, Mahmoud MA, Berge G, Paulsen BS, Maiga A: An ethnobotanical survey of herbal drugs of Gourma district, Mali. Pharma Bio. 37:80-91(1999).

Gazzaneo LR, Paiva de Lucena RF, Paulino de Albuquerque U: Knowledge and use of medicinal plants by local specialists in a region of Atlantic Forest in the state of Pernambuco (Northeastern

Brazil). J Ethnobio and Ethnomed. 1:9, (2005).

Hanazaki N, Tamashiro JY, Leitao-Filho H, Gegossi A: Diversity of plant uses in two Caicaras communities from the Atlantic forest coast, Brazil. Biodiv and Conser. 9:597-615, (2000).

Harsha VH, Hebbar SS, Hegde GR, Shripathi V: Ethnomedical knowledge of plants used by Kunabi Tribe of Karnataka in India. Fitoterapia, 73:281-287, (2002).

Hebbar SS, Harsha VH, Shripathi V, Hegde GR: Ethnomedicine of Dharwad district in Karnataka, India–plants used in oral health care. J Ethnopharmacol. 94:261-266, (2004).

Jain SK: Dictionary of Indian Folk Medicine and Ethnobotany. (1991). Deep publications, Paschim Vihar, New Delhi.

Kala CP: Ethnomedicinal botany of the Apatani in the Eastern Himalayan region of India. J Ethnobio and Ethnomed. 1:11, (2005).

Khan AU: History of decline and present status of natural tropical thorn forest in Punjab. Pak Biologi Conser. 63:210-250, (2002).

Kurup PNV. Traditional Medicine and Health Care Coverage. World Health Organization Geneva. 50-58, (1983).

Lev E: Ethno-diversity within current ethno-pharmacology as part of Israeli traditional medicine – A review. J Ethnobio and Ethnomed. 2:4, (2006).

Maruthi KR, Krishna V, Manjunatha BK, Nagaraja VP: Traditional medicinal plants of Davanagere district, Karnataka with reference to cure skin diseases. Environ and Eco. 18:441-446, (2000).

Natarajan B, Paulsen BS: An ethnopharmacological study from Thane district, Maharashtra, India: Traditional knowledge compared with modern biological science. Pharma Bio. 38:139-151, (2000).

Pei S J: Ethnobotanical approaches of traditional medicine studies: Some experiences from Asia. Pharma Bio. 39:74-79, (2001).

Principe P: Monetising the pharmacological benefits of plants. (1991). US Environmental protection Agency, Washington, D.C.

Rossato SC, Leitao-Filho H, Gegossi A: Ethnobotany of Caicaras of the Atlantic forest coast (Brazil). Eco bot. 53:387-395, (1999).

Sachidananda S. Integra Yoga: the yoga sutras of Patanjali. Pomfret, CT, USA, Integral Yoga Publicatios, (1978).

Said SM. Traditional Medicine and Health Care Coverage. World Health Organization Geneva. 61-67, (1983).

Saikia AP, Ryakala VK, Sharma P, Goswami P, Bora U: Ethnobotany of medicinal plants used by Assamese people for various skin ailments and cosmetics. J Ethnopharmacol. (2006).

Samvatsar S, Diwanji VB: Plant sources for the treatment of jaundice in the tribals of Western Madhya Pradesh of India. J Ethnopharmacol. 73:313-316, (2000).

Vithoulkas G. Traditional Medicine and Health Care Coverage. World Health Organization Geneva. 110-114, (1983).

chapter 20

Plant Metabolomics

S. Mohana Lakshmi, Ashok Kumar C.K. and Subhash C Mandal

INTRODUCTION

Metabolomics aims to quantify and identify all metabolites in a given biological context an aim that admittedly is as challenging as full-scale proteomics. It is thus a manifestation of the endpoint of metabolic and physiological processes. Taken individually, measurements of the metabolome in different physiological conditions are likely to be more indicative for the purposes of systems biology studies than transcriptome profilings (Fiehn, 2001; Sumner, 2003).

The metabolome is a complete set of metabolites in a cell or tissue (Fiehn, 2001; Goodacre et al., 2004) consists of low-molecular weight chemical intermediates (Oliver et al., 1998) which are the end products of gene expression. For fundamental reasons based on metabolic control analysis http://dbk.ch.umist.ac.uk/ mca_home.htm (reviews: (Kell and Westerhoff, 1986; Fell, 1996; Heinrich and Schuster, 1996). It is understood that any change in gene (protein) expression levels will have only small effects on metabolic fluxes, they must have large effects on metabolite concentrations.

Metabolomic approaches seek to profile metabolites in a nontargeted way, i.e. to effectively separate and detect as many metabolites as possible in a single analysis. Eventually, the information on transcript and protein abundance was combined and this would ideally lead to a nearly complete molecular picture of the state of a particular biological system at a given time. Plant metabolomics is essentially a comprehensive, high-throughput analyses of complex metabolite mixtures typical of plant extracts.

To achieve the overview of metabolic composition it is essential to establish a multifaceted, fully integrated strategy for optimal sample extraction, metabolite separation, detection, identification, automated data gathering systems, handling and analysis system and finally quantification. Both analytical and computational developments are essential to achieve this aspect. And moreover these data also require proper storage in suitably configured databases.

It is very apparent that large quantities of metabolomic or metabolic profiling data if generated will help to open up many previously inaccessible areas of plant drug research. The objective of metabolomics targets at assessing metabolic changes in a comprehensive and global manner in order to check the biological functions or provide detailed biochemical responses of cellular systems.

The Metabolomics Society (2005) is to promote the international growth and development of the field of metabolomics, to provide the opportunity for collaboration among researchers in metabolomics, including connections between academia, government and industry, regulators and vendors in the field of metabolomics, and to provide opportunities for dissemination of research achievements in workshops, conferences, and journal publications.

The First International Congress on Plant Metabolomics was held in Wageningen, The Netherlands, in April 2002, with the primary goal of bringing together those scientists who are actively involved in this field and those who soon plan to be in future. In such instances, opportunities are created for collaboration and joint strategies can be determined to meet the metabolomics challenge. Selected abstracts from the oral and poster presentations at the meeting are now accessible at www. metabolomics.nl and this site will continue to be used as an aid for information exchange and collaboration.

Although microbes prove to be the richest overall source of metabolites, plants are the source of the most complex individual mixtures. Mariet van der Werf (TNOFood, Zeist, The Netherlands) reported that it has been predicted that bacterial genomes, which were already been sequenced can support the biosynthesis of just a few hundred metabolites (e.g. 580 for *Bacillus subtilis* and 800 for *Escherichia coli*), but for individual plants, this value is likely to be in the tens of thousands.

Approximately 50,000 different phytoconstituents have been elucidated in plants and it is predicted that the final figure for the plant kingdom will approach or even exceed 200,000 (Fiehn, 2001) Thus, metabolomics exerts a considerable challenge for plant scientists.

Metabolomics information not only will assist in the deeper insights in understanding of the complex interactive nature of plant metabolic networks and their responses to environmental and genetic change but also will provide information regarding the fundamental nature of plant phenotypes in relation to development, physiology, tissue identity, resistance, biodiversity, etc.

The instrumental tools in use for metabolomics studies are element analysis via ICP-AES, ion analysis via HPLC or CE, specific HPLC (for amino acids and thiols) and highly random, high throughput approaches mainly based on mass spectrometry combined with various initial separation tools such as GC-MS, GC-TOF, LC-MS (Fiehn, 2003; Wagner, 2003) or others as NMR techniques Harris, (2003; Ott et al., 2003; Defernez, and Colquhoun, 2003; Davis et al., 2003). Furthermore, the coupling of electrospray ionization (ESI) MS with CE (Soga, et al., 2002) and hydrophilic interaction chromatography (Tolstikov and Fiehn, 2002) has been successfully used to analyse metabolomics problems. Metabolome (Goodacre et al., 2004; Harrigan and Goodacre, 2003) is a complex mixture of chemical compounds with broadly differing chemical and physical properties which presents limitations to all analytical technologies. Instrumentation utilized in measurement of the metabolome includes mass spectrometry (Roessner, 2000; Soga T, et al., 2003; Wilson et al., 2003), Fourier transform infra red spectroscopy (Johnson et al., 2003; Kaderbhai et al., 2003) nuclear magnetic resonance spectroscopy (NMR) (Lindon et al., 2000; Solanky et al., 2003), A number of analytical strategies are employed (Harrigan and Goodacre, 2003; Goodacre et al., 2004) ranging from the study of a few metabolites common to a specific metabolic pathway or chemical class such as amino acids to the comprehensive analysis of hundreds of chemically diverse metabolites (metabolite profiling, metabolic finger printing, metabolomics, metabonomics). Currently no single technique can provide non-biased detection of all compounds present in a metabolome and in future applications it is expected that a number of different technologies will be employed to fulfil this objective. Metabolite profiling involves separation of metabolites, using gas chromatography, liquid chromatography (Plumb et al., 2003) or capillary electrophoresis (Soga et al., 2003), prior to detection of individual compounds and with metabolite identification by comparison to already available mass spectral/retention index libraries (Wagner et al., 2003). However, for large studies sample preparation and analysis are both time consuming and laborious. Typical runtimes of 10-20 min gives detection of more than 900 metabolite peaks (Hagan, 2005; Plumb et al., 2004; Soga et al., 2003). To overcome problems of long runtimes when analysing large sample sets metabolic fingerprinting can be employed. This involves analysis at the expense of lower sensitivity and a reduced ability to identify metabolites. The objective is to provide high-throughput (1–3 min analysis time) analyses with the objective of screening samples to enable discrimination between samples of differing biological origin or status.

Plant metabolomics aims at providing comprehensive information that could help to optimise metabolic engineering strategies by providing more information about biosynthetic pathways and the interactions between them (Hall et al., 2002; Fernie, 2003). Metabolomics is the study of all the metabolites of a given biological sample but since no single technique provides such comprehensive detection, numerous analytical tools such as gas chromatography (GC), liquid chromatography (LC), mass spectrometry (MS) and nuclear magnetic resonance (NMR) have been used to investigate the metabolome. Notable advances have been made with single techniques such as GC/MS (Fiehn et al., 2000; Roessner et al., 2000) and LC/MS (Tolstikov et al., 2003). Studies that involve multiple techniques such as NMR, LC/UV and LC/MS have also appeared (Le Gall et al., 2003a, 2003b).

Estimating and monitoring the metabolome are perhaps two of the most important analytical challenges of the twentyfirst century. While methodologies for genomic and proteomic analyses have stabilized into several well-characterized approaches, analytical methods for metabolomic analysis remain in a considerable flux. The problem rests with the entire diversity of the metabolome. Estimates for the number of metabolites in the human and plant metabolomes range from 2,766 to about 200,000 (Duarte et al. 2007; Fiehn 2002). The polarity of these metabolites varies from nonpolar lipids to extremely polar inorganic ions. Functional groups occurs in metabolites include alcohols, amines, organic acids, aromatic alcohols, esters, aldehydes, ethers, phosphates and many others. Some metabolic sub-groups are so large they have their own classification such as the lipidome and the glycome. Also, because the metabolome encompasses a relatively narrow band of molecular weights numerous isomers exist. Compound chirality is also a concern and a challenge to analysis. In addition to the chemical complexity of the metabolome, physiological concentrations of metabolites in the plant tissues range between millimolar to picomolar levels.

Metabolomics technologies and applications

The development of atomic theory at the beginning of the twentieth century served as a platform for the early forms of spectrometry. The construction of the first mass spectrometer by J.J. Thomson in 1912 was soon followed by a series of technological approaches, leading to the first application of ICR-MS by 1949 and the first spectrometers coupled with gas chromatographs was performed in the late 1950s (De Hoffmann and Stroobant, 2002). Although the phenomenon of NMR was not described until the mid-1940s, it was not long before this property was being used for the structural elucidation and determination of molecules. The application of these analytical methods to metabolomics is more recent, and has been accompanied by rapid and extensive improvements in data-processing technologies.

Mass spectrometry in Metabolomics study

Instrumental methods in different fields (especially plants and microbes versus animals) varies, largely for historical reasons, but there is increasing convergence to use as many as possible for all samples due to their complementarity. As well as increasingly refined gas chromatography-mass spectrometry (GC-MS) methods, especially those using gas chromatography time-of-flight mass spectrometry (GCTOF) instruments that allow much better deconvolution than by most GC-MS instruments because they can record spectra, and thus sample, very quickly. Fourier transform ion cyclotron resonance (FT-ICR) mass spectrometry [Marshall AG, Hendrickson CL, 2002; Aharoni A, et al, 2002) is a very high-resolution mass spectral method (10^5–10^6), with mass accuracy better than 1 ppm), which allows separation and empirical formula measurement of potentially thousands of metabolites.

The potentially holistic approach to metabolome analysis is done primarily by recent advances in mass spectrometry (MS) technology and by the efforts of functional genomics research. Most technology for metabolomics is based on MS. Gas chromatography– MS (GC-MS) and HPLC–photodiode array–MS remain the methods of choice for quantitative and qualitative metabolite profiling. The ultimate goal of metabolomics— the ability to efficiently detect and quantify every metabolite in a plant extract—is difficult to be attained by any single analytical method available at present. Some metabolite selection occurs in all methodologies, from initial different solvent extraction process through chromatography to MS ionization.

Oliver Fiehn (Max Planck Institute for Molecular Plant Physiology, Potsdam, Germany) reported (The First International Congress on Plant Metabolomics was held in Wageningen, The Netherlands, in April 2002) the use of rapid scanning time-of-flight (TOF) MS coupled with GC separation and also integrated with peak deconvolution software. This technique increased the number of metabolites detectable by GC-MS in crude plant extracts to 500 to 1000.

Direct infusion of extracts into MS instruments using "soft" electrospray or atmospheric pressure chemical ionization sources is an attractive way to obtain "fingerprints" of the molecular ions of the metabolites present in plant extracts. Such use of FT-MS was demonstrated in presentations by Asaph Aharoni and Dayan Goodenowe (Phenomenome Discoveries, Saskatoon, Canada) in the same conference. This powerful, and relatively expensive, mass analyzer has the ability to generate mass data of sufficient accuracy for the determination definitive empirical formula. Several hundred ions were observed in this for each ionization method in both positive and negative modes.

Metabolomic analysis is supposed to avoid bias against certain compound classes and to allow for the analysis of every metabolite individually. Although this aim has not been reached but clear progress in this direction was reported. For example, a combination of different metabolite-profiling tools was used by Ric de Vos (Plant Research International, Wageningen, The Netherlands, 2002) for the analysis of metabolic effects in high-flavonoid genetically modified tomatoes. Using LC/photodiode array detection as well as LC-QTOF-MS and direct infusion– QTOF-MS, it was found that flavonoid contents were up to 70-fold more when compared with those of common cultivars, and glycosidic structures were presented for all aglycone intermediates that accumulated.

These analyses were performed in tandem with GC-MS profiling of volatile compounds using headspace solid-phase microextraction. In this, in addition to an increase in flavonoids, the methylsalicylate a volatile compound was found to be increased in transgenic plants over expressing the Lc/C1 transcription factor. Sumner, in the same conference provided specific examples, including LCUV- MS of flavonoids and saponins, GCMS of polar and lipophilic extracts, and capillary electrophoresis-MS of anions and amino acids.

Nuclear magnetic spectrophotometry in metabolomic probing

In addition to MS, NMR also plays an important role in recording the metabolic profiling datas. For the more concentrated metabolites, nuclear magnetic resonance (NMR) has provided both qualitative and quantitative information however; NMR is not sufficiently sensitive for use with metabolites at low concentrations (Dunn et al. 2005; Dunn and Ellis 2005).

Marianne Defernez (Institute of Food Research, Norwich; Mike Beale, Institute of Arable Crops Research-Long Ashton; Nigel Bailey, Imperial College, London) and Adrian Charlton (Central Science Laboratory, York) presented the use of proton NMR of crude plant extracts, followed by multivariate analysis, to cluster data sets to highlight differences. This method of analysis gives a comprehensive summation fingerprint of all (hydrogen-containing) metabolites extracted and can give direct structural information regarding individual metabolites in the mixture, particularly when two-dimensional techniques are used. Therefore, it is suitable for high-throughput, rapid, first pass screening. Subtraction of these data sets generates virtual NMR spectra and hence important structural data on compound(s) contributing to differences between samples.

Fourier transform-infrared spectroscopy (FT-IR) in metabolomic study

Fourier transform-infrared spectroscopy (FT-IR) has also been used to spectroscopically analyse the metabolome (Harrigan et al., 2004; Johnson et al., 2004). This method detects even small phenotypic differences, which cannot be measured by other methods. Because FT-IR is chemically non-selective, it is very much suited for the rapid fingerprinting of a metabolome rather than the identification of specific metabolites (Aharoni et al., 2002; Brown Stephen et al., 2005).

Gas chromatography in metabolomic study

At lower concentrations in metabolomic study, sequential approaches of concentration, separation, and detection methods are commonly employed. Those metabolites which have vapor pressures or can be converted into volatile products can be separated by gas chromatography (GC). The major disadvantage of GC for metabolic profiling is that non-volatile compounds cannot be probed unless time-consuming sample derivatization is employed (Fiehn et al., 2000; Koek et al., 2006).

HPLC in metabolomic study

Separation of non-volatile metabolites, which make up most of the metabolome concentration, can be achieved by liquid chromatographic techniques. Reverse phase high performance liquid chromatography (HPLC) has been used for the separation of non-volatile metabolites at low concentrations and varying polarities (Buchholz et al., 2002; Kell 2004; Wilson et al., 2005). HPLC, however, is not ideal for a rapid screening process because of its low resolution and slow analysis time as compared to gas phase separations (Asbury and Hill, 2000a). Recently ultra performance liquid chromatography (UPLC) has been introduced for metabolic probing (Nordstrom et al., 2006). Due to the small diameter (2 μm) of the packing material in UPLC and the novel silicoethyl boded phase, linear mobile phase velocities of up to 10 mm/s can be achieved without much change in resolution.

Capillary electrophoresis (CE) in metabolomic profiling

Capillary electrophoresis (CE) can also be used in metabolomic profiling especially to separate cations and anions in the metabolome but is slow, in some cases requiring up to 16 h for a complete analysis (Soga et al., 2003). After chromatographic or electrophoresis separation, identification of metabolites is normally achieved by mass spectrometry. Time-of-flight, quadrupole, and ion trap mass spectrometers have also been used after chromatographic separation to identify metabolites (Hollywood et al., 2006).

Electrospray Ionisation Time-of-Flight Mass Spectrometry (ESI-TOF-MS) in metabolomic studies

Electrospray Ionisation Time-of-Flight Mass Spectrometry (ESI-TOF-MS) can be employed in metabolomic studies and is generally referred to as Direct Injection (or infusion) Mass Spectrometry (DIMS). Electrospray ionisation is applied to metabolites containing polar moieties in their molecular structure. Ionisation provides minimal fragmentation of molecular ion and a less complex mass spectrum when compared to the mass spectra of electron impact ionisation of multi-component samples. Although the techniques of mass spectra are still complex the presence of molecular ions enhances the ability to identify metabolites. Therefore chromatographic separation of complex samples is not required (Schroder, 1996). Commercially available Time-of-Flight (TOF) instruments can provide a greatly improved mass resolution (FWHM = 5000+ at mass 500 Da) compared to aditional quadrupole instruments.

Plant metabolomics studies have also been useful for the characterization of olive oils and of vegetable oils used in its adulteration (Goodacre et al., 2002). Also separation and characterization of medicinal plant extracts (Mauri and Pietta, 2000) by detection of a wide range of secondary metabolites have been reported, with subsequent metabolite identification by tandem mass spectrometry. It is now known that Fourier Transform Ion Cyclotron Resonance Mass Spectrometry (FT-ICR-MS) provides many advantages over other mass spectrometers in terms of sensitivity, resolving power and metabolite identification (Brown, 2005). A metabolome analysis of strawberry fruits and tobacco flowers has been conducted and showed its potential by identification of metabolites differing between developmental stages of strawberry fruit (Aharoni, 2002).

Experimental and instrumental parameters highly influence the mass spectra of biological samples. Reliable metabolic fingerprints therefore require reliable standardisation and verification. Thus high standards now employed for analysis of microarray experiments (Minimum Information about a Microarray Experiment – MIAME) required for publication in peer-reviewed journals (Brazma et al., 2001) should be established for metabolomics (Bino et al., 2004; Jenkins et al., 2004).

Hyphenation techniques of chromatography and spectroscopy in metabolite profiling

Through the years many analytical methods have been developed that are not restricted to the selective analysis of one or a few compounds. With the improved performance of chromatography methods in the late 1960s and early 1970s (improvements in reliability, selectivity and resolution), peak identification and detection in complex matrices were made possible based purely on retention times. These separation techniques were then coupled to highly sensitive detectors that also had high effective ranges of quantification, such as flame ionization coupled to gas chromatography (GC/FID) or fluorescence and UV detectors to liquid chromatography (LC). These analytical methods were soon applied to plant tissues to profile important compound classes such as amino acids (Adams, 1974). Also in the late 1960s, mass spectrometry (MS) was improved to make it as universal as flame ionization, in addition of offering a completely independent method for compound identification and classification when coupled to gas chromatography (de Jongh et al., 1969). Halket et al. (1999) utilized mass spectral deconvolution software to increase reliability of metabolite detections. For the first time, peak identification of 68 pre-selected target compounds was based on both purified mass spectra and retention time indices in an automated and robust way.

In the plant field, less effort has been put into profiling compound classes. Sauter et al. (1991) chose peaks that apparently detect major compounds in GC/MS chromatograms in order to get an overview of major steps in metabolism before and after pesticide spraying. Derivatization conditions for metabolité profiling were optimized by selecting 12 compounds representing plant primary metabolism (Adams *et al.*, 1999), and were applied to profile polar organics (sugars, polyols, acids and amino acids) in apricots (Katona et al., 1999). Another step in elucidating metabolism was conducted by Christensen and Nielsen (2000), who used GC/MS to profile the fractional enrichment of 13C-labelled substrates in order to study biochemical pathways for production of secondary metabolites. Metabolite profiling was extended to cellular by combining GC/MS, HPLC analysis of nucleotides, enzyme assays and pyrophosphate target analysis solvents fractionation (Farré et al., 2001). Such compartmental analysis is clearly needed for understanding plant metabolism. Using LC/MS it was possible to detect and identify more secondary metabolites from plants than by NMR. These were semi-quantified by LC/MS for sample to sample variation.

GC-MS/ LC-MS

In general GC-MS is effective for the profiling of relatively low molecular weight, hydrophobic compounds such as essential oils, hydrocarbons, esters and metabolite derivatives with less polarity. LC-MS equipped with atmospheric pressure chemical ionization (APCI) is useful for the profiling of polar and low to moderate molecular weight (i.e. MW \2000) metabolites, those of sterols, fatty, organic and amino acids, metal ions, and alkaloids. Polar molecules within a molecular weight range (i.e. from 10 to 300,000), including proteins and DNA, can be probed by electrospray ionization (ESI)-LC-MS. An alternative ionization method for the analysis of high molecular weight molecules and other compounds like carotenoid is matrix-assisted laser desorption/ionization (MALDI) coupled with time-off light (TOF) MS (Fraser et al. 2007). GC-MS, which has been enumerated as the 'gold standard' of metabolomics (Harrigan and Goodacre 2003), involves the separation of volatile, thermally stable compounds by GC and subsequent detection by electron ionization (EI) MS. An attractive feature of GC-MS is the direct measurement of volatile compounds. The situation for LC-MS is more complex since the presence of acidic groups or electronegative atoms, such oxygen and nitrogen, can facilitate the formation of negative ions. However, many compounds in plant extracts will not fully ionize, if at all, under the conditions used for a single analysis. For this reason, LC-MS is better suited to the targeted profiling of specific types of compounds that shows similar ionizing behavior (e.g. alkaloids) and is generally not useful for broad-scope metabolomics studies. However, the combination of LC-MS and GC-MS data certainly provides a more complete picture of a plant metabolome.

Metabolomic sample preparation

When attempting for simultaneous detection of all metabolites in plant tissues, the applied methods cannot be restricted to the technical question which type of data acquisition might be most suitable but also must seriously consider adequate methods for sample preparation. As an initial step for such methods, plant physiologists were long been aware of the importance of readily stopping the inherent enzymatic activity of biological samples. This has been achieved by freeze clamping, immediate freezing in liquid nitrogen, or by acidic treatments using perchloric or nitric acid (ap Rees and Hill, 1994). Although advantageous for extraction of amines (Bouchereau et al., 2000) acidic treatments renders severe problems for many analytical methods that follow, and harvesting and keeping plant tissues into tubes for liquid nitrogen freezing may take up to 15 s. Compared to freeze clamping techniques, freezing samples in liquid nitrogen is a slower process that could potentially produce artefacts caused by pathological wound responses, rapid activation of touch-inducible genes, etc. This might occur in case if samples are weighed before freezing, and if no attention is paid to this special problem. Since freeze clamping is not easily applicable in cases were lots of samples have to be harvested, freezing in liquid nitrogen remains a reasonable way to stop enzymatic activity.

Certainly, great care must be also taken to avoid incomplete thawing tissues before extracting metabolites. One way to do this is to freeze-dry biological samples resulting in completely dried samples. In the absence of water in the samples, enzymes or transporters are inactive. If stored before sample extraction, samples have to be maintained in dry environments like evacuated desiccators, since tissues are highly hygroscopic. Alternatively, frozen tissues can be directly extracted by adding organic solvents and applying heat, thereby also inhibiting the enzymatic activity. Extracting frozen tissues that still contain the original amount of water in them might be advantageous for metabolomic studies when compared to extracting freeeze-dried samples, since freeze-drying may cause irreversible adsorption of metabolites on cell walls and membranes. If metabolomic analysis sets out to distinguish between metabolite levels in different compartments, samples need to be freeze-dried prior to non-aqueous fractionation methods (Gerhardt and Heldt, 1984; Farré et al., 2001). An alternative method to non-aqueous fractionation is the use of nuclear magnetic resonance analysis (NMR) to distinguish steady-state concentrations of metabolites in different compartments *in vivo* (Roberts, 2000). Such approaches will become increasingly important as it is recognized that gene function cannot be assigned without understanding the essential role of biochemical pathway and without the help of thc plant physiology.

Prior to sample extraction, different types of sample homogenization is done, depending on the number of samples to be treated, and on the type of tissue. Leaf tissues may be ground under liquid nitrogen using mortar and pestle, or using a ball mill with pre-chilled holders (Fiehn et al., 2000a), or together with the extraction solvent by ultraturrax devices (Orth et al., 1999). Other plant organs such as roots, sometimes to be too hard to use ball mills, whereas potato tubers are too soft for homogenization (Roessner *et al.*, 2000). After homogenization, different methods of metabolite extraction can be used but, again, no systematic study is available that directly compares the results of these techniques. Most frequently, polar organic solvents like ethanol, methanol, methanol-water mixtures are directly added to freshly frozen tissues (Johansen *et al.*, 1996; Streeter and Strimbu, 1998), with an additional step of using non-polar solvents such as chloroform to exhaustively extract lipophilic components. In order to increase the extraction efficiency, additional energy is put into the system either directly by heat (e.g. 70°C), or by other techniques such as pressurized liquid extraction (Benthin et al., 1999), supercritical fluid extraction (Castioni et al., 1995; Jarvis and Morgan, 1997; Blanch *et al.*, 1999), sonication (Sargenti and Vichnewski, 2000), subcritical water extraction (Gámiz-Gracia and de Castro, 2000), microwave techniques (Namiesnik and Gorecki, 2000), or pervaporation (Starmans and Nijhuis, 1996). Rarely data are available that compare these techniques and few systematic studies have been carried out on the occurrence of possible metabolite breakdown reactions caused by oxidation (Peng and Jayallemand, 1991). It is similar for sample storage, although it is generally assumed that alterations of metabolite content can be excluded during storage at –80°C.

Tentative metabolite probe

In order to provide preliminary identification for metabolites, a list of over 700 metabolites with their metabolic pathways are known to be present in plant and microbial metabolomes, was compiled which were available from several databases including the KEGG database (http://www.genome.ad.jp/kegg/kegg2.html). The monoisotopic masses of molecular ions are present in plant extracts as [M+H]+, [(M)H], [M+NH4]+, [M+Na]+ or [M+K]+ ions and were calculated and tabulated by metabolite name vs. monoisotopic mass for each molecular ion; for example lactic acid, [M+H]+, 91.0395. The metabolite identification table is available on request from various sources. Metabolites were identified by searching, the "lookup" function in Microsoft Excel, of determined accurate masses against monoisotopic masses of known metabolites. W.B. Dunn et al./ conducted and recorded Automated electrospray-TOF mass spectrometry for metabolic fingerprinting of the plant metabolome.

Data processing

Metabolite target analysis is a combination of techniques to prepare and analyse samples for one or a small number of compounds from a complex mixture. Often, the sample preparation techniques aim at preconcentration and purification of the metabolite under study, before analysing it with a hyphenation of chromatography and a selective detector (such as liquid chromatography coupled to fluorescence detection, or gas chromatography coupled to sulfur chemiluminescence detector). Metabolite target analysis is clearly the most widely used technique, and it is applied in all areas of plant research such as phytohormone analysis.

Data analysis

Irrespective of the analytical technique used, the analysis of the data is usually performed in three stages. Firstly the raw data need to be preprocessed to convert them to a suitable form. Secondly these modified data's may be subjected to data reduction so that only the most relevant input variables are used in the subsequent data analysis (Seasholtz and Kowalski, 1993). Thus normalizing to a constant total signal introduces dependencies between the variables that would not exist without this step. Similarly the missing variables can have significant effects on the position of individual samples in clustering diagrams. Missing values may arise because they are below the limit of detection or because they were not collected. Deconvolution and further processing of hyphenated data to establish the contribution of each eluting component is a very difficult, active and vital area, which needs to begin by "registering" (Woodward et al., 2004) or aligning datasets (Duran et al., 2003). Automating this step reliably is a high priority for metabolomics. The objective of the third stage of the data analysis is to record patterns within the data which give useful biological information that may be useful to generate hypotheses that can be further tested and refined. The methods available for metabolome analysis can be placed in four main (partly overlapping) categories – univariate and multivariate statistical, unsupervised learning (which looks at the overall pattern or structure of the data), supervised learning (which uses known information to help to study the classification of the data (Duda et al., 2001; Hastie et al., 2001), and system-based analyses which use theories such as MCA (Fell, 1996) to help interpret the data in terms of the biological networks (Kell, 2004). Many unsupervised learning methods are equivalent to clumping methods and are often statistically based, while supervised methods are from many varieties (Weiss and Kulikowski 1991; Michie et al., 1994; Mitchell, 1997), including statistical, neural, rule-based, evolutionary and so on.

CONCLUSION

The combination of analytical results from all levels of gene products (transcriptome, proteome, and metabolome) remains more vision than reality. Metabolomics is a rapidly developing area in plant biology and has become an integral part of many functional genomics programs. Metabolomic profiling of plant is helpful not only in identification and quantification of the various metabolites present in the plant tissues but also helps in understanding the biosynthetic pathways in the production of these metabolites and also their response to genetic and environmental change. The plant metabolome is large and diverse, and although the technologies reviewed here are sufficient to generate extensive datasets, the ability to identify individual metabolites remains a general limitation. Even though metabolomic analysis is comparably fast and cheap, reliable and precise, the unambiguous and simultaneous identification of all metabolites in a biological system is a challenge. Finally, if metabolomic profiling is to be used to its fullest, it is imperative that publicly available metabolomic databases be created. Metabolomic data are rich in information, and there is considerable interest in re-assessing previously acquired data under different perspectives. Through this progress, the responses of plants to genetic manipulations and environmental perturbations will become increasingly predictable. This will make systems biology attractive as a tool for the creation of hypotheses.

BIBLIOGRAPHY

Adams MA, Chen ZL, Landman P. and Colmer D. Simultaneous determination by capillary gas chromatography of organic acids, sugars, and sugar alcohols in plant tissue extracts as their trimethylsilyl derivatives. Anal. Biochem. 266, 77-84, (1999).

Adams RF. Determination of amino acid profiles in biological samples by gas chromatography. J. Chromatogr, 95, 189-212, (1974).

Aharoni A, Ric de Vos CH, Verhoeven HA, Maliepaard CA, Kruppa G, Bino R, Goodenowe DB: Nontargeted metabolome analysis by use of Fourier Transform Ion Cyclotron Mass Spectrometry. OMICS, 6, 217-234, (2002).

Aharoni A, Ric de Vos CH, Verhoeven Harrie A, Maliepaard Chris A, Kruppa G, Bino R, & Goodenowe Dayan B. Nontargeted metabolome analysis by use of Fourier Transform Ion Cyclotron Mass Spectrometry. Omics : A Journal of Integrative Biology, 6, 217-234, (2002).

Aharoni A, RicDe Vos CH, Verhoeven HA, Maliepaard CA, Kruppa G, Bino R. and Goodenowe DB (2002). Nontargeted metabolome Analysis by Use of Fourier Transform Ion Cyclotron Mass Spectrometry. OMICS, 6, 217-234, (2005).

Asbury GR & Hill HH. Evaluation of ultrahigh resolution ion mobility spectrometry as an analytical separation device in chromatographic terms. Journal of Microcolumn Separations, 12, 172-178, (2000a).

Benthin B, Danz H. and Hamburger M. Pressurized liquid extraction of medicinal plants. J. Chromatogr. A 837, 211-219, (1999).

Bino RJ, Hall RD, Fiehn O, Kopka J, Saito K, Draper J, Nikolau BJ, Mendes P, Roessner-Tunali U, Beale MH, Trethewey RN, Lange BM, Wurtele ES. and Sumner LW. Potential of metabolomics as a functional genomics tool. Trends Plant Sci. 9, 418-425, (2004).

Blanch GP, Caja MM, Castillo MLR, Santa-Mariá G, Herraiz M. Fractionation of plant extracts by supercritical fluid extraction and direct introduction in capillary gas chromatography using a programmable temperature vaporizer. J. Chromatogr. Sci. 37, 407-410, (1999).

Bouchereau A, Guénot P. Larher F. Analysis of amines in plant materials. J. Chromatogr. B, 747, 49-67, (2000).

Brazma A, Hingamp P, Quackenbush J, Sherlock G, Spellman P, Stoeckert C, Aach J, Ansorge W, Ball CA, Causton HC, Gaasterland T, Glenisson P, Holstege FCP, Kim IF, Markowitz V, Matese JC, Parkinson H, Robinson A, Sarkans U, Schulze-Kremer S, Stewart J, Taylor R, Vilo J. and Vingron, M. Minimum information about a microarray experiment (MIAME) - toward standards for microarray data. Nat. Genet. 29, 365-371, (2001).

Brown Stephen C, Kruppa G, & Dasseux J-L. Metabolomics applications of FT-ICR mass spectrometry. Mass Spectrometry Reviews, 24, 223-231, (2005).

Brown SC, Kruppa G. and Dasseux J-L. Metabolomics applications of FT-ICR mass spectrometry. Mass Spectrom. Rev. 24, 223-231, (2005).

Buchholz A, Hurlebaus J, Wandrey C, & Takors R. Metabolomics: Quantification of intracellular metabolite dynamics. Biomolecular Engineering, 19, 5-15, (2002).

Castioni P, Christen P. and Veuthey JL. Supercritical fluid extraction of compounds from plant origin. Analusis 23, 95-106, (1995).

Christensen B, Nielsen J. Metabolic network analysis of Penicillium chysogenum using 13C-labelled glucose. Biotechnol. Bioeng. 68: 652-659, (2000).

De Hoffmann E, Stroobant V. Mass spectrometry. Principles and Applications, 2nd ed. Wiley, (2002).

De Jongh DC, Radford T, Hribar JD, Hanessian S, Bieber M, Dawson G. and Sweeley CC. Analysis of trimethylsilyl derivatives of carbohydrates by gas chromatography and mass spectrometry. J. Am. Chem. Soc, 91, 1728-1740, (1969).

Defernez M. and Colquhoun IJ. Factors affecting the robustness of metabolite fingerprinting using 1H-NMR spectra. Phytochemistry; 62, 1009-1017, (2003).

Duarte NC, Becker SA, Jamshidi N, Thiele I, Mo M. L, Vo TD, Śrivas R, & Palsson BO. Global reconstruction of the human metabolic network based on genomic and bibliomic data. Proceedings of the National Academy of Sciences of the United States of America, 104, 1777-1782, (2007).

Duda RO, Hart PE, Stork DE. Pattern Classification, 2nd ed. John Wiley, London, (2001).

Dunn WB, & Ellis DI. Metabolomics: Current analytical platforms and methodologies. Trac-Trends in Analytical Chemistry, 24, 285–294, (2005)

Dunn WB, Bailey NJC & Johnson HE. Measuring the metabolome: Current analytical technologies. Analyst, 130, 606-625, (2005).

Duran AL, Yang J, Wang L, Sumner LW. Metabolomics spectral formatting, alignment and conversion tools (MSFACTs). Bioinformatics 19, 2283-2293, (2003).

Farré EM, Tiessen A, Roessner U, Geigenberger P, Trethewey RN. and Willmitzer L. Analysis of the compartmentation of glycolytic intermediates, nucleotides, sugars, organic acids, amino acids and sugar alcohols in potato tubers using a non-aqueous fractionation method. Plant Physiol., (2001) in press.

Farré EM, Tiessen A, Roessner U, Geigenberger P, Trethewey RN. and Willmitzer L. Analysis of the compartmentation of glycolytic intermediates, nucleotides, sugars, organic acids, amino acids and sugar alcohols in potato tubers using a non-aqueous fractionation method. Plant Physiol., (2001) in press.

Fell DA. Understanding the Control of Metabolism. Portland Press, London, (1996).

Fell DA. Understanding the Control of Metabolism. Portland Press, London. (1996).

Fernie AR. Metabolome characterisation in plant system analysis. Funct. Plant Biol. 30, 111-120, (2003).

Fiehn O. and Weckwerth, W. Deciphering metabolic networks. Eur. J. Biochem, 270 579-588, (2003).

Fiehn O. Combining genomics, metabolome analysis, and biochemical modelling to understand metabolic networks. Comp. Func. Genomics, 2, 155-168, (2001).

Fichn O. Mctabolomics–the link between genotypes and phenotypes. Plant Mol. Biol 48, 155-171, (2002).

Fiehn O. Metabolomics–the link between genotypes and phenotypes. Plant Molecular Biology, 48, 155-171, (2002).

Fiehn O. Metabolomics–the link between genotypes and phenotypes. Plant Molecular Biology, 48, 155-171, (2002).

Fiehn O, Kopka J, Dörmann P, Altmann T, Trethewey RN and Willmitzer L. Metabolite profiling for plant functional genomics. Nat. Biotechnol, 18, 1157-1161, (2000).

Fiehn O, Kopka J, Dormann P, Altmann T, Trethewey RN, & Willmitzer L. Metabolite profiling for plant functional genomics. Nature Biotechnology, 18, 1157-1161, (2000).

Fiehn O, Kopka J, Dormann P, Altmann T, Trethewey R N, & Willmitzer L. Metabolite profiling for plant functional genomics. Nature Biotechnology, 18, 1157-1161, (2000).

Fiehn O, Kopka J, Trethewey RN. and Willmitzer L. Identification of uncommon plant metabolites based on calculation of elemental compositions using gas chromatography and quadrupole mass spectrometry. Anal. Chem. 72, 3573-3580, (2000a).

Fraser PD, Enfissi EMA, Goodfellow M. Metabolite profiling of plant carotenoids using the matrix-assisted laser desorption ionization time-of-flight mass spectrometry. Plant J, 49, 552-564, (2007).

Gámiz-Gracia L, Castro MDL. Continuous subcritical water extraction of medicinal plant essential oil: comparison with conventional techniques. Talanta, 51, 1179-1185, (2000).

Gerhardt R, Heldt HW. Measurement of subcellular metabolite levels in leaves by fractionation of freeze-stopped material in nonaqueous media. Plant Physiol, 75, 542-547, (1984).

Goodacre R. and Kell DB. Evolutionary computation for the interpretation of metabolome data in Harrigan GG. and Goodacre R. (Eds), Metabolic profiling: its role in biomarker discovery and gene function analysis. (2003).

Goodacre R, Vaidyanathan S, Bianchi G. and Kell DB. Metabolic profiling using direct infusion electrospray ionization mass spectrometry for the characterisation of olive oils. Analyst 127, 1457-1462, (2002).

Goodacre R, Vaidyanathan S, Dunn WB, Harrigan GG. and Kell DB. Metabolomics by numbers: acquiring and understanding global metabolite data. Trends Biotechnol, 22, 245-252, (2004).

Goodacre R, Vaidyanathan S, Dunn WB, Harrigan GG. and Kell DB. Metabolomics by numbers: acquiring and understanding global metabolite data. Trends Biotechnol, 22, 245-252, (2004).

Goodacre R, Vaidyanathan S, Dunn WB, Harrigan GG. and Kell DB. Metabolomics by numbers: acquiring and understanding global metabolite data. Trends Biotechnol, 22, 245-252, (2004).

Halket JM, Przyborowska A, Stein SE, Mallard WG, Down S. and Chalmers RA. Deconvolution gas chromatography mass spectrometry of urinary organic acids. Potential for pattern recognition and automated identification of metabolic disorders. Rapid Commun. Mass Spectrom. 13, 279-284, (1999).

Hall R, Beale M, Fiehn O, Hardy N, Sumner L. and Bino R. Plant metabolomics: the missing link in functional genomics strategies. Plant Cell, 14, 1437–1440, (2002).

Harrigan GG, Goodacre R. Metabolic profiling: its role in biomarker discovery and gene function analysis. Kluwer Academic Publishers, (2003).

Harrigan GG, LaPlante RH, Cosma GN, Cockerell G, Goodacre R, Maddox JF, Luyendyk JP, Ganey PE, & Roth RA. Application of high-throughput Fouriertransform infrared spectroscopy in toxicology studies: Contribution to a study on the development of an animal model for idiosyncratic toxicity. Toxicology Letters, 146, 197–205, (2004).

Harrigan GG. and Goodacre R. Metabolic Profiling: Its Role in Biomarker Discovery and Gene Function Analysis. Kluwer Academic Publishers, Boston. (2003).

Hastie T, Tibshirani R, Friedman J. The Elements of Statistical Learning: Data Mining, Inference and Prediction. Springer-Verlag, Berlin, (2001).

Heinrich R, Schuster S. The Regulation of Cellular Systems. The Plant Cell, 14, 1437, (2002).

Hollywood K, Brison DR, & Goodacre R. Metabolomics: Current technologies and future trends. Proteomics, 6, 4716–4723, (2006).

Jarvis AP, Morgan ED. Isolation of plant products by supercritical fluid extraction. Phytochem. Anal. 8, 217–222, (1997).

Jenkins H, Hardy N, Beckmann M, Draper J, Smith AR, Taylor J, Fiehn O, Goodacre R, Bino RJ, Hall R, Kopka J, Lane GA, Lange BM, Liu JR, Mendes P, Nikolau BJ, Oliver SG, Paton NW, Rhee S, Roessner-Tunali U, Saito K, Smedsgaard J, Sumner LW, Wang T, Walsh S, Wurtele ES. and Kell DB. A proposed framework for the description of plant metabolomics experiments and their results. Nat. Biotechnol, 22, 1601–1606, (2004).

Johansen HN, Glitso V, Knudsen KEB. Influence of extraction solvent and temperature on the quantitative determination of oligosaccharides from plant materials by high performance liquid chromatography. J. Agric. Food Chem, 44, 1470–1474, (1996).

Johnson HE, Broadhurst D, Kell DB, Theodorou MK, Merry RJ, & Griffith GW. High-throughput metabolic fingerprinting of legume silage fermentations via Fourier transform infrared spectroscopy and chemometrics. Applied and Environmental Microbiology, 70, 1583–1592, (2004).

Johnson HE, Broadhurst D, Goodacre R. and Smith, A.R. Metabolic fingerprinting of salt-stressed tomatoes. Phytochemistry, 62, 919–928, (2003).

Kaderbhai NN, Broadhurst DI, Ellis DI, Goodacre R. and Kell DB. Functional genomics via metabolic footprinting: monitoring metabolite secretion by Escherichia coli tryptophan metabolism mutants using FT-IR and direct injection electrospray mass spectrometry. Comp. Funct. Genom, 4, 376–391, (2003).

Katona ZF, Sass P. and Mɑlnár-Perl I. Simultaneous determination of sugars, sugar alcohols, acids and amino acids in apricots by gas chromatography-mass spectrometry. J. Chromatogr. A, 847, 91–102, (1999).

Kell DB, Oliver SG. Here is the evidence, now what is the hypothesis? The complementary roles of inductive and hypothesis-driven science in the post-genomic era. Bioessays, 26, 99–105, (2004).

Kell DB. and Westerhoff HV. Metabolic control theory–its role in microbiology and biotechnology. FEMS Microbiol Rev, 39, 305–320, (1986).

Kell DB. Metabolomics and systems biology: Making sense of the soup. Current Opinion in Microbiology, 7, 296-307, (2004).

Koek MM, Muilwijk B, van der Werf MJ, & Hankemeier, T. Microbial metabolomics with gas chromatography/mass spectrometry. Analytical Chemistry, 78, 1272-1281, (2006).

Le Gall G, Colquhoun IJ, Davis AL, Collins GJ. and Verhoeyen, M.E. Metabolite profiling of tomato (Lycopersicon esculentum) using 1H-NMR spectroscopy as a tool to detect potential unintended effects following a genetic modification. J. Agric. Food Chem, 51, 2447-2456, (2003).

Le Gall G, Colquhoun IJ, Davis AL, Collins GJ. and Verhoeyen, M.E. Metabolite profiling of tomato using 1H NMR spectroscopy as a tool to detect potential unintended effects following a genetic modification. J. Agric. Food Chem, 51, 2447-2456, (2003b).

Le Gall G, DuPont MS, Mellon FA. Characterization and content of flavonoid glycosides in genetically modified tomato (Lycopersicon esculentum) fruits. J. Agric. Food Chem, 51, 2438-2446, (2003a).

Lindon JC, Nicholson JK, Holmes E. and Everett JR. Metabonomics: metabolic processes studied by NMR spectroscopy of biofluids. Concepts Magn. Reson. 12, 289-320, (2000).

Marshall AG, Hendrickson CL: Fourier transform ion cyclotron resonance detection: principles and experimental configurations Int J Mass Spectrom, 215, 59-75, (2002).

Mauri P. and Pietta P. Electrospray characterization of selected medicinal plant extracts. J. Pharmaceut. Biomed. Anal, 23, 61-68, (2000).

Michie D, Spiegelhalter DJ, Taylor CC. Machine Learning: Neural and Statistical Classification. Ellis Horwood, Chichester, (1994).

Mitchell TM. Machine Learning. McGraw Hill, New York, (1997).

Namiesnik J, Gorecki T. Sample preparation for chromatographic analysis of plant material. J. Plan. Chromatogr, 13, 404-413, (2000).

Nordstrom A, O'Maille G, Qin C, & Siuzdak G. Nonlinear data alignment for UPLC-MS and HPLC-MS based metabolomics: Quantitative analysis of endogenous and exogenous metabolites in human serum. Analytical Chemistry, 78, 3289-3295, (2006).

Oliver SG, Winson MK, Kell DB. Baganz F. Systematic functional analysis of the yeast genome. Trends Biotechnol, 16, 373-378, (1998).

Orth HCJ, Rentel C. and Schmidt PC. Isolation, purity analysis and stability of hyperforin as a standard material from Hypericum perforatum L. J. Pharm. Pharmcol. 51: 193-200, (1999).

Ott K-H, Aranibar N, Singh B, Stockton G. Metabolomics classifies pathways affected by bioactive compounds. Artificial neural network classification of NMR spectra of plant extracts. Phytochemistry 62, 971-985, (2003).

Peng S, Jayallemand C. Use of antioxidants in extraction of tannins from walnut plants. J. Chem. Ecol. 17: 887-895, (1991).

Rees T, Hill SA. Metabolic control analysis of plant metabolism. Plant Cell Envir, 17, 587-599, (1994).

Roberts JKM. NMR adventures in the metabolic labyrinth within plants. Trends Plant Sci. 5: 30-34, (2000).

Roessner U, Wagner C, Kopka J, Trethewey RN. and Willmitzer L. Simultaneous analysis of metabolites in potato tuber by gas chromatography–mass spectrometry. Plant J, 23, 131-142, (2000).

Roessner U, Wagner C, Kopka J, Trethewey RN. and Willmitzer L. Simultaneous analysis of metabolites in potato tuber by gas chromatography-mass spectrometry. Plant J, 23, 131-142, (2000).

Roessner U, Wagner C, Kopka J, Trethewey RN. and Willmitzer L. Simultaneous analysis of metabolites in potato tuber by gas chromatography-mass spectrometry. Plant J, 23, 131-142, (2000).

Sargenti SR. Vichnewski W. Sonication and liquid chromatography as a rapid technique for extraction and fractionation of plant material. Phytochem. Anal, 11, 69-73, (2000).

Sauter H, Lauer M. and Fritsch H. Metabolic profiling of plants: a new diagnostic technique. ACS Symp. Ser, 443, 288-299, (1991).

Schroder HF. Polar organic pollutants from textile industries in the wastewater treatment process - Biochemical and physicochemical elimination and degradation monitoring by LC-MS, FIA-MS and MS- MS. Trac-Trends Anal. Chem, 15, 349-362, (1996).

Seasholtz MB, Kowalski B. The parsimony principle applied to multivariate calibration. Anal. Chim. Acta 277, 165-177, (1993).

Soga T, Ohashi Y, Ueno Y, Naraoka H, Tomita M, & Nishioka T. Quantitative metabolome analysis using capillary electrophoresis mass spectrometry. Journal of Proteome Research, 2, 488-494, (2003).

Soga T, Ueno Y, Naraoka H, Ohashi Y, Tomita M. and Nishioka T. Simultaneous determination of anionic intermediates for Bacillus subtilis metabolic pathways by capillary electrophoresis electrospray ionization mass spectrometry. Anal. Chem, 74, 2233-2239, (2002).

Solanky KS, Bailey NJC, Beckwith-Hall BM. Application of biofluid 1H nuclear magnetic resonance-based metabonomic techniques for the analysis of the biochemical effects of dietary isflavones on human plasma profile. Anal. Biochem, 323, 197-204, (2003).

Starmans DAJ, Nijhuis HH. Extraction of secondary metabolites from plant material: a review. Trends Food Sci. Technol, 7, 191-197, (1996).

Streeter JG, Strimbu CE. Simultaneous extraction and derivatization of carbohydrates from green plant tissues for analysis by gas-liquid chromatography. Anal. Biochem, 259, 253-257, (1998).

Sumner LW, Mendes P, Dixon RA. Plant metabolomics: large-scale phytochemistry in the functional genomics era. Phytochemistry, 62, 817-836, (2003).

Tolstikov VV. and Fiehn O. Analysis of highly polar compounds of plant origin: combination of hydrophilic interaction chromatography and electrospray ion trap mass spectrometry. Anal. Biochem, 301, 298-307, (2002).

Tolstikov VV, Lommen A, Nakanishi N, Tanaka N. and Fiehn O. Monolithic silica-based capillary reversed-phase liquid chromatography/electrospray mass spectrometry for plant metabolomics. Anal. Chem. 75, 6737-6740, (2003).

Wagner C, Sefkow M, Kopka J. Construction and application of a mass spectral and retention time index database generated from plant GC/EITOF-MS metabolite profiles. Phytochemistry, 62, 887-900, (2003).

Ward JL, Harris C, Lewis J. and Beale MH. Assessment of 1H-NMR spectroscopy and multivariate analysis as a technique for metabolite fingerprinting of Arabidopsis thaliana. Phytochemistry, 62, 949-957, (2003).

Weiss SH, Kulikowski CA. Computer Systems that Learn: Classification and Prediction Methods from Statistics, Neural networks, Machine Learning, and Expert Systems. Morgan Kaufmann Publishers, San Mateo, CA, (1991).

Wilson ID, Plumb R, Granger J, Major H, Williams R, & Lenz EA. HPLC-MS-based methods for the study of metabonomics. Journal of Chromatography B-Analytical Technologies in the Biomedical and Life Sciences, 817, 67-76, (2005).

Wilson ID. and Brinkman UA. Hyphenation and hypernation the practice and prospects of multiple hyphenation. J. Chromatogr. A, 1000, 325-356, (2003).

Woodward AM, Rowland JJ, Kell DB. Fast automatic registration of images using the phase of a complex wavelet transform: application to proteome gels. Analyst 129, 542-552, (2004).

Woodward AM, Rowland JJ, Kell DB. Fast automatic registration of images using the phase of a complex wavelet transform: application to proteome gels. Analyst 129, 542-552, (2004).

www.plantcell.org©2002 American Society of Plant Biologists MEETING REPORT Plant Metabolomics: The Missing Link in Functional Genomics Strategies.

chapter 21

Chemistry and Biological Significance of Xanthones

Deepak P. Belsare, Dinesh D. Rishipathak, S.C. Pal and Subhash C. Mandal

INTRODUCTION

During last few decades there has been a tremendous growth in the study of various aspects of naturally occurring and synthetic xanthones. This development in the field of chemistry and biology of xanthones was possible due to increase in number of naturally occurring xanthones, successful synthesis involving newer methods, availability of physical and spectral data, and an extensive research work on their biological and biochemical aspects.

Xanthones are widely distributed as polyoxygenated, prenylated, methylated, furano, and chloro substituted derivatives in nature. The number of families of higher plants notably, Guttiferae, Gentinaceae, Polygalaceae, Moraceae and Leguminosae has been reported to produce xanthones as secondary metabolites. Furano and chloro substituted xanthones have been found only in lower organisms, such as moulds and fungi as metabolites.

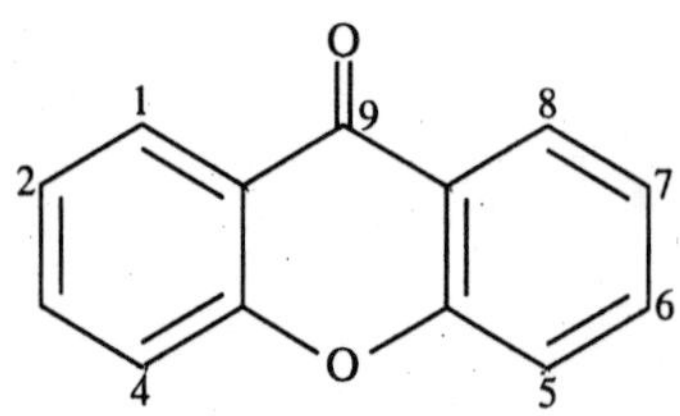

General structure of xanthone

Although xanthone structure contains only four different locations for substituents, which are duplicated symmetrically. This unique backbone along with type and position of the attached chemical groups define specific xanthones. The oxygenation pattern of xanthones is important chemotaxonomically. There is a correlation between the type and position of substituents in xanthone nucleus, plant family and species. The two families *Gentianaceae* and *Guttiferae* are the important sources of substituted xanthones. Number of xanthone compounds has been identified in species of *Gentianaceae*. Canscora, Gentiana, Polygala, Swertia, Halenia, Hopcea, Enieostemna and Frasera are some important xanthone yielding genera.

Biosynthesis of Xanthones

Xanthones are biosynthesized in higher plants by a mixed shikimate-acetate pathways. Studies indicated that m-hydroxy benzoic acid acts as an important precursor of xanthone biosynthesis, indicating that a C_6-C_1 unit and three acetate unit forms the intermediate benzophenone. This intermediate is further hydroxylated enzymatically to form 2, 3, 4, 6-tetrahydroxy benzophenone which acts as a main intermediate in xanthone biosynthesis (Attkinnson et al., 1968; Berrhues, 1996).

Tracer studies (Lewis, 1963; Attkinnson et al., 1969) have suggested the fact that the benzophenone intermediates react intramoleculary (oxidative coupling) to form xanthones. The enzyme catalyzing this reaction is xanthone synthase (Barillas, 1997). The c-glycosides are limited as compared to O-glycosides. There is a biogenetic relationship between flavonoid and xanthones. Mangiferin is derived from a p-coumarate and two acetate units (Bennett et al., 1989).

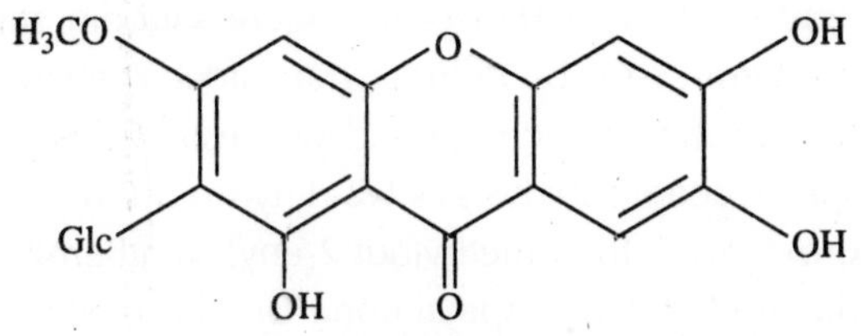

Mangiferin

Isolation of xanthone derivatives

Bioactivity-guided fractionation of a dichloromethane-soluble extract of *Garcinia mangostana* fruits has led to the isolation and identification of five compounds, including two xanthones, 1,2-dihydro-1, 8,10-trihydroxy-2-(2-hydroxypropan-2-yl)-9-(3-methylbut-2-enyl)furo[3,2-a]xanthen-11-one and 6-deoxy-7-demethylmangostanin, along with three known compounds, 1,3,7-trihydroxy-2,8-di-(3-methylbut-2-enyl)xanthone , mangostanin , and alpha-mangostin. (Chin et al. 2008) Bioactivity guided fractionation of *polygala alpestris* L. (Rchb) extracts lead to the identification of two new xanthones, 1,3,7- trihydroxy 2,7- dimethoxy xanthones and 2,3-methylenedioxy-4,7-dihydroxyxanthones. In addition five known compounds 3,4-dimethoxy- 1,7-dihydroxyxanthone, 1,3-dihydroxy-7-methoxyxanthone, 1,7-dihydroxy-2,3-dimethoxyxanthone, 3-,6-*O*- disinapoyl sucrose, 3-5-dimethoxybiphenyl-4-ol were isolated (Dall'Acquaa et al., 2004).

Kielcorin and the Cadensins *A* and *B*, isolated respectively from *Kielmeyera coriacea* and *Caraipa densiflora* (Guttiferae), were shown to be xanthonolignoids. Three xanthones, polyanxanthone A, B and C have been isolated from the methanol extract of the wood trunk of *Garcinia polyantha*, along with five known xanthones 1,3,5-trihydroxyxanthone;1,5-dihydroxyxanthone;1,3,6,7-tetrahydroxyxanthone;1,6-dihydroxy-5-dethoxyxanthoneand1,3,5,6-tetrahydroxyxanthone (Oliv et al., 2008).

A new xanthone 1, 4, 8-trihydroxyxanthone (1,4,8-trihydroxy-9*H*-xanthen-9-one) was isolated from the roots of *Vismia latifolia* (Guttiferae). Four other known xanthones were isolated: 1, 5-dihydroxy-8-methoxyxanthone, 1,7-dihydroxyxanthone, 1,6-dihydroxy-7-methoxyxanthone and 1,3,5,6-tetrahydroxyxanthone. The structures were established by UV, IR, MS, 1D and 2D NMR spectroscopic techniques. A marine fungal isolate, identified as *Wardomyces anomalus*, on cultivation found to produce two new xanthone derivatives 2,3,6,8-tetrahydroxy-1-methylxanthone and 2,3,4,6,8-pentahydroxy-1-methylxanthone in addition to the known xanthone derivative 3,6,8-trihydroxy-1-methylxanthone (Abdel-Lateff et al., 2000).

Biological activities of xanthones

Many naturally occurring xanthones, their xanthone-O-glucosides, xanthone-C-glucosides and synthetic polyoxygenated xanthones have been found to possess a number of significant biological activities. Many plants of medicinal importance have shown the presence of xanthonic constituents to which their therapeutic properties may be attributed. The plants containing xanthones are used mainly as laxative, as diuretic, for liver troubles, in mental disorders- insanity, epilepsy, and nervous debility and also in tuberculosis.

Antimalarial activity

The antimalarial activity of 22 xanthones against chloroquine resistant strains of *Plasmodium falci-*

parum was evaluated. Natural caloxanthone-C, Demethylcalabaxanthone, Calothwaitesixanthone, Calozeyloxanthone, dombakinaxanthone, macluraxanthone, and 6-deoxy-gamma-mangostin were isolated from *Calophyllum caledonicum*. The relationship between antimalarial activity and molecular structure of xanthones has also been explored. The most potent xanthones, and (IC_{50} = c.a. 1.0 mg/mL) are 1,3,7 trioxygenated and prenylated on the 2 and 8 positions. (Hay et al, 2004) Five xanthones from the bark of *Garcinia cowa*, namely 7-O-methylgarcinone E, cowanin, cowanol, cowaxanthone, and beta-mangostin, were found to possess *in vitro* antimalarial activity against *Plasmodium falciparum* with IC_{50} values ranging from 1.50 to 3.00 μg/ml. (Likhitwitayawuid et al., 1998; Shen et al., 2006).

A series of 3, 6-bis-ω-diethylaminoalkoxyxanthones with side chains ranging from 2 to 8 carbon atoms were prepared and evaluated. Measurement of heme affinity for each of the derivatives revealed a strong correlation (R^2 = 0.97) between affinity and antimalarial potency. The two most active compounds in the series contained 5- and 6-carbon side chains and exhibited low nanomolar 50% inhibitory concentration (IC_{50}) values against strains of chloroquine-susceptible and multidrug-resistant *Plasmodium falciparum in vitro*. Both of these xanthones exhibit stronger heme affinity (8.26 x 10^5 and 9.02 x 10^5 M^{-1}, respectively) than either chloroquine or quinine under similar conditions and appear to complex heme in a unique manner. (Kelly et al., 2002) Xanthones with a hydroxyl group in the peri-position exhibited decreased antimalarial activity, possibly due to intramolecular hydrogen bonding with the carbonyl and consequent reduced affinity for heme. Paired hydroxyls attached to the lower half of the xanthone greatly enhanced drug potency. (Ignatushchenko et al., 2002). The synthesis and antimalarial properties of twelve new chlorinated 9H-xanthones, carrying a [2-(diethylamino) ethyl] amino group in position 1 are reported. All compounds were found to be active towards the chloroquine-susceptible and chloroquine-resistant strains 3D7 and Dd2, of *Plasmodium falciparum*. (Portela et al., 2007).

The phytochemical study of the methanol extract of the stem bark of *Allanblackia monticola* STANER L.C. resulted in the isolation of a new prenylated xanthenedione, designated as allanxanthone C, together with the five known xanthones, garciniafuran, tovophyllin A, rubraxanthone, norcowanin and mangostin and one saponin, stigmasterol- 3-*O*- b-D-glucopyranoside. The structure of the new compound was established by spectroscopic analysis as 1,2-dihydro-3,6,8-trihydroxy-1,1,7-tri (3-methylbut-2-enyl) xanthen-2,9-dione (3- hydroxyapetalinone C). The methanol extract and pure compounds were tested on two strains of *Plasmodium falciparum*, F32 (chloroquine sensitive) and FcM29 (chloroquine resistant). The IC_{50} values obtained ranged from 0.6 to 8.9 mg/ml (Blaise et al., 2006).

Antitumor activity

The effects of six xanthones from the pericarps of mangosteen, *Garcinia mangostana*, on the cell growth inhibition of human leukemia cell line HL60 were examined. All xanthones displayed growth inhibitory effects. Among them, alpha-mangostin showed complete inhibition at 10 microM through the induction of apoptosis. (Matsumoto et al., 2003). This finding that crude alpha-mangostin has potent chemopreventive effects in our short-term colon carcinogenesis bioassay system suggests that longer exposure might result in suppression of tumor development. (Nabandith et al., 2004).

Xanthones bearing different functionalities, namely-hydroxyxanthone, 3-hydroxyxanthone, 1,4-dihydroxyxanthone, 2,6-dihydroxyxanthone, 1,2-diacetoxyxanthone, 2,6-diacetoxyxanthone,3-methoxyxanthone,1,3,7-trimethoxyxanthone and

1,5-dihydroxy-6-methoxyxanthone were synthesized and examined for their effect on nicotinamide adenine dinucleotide phosphate (NADPH)-catalyzed liver microsomal lipid peroxidation and on tumour necrosis factor-α (TNF-α) induced expression of intercellular adhesion moledule-1 (ICAM-1) on endothelial cells, with a view to establish structure–activity relationship. Hydroxy- and acetoxyxanthones showed potent inhibitory effects on NADPH-catalyzed lipid peroxidation and TNF-α induced expression of ICAM-1 on endothelial cells. (Madan et al., 2002). Results have shown that one of the xanthone derivatives which could be identified as garcinone E has potent cytotoxic effect on all HCC cell lines as well as on the other gastric and lung cancer cell lines included in the screen.(Ho et al., 2002). The chemopreventive action of xanthone derivatives bellidifolin, gentiacaulein, norswertianin and swerchirin on DNA damage photosensitized by riboflavin was demonstrated using [^{32}P]-5′-end-labeled DNA fragments obtained from genes relevant to human cancer. gentiacaulein and norswertianin effectively inhibited the formation of piperidine-labile products at consecutive G residues by photoexcited riboflavin.(Kazutaka et al., 2005) Xanthone derivatives have been shown to be potent inhibitors of tumour growth. Oxygenated Xanthones and [3-(dialkylamino)-2-hydroxypropoxy]s have been prepared and tested for in-vitro inhibition of human PLC/PRF/5, KB and 212 cells. Structure-activity analysis indicated epoxidation of the hydroxyxanthone increased cytotoxicity against tumour cells but ring-opening of the epoxide group with dialkylamine did not enhance the anti-tumour activity. Further evaluation of three of the most active compounds 2, 6-, 3, 6-, and 3, 5-di (2,3-epoxypropoxy) xanthone in DNA, RNA and protein synthesis of tumour cells showed potent inhibitory activity. (Lin et al., 1996).

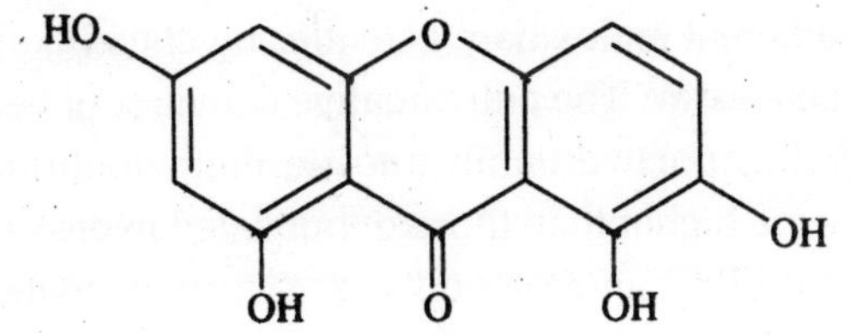

Norswertianin

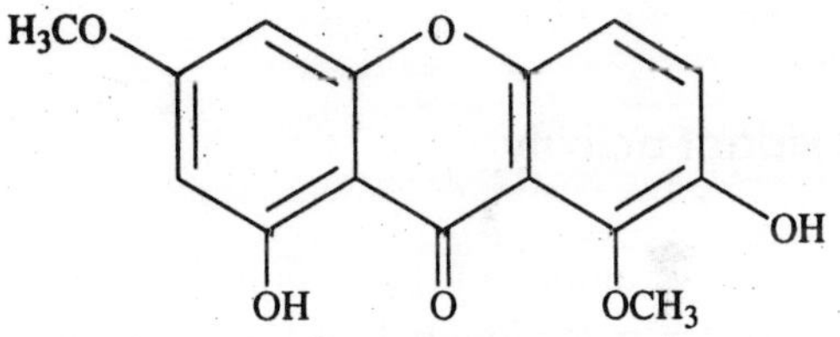

Gentaicaulein

The new benzopyranoxanthone derivatives only displayed marginal antiproliferative activity when tested against L1210 and KB-3-1 cell lines. The only compounds found significantly active against L1210 cell line, 16 and 20, belong to the benzo [*a*] pyrano [3,2-*h*] xanthen-7-one series, which possess a pyran ring fused angularly onto the xanthone basic core. (Sylvie et al. 2006). The effects of the prenylated xanthonic derivatives on the *in vitro* growth of four human tumour cell lines: MCF-7 (breast), NCI- H460 (non-small cell lung), SF-268 (central nervous system) and UACC-62 (melanoma) were evaluated and found to be selective and highly potent against the MCF-7 cell line. (Castanheiro et al. 2005) Two new xanthone derivatives were isolated from *Polygala vulgaris and were* tested for *in vitro* cytotoxic activity using two cell lines, LoVo and its strain, which express resistance to common antitumor agents. (Dall'Acqua et al. 2002).

Two new xanthones 1,5,6-trihydroxy-6′,6′-dimethyl-2*H*-pyrano(2′,3′:3,4)-2-(3-methylbut-2-enyl) xanthone and 1,6,7-trihydroxy-6′,6′-dimethyl-2*H*-pyrano(2′,3′:3,2)-4-(3-methylbut-2-enyl)xanthone , have been isolated from the stem bark of *Garcinia lancilimba* (Guttiferae), together with six known xanthones. Their structures were identified on the basis of extensive spectral evidence including detailed 2D NMR and HR-MS data. Two new compounds showed moderate inhibitory effect on human breast cancer MDA-MB-435S cell line. (Yang et al., 2007).

Antimicrobial activity

Calozeloxanthone, a xanthone which has been isolated from *Calophyllum moonii* and *Calophyllum lankensis*, showed the highest activity against methicillin-resistant *S. aureus* (MRSA) strains at a concentration of 8.3 μg/ml. (Dharmaratne et al., 1999).

A number of flavone and xanthone derivatives bearing some characteristic features of fluoroquinolones such as the fluorine atom and an ortho piperazine ring are described. The new compounds have been tested for possible cytotoxic and antimicrobial activities. Cytotoxicity of both groups of compounds is rather poor, while the antibacterial activity is restricted to xanthones. (Mari et al., 1999).

Antioxidant activity

Two xanthones, alpha- and gamma-mangostins, were isolated from the fruit hull of *Garcinia mangostana*, and both significantly inhibited nitric oxide (NO) and PGE_2 production from lipopolysacchride (LPS)-stimulated RAW 264.7 cells. The IC_{50} values for the inhibition of NO production by alpha- and gamma-mangostins were 12.4 and 10.1muM, respectively. (Chen et al., 2008) Chemical investigation of the n-butanol extract from the methanol extract of the root bark of *Artocarpus nobilis* furnished four new prenylated flavonoids together with Artonin E 2'-methylether, isoartonin E 2'-methylether, dihydroisoartonin E 2'-methylether, Artonin V 2'-methylether artobiloxanthone, artonin E and cycloartobiloxanthone. All these compounds showed strong radical scavenging properties towards DPPH radical. (Jayasinghe et al., 2008) Substances with antioxidative properties were obtained from an ether extract of *Swertia japonica* Makino. Six active components of the extract were isolated and identified as methylbellidifolin, methylswertianin, swertianin, bellidifolin, norswertianin and desmethylbellidifolin. These six xanthone derivatives were shown to possess different antioxidant activities by chemiluminescent assay. The antioxidative activities of bellidifolin, norswertianin and desmethylbellidifolin were higher than those of butylated hydroxytoluene (BHT) and α-tocopherol. On autooxidation of methyl linoleate, bellidifolin had activity similar to that of BHT. (Ashida et al., 1994).

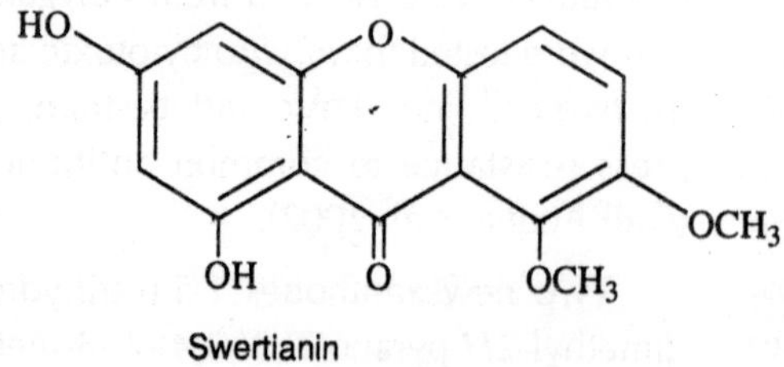

Swertianin

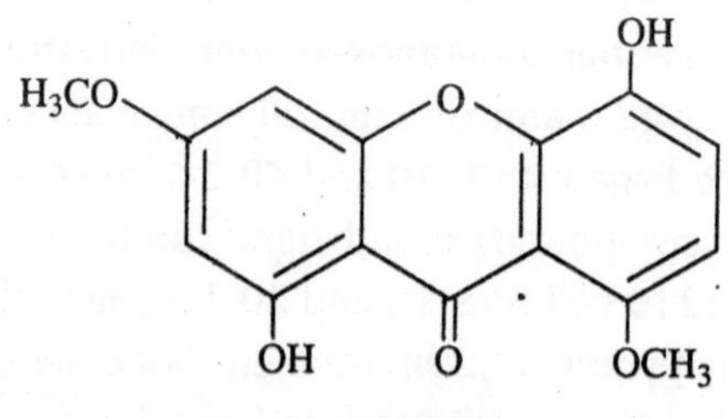

Bellidifolin

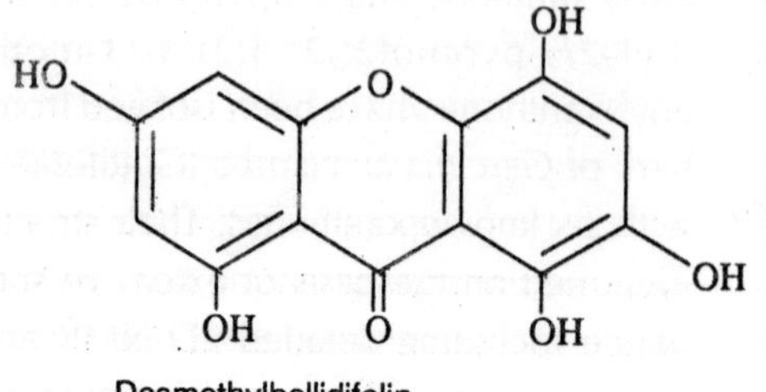

Desmethylbellidifolin

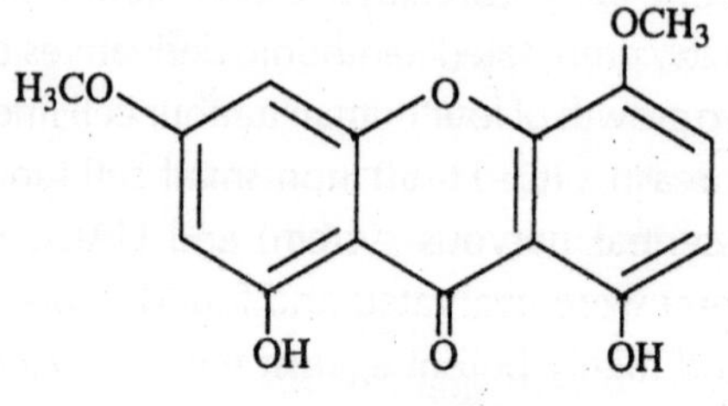

Methylbellidifolin

Antiinflammatory activity

1,5-dihydroxy-3, 8-dimethoxy xanthone of *Swertia chirata* showed significant antiinflammatory action in acute, sub-acute and chronic experimental models in rats. (Banerjee et al., 2000) Gamma-Mangostin had a potent inhibitory activity of prostaglandin E_2 (PGE_2) release induced by A23187, a Ca2+ ionophore with the IC50 value of about 5 microM. In enzyme assay *in vitro*, gamma-mangostin inhibited the activities of both constitutive COX-I and inducible COX-II in a concentration-dependent manner, with the IC_{50} values of about 0.8 and 2 microM, respectively. (Nakatani et al., 2002).

2-Hydroxyacetyl-7-acetylxanthone, a new xanthone derivative, was synthesized in four steps starting from xanthene, by two synthetic approaches. The new compound displayed antianaphylactic activity in the PCA test and in the anaphylaxis shock test in rats. It also displayed analgesic activity in the writhing test in mice, and antiinflammatory activity in the carrageenan edema test in rats. (Mari et al., 1999).

Xanthones as MAO inhibitors and CNS depressants

1, 6-Dihydroxyxanthone and 1, 3, 6-trihydroxyxanthone exhibited much potent inhibitory activity toward rat brain mitochondrial MAO (type A). On the other hand, 1, 3, 7-trihydroxyxanthone showed great potency for inhibition of mouse liver mitochondrial MAO (type B). These results indicate that 1, 3, 6-trihydroxyxanthone and 1, 3, 7-trihydroxyxanthone were rather specific inhibitors of type MAO-A and type MAO10-B, respectively. 1, 3-Dihydroxy-6-alkoxyxanthones containing alkoxy residues with carbon number 1 to 8 were synthesized and compared for their inhibitory activity toward rat brain mitochondrial MAO. Among them, 6-ethoxy-, 6-propyloxy-, and 6-butyloxy-derivatives were potent inhibitors, and especially, 1, 3-dihydroxy-6-propyloxyxanthone was the most inhibitory. The xanthone aglycone produces signs of dose dependent weak CNS stimulant activities. This effect may be due to MAO inhibition. The inhibition of type A and type B MAO by number of xanthones has been reported. Bellidifolin and 1,3,5,8- tetra substituted xanthones has been shown to be selective inhibitor of type A MAO *in vitro*, but the glucosides (Bellidifolin-8-O glucoside and desmethylbellidifolin-8-Oglucoside) showed no activity. (Suzuki et al., 1981).

The significant CNS depressant action has been shown by tetraoxygenated xanthones and their O-glucosides of *Swertia chirata* and *S. purpurascens* (Ghosal et al., 1974).

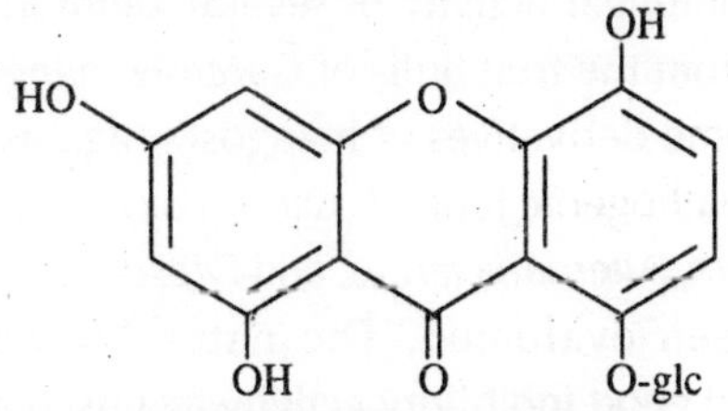

Desmethylbellidifolin-8-Oglucoside

Vasorelaxant activity

1, 5-Dihydroxy-2, 3-dimethoxy-xanthone (HM-5) is one of the naturally occurring xanthones of a Tibetan medicinal herb *Halenia elliptica*. Recently, it has been shown that HM-5 is one of the phase I metabolites of 1-hydroxy-2, 3, 5-trimethoxy-xanthone (HM-1), the major active component of *H. elliptica* with potent vasorelaxant actions. (Wang et al., 2008). A series of xanthones and xanthonoxypropanolamines have been synthesized. The activity of compounds on cardiovascular system was evaluated. All the compounds tested exhibited effective hypotensive activity in anesthetized rats. An oxypropanolamine side chain substituted at the C-3 position of xanthone nucleus significantly enhanced the hypotensive activity. (Wang et al., 2002) Xanthones and xanthone derivatives have been shown to have beneficial effects in some cardiovascular diseases, including ischemic heart disease, atherosclerosis, hypertension and thrombosis. The protective effects of xanthones in the cardiovascular system may be due to their antioxidant, antiinflammatory, platelet aggregation inhibitory, antithrombotic and/or vasorelaxant activities. In particular, the antagonism of endogenous nitric oxide synthase inhibitors by xanthones may represent the basis for improved endothelial function and for reduction of events associated with atherosclerosis. (Ashida et al., 1994).

The antifungal activity

The antifungal activity of several xanthones isolated from the fruit hulls of *Garcinia mangostana* and some derivatives of mangostin against three phytopathogenic fungi, *Fusarium oxysporum vasinfectum*, *Alternaria tenuis*, and *Dreschlera oryzae*, has been evaluated. The natural xanthones showed good inhibitory activity against the three fungi. Substitution in the A and C rings has been shown to modify the bioactivities of the compounds. (Gopalakrishnan et al., 1997).

Alpha-glucosidase inhibitory activity

The results indicated that these xanthone derivatives were capable of inhibiting *in vitro* alpha-glucosidase with moderate to good activities. Among them, polyhydroxylxanthones exhibited the highest activities and thus may be exploitable as a lead compound for the development of potent alpha - glucosidase inhibitors. (Liu et al., 2006) A series of novel xanthone derivatives with extended π-systems, that is, benzoxanthones and their structurally perturbed analogs have been designed and synthesized as α-glucosidase inhibitors. Their inhibitory activities toward yeast α-glucosidase were evaluated with the aim to enrich the structure – activity relationship. The results indicated that benzoxanthones were capable of inhibiting *in vitro* yeast α-glucosidase. (Liu et al., 2007).

Antitubercular activity

Alpha- and beta-mangostins and garcinone B exhibited strong inhibitory effect against *Mycobacterium tuberculosis* with the minimum inhibitory concentration (MIC) value of 6.25 μg/ml. (Suksamrarn et al., 2003).

Trypanocidal activity

The constituents of the stem bark of *Garcinia subelliptica* (Guttiferae) were investigated based on its trypanocidal activity against epimastigotes of *Trypanosoma cruzi*, the etiologic agent for Chagas' disease. As the active components, nine xanthones were isolated including two new ones, 4-hydroxybrasilixanthone B and 1,3,5,6- tetrahydroxy-4,7,8-tri (3-methyl-2-butenyl) xanthone. (Abe et al., 2003).

CONCLUSION

Literature studies show varieties of activities associated with natural as well as synthetic xanthones. Xanthones are present in different plant famIlies like Guttiferae, Gentinaceae, Polygalaceae, Moraceae and Leguminosae. Different species of genus Garcinia and Swertia contain number of xanthones which are biologically active. Xanthones are more potent than vitamin C and vitamin E as antioxidant. Considering the lead molecule xanthones from natural sources chemists shall try to synthesize the related molecules and their derivatives which may result in promising medicinally useful drugs.

Naturally occurring xanthones and their biological activities

Activity	*Plant source*	*Isolated compounds showing the activity*
Antimalarial	*Calophyllum Caledonicum* *Garcinia cowa* *Allanblackia monticola*	1. 1,3,7 trioxygenated and prenylated on the positions 2 and 8 (Hay et al., 2004) 2. 7-O-methylgarcinone E, cowanin, cowanol, cowaxanthone, and beta-mangostin, (Likhitwitayawuid et al., 1998; Shen et al., 2006) 3. 6-bis-w-diethylaminoalkoxyxanthones (Kelly et al. 2002) 4. 9H-xanthones, carrying a [2-(diethylamino) ethyl] amino group in position 1 (Portela et al., 2007)
Antitumor	*Garcinia mangostana* *Polygala vùlgaris* *Garcinia lancilimba*	1. Alpha-mangostin (Chin et al, 2008) 2. Hydroxy- and acetoxyxanthones (Madan et al. 2002) 3. Garcinone E (Ho et al., 2002) 4. bellidifolin , gentiacaulein , norswertianin and swerchirin (Kazutaka et al., 2005) 5. 2, 6-, 3, 6-, and 3, 5-di (2,3-epoxypropoxy) xanthone (Lin et al., 1996) 6. 1,5,6-trihydroxy-6', 6'-dimethyl-2*H*-pyrano(2',3':3,4)-2-(3-methylbut-2-enyl) xanthone and 1,6,7-trihydroxy-6',6'-dimethyl-2*H*-pyrano(2',3':3,2)-4-(3-methylbut-2-enyl) xanthone(Yang et al., 2007)
Antimicrobial	*Calophyllum moonii* *Calophyllum Lankensis*	Calozeloxanthone (Dharmaratne et al., 1999)
Antioxidant	*Garcinia mangostana* *Artocarpus nobilis* *Swertia japonica* *Swertia davidi*	1. Alpha- and gamma-mangostins (Chen et al., 2008) 2. Artonin E 2'-methylether, isoartonin E 2'-methylether, dihydroisoartonin E 2'-methylether, Artonin V 2'-methylether artobiloxanthone, artonin E and cycloartobiloxanthone (Jayasinghe et al., 2008) 3. Methylbellidifolin, methylswertianin, swertianin, bellidifolin, norswertianin and Desmethylbellidifolin (Ashida et al., 1994)
Antiinflammatory	*Swertia chirata*	1. 1,5-dihydroxy-3,8-dimethoxy xanthone (Banerjee et al., 2000)
Vasorelaxant	*Halenia elliptica* *Swertia davidi*	1. 1, 5-Dihydroxy-2, 3-dimethoxy-xanthone (Wang et al., 2008) 2. Xanthonoxypropanolamines (Wang et al., 2002)
Alpha glucosidase inhibitors		Benzoxanthones (Liu et al., 2007)
Antifungal	*Garcinia mangostana*	Substitution in the A and C rings of xanthones (Gopalakrishnan et al., 1997)
Antitubercular	*Garcinia mangostana*	Alpha- and beta-mangostins (Suksamrarn et al., 2003)

REFERENCES

Abdel-Lateff A, Klemke C, König GM, and Wright AD. 'Two New Xanthone Derivatives from the Algicolous Marine Fungus *Wardomyces anomalus' Journal of Molecular Catalysis B: Enzymatic* 10 (1-3), 291-294 (2000).

Abe Fumiko, Nagafuji Shinya, Okabe Hikaru, Higo Hiroo, and Akahane Hiroshige 'Trypanocidal Constituents in Plants 2 - Xanthones from the Stem Bark of *Garcinia subelliptica' Biol. Pharm. Bull.* 26(12), 730-1733 (2003).

Ashida S, Suzuki T.'Antioxidative components, xanthone derivatives', in *Swertia japonica* Makino *Journal of the American Oil Chemists' Society* 71(10), October, (1994).

Attkinnson JE, Gupta P, Lewis JR, 'Benzophenone participation in xanthone biosynthesis (*Gentianaceae*)' *Chem. Commun.* 1386-1387. (1968).

Attkinnson JE, Gupta P, Lewis JR, 'Some phenolic constituents of *Gentiana lutea*' *Tetrahedron*, 25, (7), 1507, (1969).

Banerjee Shivaji, Sur Tapas Kumar, Mandal Suvra, Das Prabhash Chandra, Sikdar Sridhar 'Assessment of the anti-inflammatory effects of *Swertia chirata* in Acute and chronic experimental models in male albino rats' *Indian Journal of Pharmacology* 32, 21-24, (2000).

Barillas W, Beerhues L, '3-Hydroxybenzoate: coenzyme A ligase and 4-coumarate: Coenzyme A ligase from cultured cells of *Centaurium erythraea' Plant Med.* 202, 112-116 (1997).

Bennett GJ, Lee HH. 'Xanthones from Guttiferae' *Phytochemistry*, 28(4), 967-998. (1989).

Berrhues L, 'Benzophenone synthase from cultured cells of *Centaurium erythraea' FEBS Letters* 383, 264-266, (1996).

Blaise A, Meyer M, Valentin A, Laure NE, Fomum ZT and Nkengfack AE. 'Prenylated xanthone derivatives with antiplasmodial activity from *Allanblackia monticola*' *Chem. Pharm. Bull.* 54(1), 111-113 (2006).

Castanheiro R, Pinto M, Silva A, Cravo S, Pedro M., Wilairat R, Nazareth N, Nascimento M, "Prenylated Xanthonic Derivatives: Synthesis, Structure Elucidation and Inhibition of Growth of Human Tumor Cell Lines", *"Joint Meeting on Medicinal Chemistry"*, Vienna, Austria, (2005).

Chen LG, Yang LL, Wang CC. 'Anti-inflammatory activity of mangostins from Garcinia mangostana' *Food Chem. Toxicol*, 46(2), 688-93, (2008).

Chin YW, Jung HA. 'Xanthones with quinone reductase-inducing activity from the fruits of Garcinia mangostana (Mangosteen).' *Pytochemistry* 69 (3), 754-758 (2008).

Dall'Acquaa Stefano, Violaa Giampietro, Cappellettib Mariella Elsa, and Innocentia Gabbriella 'Xanthones from *Polygala alpestris* (Rchb.)', *Zeitschrift für Naturforschung*. C. A journal of biosciences, 59, 335-338 (2004).

Dall'Acqua Stefano, Innocenti Gabbriella, Viola Giampietro, Piovan Anna, Caniato Rosy and Cappelletti Mariella Elsa 'Cytotoxic Compounds from *Polygala vulgaris' Chem Pharm Bull.* 50(11), 1499-1501 (2002).

Dharmaratne HRW, Wijesinghe WMNM. and Thevanasem V. 'Antimicrobial activity of xanthones from Calophyllum species, against methicillin-resistant *Staphylococcus aureus* (MRSA)' *Journal of Ethnopharmacology* 66(3), 339-342 (1999).

Ghosal S, Sharma PV, Chaudhuri RK, 'Chemical constituents of gentianaceae X: Xanthone-O-glucosides of *Swertia purpurascens* wall' *J. Pharm. Sci.* 63, 1286-1289 (1974).

Gopalakrishnan G, Banumathi B, Suresh G. 'Evaluation of the antifungal activity of natural xanthones from *Garcinia mangostana* and their synthetic derivatives.' *J Nat Prod.* 60(5), 519-24 (1997).

Hay AE, He´lesbeux J, Duval O, LabaRed M, Grellier P, Richomme P. 'Antimalarial xanthones from

Calophyllum caledonicum and *Garcinia vieillardii*', *Life Sciences*, 75, 3077-3085 (2004).

Ho CK, Huang YL, Chen CC. 'Garcinone E, a xanthone derivative, has potent cytotoxic effect against hepatocellular carcinoma cell lines' *Planta Med.* 68(11), 975-9 (2002).

Ignatushchenko MV, Winter RW, and M Riscoe' 'Xanthones as antimalarial agents: stage specificity *Am. J. Trop. Med. Hyg* 62(1), 77-81 (2000).

Jayasinghe UL, Samarakoon TB, Kumarihamy B.M., Hara N, Fujimoto Y. 'Four new prenylated flavonoids and xanthones from the root bark of *Artocarpus nobilis*'. *Fitoterapia.* 79(1), 37-41 (2008).

Kazutaka H, Mami Y, Akito N, Hajime M, Virendra R, Singh M, Rawat M, Shinji O, Shosuke K. 'Chemopreventive action of xanthone derivatives on photosensitized DNA damage' *Photochemistry and Photobiology* 81 (2) 314-319 (2005).

Kelly Jane Xu, Winter Rolf, Peyton David H., Hinrichs David J, and Riscoe Michael 'Optimization of Xanthones for Antimalarial Activity: the 3,6-Bis- Diethylaminoalkoxyxanthone Series' *Antimicrobial Agents and Chemotherapy*, 46 (1), 144-150, (2002).

Likhitwitayawuid, Phadungacharo, Krungkrai 'Antimalarial xanthones from *Garcinia cowa.*' *Planta Med.* 64(1), 70-2 (1998).

Lin CN, Liou SJ, Lee TH, Chuang YC, Won SJ. 'Xanthone derivatives as potential anti-cancer drugs' *J Pharm Pharmacol* 48 (5) 539-44 (1996).

Liu Y, Zou L, Ma L, Chen WH, 'Synthesis and pharmacological activities of xanthone derivatives as alpha-glucosidase inhibitors'. *Bioorg Med Chem.* 14(16) 5683-90 (2006).

Madan B, Singh I, Ajit Kumar, Prasad AK, Raj Hanumantharao G, Parmar VS. and Ghosh B. 'Xanthones as inhibitors of microsomal lipid peroxidation and TNF-α induced ICAM-1 expression on human umbilical vein endothelial cells (HUVECs) *Bioorg Med Chem* 10(11), 3431-3436 (2002).

Mari S, Rossi M, Valenti P, Da Re 'Flavone and xanthone derivatives related to fluoroquinolones', *Farmaco.* 54(6), 411-5 (1999).

Matsumoto K, Akao Y, Kobayashi E, Ohguchi K, Ito T, Tanaka T, Iinuma M, Nozawa Y. 'Induction of apoptosis by xanthones from mangosteen in human leukemia cell lines', *J Nat Prod.* 66(8), 1124-7, (2003).

Sylvie Michel, Koch Michel, Tillequin François, Pfeiffer Bruno, and Pierré Alain 'Synthesis and Cytotoxic Activity of Benzo [*a*] pyrano [3,2-*h*] and [2,3-*i*] xanthone Analogues of Psorospermine, Acronycine, and Benzo [*a*] acronycine', *Chem. Pharm. Bull.* 54 (8), 1113-1118 (2006).

Nabandith V, Suzui M, Morioka T, Kaneshiro T, Kinjo T, Matsumoto K, Akao Y, Iinuma M, Yoshimi N. 'Inhibitory effects of crude alpha-mangostin, a xanthone derivative, on two different categories of colon preneoplastic lesions induced by 1, 2-dimethylhydrazine in the rat. *Asian Pac J Cancer Prev.* 5 (4), 433-8, (2004).

Nakatani K, Nakahata N, Arakawa T, Yasuda H, Ohizumi Y. 'Inhibition of cyclooxygenase and prostaglandin E_2 synthesis by gamma-mangostin, a xanthone derivative in mangosteen, in C6 rat glioma cells.' *Biochem Pharmacol.* 63 (1), 73-9 (2002).

Oliv Louh GN, Lannang AM, Mbazoa CD, Tangmouo JG, Komguem J, Castilho P, Ngninzeko FN, Qamar N., Lontsi D, Choudhary MI, Sondengam BL. 'Polyanxanthone A, B and C, three xanthones from the wood trunk of *Garcinia polyantha*' *Phytochemistry*, 69(4), 1013-1017 (2008).

Portela C, Afonso CM, 'Synthesis and antimalarial properties of new chloro-9H-xanthones with an aminoalkyl side chain.' *Chem Biodivers* 4(7); 1508-19 (2007).

Shen Jie and Yang Jun-Shan 'Two New Xanthones from the Stems of *Garcinia cowa*' *Chemical & Pharmaceutical Bulletin* 54 (1), 126 (2006).

Suksamrarn S, Suwannapoch N, Phakhodee W, Thanuhiranlert J, Ratananukul P, Chimnoi N, Suksamrarn A. 'Antimycobacterial activity of prenylated xanthones from the fruits of Garcinia mangostana' *Chem Pharm Bull (Tokyo).* 51(7), 857-9, (2003).

Suzuki O, Katsumata Y, Oya M, Chari VM, Klapfenberger R, Wagner H, Hostettmann K, 'Inhibition of type A and type B monoamine oxidases by naturally occurring xanthones', *Plant Med.* 42, 17-21 (1981).

Wang Li-Wen, Kang Jaw-Jou, Chen Ing-Jun, Tengand Che-Ming, Lin Chun-Nan 'Antihypertensive and vasorelaxing activities of synthetic xanthone derivatives' *Bioorg Med Chem* 10(3), 567-572, (2002).

Wang Y, Shi JG, Wang MZ, Che CT, Yeung JH. 'Mechanisms of the vasorelaxant effect of 1, 5-dihydroxy-2, 3-dimethoxy-xanthone, an active metabolite of 1-hydroxy-2, 3, 5-trimethoxy-xanthone isolated from a Tibetan herb, *Halenia elliptica*, on rat coronary artery.' *Life Sci.* 82(1-2), 91-82, (2008).

Liu Y, Ma L, Chen Wen-Hua, Wang, Bo and Xu Zun-Le 'Synthesis of xanthone derivatives with extended π-systems as α-glucosidase inhibitors: Insight into the probable binding mode' *Bioorg Med Chem* 15(8), 2810-2814 (2007).

Yang Nian-Yun, Han Quan-Bin, Cao Xin-Wei, Qiao Chun-Feng, Song Jing-Zheng, Chen Shi-Lin, Yang Da-Jian, Yiu Hillary, Xu Hong-Xi Two New Xanthones Isolated from the Stem Bark of Garcinia lancilimba *Chem Pharm Bull* (Tokyo). 55 (6) 950-2 (2007).

chapter 22

BIOACTIVE FLAVONOIDS

S.A. Nirmal, S.C. Pal, Mostafa Elachouri and Subhash C Mandal

INTRODUCTION

Nutrition is an era of alteration, which defined the role of bioactive compounds present in the foods materials. These compounds are defined as components of foods that influence physiological or cellular activities resulting in a beneficial health effect. This definition distinguishes these compounds from many others that are bioactive, but have detrimental effects and are considered as toxic e.g. few plant secondary metabolites. The purpose of this review is to provide an overview of the scientific evidences to straighten out the biological and a health effect of these bioactive compounds. Above all flavonoids (quercetin, kaempferol, myricetin etc.) one of the groups, which plays diverse role in different way in our biological system. These compounds are typically occurring in small amounts in different foods. Here we tried to pull together some activities of major flavonoids, which are proved scientifically at cellular level laboratory research studies. Flavonoids are nearly ubiquitous in plants and are recognized as the pigments responsible for the colors of leaves, especially in autumn. They are rich in seeds, citrus fruits, olive oil, tea, and red wine. They are low molecular weight compounds composed of a three-ring structure with various substitutions. This basic structure is shared by tocopherols (vitamin E).

Flavonoid

"Flavonoid is a colorless crystalline compound, $C_{15}H_{10}O_2$, the parent substance of a number of important yellow pigments, occurring in the leaves or in the stems and seed capsules of many primroses." The term flavonoid refers to a class of plant secondary metabolites. According to the IUPAC nomenclature, they can be classified into:

i. *flavonoids*, derived from 2-phenylchromen-4-one (2-phenyl-1,4-benzopyrone) structure.

ii. *isoflavonoids*, derived from 3-phenylchromen-4-one (3-phenyl-1,4- benzopyrone) structure.

iii. *neoflavonoids*, derived from 4-phenylcoumarine (4-phenyl-1,2- benzopyrone) structure.

Flavonoids can be regarded as C_6-C_3-C_6 compounds where C6 moiety is benzene ring and it is classified according to the state of oxygenation of the C_3 unit i.e. C-2, 3, 4 (Evans, 2005).

Table 22.1. Various classes of flavonoids along with their examples

Type	Nature	Examples
Flavone	Dihydroxy 5,7	Chrysin
	Trihydroxy 7,3',4'	Butin
	Trihydroxy 5,7,4'	Apigenin
	Tetrahydroxy 5,7,3',4'	Luteolin
	Tetrahydroxy 5,7,3',4'	Fisetin

Contd. to next page.

Flavonol	Pentahydroxy 3,5,7,3',4'	Quercetin
	Tetrahydroxy 3,5,7,4'	Kaempferol
Flavonone	Tetrahydroxy 5,7,3',4'	Eriodictyol
	Dihydroxy 7,4'	Liquiritigenin
Xanthone	1,7-Dihydroxy-3-methoxy	Gentisin
Isoflavone	Dihydroxy 7,4'	Formononetin
	Trihydroxy 5,7,4'	Genistein
Biflavone	Hexahydroxy 2 X (5,7,4')	Amentoflavone

Flavonoids are most commonly known for their antioxidant activity. However, it is now known that the health benefits they provide against cancer and heart disease are the result of other mechanisms. Flavonoids are also commonly referred to as bioflavonoids in the media–the terms are equivalent and interchangeable, for flavonoids are biological in origin. The flavonoids are polyphenolic compounds possessing 15 carbon atoms; two benzene rings joined by a linear three-carbon chain.

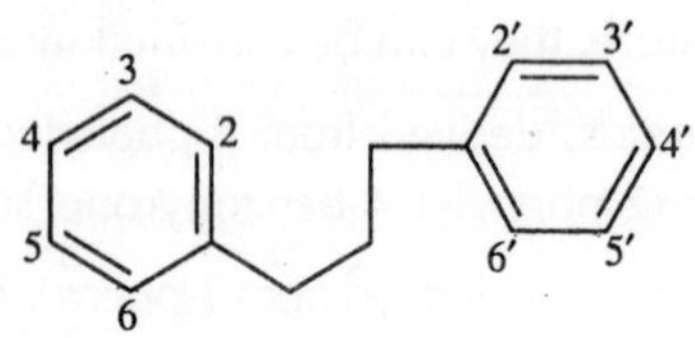

Fig. 22.1. The skeleton above can be represented as the C_6-C_3-C_6 system

Flavonoids constitute one of the most characteristic classes of compounds in higher plants. Many flavonoids are easily recognized as flower pigments in most angiosperm families (flowering plants). However, their occurrence is not restricted to flowers but include all parts of the plant.

The chemical structure of flavonoids are based on a C_{15} skeleton with a chromane ring bearing a second aromatic ring B in position 2, 3 or 4.

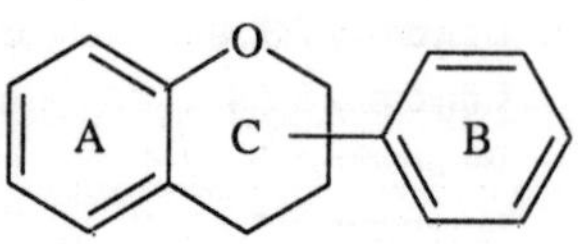

Fig. 22.2. C_{15} skeleton of flavonoids

In few cases, the six-membered heterocyclic ring C occurs in an isomeric open form or is replaced by a five-membered ring. Biogenetically, the A ring usually arises from a molecule of resorcinol or phloroglucinol synthesized from the acetate pathway and has a characteristic hydroxylation pattern at the 5 and 7 position. The B ring comes from the Shikimate pathway and is usually 4,3,4′ or 3,4,5-hydroxylated. Based on their chemical structure, flavonoids are divided into several subclasses, of which flavonols are the most abundant in the plant kingdom.

Biosynthesis

Flavonoids are synthesized by the phenylpropanoid metabolic pathway in which the amino acid phenylalanine is used to produce 4-coumaroyl-CoA. This can be combined with malonyl-CoA to yield the true backbone of flavonoids, a group of compounds called chalcones, which contain two phenyl rings. Conjugate ring-closure of chalcones results in the familiar form of flavonoids, the three-ring structure of a flavone. The metabolic pathway continues through a series of enzymatic modifications to yield flavanones, dihydroflavonols, anthocyanins. Along this pathway, many products can be formed, including the flavonols, flavan-3-ols, proanthocyanidins (tannins) and a host of other polyphenolics.

Biological effects

1. CNS activity

Some synthetic flavonoids possess anxiolytic like properties similar or superior to that of diazepam (Griebel et al., 1999). e.g. 6-bromoflavone and 6-bromo-3′-nitro- flavones, latter is very potent than 6-bromoflavone.

2. Cardiotonic activity

Flavonoids are having cardioprotective effects (Huesken et al., 1995). The unsubstituted parent flavone exerts coronary dilatory activity and its combination with rutin and isoquercetin is useful in the treatment of atherosclerosis. 3-methyl quercetin has positive chronotropic effect on guinea pig right atrium and antiarrhythmic effect on left atrium (Lackeman et al., 1986). In recent report the cardiotoxicity (negative inotropic effect) of doxorubicin on the mouse left atrium has been inhibited by flavonoids, 7-monohydroxy ethyl rutoside and 7,3',4'- trihydroxyethyl rutoside. The glycosides of luteolin, apigenin and genistein produced antihypertensive activity even more than the reference drug papaverine. Three flavonoids showed vasorelaxant effect in order of potency, luteolin > eriodictyol > naringenin on rat thoracic aorta. Quercetin is having stronger inotropic responses among the different flavonoids. The relative order of potency of the tested flavonoids is, quercetin > morin = kaempferol > luteolin = apigenin > fisetin = galangin (Itoigawa et al., 1999).

3. Lipid lowering activity

Oxidative modification of low-density lipoproteins (LDL) by free radicals is an early event in the pathogenesis of atherosclerosis. A number of mechanisms are likely to contribute to inhibition of LDL oxidation by flavonoids. Flavonoids may directly scavenge some radical species by acting as chain breaking antioxidants (De-Whalley et al., 1990). In addition, they may recycle other chain-breaking antioxidants such as a-tocopherol by donating a hydrogen atom to the tocopheryl radical (Francel et al., 1993). Transition metals such as iron and copper are important pro-oxidants, and some flavonoids can chelate divalent metal ions, hence preventing free radical formation. The ability of quercetin, and the quercetin glycosides, to protect LDL against oxidative modification has shown a significant protective effect (Mc Anlis et al., 1997). Liquiritigenin showed a significant fall in serum cholesterol, LDL-cholesterol and atherogenic index.

4. Antiulcer activity

Some recent reports have indicated that many flavonoids possess antiulcerogenic activity. â Hydroxy ethyl rutosides, gossypin, naringin, naringenin and (+)-Cyanidanol-3 were shown to exhibit anti-ulcer activity (Parmar & Shikha Parmar, 1998). Quercetin, rutin and kaempferol administered intraperitoneally (25- 100 mg/kg) inhibited dose-dependent gastric damage produced by acidified ethanol in rats. Flavone was inactive while naringin was active at a higher dose (200 mg/kg). Lorenz et al, 1973 showed that (+) - Cyanidanol-3 has histidine decarboxylase inhibitory activity and hence anti-ulcer activity. 3-Methoxy-5,7,3',4'-tetra hydroxy flavan (Meciadanol), a congener of (+)-cyanidanol-3 exhibited significant anti-ulcer activity in pylorus ligated rats, restraint ulcers and gastric mucosal damage induced by aspirin models (Parmar and Shikha Parmar, 1998).

5. Hepatoprotective activity

Many flavonoids have also been found to possess hepatoprotective activity. In a study carried out to investigate silymarin, apigenin, quercetin and naringenin as putative therapeutic agents against microcrystin LR-induced hepatotoxicity, silymarin was found to be the most effective one (Carlo et al., 1993). Rutin and venorutin showed regenerative and hepatoprotective effects in experimental cirrhosis (Lorenz et al., 1973).

6. Antioxidant activity

Free radical production in animal cells can either be accidental or deliberate. With the increasing acceptance of free radicals as common place and important biochemical intermediates, they have been implicated in a large number of human diseases (Wegener & Fintelmann, 1999). Quercetin, kaempferol, morin, myricetin and rutin by acting as antioxidants exhibited several beneficial effects, such as antiinflammatory, antiallergic, antiviral as well as an anticancer activity. They have also been suggested to play a protective role in liver diseases, cataracts, and cardiovascular diseases. Quercetin and silybin acting as free radical scavengers were shown to exert a protective effect in reperfusion ischemic tissue damage (Santos et al., 1998). The scavenging activity of flavonoids has been reported to be in the order: myricetin > quercetin > rhamnetin > morin >diosmetin > naringenin > apigenin > catechin > 5,7-dihydroxy-3',4',5'-trimethoxyflavone > robinin >kaempferol > flavone (Ratty, 1988). Morin, myricetin, kaempferol and quercetin have also been suggested as stabilizers for fish oil as an alternative to synthetic antioxidants (Husain et al., 1987).

7. Effect on heat shock proteins

Heat shock proteins (HSP) have been recognized against physiological stress such as heat shock, heavy metals and glucose starvation. Recent progress has revealed the role of HSPs in various diseases. HSP27 has been shown to be involved in the acquired resistance of tumor cells, hyperthermic and chemotherapeutic treatment. Aberrant expression of HSP could cause various autoimmune diseases. Flavonoids inhibited the expression of HSP27, HSP47, and HSP72/73 (Laughton et al., 1989). The results suggested the pharmacological possibilities of flavonoids in diseases derived from abnormal expression of JISPs.

8. Anti-inflammatory activity

A number of flavonoids are reported to possess anti-inflammatory activity. Hesperidin, a citrus flavonoids possesses significant antiinflammatory and analgesic effects (Shahidi et al., 1998). Recently, apigenin, luteolin and quercetin have been reported to exhibit anti-inflammatory activity. Quercetin, gallic acid ethyl ester and some as yet unidentified flavonoids might account for the antinociceptive action reported for the hydroalcoholic extract of *Phyllanthus caroliniensis*.

9. Antineoplastic activity

Quite a number of flavonoids have exhibited antineoplastic activity. Study showed that the flavonoids quercetin, kaempferol, catechin, toxifolin and fisetin suppressed cell growth (Kim et al., 1993; Gill et al., 1994). On screening antileukaemic efficacy of 28 naturally occurring and synthetic flavonoids on human promyelocytic leukaemic HL-60 cells, genistein, an isoflavone was found to have strong effect. Genistein is also reported to inhibit in a dose dependent manner the growth of HGC-27 cells derived from human gastric cancer. Of the 14 flavonoids tested against murine and human cancer cell lines, 2',6'-diacetoxy -4,4' -dimethoxydihydro chalcone was the most potent and showed selectivity for the cell line P-388 (Hirano et al., 1994). Trifolirhizin tetraacetate showed greater selectivity for the human cell lines.

10. Effects on blood vessels

Quercetin and rutin have been used as effective constituents of several pharmaceuticals used for treatment of capillary fragility and phlebosclerosis. The activities of certain flavonoids in inhibiting capillary permeability and Arthus phenomenon were found to be in the following order, hesperitin > rutin > quercetin > naringenin > kaempferol > isoquercitol (Paul et al., 1997; Fritz et al., 1996). Flavonoids tangeratin, hesperidin, quercetin, and rutin have been found to reduce aggregation of horse erythrocytes. The decrease in blood cell aggregation produced by most of the flavonoids may explain the reported beneficial effects of these compounds on abnormal capillary permeability and fragility, the reduction of disease symptoms and their protection against various traumas and stresses (Versantvoort et al., 1993). The flavonoids O- (beta-hydroxyethyl) rutoside, (+)-catechol, trihydroxyethyl rutoside increased the negative charge density of the blood vessel wall *in vitro* and were markedly antithrombogenic (Griffith and Ballow, 1972). Quercetin also has been reported to inhibit aggregation of human platelets. Other antiaggregatory flavonoids reported were 3-methyl quercetin, toxerutin, fisetin, dihydroquercetin and flavone. Nobeletin and sinensetin decreased erythrocyte aggregation and sedimentation *in vitro* and might be useful in dietary control of high blood viscosity syndrome (Wenner et al., 1980). Orally administered flavonoids weakly inhibit the vascular permeability and prevent pulmonary haemorrhage.

11. Antimicrobial activity

1. *Antibacterial Activity*

Most of the flavonoids studies were found to be active against many bacteria. Most of the flavonones having no sugar moiety showed antimicrobial activities where as none of the flavonols and flavonolignans tested showed inhibitory activity on the microorganisms (Wild & Fasel, 1969). e.g. Quercetin, Baicalin, Quercetogetin, Hespertin, Fisetin, iso-liquiritigenin,Naringin, Rutin, Apigenin, Chrysin, Baicalin, Hydroxyethylrutosine, Datisetin, Hydroxyethylrutoside.

2. *Antifungal Activity*

Number of flavonoids isolated from peel of tangerine orange, when tested for fungistatic activity towards Deuterophoma tracheiphila showed promising activity. Chlorflavonin was the first chlorine-containing flavonoid type antifungal antibiotic produced by strains of *Aspergillus candidus* (Tencate et al., 1973). e.g. Chloroflavonin, Quercetin, Chrysoeriol, Rutin, Epicathenin, Apigenin, Echinacin, Phaseolinisoflavan.

3. *Antiviral Activity*

Flavonoids also displayed antiviral, including anti-HIV activity. It has been found that flavonols are more active than flavones against herpes simplex virus type 1 and the order of importance was galangin > kaempferol > quercetin (Thomas et al., 1988). e.g. Quercetrin, Rutin, Galangin, Kempferol, Apigenin, Chrysin, Morin, Naringin, Luteolin.

Classification of flavonoids

Table 22.2. Various classes of flavonoids along with their examples.

Type	*Examples*
Flavones	Luteolin, Apigenin, Tangeritin, Diosmin, Flavoxate
Isoflavone	Genistein, Daidzein, Biochanin A, Formononetin, Coumestrol, Daidzin, Puerarin
Flavonols	Myricetin, Quercetin, Kaempferol, Fisetin, Isorhamnetin, Pachypodol, Rhamnazin
Flavanones	Hesperetin, Naringenin, Eriodictyol, Homoeriodictyol
3-Hydroxyflavanones	Dihydroquercetin, Dihydrokaempferol
Flavan-3-ols	Catechins, Epicatechins, Epigallocatechin
Anthocyanidins	Cyanidin, Malvidin, Delphinidin, Pelargonidin, Peonidin, Petunidin

Flavones

Flavones are a class of flavonoids based on the backbone of 2-phenylchromen-4-one (2-phenyl-1-benzopyran-4-one) shown on the right. Natural flavones include Apigenin (4′,5,7-trihydroxyflavone), Luteolin (3′,4′,5,7-tetrahydroxyflavone) and Tangeritin (4′,5,6,7,8-pentamethoxyflavone). Synthetic flavones are Diosmin and Flavoxate.

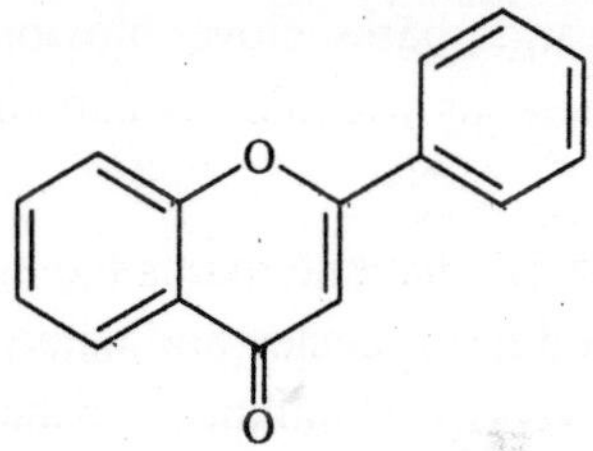

Fig. 22.3. Molecular structure of the flavone backbone (2-phenylchromen-4-one/2-phenyl-1-benzopyran-4-one).

Examples of flavone: Luteolin, Apigenin, Tangeritin, Diosmin, Flavoxate.

Luteolin is a flavonoid, more specifically it is one of the commonly available flavones (Mann, 1992).

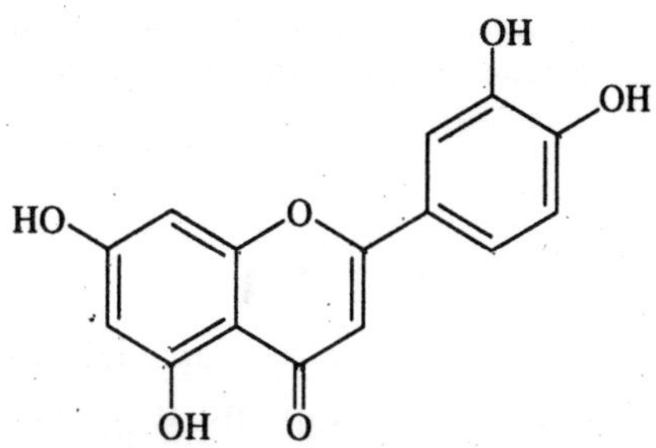

Fig. 22.4. Luteolin

Functions

i. Play an important role in the human body as an antioxidant.
ii. A free radical scavenger.
iii. An agent in the prevention of inflammation.
iv. A promoter of carbohydrate metabolism.
v. An immune system modulator.
vi. Play an important part in the prevention of cancer.
vii. It can dramatically reduce inflammation and the symptoms of septic shock.

Occurrence

Luteolin is most often found in leaves, but it is also seen in rinds, barks, clover blossom and ragweed pollen. It has also been isolated from *Salvia tomentos*.

Apigenin is a flavone that is the aglycone of apiin, isolated from parsley and celery, and apigetrin. It is a yellow crystalline solid that has been used to dye wool.

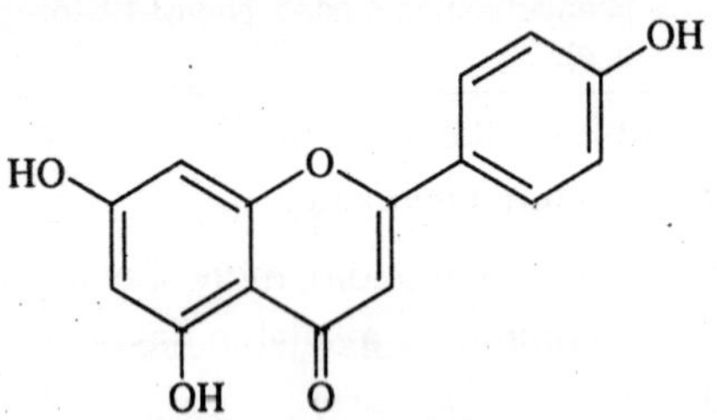

Fig. 22.5. Apigenin; 5,7-dihydroxy-2-(4-hydroxyphenyl)-4H-1-benzopyran-4-one.

Function

Inhibition of adenylate cyclase and decreased the platelet cyclic AMP response to prostacyclin (Nikaidou et al., 2005).Tangeritin is a polymethoxylated flavone.

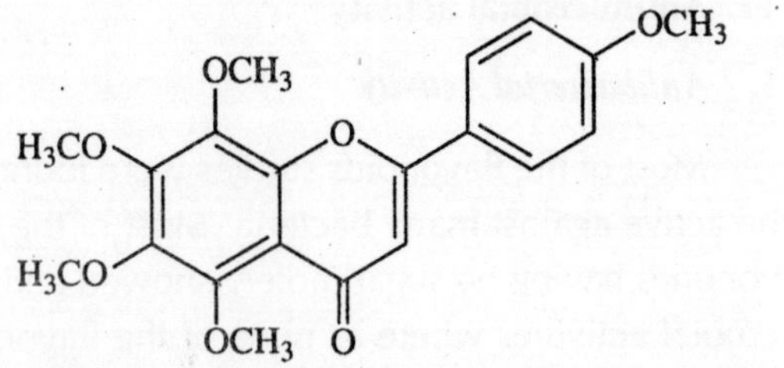

Fig. 22.6. 5,6,7,8-tetramethoxy-2-(4-methoxyphenyl)-4H-1-benzopyran-4-one

Occurrence

Tangerine, citrus peels, commercially available as a dietary supplement.

Functions

i. Strengthens the cell wall and protects it from invasion.
ii. Cholesterol lowering agent.
iii. Potential protective effect against Parkinson's disease.
iv. Potential as an anti cancer agent.
v. *In vitro* studies showed antimutagenic, anti-invasive, and antiproliferative effects.

Diosmin is a semisynthetic phlebotropic drug, a member of the flavonoid family (Danielsson et al., 2002).

Functions

i. It is used with Hesperidin to control internal symptoms of hemorrhoids (piles).
ii. It is an oral phlebotropic drug used in the treatment of venous disease, i.e. chronic venous insufficiency (CVI) and hemorrhoidal disease (HD), in acute or chronic hemorrhoids, in place of rubber-band ligatino, in combination with fiber supplement, or as an adjuvant therapy to hemorrhoidectomy, in order to reduce secondary bleeding.

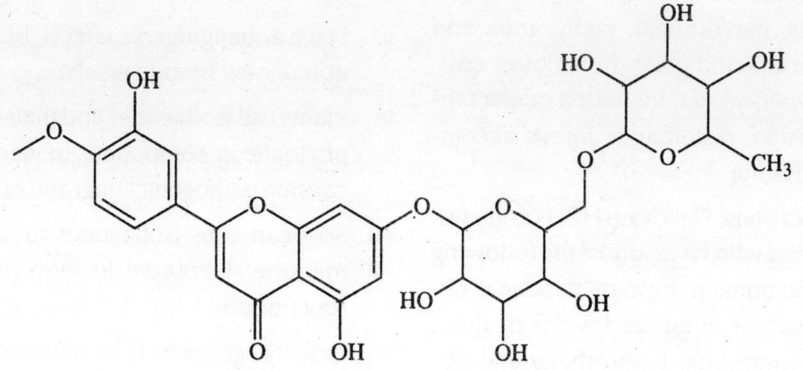

Fig. 22.7. Diosmin

iii. Diosmin prolongs the vasoconstrictor effect of noradrenaline on the vein wall, increasing venous tone, and therefore reducing venous capacitance, distensibility, and stasis. This increases the venous return and reduces venous hyperpressure present in patients suffering from CVI.

iv. Diosmin improves lymphatic drainage by increasing the frequency and intensity of lymphatic contractions, and by increasing the total number of functional lymphatic capillaries. Furthermore, Diosmin (with Hesperidine) decreases the diameter of lymphatic capillaries and the intralymphatic pressure.

v. At the microcirculation level, Diosmin reduces capillary hyperpermeability and increases capillary resistance by protecting the microcirculation from damaging processes.

vi. Diosmin reduces the expression of endothelial adhesion molecules (ICAM1, VCAM1), and inhibits the adhesion, migration, and activation of leukocytes at the capillary level. This leads to a reduction in the release of inflammatory mediators, principally oxygen free radicals and prostaglandins (PGE2, PGF2a).

Flavoxate is a semisynthetic drug, a member of the flavonoid family having anticholinergic with antimuscarinic effects (Brenner, 2000).

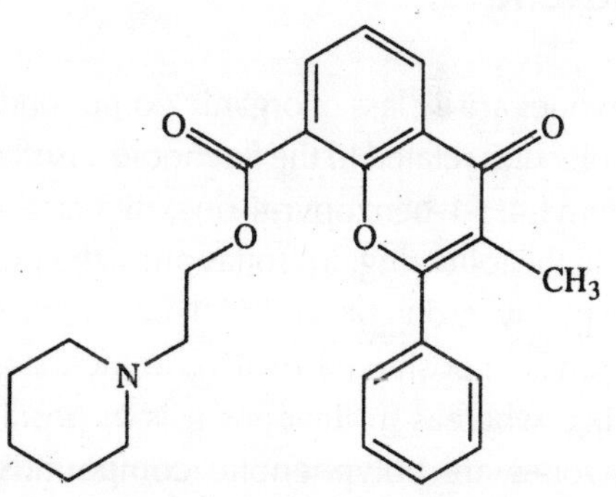

Fig. 22.8. 2-(1-piperidyl)ethyl 3-methyl-4-oxo-2-phenyl-chromene-8-carboxylate

Functions

i. Muscle relaxant properties may be due to direct action on the smooth muscle rather than by antagonizing muscarinic receptors.

ii. Used to treat urinary bladder spasms.

iii. Flavoxate HCl is indicated for symptomatic relief of intestinal cystitis, dysuria, urgency, nocturia, suprapubic pain, frequency and incontinence as may occur in cystitis, prostatitis, urethritis, urethrocystitis, urethrotrigonitis.

Adverse Reactions: The following adverse reactions have been observed, but there are not enough data to support an estimate of their frequency. Nausea, vomiting, dry mouth vertigo, headache, mental confusion, especially in the elderly, drowsiness, nervousness. tachycardia and palpitation, urticaria and other dermatoses, eosinophilia and hyperpyrexia, increased ocular tension, blurred vision, disturbance in eye accommodation and dysuria.

Contraindications: Flavoxate HCl is contraindicated in patients who have any of the following obstructive conditions: pyloric or duodenal obstruction, obstructive intestinal lesions or ileus, achalasia, gastrointestinal hemorrhage and obstructive uropathies of the lower urinary tract.

Isoflavone

Isoflavones are a class of organic compounds and biomolecules related to the flavonoids. Isoflavone (3-phenyl-4*H*-1-benzopyr-4-one) differs from flavone in the following: in isoflavones, the position of the phenyl group on the 4H-1-benzopyr-4-one skeleton is in position 3 relative to the oxygen of the ring, whereas in flavones it is in position 2. Isoflavones are polyphenolic compounds produced almost exclusively by the members of the Fabaceae/*Leguminosae* (bean) family. Early evidence that plants produced estrogen-like compounds was observed in the infertility among sheep eating large amounts of clover in Australia. Similarly, Californian Quails were thought to feed on high-isoflavone legume seeds during periods of food shortage to reduce their fertility (Danielsson et al., 2002).

Examples of isoflavone: Genistein, Daidzein, Biochanin A, Formononetin, Coumestrol, Daidzin, Puerarin.

Functions

i. Act as phytoestrogens in mammals.
ii. Very strong antioxidants.
iii. Useful in treating cancer.
iv. Significant cholesterol-reducing effects.
v. Have antiangiogenic effects (blocking formation of new blood vessels).
vi. Plants use isoflavones and their derivatives as phytoalexin compounds to ward off disease-causing pathogenic fungi and other microbes.
vii. Soybean uses isoflavones to stimulate soil-microbe rhizobium to form nitrogen-fixing root nodules.
viii. Activity against enzyme aldose reductase (Gugler and Dengler, 1973).

Critics claim that isoflavones increase the incidence of epithelial hyperplasia, which precedes cancerous tumors, and that they cause goiter and hyperthyroidism. Phytoestrogens may actually promote cancer.

Biosynthesis

Isoflavones are produced from a branch of the general phenylpropanoid pathway which produces all flavonoid compounds in higher plants. The phenylpropanoid pathway begins from the amino acid phenylalanine, and an intermediate of the pathway, naringenin, is sequentially converted into the isoflavone genistein by two legume-specific enzymes, isoflavone synthase and a dehydratase. Similarly, another intermediate naringenin chalcone is converted to the isoflavone daidzein by sequential action of three legume-specific enzymes: chalcone reductase, type II chalcone isomerase, and isoflavone synthase.

Occurrence

Most members of the *Fabaceae* family contain significant quantities of isoflavones. Analysis of levels in various species has found that the highest levels of genistein and daidzein were found in psoralea (*Psoralea corylifolia*). Various legumes including kudzu (*Pueraria lobata*), lupine (*Lupinus spp*), fava bean (*Vicia faba*), and soy (*Glycine max*) contained substantial amounts of isoflavones according to this analysis. Highly processed foods made from legumes, such as tofu, retained most of their isoflavone content, with the exception of fermented miso, which actually has increased levels. Other dietary sources of isoflavones include chick pea (biochanin A), alfalfa (formononetin and coumestrol), and peanut (genistein).

Research

Isolated phytoestrogen-like isoflavones are an active research area. A research studied the effect of the isolated soy isoflavones genistein and daidzein (commonly found in dietary supplements and infant formulas) on adult mice with their ovaries removed. The study found the mice had thymic and immune system abnormalities and reduction in immune system activity. The article suggests further research into human phytoestrogen response is warranted. Other research showed a link between soy and health problems in certain animals.

Genistein is one of several known isoflavones.

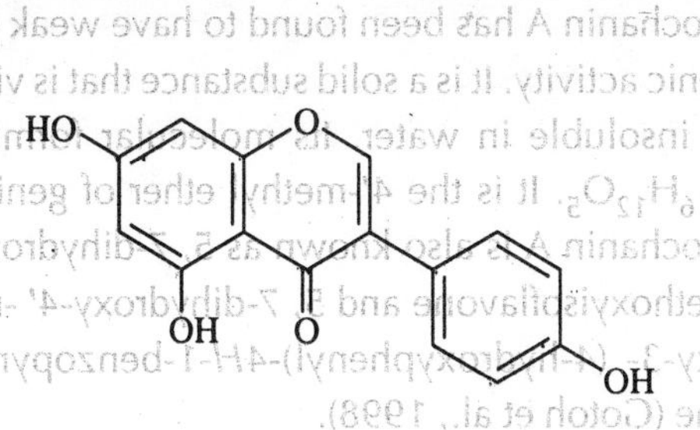

Fig. 22.9. Genistein

Source

Soybeans and soy products like tofu and textured vegetable protein being the primary food source.

Functions

i. As antioxidant.
ii. Many isoflavones have been shown to interact with animal and human estrogen receptors, causing effects in the body similar to those caused by the hormone estrogen in stimulating development and maintenance of female characteristics or they can block cells from using other forms of estrogen.
iii. Have antiangiogenic effects (blocking formation of new blood vessels).
iv. Block the uncontrolled cell growth associated with cancer, most likely by inhibiting the activity of substances in the body that regulate cell division and cell survival (growth factors).
v. Studies show that groups of people who eat large amounts of soy-based products have lower incidences of breast, colon, endometrial, and prostate cancers than the general (US) population.
vi. Inhibition of protein tyrosine kinases (PTK) (Srivastava, 1985).
vii. Blocking the PLC activation and formation of inositol trisphosphate (IP3) and diacylglycerol (DAG) (Gil et al., 1994).

Research

i. Initial studies of soy isoflavone mixtures containing genistein, daidzein, and glycitein have found them safe for human use. Laboratory studies using animals models have shown that both soy and isoflavones can be protective against cancer when given during early life but can stimulate response to cancer-causing chemicals when given during fetal development or when circulating levels of estrogen are low (menopause).
ii. Some recent studies have raised the concern that genistein might potentially increase the

risk of leukemia, because it can inhibit an enzyme topoisomerase that protects DNA from mutation.

iii. Genistein influences several targets in living cells. One important function is the inhibition of several tyrosine kinase.

iv. Genistein inhibits the mammalian hexose transporter GLUT1 and contraction of several types of smooth muscles.

v. Genistein can bind to CFTR receptors. This binding causes the channel to become permanently open causing "free-flow" of chloride ions through the channel.

Daidzein is one of several known isoflavones.

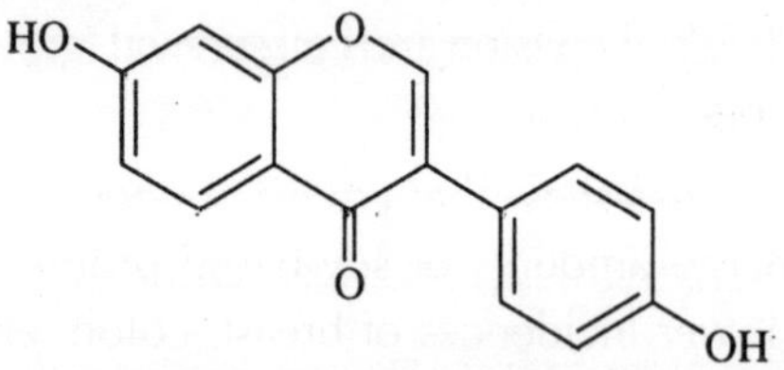

Fig. 22.10. Daidzein; 7-Hydroxy-3- (4-hydroxyphenyl) chromen-4-one (4′, 7-Dihydroxyisoflavone, Daidzeol, Isoaurostatin)

Source

Soybeans and soy products like tofu, and textured vegetable protein.

Coumestrol is a natural organic compound in the class of phytochemicals known as coumestans. It has garnered research interest because of its estrogenic activity and its prevalence in some foods, such as soybeans. Coumestrol was first identified by E. M. Bickoff in alfalfa in 1957.

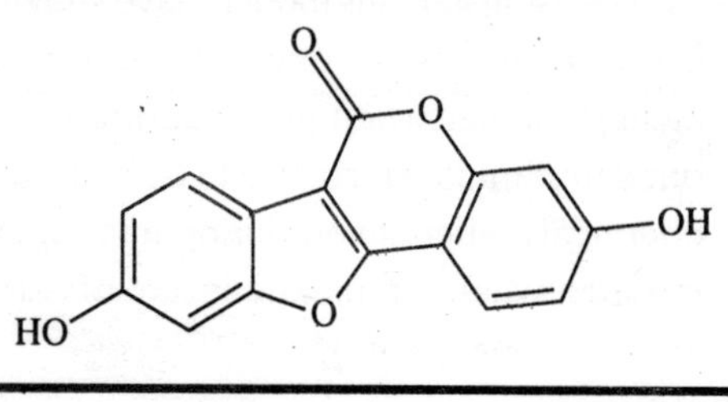

Fig. 22.11. Coumestrol; 3,9-Dihydroxy-6-benzofurano [3,2-c] chromenone

Source

Legumes, soybeans, brussel sprouts, spinach and clover.

Functions

i. Coumestrol is a phytoestrogens, mimicking the biological activity of estrogens.

ii. The chemical shape of coumestrol orients its two hydroxy groups in the same position as the two hydroxy groups in estradiol, allowing it to inhibit the activity of aromatase and hydroxysteroid dehydrogenase. These enzymes are involved in the biosynthesis of steroid hormones, and inhibition of these enzymes results in the modulation of hormone production.

Biochanin A

Biochanin A belongs to the isoflavone class of flavonoids. It is also classified as a phytoestrogen since it is a plant-derived nonsteroidal compound that possesses estrogen-like biological activity. Biochanin A has been found to have weak estrogenic activity. It is a solid substance that is virtually insoluble in water. Its molecular formula is $C_{16}H_{12}O_5$. It is the 4′-methyl ether of genistein. Biochanin A is also known as 5, 7-dihydroxy-4′-methoxyisoflavone and 5, 7-dihydroxy-4′ -methoxy-3- (4-hydroxyphenyl)-4*H*-1-benzopyran-4-one (Gotoh et al., 1998).

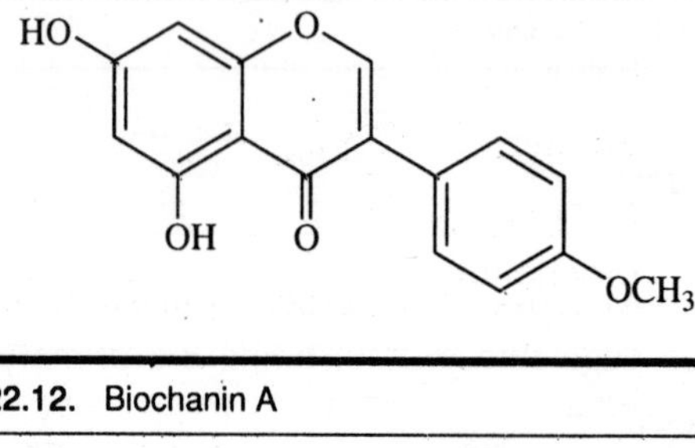

Fig. 22.12. Biochanin A

Sources

Soy products and certain legumes, most notably red clover or *Trifolium pratense*. Red clover contains, in addition to biochanin A, the isoflavones genistein, daidzein and formononetin (methoxy daidzein). These isoflavones are present in red clover in the form of glycosides. However, when the leaves are crushed during the preparation of red clover isoflavone extracts, the glycosides undergo enzymatic hydrolysis, and the final preparation principally contains the aglycones.

Actions

i. Estrogenic
ii. Antioxidant
iii. Anticarcinogenic
iv. Anti-atherogenic
v. Anti-osteoporotic
vi. In comparison with other isoflavones, such as genistein and daidzein, biochanin A might be expected to have possible anti-osteoporotic activity. This might be due, in part, to its weak estrogenic activity.

Precautions

i. Pregnant women and nursing mothers should avoid the use of biochanin A-containing supplements.
ii. Women with estrogen receptor-positive tumors should exercise caution in the use of biochanin A-containing supplements and should use them only if they are recommended and monitored by a physician.

Puerarin

8-beta-D-Glucopyranosyl-7-hydroxy-3-(4-hydroxyphenyl)-4H-1-benzopyran-4-one

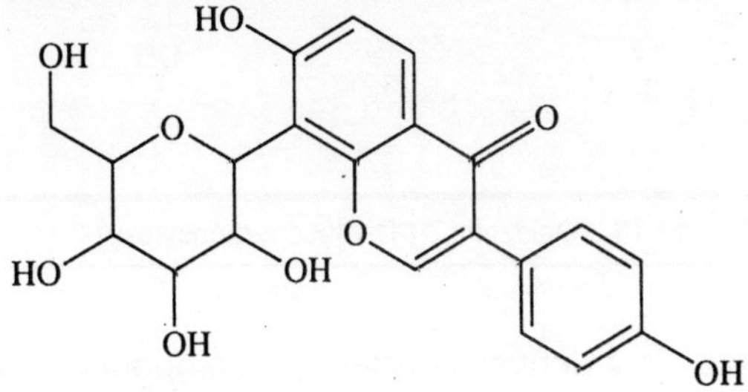

Fig. 22.13. Puerarin

Formononetin

7-Hydroxy-3-(42-methoxyphenyl)-4H-benzopyran-4-one; 7-Hydroxy-3-(4-methoxyphenyl) chromone; 7-Hydroxy-4'-methoxyisoflavone; Dadein 4'-methyl ether. A non-steroidal phytoestrogenic isoflavone found in soy-based food products. Has been shown to interact with human estrogen receptor with relatively low potency. Induces mammary gland proliferation in mice. Inhibits lecithin peroxidation induced by hydroxyl radicals. Also acts as a selective inhibitor of g-isoform of alcohol dehydrogenase.

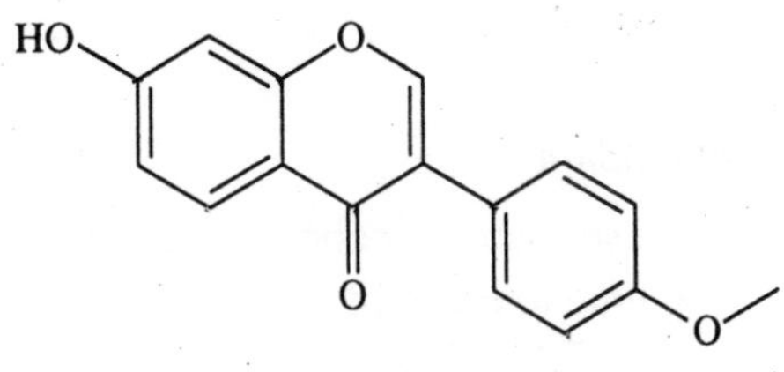

Fig. 22.14. Formononetin

Daidzein

Daidzein is the aglycone (aglucon) of daidzin. Daidzein is an isoflavone and a phytoestrogen. It

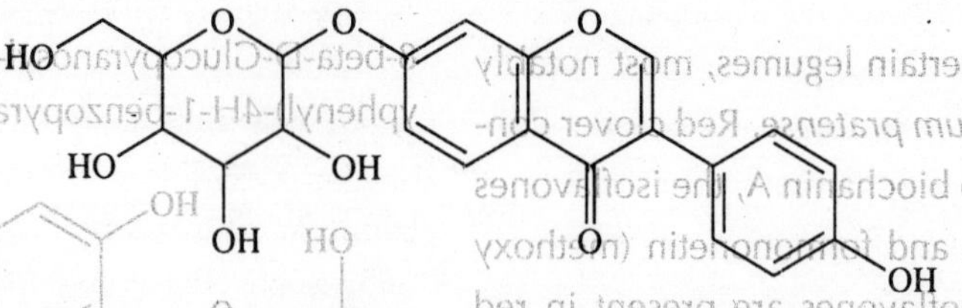

Fig. 22.15. Daidzein; 7-(-D-Glucopyranosyloxy)-3-(4-hydroxyphenyl)-4H-1-benzopyran-4-one; Daidzein-7-*O*-glucoside

is a plant-derived nonsteriodal compound. Daidzein is found naturally as the glycoside daidzin and as the glycosides 6″-O-malonylgenistin and 6″-O-acetyldaidzin. Daidzein is a solid substance that is insoluble in water whereas daidzin demonstrates some water solubility. When in nutritional supplements, Daidzein often appears as daidzin, in a beta-glucoside form. White to beige powder, which is soluble in DMSO or dilute aqueous base and insoluble in water.

Sources

Legumes, such as soybeans and chickpeas and *Radix puerariae*, an old Chinese herbal medicine made from the roots of Kudzu.

Uses

i. Antioxidant
ii. Decreases blood alcohol levels and shortens sleep time induced by ethanol intoxication.

Flavonols (3-hydroxyflav*ones*) are a class of flavonoids that use the 3-hydroxyflavone backbone (3-hydroxy-2-phenylchromen-4-one (IUPAC)). Their diversity stems from the different positions of the phenolic -OH groups. It inhibits phosphodiesterases activity and involved in regulation of many cellular processes, such as cell division (Beretz et al., 1986).

Myricetin is a naturally-occurring flavonoid. It is commonly found in the form of glycosides, such as myricitrin.

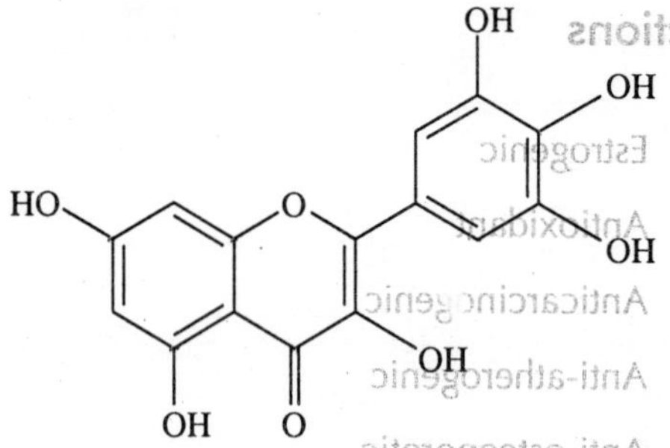

3,5,7-Trihydroxy-2-(3,4,5-trihydroxyphenyl)-4-chromenone

Fig. 22.16. Myricetin

Sources

Grapes, berries, fruits, vegetables, and walnuts

Functions

i. Antioxidant properties.
ii. In vitro research suggests that myricetin in high concentrations can modify LDL cholesterol such that uptake by white blood cells is increased.
iii. A Finish study correlated high myricetin consumption with lowered rates of prostate cancer.

iv. Increasing the DNA-enzyme complex in L1210 cells and interfering with enzyme-induced DNA relaxation (Wei et al., 1995).

Quercetin is a flavonoid and, to be more specific, a flavonol. It is the aglycone form of a number of other flavonoid glycosides, such as rutin and quercitrin, found in citrus fruit. Quercetin forms the glycosides quercitrin and rutin together with rhamnose and rutinose, respectively. Quercetin is found to be the most active of the flavonoids in studies, and many medicinal plants owe much of their activity to their high quercetin content.

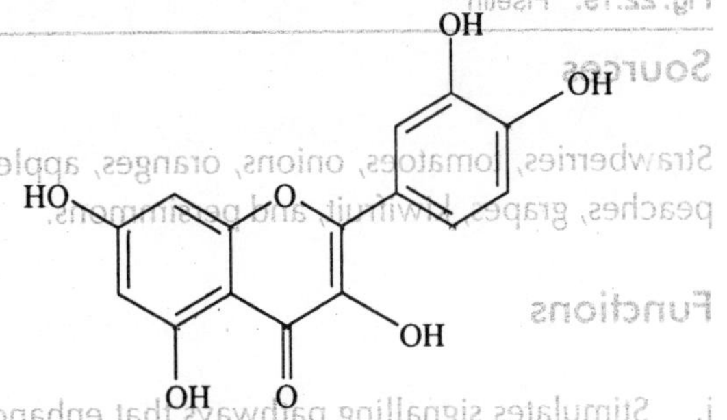

3,3′,4′,5,7-pentahydroxy-2-phenylchromen-4-one

Fig. 22.17. Quercetin

Functions

i. Quercetin has demonstrated significant anti-inflammatory activity because of direct inhibition of several initial processes of inflammation by inhibiting both the synthesis and release of histamine and other allergic/inflammatory mediators.
ii. It exerts potent antioxidant activity and vitamine C-sparing action.
iii. Quercetin also shows anti-tumour properties.
iv. A study showed that, when treated with a combination of quercetin and ultrasound at 20 kHz for 1 minute duration, skin and prostate cancers show a 90% mortality within 48 hours with no visible mortality of normal cells. Ultrasound promotes topical absorption by up to 1,000 times making the use of topical quercetin.
v. Recent studies have supported that quercetin can help men with chronic prostatitis, and both men and women with interstitial cystitis, possibly because of its action as a mast cell inhibitor.
vi. Quercetin may have positive effects in combating or helping to prevent cancer, prostatitis, heart disease, cataracts, allergies/inflammations, and respiratory diseases such as bronchitis and asthma.
vii. In plants, it is a naturally-occurring polar auxin transport inhibitor.
viii. Inhibitory action on both xanthine oxidase and xanthine dehydrogenase activity and reduced brain tumor (Klopman & Dimayuga, 1988; Hayashi et al., 1988).

Occurrence

Capers (1800mg/kg), lovage (1700mg/kg), apples (440mg/kg), tea (*Cemellia sinensis*), onions (higher concentrations of quercetin occur in the outermost rings), red grapes, citrus fruits, leafy green vegetables, cherries, raspberry, bog whortleberry (158 mg/kg, fresh weight), lingonberry (cultivated 74mg/kg, wild 146 mg/kg), cranberry (cultivated 83 mg/kg, wild 121 mg/kg), chokeberry (89 mg/kg), sweet rowan (85 mg/kg), rowanberry (63 mg/kg), sea buckthorn berry (62 mg/kg), crowberry (cultivated 53mg/kg, wild 56 mg/kg), fruit of the prickly pear cactus, a recent study found that organically grown tomatoes had 79% more quercetin than conventionally grown, honey, including honey derived from eucalyptus and tea tree flowers.

Drug interactions

i. ***Quercetin*** is contraindicated with antibiotics; it may interact with fluoroquinolones, as quercetin competitively binds to bacterial DNA gyrase. Whether this inhibits or enhances the effect of fluoroquinolones is not entirely clear.

ii. Quercetin is also a potent inhibitor of CYP3A4, an enzyme that breaks down most drugs in the body.

Kaempferol is a natural flavonoid, which is a yellow crystalline solid with a melting point 276-278 °C. It is slightly soluble in water but soluble in hot ethanol and diethyl ether. Many glycosides of kaempferol, such as kaemferitin and astragalin, have been isolated as natural products from plants.

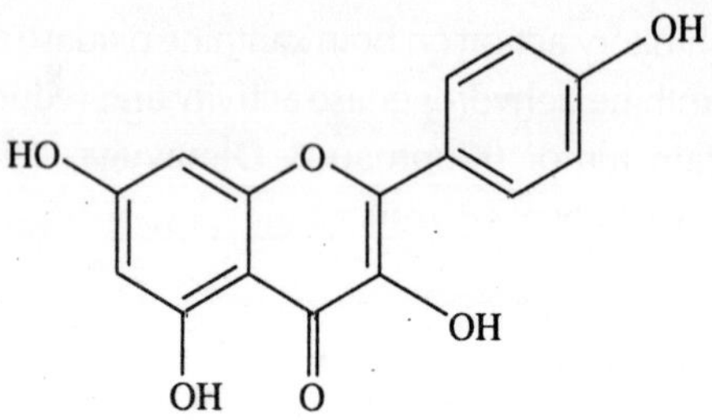

Fig. 22.18. Kaempferol; 3,5,7-trihydroxy-2-(4-hydroxyphenyl)-4H-1-benzopyran-4-one

Sources

Tea, broccoli, delphinium, witch-hazel, and grapefruit.

Functions

i. Kaemphferol consumption in tea and broccoli has been associated with reduced risk of heart disease.
ii. Kaempferol is what gives the flowers of Acacia decurrens and Acacia longifolia their color.
iii. Inhibit the aromatase enzyme activity competitively in a human Glyoxalase cell culture system (Kellis & Vickery, 1984).
iv. Tumor cell inhibition by breaking glucosaminidic bonds (Thull & Testa, 1994).

Fisetin: Naturally occurring flavonoids.

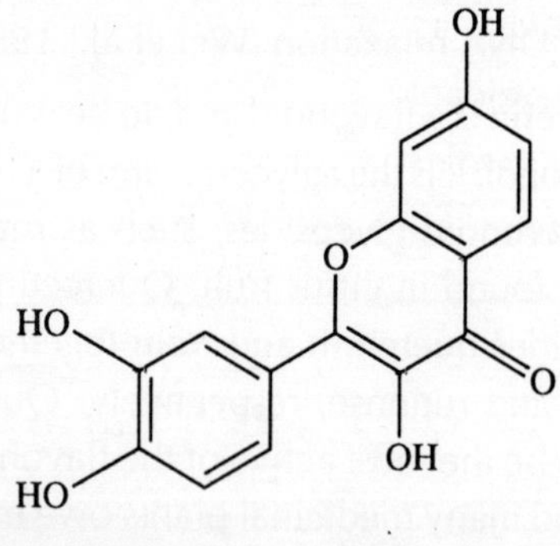

Fig. 22.19. Fisetin

Sources

Strawberries, tomatoes, onions, oranges, apples, peaches, grapes, kiwifruit, and persimmons.

Functions

i. Stimulates signalling pathways that enhance long-term memory.
ii. Nevertheless, memory-enhancing drugs can improve Alzheimer's disease symptoms.
iii. Replication of HIV-I inhibited by inhibiting enzyme activity (Varma, 1986).
iv. Inhibition of nonactivated phosphorylase kinase (Alexandrakis et al., 1999).

Isorhamnetin: Naturally occurring flavonoids. It is a yellow solid which is soluble in acetone, methanol, ethylacetate, DMSO and water.

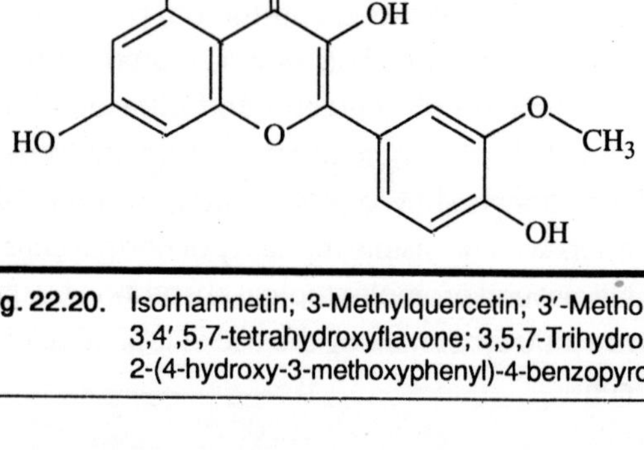

Fig. 22.20. Isorhamnetin; 3-Methylquercetin; 3′-Methoxy-3,4′,5,7-tetrahydroxyflavone; 3,5,7-Trihydroxy-2-(4-hydroxy-3-methoxyphenyl)-4-benzopyrone

Uses

i. Antiviral agent

ii. Antioxidant

iii. Antitumor compound

iv. Apoptosis inducer

Rhamnazin

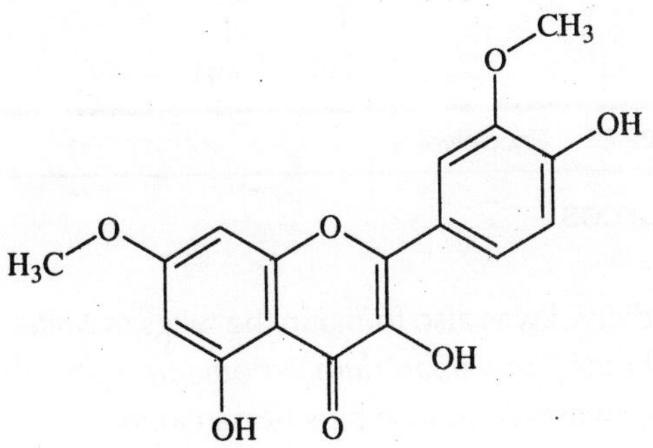

Fig. 22.21. Rhamnazin

Pachypodol

4H-1-Benzopyran-4-one, 5-hydroxy-2-(4-hydroxy-3-methoxyphenyl)-3,7-dimethoxy

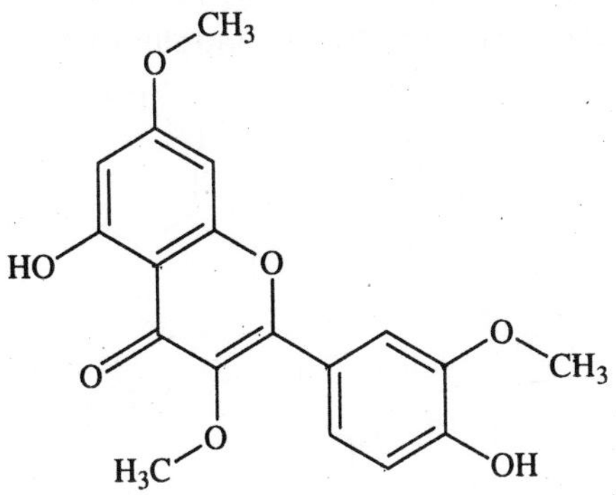

Fig. 22.22. Pachypodol

Flavanones: Flavan*ones* use the 2,3-dihydro-2-phenylchromen-*4-one* skeleton. Examples: Hesperetin, Naringenin, Eriodictyol, Homoeriodictyol (Gotoh et al., 1998).

Hesperetin: Hesperetin belongs to the flavanone class of flavonoids. Hesperetin, in the form of its glycoside hesperidin, is the predominant flavonoid in lemons and oranges.

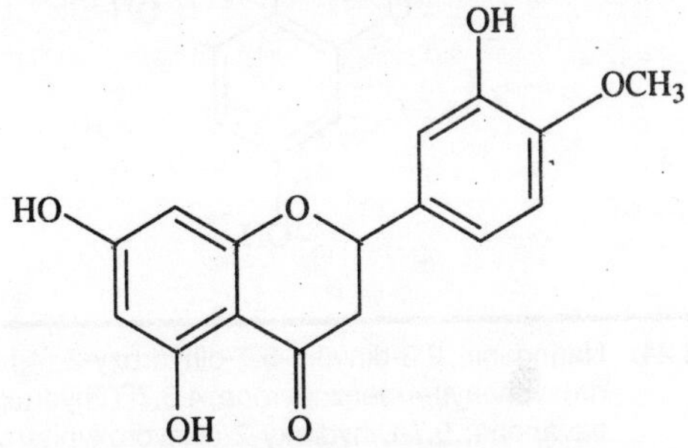

Fig. 22.23. Hesperetin; (S)-2,3-dihydro-5,7-dihydroxy-2-(3-hydroxy-4-methoxyphenyl)-4H-1-benzopyran-4-one

Sources

Number of citrus juices.

Uses

i. Antioxidant

ii. Anti-aromatase activity

iii. Cholesterol lowering

iv. Anti-allergic

v. Hypolipidemic

vi. Vasoprotective

vii. Anticarcinogenic

viii. Vasodilator effects of hesperetin is basically due to the inhibition of PDE1 and PDE4 activities, which may be useful in hypertension

Naringenin: Naringenin is a flavonone. It is a yellow crystalline powder having melting point:

247–250 C. Naringin is the aglycones of naringenin. Naringin is known as an antioxidant in the body. Unfortunately, this bioflavonoid is difficult to absorb on oral ingestion.

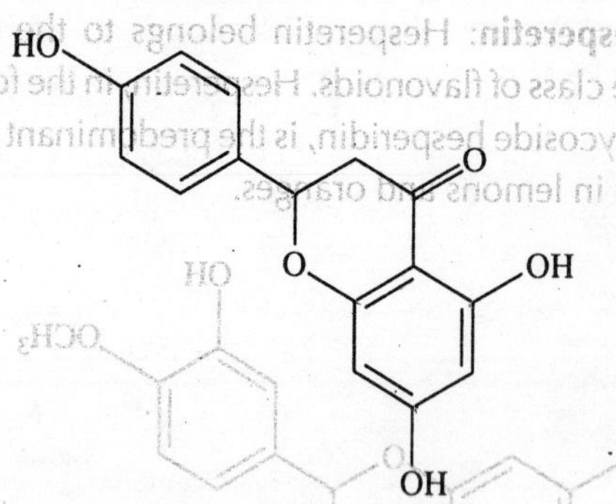

Fig. 22.24. Naringenin; 2,3-dihydro-5,7-dihydroxy-2-(4-hydroxyphenyl)-4-benzopyrone; 4,5,7-Trihydroxyflavanone; 5,7-Dihydroxy-2-(4-hydroxyphenyl) chroman-4-one

Sources

Grapefruit juice.

Functions

i. Antioxidant
ii. Free radical scavenger
iii. Anti-inflammatory
iv. Carbohydrate metabolism promoter
v. Immunity system modulator
vi. Anti-ulcer agent
vii. Estrogen antagonist, which inhibit the action or biosynthesis of estrogenic compounds
viii. Antihypertensive
ix. In treatment of Alzheimer's disease
x. Reduce oxidative damage to DNA in vitro

Eriodictyol: A colorless crystalline compound $C_{15}H_{12}O_6$ derived from flavanone and found especially in the leaves of some resinous shrubs of the genus *Eriodictyon*. Eriodictyol is one of the 4 flavanones identified by Symrise in this plant eliciting taste-modifying properties: homoeriodictyol, its sodium salt and sterubin.

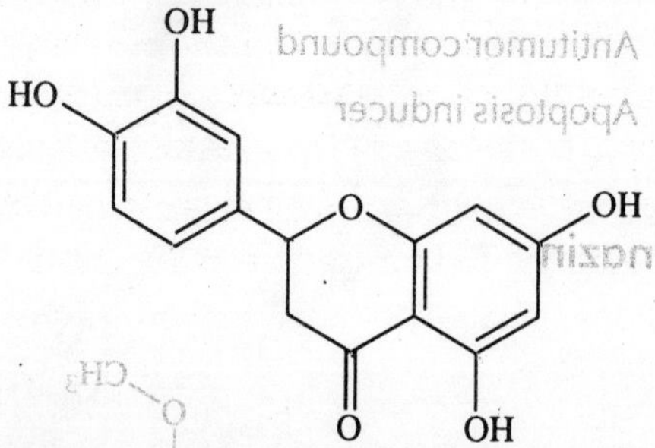

Fig. 22.25. Eriodictyol

Sources

Eriodictyol was also found in the twigs of *Millettia duchesnei*, in *Eupatorium arnottianum* and one of its glycoside in rose hips (*Rosa canina*).

Uses

Bitter-masking.

Homoeriodictyol is a bitter-masking flavanones extracted from Herba Santa (*Eriodictyon californicum*) a plant growing in America. Homoeriodictyol (3′-methoxy-4′,5,7-trihydroxyflavanone) is one of the 4 flavanones identified by Symrise in this plant eliciting taste-modifying: homoeriodictyol sodium salt, eriodictyol and sterubin.

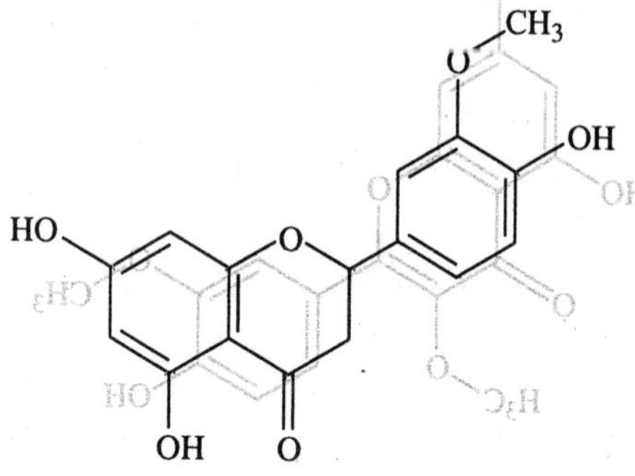

Fig. 22.26. Homoeriodictyol; (2S)-5,7-dihydroxy-2-(4-hydroxy-3-methoxy-phenyl) chroman-4-one

Uses

Homoeriodictyol Sodium salt elicited the most potent bitter-masking activity by reducing from 10 to 40% the bitterness of salicin, amarogentin, paracetamol and quinine. However no bitter-masking activity was detected with bitter linoleic acid emulsions. According to Symrise's scientists homoeriodictyol sodium salt seems to be a taste-modifier with large potential in food applications and pharmaceuticals.

Flavan-3-ols

Flavan-3-ols use the 2-phenyl-3, 4-dihydro-2H-chromen-3-ol skeleton.

Examples: Catechins (C), Gallocatechin (GC), Catechin 3-gallate (Cg), Gallocatechin 3-gallate (GCg), picatechins (EC), Epigallocatechin (EGC), Epicatechin 3-gallate (ECg), Epigallocatechin 3-gallatc (EGCg).

Catechins are polyphenolic antioxidant plant metabolites, specifically flavonoids called flavan-3-ols.

Source

Various teas derived from the tea-plant *Camellia sinensis* including white tea, green tea, black tea and Oolonga tea, chocolate, fruits, vegetables and wine.

Catechin, epicatechin, gallocatechin, epigallocatechin, and the gallates

i. Catechin and epicatechin are epimers, with (-)-epicatechin and (+)-catechin being the most common optical isomers found in nature. Catechin was first isolated from the plant extract catechu, from which it derives its name. Heating catechin past its point of decomposition releases pyrocatechol, which explains the common origin of the names of these compounds.

ii. Epigallocatechin and gallocatechin contain an additional phenolic hydroxyl group when compared to epicatechin and catechin, respectively, similar to the difference in pyrogallol compared to pyrocatechol.

iii. Catechin gallates are gallic acid esters of the catechins; such as EGCG (epigallocatechin gallate), which is commonly the most abundant catechin in tea.

Uses

i. Reduction in atherosclerotic plaques was seen in animal models.

ii. Reduction in carcinogenesis was seen *in vitro*.

iii. Epicatechin can reduce the risk of four of the major health problems: stroke, heart failure, cancer and diabetes.

iv. Epigallocatechin-3-gallate is an antioxidant that helps protect the skin from UV radiation-induced damage and tumor formation.

v. Green tea catechins have also been shown to possess antibiotic properties due to their role in disrupting a specific stage of the bacterial DNA replication process.

vi. The simultaneous induction of CYP1A2 and UGT activities (Ferrandiz et al., 1990).

vii. Inhibited the activity of histidine decarboxylase (Kuppusamy et al., 1990).

viii. Inhibit NO synthase isomer enzymes activity (Lowenstein & Snyder, 1992).

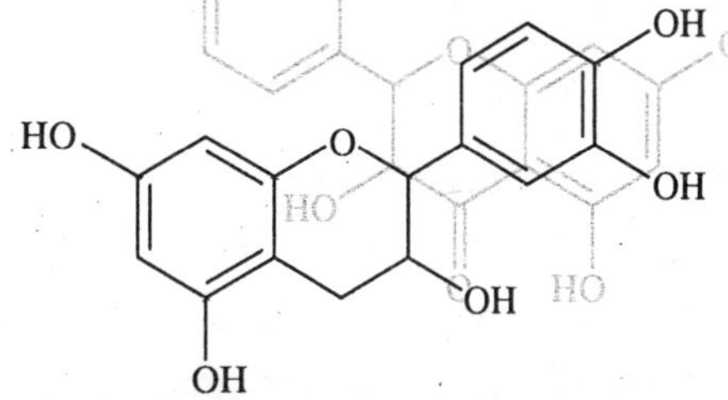

Fig. 22.27. Epicatechin (EC)

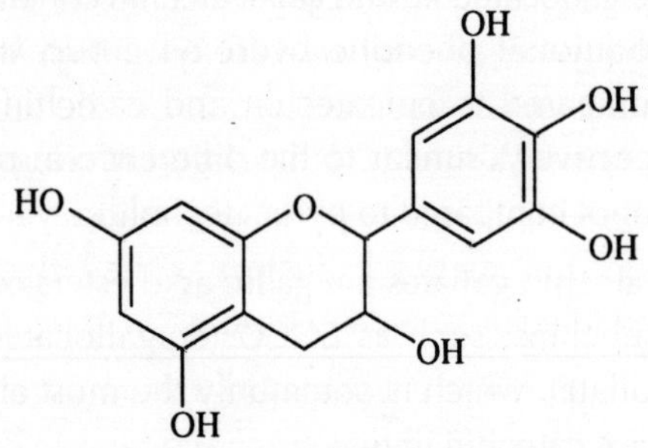

Fig. 22.28. Epigallocatechin (EGC)

3-Hydroxyflavanones

Dihydroquercetin

Uses

i. Two directions of use dihydroquercetin in food industry: as antioxidant and as biologically active supplement for creation different types of parapharmaceutical production is shown.
ii. High antioxidant activity of dihydroquercetin is combined with absence embryotoxicity, teratogenicity, allergenicity and mutability.
iii. Parapharmaceutical production with dihydroquercetin is intended for prophylactic of "oxidative stress" diseases (cardiovascular, bronchopulmonary, etc.).

Dihydrokaempferol

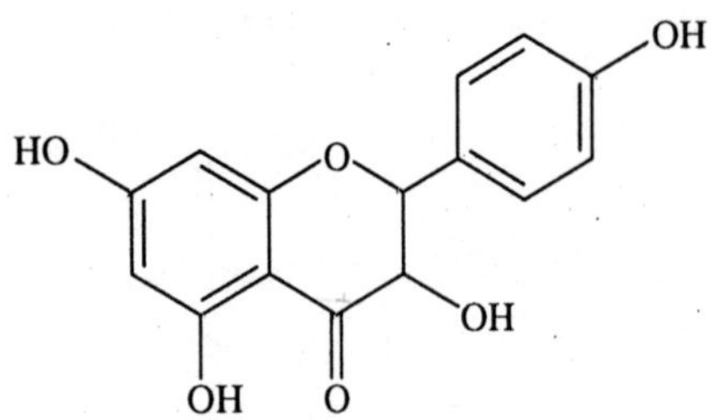

Fig. 22.29. Dihydrokaempferol

Anthocyanins

Anthocyanins (from Greek: *anthos* = flower + *kyanos* = blue) are water soluble vacuolar favonoid pigments that appear red to blue, according to pH. They are synthesized by organisms of the plant kingdom, and have been observed to occur in all tissues of higher plants, providing color in leaves, stems, roots, flowers and fruits.

Functions

i. In flowers, bright reds and purples due to anthocyanin pigments help attract pollinators. In fruits, the colorful skins also attract the attention of animals, which may eat the fruits and disperse the seeds.
ii. In photosynthetic tissues (such as leaves and sometimes stems), anthocyanins have been shown to act as a "sunscreen", protecting cells from high-light damage by absorbing blue-green light, thereby protecting the tissues from photoinhibition, or high-light stress. This has been shown to occur in red juvenile leaves, autumn leaves, and broad-leaved evergreen leaves that turn red during the winter.
iii. It has also been proposed that red coloration of leaves may camouflage leaves from herbivores blind to red wavelengths, or signal unpalatability, since anthocyanin synthesis often coincides with synthesis of unpalatable phenolic compounds.
iv. In addition to their role as light-attenuators, anthocyanins also act as powerful antioxidants.

Anthocyanidins: Flavylium cation derivatives

Occurrence

i. Anatomically, anthocyanins are found in the cell vacuole, mostly in flowers and fruits and also in leaves, stems, and roots. In these parts they are found predominantly in outer cell layers such as the epidermis and peripheral mesophyll cells.

ii. Other plants rich in anthocyanins are black-current, chokeberry, cherry, eggplant, blue grape, Vaccinium and red cabbage and also the Usambara-violet.

iii. Anthocyanins are less abundant in banana, asparagus, pea, fennel, pear and potato.

iv. Most frequent in nature are the glycosides of cyanidin, delphinidin, malvidin, pelargonidin, peonidin and petunidin.

v. Roughly 2% of all hydrocarbons fixated in photosynthesis are converted into flavonoids and their derivatives such as the anthocyanins. This is not less than 10^9 tons per year.

The pigment components of anthocyanidins, the sugar-free anthocyanins, can be identified based on the structure of a large group of polymethine dye, the benzopyrylium (chromenylium) ion. In particular anthocyanidins are salt derivatives of the 2-phenylchromenylium cation also known as flavylium cation. As shown in the figure below, the phenyl group at the 2-position, can carry different substituents. The counterion of the flavylium cation is mostly chloride. With this positive charge the anthocyanins differ from other flavonoids.

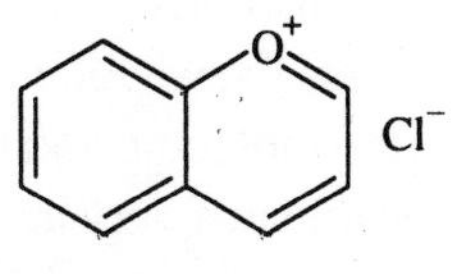

Fig. 22.30. Benzopyrylium (chromenylium) salts with chloride as the counterion

Anthocyanins: Glucosides of anthocyanidins

The anthocyanins, and anthocyanidins with sugar group, are mostly 3-glucosides of the anthocyanidins. The anthocyanins are subdivided into the sugar-free anthocyanidin aglycones and the anthocyanin glycosides. As of 2006 more than 550 anthocyanins had been reported. The difference in chemical structure that occurs in response to changes in pH is the reason why anthocyanins are often used as pH indicator, as they change from red in acids to blue in bases.

More than five enzymes are thus required to synthesize these pigments, each working in concert. Any even minor disruption in any of the mechanism of these enzymes by either genetic or environmental factors would halt anthocyanin production.

Uses

i. Food additives

ii. Powerful antioxidants

iii. Scientists provided laboratory evidence for potential health effects against
   - cancer
   - aging and neurological diseases
   - inflammation
   - diabetes
   - bacterial infections

Cyanidin is a natural organic compound which is classified as a flavonoid and an anthocyanin.

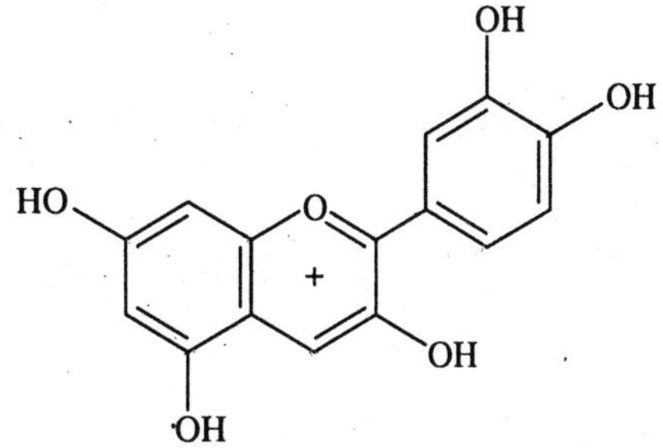

Fig. 22.31. Cyanidin

Sources

Grapes, bilberry, blackberry, blueberry, cherry, cranberry, elderberry, hawthorn, loganberry, raspberry, apples, plums, red cabbage, the highest concentrations of cyanidin are found in the skin of the fruit, and biosynthesis of cyanidin 3-O-glucoside in *Escherichia coli* was demonstrated.

Uses

i. antioxidant effects which protect cells from oxidative damage and reduces the risk of heart diseases and cancer.

ii. cyanidin may aid in preventing obesity and diabetes

iii. anti-inflammatory effects

iv. important future role in cancer therapy

Malvidin is an anthocyanidin. As a primary plant pigment, its glycosides are highly abundant in nature. Slightly acidic and neutral solutions of malvidin are characteristically of a red color, while basic solutions of malvidin yield a blue color.

Sources

It is primarily responsible for the color of red wine, *Vitis vinifera* being one of its sources. It is also one of the anthocyanidins responsible for the blue pigment found in the *Primula polyanthus* plant.

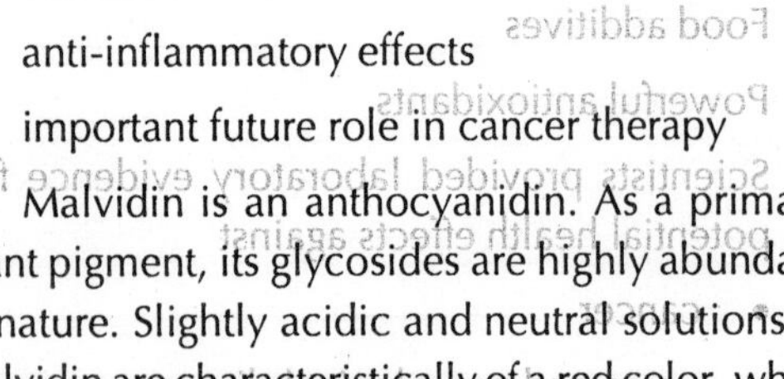

Fig. 22.32. Malvidin; 2-(4-hydroxy-3,5-dimethoxyphenyl) chromenylium-3,5,7-triol

Delphinidin is an anthocyanidin and a primary plant pigment. Delphinidin gives blue hues to flowers like violas and delphiniums. It also gives the blue-red color of the grape and can be found in cranberries and concord grapes.

Delphinidin, like nearly all other anthocyanidins is pH sensitive, and changes from blue in basic solution to red in acidic solution.

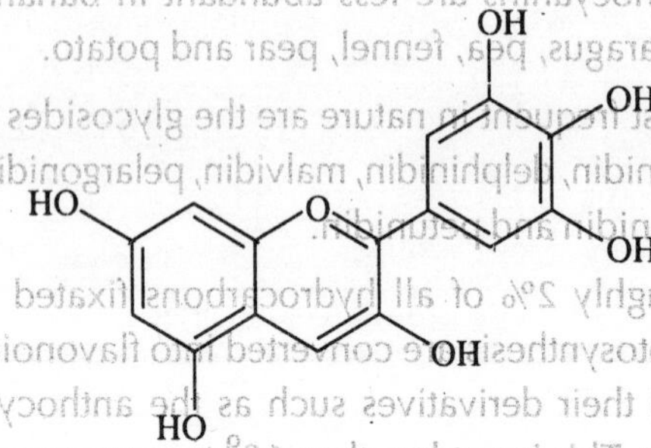

Fig. 22.33. Delphinidin

Peonidin is an anthocyanidin and a primary plant pigment. Peonidin gives purplish-red hues to flowers such as the peony, from which it takes its name, and roses. It is also present in some blue flowers, such as the morning glory.

Like most anthocyanidins it is pH sensitive, and changes from red to blue as pH rises. This happens because anthocynaidins are highly conjugated chromophores. When the pH is changed, the extent of the conjugation (of the double bonds) is altered, which alters the wavelength of light energy absorbed by the molecule. (Natural anthocyanidins are most stable in a very low pH environment; at pH 8.0, most become colorless.) At pH 2.0, peonidin is cherry red; at 3.0 a strong yellowish pink; at 5.0 it is grape red-purple; and at 8.0 it becomes deep blue; unlike many anthocyanidins, however, it is stable at higher pH, and has in fact been isolated as a blue colorant from the brilliant "Heavenly Blue" morning glory (*Ipomoea tricolor Cav cv*). A very large question, however, has been raised about anthocyanidins' penetration and retention in human cells *in vivo*, due to their rapid elimination from the human body.

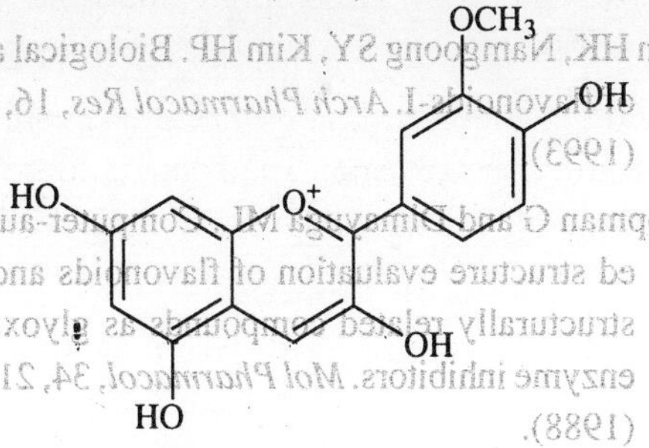

Fig. 22.34. Peonidin

Use

Peonidin, like many anthodcyanidins, has show potent inhibitory and apoptotic effects on cancer cells *in vitro*, notably metastatic human breast cancer cells.

Source

i. Cranberries, Blueberries, plums, grapes, and cherries also contain significant amounts, ranging from 5 to 12 mg/100g.

ii. Only fresh fruit has been shown to contain significant peonidin.

iii. It has also been isolated from raw black rice and black bananas.

BIBLIOGRAPHY

Alexandrakis M, Singh L, Boucher W, Letourneau R, Theoflopoulos P. and Theoharides TC. Differential effects of flavonoids on inhibition of secretion and on accumulation of secretory granules in rat basophilic leukemia cells. Int J Immunopharmacol, 21, 379-390 (1999).

Beretz A, Anton R, Cazenave JP. The effects of flavonoids on cyclic nucleotide phosphodiesterases. In: Cody V, Middleton E and Harborne JB: Plant Flavonoids in Biology and Medicine: Biochemical, Pharmacological and Structure-Activity Relationships. Alan R. Liss, Inc., New York, Vol. 1, 281-296, (1986).

Brenner GM. Pharmacology WB. Saunders Company, Philadelphia, (2000).

Carlo GD, Autore G, IZZOAA, Moiolino P, Mascolo N, Viola P, Diurno MV, Capawa F. Inhibition of intestinal motility and secretion by flavonoids in mice and rats; structure-activity relationships. *J Pham Pharmacol*, 45, 1045-1059, (1993).

Danielsson G, Jungbeck C, Peterson K, Norgren L. A randomized controlled trial of micronized purified flavonoid fraction vs placebo in patients with chronic venous disease. *Eur J Vasc Endovasc Surg*, 23, 73-76 (2002).

De-Whalley C, Rankin SM, Houct JRS, Jessup W, Leake DS. Flavonoids inhibit the oxidative modification of low density lipoproteins by macrophages. *Biochem Pharmacol*, 39, 1743-1750, (1990).

Evans WC. Pharmacognosy, Saunders Publishers, China, 15th Edn., pp. 246-247, (2005).

Ferrandiz ML, Ramachandran Nair AG. and Alcaraz MJ. Effect of flavonoids from Spanish and Indian medicinal herbs on arachidonate metabolism in rat peritoneal leukocytes. Pharmazie, 45, 444-445, (1990).

Francel EN, Kanner J, German JB, Packs E, Kinsella JE. Inhibition of oxidation of human low-density lipoprotein by phenolis substances in red wine. *Lancet*, 341, 454-457, (1993).

Fritz B, Tobias S, Albrecht K, Chaelotte B, Kent C, *et al.* Selected novel flavones inhibit the DNA binding or the DNA religation step of eukaryotic topoisomerase-I. *J Biol Chem*, 271. 2262-2270, (1996).

Gil B, Sanz MJ, Terencio M, Ferrandiz ML, Bustos G, Paya M, Gunasegaran R. and Alcaraz MJ. Effects of flavonoids on Naja naja and human recombinant synovial phospholipase A2 and inflammatory responses in mice. *Life Sci*, 54, 333-338 (1994).

Gill B, Sanz MJ, Terencio MC, Ferrandiz ML, Bustos G, Paya M. The flavonoids. *Life Sci*, 54, 333-339, (1994).

Gotoh T, Yamada K, Yin H, et al. Chemoprevention of N-nitroso-N-methylurea-induced rat mammary carcinogenesis by soy foods or biochanin *A. Jpn J Cancer Res*, 89, 137-142, (1998).

Griebel G, Perrault G, Tan S, Schoemarker H, Sanger DJ. Pharmacological studies on synthetic flavonoids: comparison with diazepam. *Neuropharmacology, 38*, 965-977, (1999).

Griffith LA, Ballow A. The fate of orally and parenterally administered flavonoids in the mammal, the significance of biliary excretion. *Angiologica*, 9, 162-174, (1972).

Gugler R and Dengler HJ. Inhibition of human liver catechol-O-methyltransferase by flavonoids. *Naunyn-Schmiedeberg's Arch Pharmacol, 276*, 223-233 (1973).

Hayashi T, Sawa K, Kawasaki M, Arisawa M, Shlmizu M and Morita N. Inhibition of cow's milk xanthine oxidase by flavonoids. *J Nat Prod*, 51, 345-348 (1988).

Hirano T, Gotoh M, Oak K. Natural flavonoids and lignans are plant cytostatic agents against Human Leukemic HL-60 cells. *Life Sci*, 55, 1061-1069, (1994).

Huesken BCP, Dejong J, Beekman B, Onderwater RCA. Flavonoids as cardio protective agents. *CancerChemother Pharmacol*, 37, 55-62, (1995)

Husain SR, Cillard J, Cillard P. Hydroxy radical scavenging activity of flavonoids. *Phytochemistry*, 26, 2489-2492, (1987).

Itoigawa M, Takeya K, Ito C, Furu Kawa H. Structure activity relationship of cardiotonic flavonoids in guinea pig papillary muscle. *J Ethnopharmacol*, 65, 267-272, (1999).

Kellis JT and Vickery LE. Inhibition of human estrogen synthetase (aromatase) by flavones. *Science*, 225, 1032-1034, (1984).

Kim HK, Namgoong SY, Kim HP. Biological actions of flavonoids-I. *Arch Pharmacol Res*, 16, 18-27, (1993).

Klopman G and Dimayuga ML. Computer-automated structure evaluation of flavonoids and other structurally related compounds as glyoxalase I enzyme inhibitors. *Mol Pharmacol*, 34, 218-222, (1988).

Kuppusamy UR, Khoo HE and Das NP. Structure-activity studies of flavonoids as inhibitors of hyaluronidase. Biochem Pharmacol, 40, 397-401, (1990).

Lackeman GM, Claeys M, Rwangabo PC, Herman AG, Vlietinck A. Chronotropic effect of quercetin on guinea pigright atrium. *J Planta Med, 52*, 433-439, (1986).

Laughton MJ, Halliwell B, Evans PJ, Hoult JRS. Antioxidant and pro-oxidant actions of the plant phenolics quercetin, morin, glossypol and myricetin effects on lipid peroxidation, hydroxy radical generation and bleomycin dependent damage to DNA. *Biochem Pharmacol, 38*, 2859-2865, (1989).

Lorenz W, Kusche J, Barth H, Mathias CH. Action of several flavonoids on enzyme of histidine metabolism *in vitro. In Histamine*, pp. 265-269 (Ed. Cz. Maslinski) Dowden, Hutchinson and Ross. Stroudsberg. Pennsylvania, (1973).

Lowenstein CJ. and Snyder SH. Nitric oxide, a novel biologic messenger. Cell, 70, 705-707 (1992).

Mann J. Secondary Metabolism. Oxford University Press, Oxford, UK, 2nd edition, pp. 279-280, (1992).

Mc Anlis GT, Mc Enany J, Pearce J, Young IY. The effect of various dietary flavonoids on the susceptibility of low-density lipoproteins to oxidation *in vitro* using both metallic and nonmetallic oxidising agents. *Biochem Soc Trans*, 25, 142-148, (1997).

Nikaidou S, Ishizuka M, Maeda Y, Hara Y, Kazusaska A, Fujita S. Effect of components of green tea extracts, caffeine and catechins on hepatic drug metabolizing enzyme activities and mutagenic transformation of carcinogens. *Jpn J Vet Res*, 52, 185-190 (2005).

Parmar NS, Shikha Parmar. Anti-ulcer potential of flavonoids. *Indian J Physiology and Pharmacology*, 42, 343-351, (1998).

Paul P, Ritra J, Ritva S, Mackku H, Lyly T, Eero P, Arpo A. Dietary flavonoids and the risk of lung cancer and other malignant neoplasms. *Am J Epidemiolo*, 146, 223-230, (1997).

Ratty AK. Effects of flavonoids on nonenzymatic lipid peroxidation: structure-activity relationship. *Biochem Med Metabol Biol*, 39, 67-79, (1988).

Santos AC, Vyemura SA, Lopes JL, Bazon JN, Mingatto FE, Curtic. Effect of naturally occuring flavonoids on lipid peroxidation and membrane permeability transition in mitochondria. *Free Radic Biol Med*, 24, 1455-1461, (1998).

Shahidi F, Yang Z, Saleemi ZO. Natural flavonoids as stabilizers. *J Food Lipids*, 1, 69-75, (1998).

Srivastava AK. Inhibition of phosphorylase kinase, and tyrosine protein kinase activities by quercetin. *Biochem Biophys Res Commun*, 131, 1-5 (1985).

Tencate JW, Van Haeringen NJ, Gerritsen J, Glasius E. Biological activity of a semisynthetic flavonoid, O-(β-Hydroxyethyl) Rutosine: Light-scattering and metabolic studies of human red cells and platelets. *Clin Chem*, 19, 31-35, (1973).

Thomas PRS, Nash GB, Dormandly JA. White cell accumulation in dependant legs of patients with venous hypertension: A possible mechanism for trophic changes in the skin. *Br Med J*, 296, 1673-1695, (1988).

Thull U and Testa B. Screening of unsubstituted cyclic compounds as inhibitors of monoamine oxidase. *Biochem Pharmacol*, 47, 2307-2310, (1994).

Varma SD. Inhibition of aldose reductase by flavonoids: Possible attenuation of diabetic complications. In: Cody V, Middleton E and Harborne JB eds Plant Flavonoids in Biology and Medicine: Biochemical, Pharmacological and Structure- Activity Relationships. Alan R. Liss, Inc., New York, pp. 343-358, (1986).

Versantvoort CH, Schuurhuis GJ, Pinedo HM, Bekman CA, Kuiper CM, *et al.* Genistein modulates the decreased drug accumulation in non-p-glycoprotein mediated multidrug resistant tumor cells. *Br J Cancer*, 68, 939-946, (1993).

Wegener T, Fintelmann V. Flavonoids and Bioactivity. *Wein Med Wochem Schr*; 149, 241-247, (1999).

Wei H, Bowen R, Cai O, Barnes S and Wang Y. Antioxidant and antipromotional effects of the soybean isoflavone genistein. *Proc Soc Exp Biol Med*, 208, 124-130, (1995).

Wenner A, Leu HJ, Spycher M, Brunner U. Ultra structural changes of capillaries in chronic venous insufficiency. *Exp Cell Biol,* 48, 1-14, (1980).

Wild C, Fasel J. Effect of a flovonoid on the capillary resistance of the rectal mucosa in hepatic cirrhosis. *Am J Proct*, 20, 60-62, (1969).

chapter 23

Flavonoids: A Dietary Bioactive Natural Product

Sharad Srivastava, Amit Srivastava and AKS Rawat

INTRODUCTION

Plants are used as a medicine from historic time and the use of plant as natural medicine has involved many biologically active phytonutrients. These phytonutrients are organic compounds of plant which are thought to promote human health and also act as a nutraceutical. In recent years the world appears to be increasingly interested in the health benefits of foods and have begun to look beyond the basic nutritional benefits of food stuffs to disease prevention and health enhancing ingredients of the same (Fahad and Wasim,2008). Traditional medicinal systems owe their importance to the bioactive components that have their origin in plant sources and most of them were associated with routine food habits. Plants have unlimited ability to synthesize aromatic substances, most of which are phenols or their oxygen substituted derivatives (Geissman, 1963). Polyphenols are widely distributed plant derived dietary constituents and have been implicated as the active components in a number of herbal and traditional medicines (Wollenweber, 1988); A potent indian ayurvedic drug 'Chyavanprash' contains large no of phenolic compounds (Rawat et. al. 2006). More than 5000 plant polyphenols have been identified and several of them are known to possess a wide spectrum of pharmacological properties (Beretz et al., 1977); flavonoids fall under this broad description and are almost ubiquitous in the plant kingdom. They are important for the normal growth, development and defense mechanism of plants. The natural source of flavonoids is fruits (in citrus fruit they may represent up to 1% of fresh material), nuts, seeds, flowers, bark, vegetables and Beverages like red wine, tea, coffee, beer also contain large amounts of flavonoids: on an average, the daily diet contains approximately 1 g of flavonoids per day (Giulia et.al,1999). Flavonoids have probably existed in the plant kingdom for over one billion years; this long interaction between plant flavonoids and humans has stimulated much interest in the biochemical and physiological activities of these chemicals. Till date, more than 6500 flavonoids and flavonoid glycosides have been reported from natural sources (Brahmachari et.al., 2006, Monbrison et.al., 2006) and displayed a wide range of biological and pharmacological activities including antioxidant, cytotoxic, anticancer, cardioprotective, hepatoprotective, neuroprotective, antibacterial and antimicrobial properties. These biological and pharmacological properties are usually attributed to their free radical scavenging efficacies, metal complexion capabilities, and their ability to bind to proteins with a high degree of specificity (Fotie, 2008); it also plays important role in management of chronic venous insufficiency (Konstantinos, 2005). Many flavonoids have shown anti inflammatory, anti-allergic, anti cancer, antibacterial, antiviral actions and some of them provide protection against cardiovascular mortality (Middleton and Kandaswami,1993; Hanasaki et.al., 1994; Hope et.al.1983; Duarte et.al.,1993; Huesken et.al., 1995). Flavonoids plays significant role in resistance of plants (Dieter, 2006); In addition flavonoids inhibit lipid peroxidation (LPO) platelet aggregation, capillary permeability, fragility, and the activity of enzyme systems including cyclo-oxygenase and lipoxygenase and also used in vasodilatory actions; flavonoids exert these effects as antioxidant, free radicals scavengers and chelators of divalent cations (Cook and Samman, 1996). In this review, focus is given to their source, chemistry, chemical structure, biosynthesis, pharmacokinetics, biochemical and pharmacological activities.

Chemistry of flavonoids

The chemistry of flavonoids is complex and at first glance can be overwhelming. In plants, flavonoids can occur with or without sugar moieties attached. The biochemical activities of flavonoids and their metabolites depend on their chemical structure and the relative orientation of various moieties onthe molecule (Cody, 1988). An overview of the chemistry of the various classifications of plant flavonoids will be given in this review well as examples for each: including flavonols, flavones, flavanones, catechins (or flavanols), anthocyanidins, isoflavones, dihydroflavonols, and chalcones.

Structure and Classification of Flavonoids

Flavonoids are low molecular weight polyphenolic substances based on the flavan nucleus (Coultate, 1990). Fig 23.1 shows the generic structure of flavonoid and the numbering system used to distinguish the carbon positions around the molecule. The three phenolic rings are referred to as the A, B, and C (or pyrane) rings (Cook and Samman, 1996), the flavonoid aglycone consists of a benzene ring (A) condensed with a six membered ring (C) which in the 2-position carries a phenyl ring (B) as a substituent. Six-member ring condensed with the benzene ring is either á pyrone (flavonols and flavonones) or its dihydro derivative (flavanols and flavanones). The position of the benzenoid substituent divides the flavonoid class into flavonoids (2-position) and isoflavonoids (3-position). Flavonols differ from flavonones by hydroxyl group at 3-position and C_2-C_3 double bonds (Harsteen, 1983). Flavonoids are often hydroxylated in position 3, 5, 7, 2′, 3′, 4′, 5′. Methylethers and acetylesters of the alcohol group are known to occur in nature. When glycosides of flavonoids are formed, the glycosidic linkage is normally located in positions 3 or 7 and the carbohydrate can be L-rhamnose, D-glucose, gluco-rhamnose, galactose or arabinose (Middleton, 1984). The skeleton (Fig. 23.1) representing as the C_6–C_3–C_6 system of flavonoids.

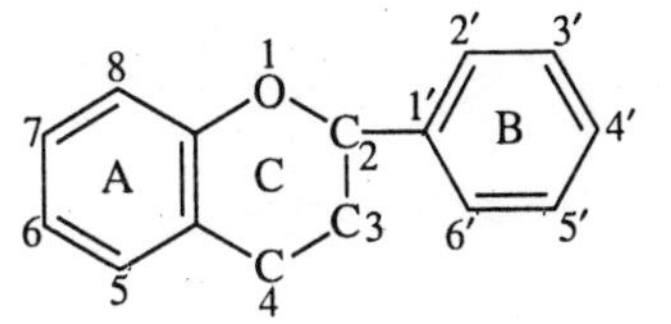

Fig.23.1: Basic Skeleton of Flavonoid

The chemical structure (Fig 23.2) and nomenclature and classification of flavonoids include flavonols, flavones, flavanones, catechins (or flavanols), anthocyanidins, isoflavones, dihydroflavonols, and chalcones are described in table 23.1 (Cook and Samman, 1996; Kevin and Michael, 1997; Giulia et.al.,1999; Tapas et.al., 2008; Hollman and Katan, 1997; Narayana et.al., 2001).

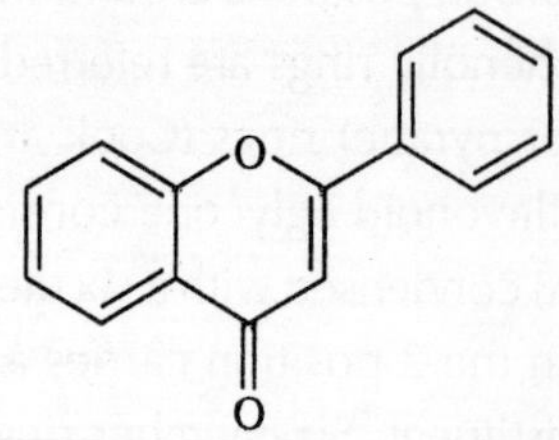

Flavone

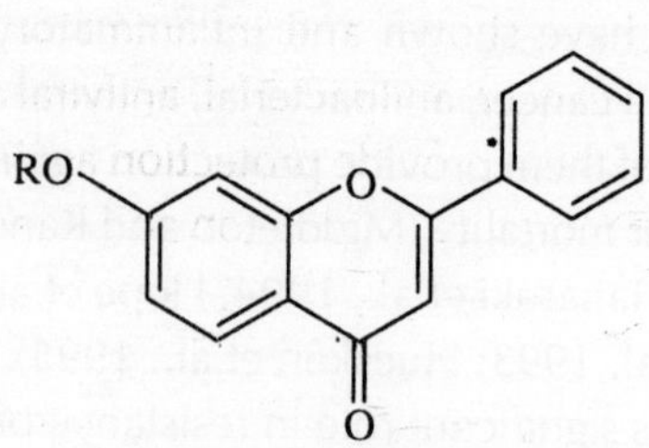

Flavone glycoside

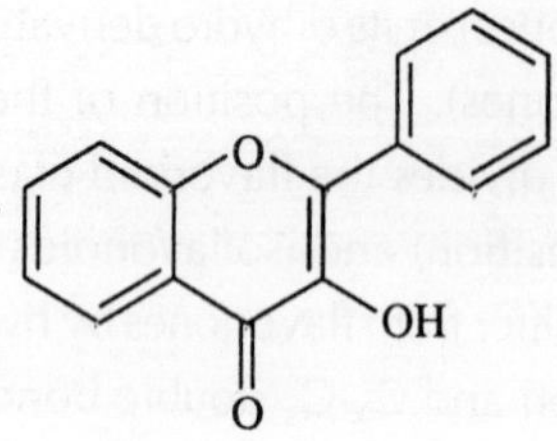

Flavonol

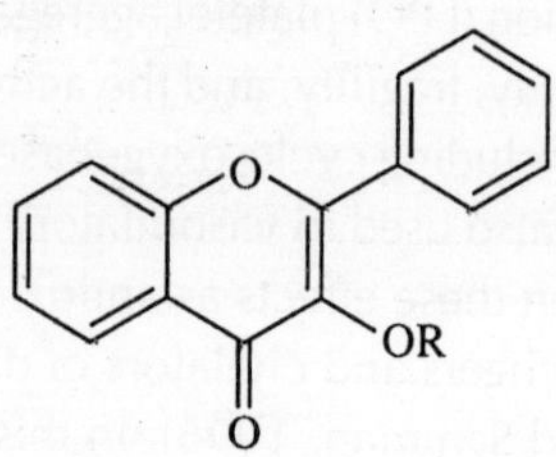

Flavonol glycoside

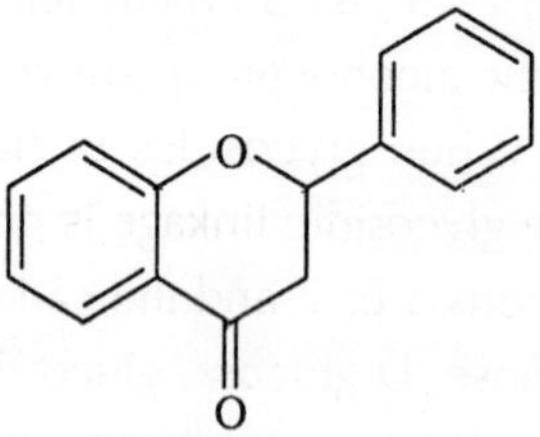

Flavanone

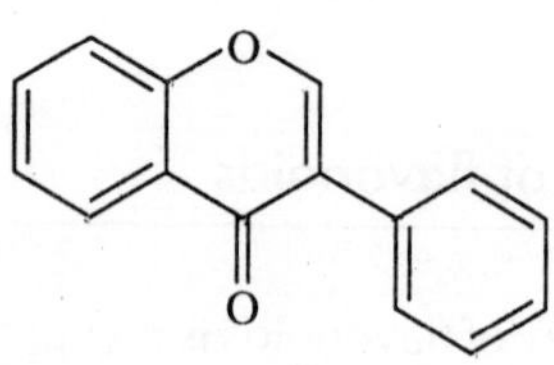

Isoflavone

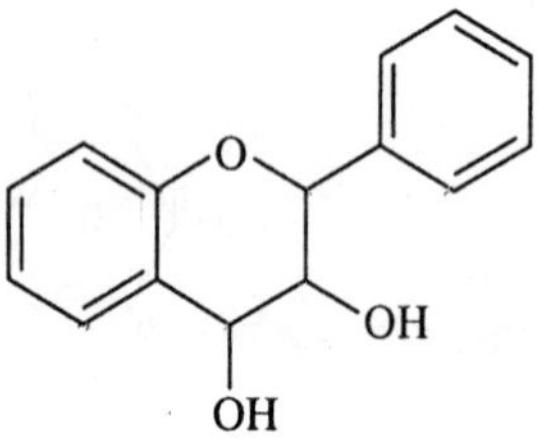

Flavan-3-ol

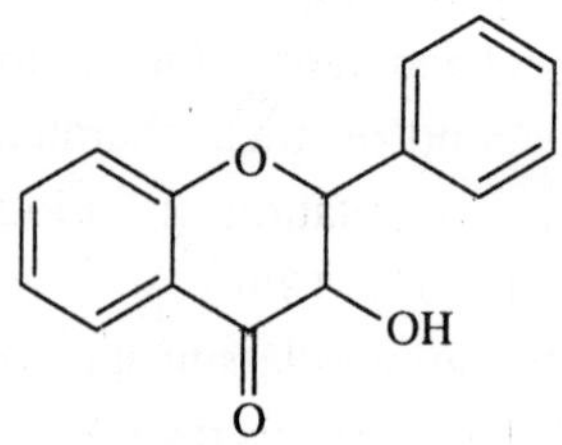

Flavanolol

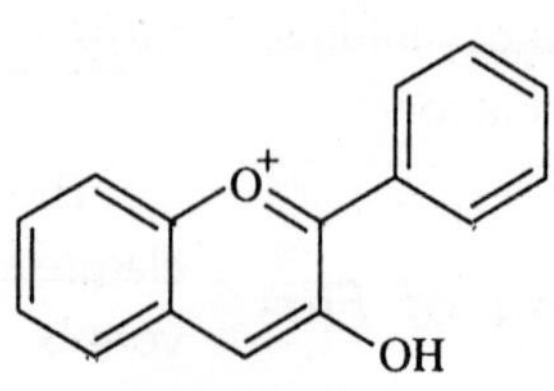

Anthrocyanidin

Fig. 23.2: Chemical structure of some representative flavonoids

Table 23.1: Nomenclature and classification of flavonoids based on the substituent at various postion in basic skelton of Flavonoid moiety.

	3	5	7	2′	3′	4′	5′
Flavones							
Rpoifolin	H	OH	O-R	H	H	OH	H
Apigenin	H	OH	OH	H	H	OH	H
Tangeretin	H	O-CH_3	O-CH_3	H	H	O-CH_3	H
Flavon	H	H	H	H	H	H	H
Baicalein	H	OH	OH	H	H	H	H
Luteolin	H	OH	OH	H	OH	OH	H
Chrysin	H	OH	OH	H	H	H	H
Techtochrysin	H	OH	O-CH_3	H	H	H	H
Diosmetin	H	OH	OH	H	OH	O-CH_3	H
Diosmin	H	OH	O-R^1	H	OH	O-CH_3	H
Isoflavones							
Genistein	-	OH	OH	H	H	OH	H
Daidzin	-	H	O-Glu	H	H	OH	H
Formononetin	-	H	OH	H	O-CH_3	H	
Flavonols							
Kaempferol	OH	OH	OH	H	H	OH	H
Morin	OH	OH	OH	OH	H	OH	H
Rutin	O-R	OH	OH	H	OH	OH	H
Myricetin	OH	OH	OH	H	OH	OH	OH
Quercetin	OH	OH	OH	H	OH	OH	H
Quercetrin	O-Rh	OH	OH	H	OH	OH	H
Myricitrin	O-Rh	OH	OH	H	OH	OH	OH
Spirenoside	OH	OH	OH	H	OH	O-Glu	H
Galangin	OH	OH	OH	H	H	H	H
Robinin	O-R1	OH	OH	H	H	OH	H
Kaempferide	OH	OH	OH	H	H	O-CH_3	H
Fisetin	OH	H	OH	H	OH	OH	H
Rhamnetin	OH	OH	O-CH_3	H	OH	OH	H
Flavones							
Hesperitin	H	OH	OH	H	OH	O-CH_3	H
Naringenin	H	OH	O-R	H	H	OH	H
Naringenin	H	OH	OH	H	H	OH	H
Eriodictyol	H	OH	OH	H	OH	OH	H
Hesperidin	H	OH	O-CH_3	H	OH	O-CH_3	H
Pinocembrin	H	OH	OH	H	H	H	H
Likvirtin	H	H	OH	H	H	O-Glu H	H
Flavanolols							
Silibinin	OH	OH	OH	H	H	O-L-O-	H
Silymarin	OH	OH	OH	H	H	O-L-O-	H
Taxifolin	OH	OH	OH	H	OH	OH	H
Pinobanksin	OH	OH	OH	H	H	H	H
Flavan-3o1s							
Catechin	OH	OH	OH	H	OH	OH	H
Epicatechin	OH	OH	OH	H	OH	OH	H
Flavyliam salts							
Cyanidis	OH	OH	OH	H	OH	OH	H
Pelargonidine	OH	OH	OH	H	H	OH	H

Rh-Rhamnose O-Glu=Glucosyl O-R= Alkoxy O-L-O=Selane

Biosynthesis of Flavonoids

The biosynthesis of flavonoid is important for understanding their diversity and to the design of sound analytical procedures. The flavonoid molecule are biosynthesized by their precursor i.e. three molecules of acetic acid and phenyl propane moiety. It involves the interaction of at least five different pathways, namely the glycolytic pathway, the pentose phosphate pathway, the shikimate pathway that synthesizes phenylalanine, the general phenylpropanoid metabolism that produces activated cinnamic acid derivatives (4-coumaroyl- CoA) and also the plant structural component lignin and finally the diverse specific flavonoid pathways (Kevin and Michael, 1997). In this scheme flavonoids are biosynthesized via a condensation of the shikimic acid and acylpolymalonate pathways. A cinnamic acid derivative (phenylpropane), synthesized from shikimic acid, acts as the starting compound in a polyketide synthesis, in which an additional three acetate residues are incorporated into the structure and this is followed by ring closure. Through subsequent hydroxylations and reductions, plants are then able to biosynthesized different classes of flavonoids like flavonols, flavones, flavanones, catechins (or flavanols), anthocyanidins, isoflavones, dihydroflavonols, and chalcones (Cook and Samman, 1996).

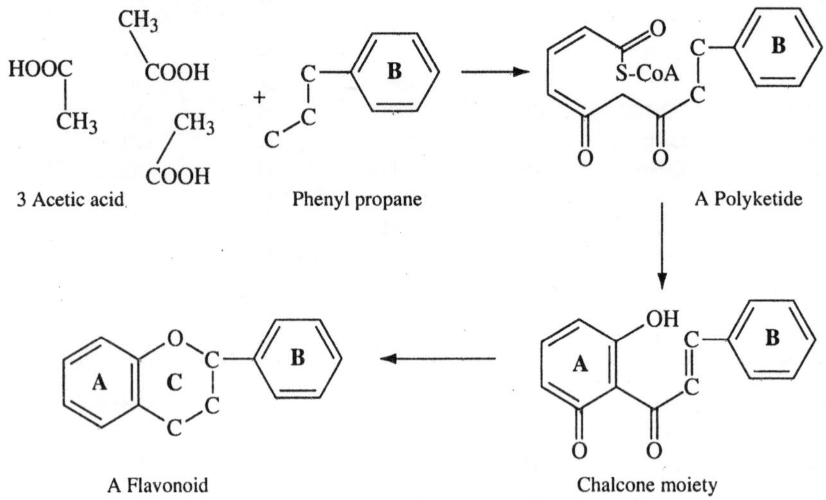

Biosynthesis of Flavonoid molecule

Dietary source of flavonoids

Flavonoids are characteristic constituents of green plants with the possible exception of algae and hornworts. They occur virtually in all parts of the plant but the quantitative distribution varies between different organs of the plant and within different populations of the same plant species (Kevin and Michael, 1997). This variability is largely controlled by genetics but other factors include maturity, climate, and position on the tree, rootstock and agricultural practices. Dietary flavonoids consist mainly of anthocyanidins, flavonols, flavones, catechins and flavanones (Hertog, 1996; Marchand et al., 2000; Hertog et al., 1993; Justesen et al., 1997; Kühnau, 1976; Hollman et al., 1999; Holden et al., 1987; Mangels,1993). Accurate data on population-wide intakes of flavonoids are not available but important dietary sources of flavonoids are—

Flavonoid Sub class	Major Food Source
Flavonols	Tea, onion, apple, kale, red wine, berry, cherry, broccoli, carrot, tomato, lettuce, nuts, walnuts, ginger
Flavones	Thyme, Parsley, citrus peels
Flavanones	Citrus fruits
Isoflavones	Soy, alfalfa sprouts, red clover, chickpeas, peanuts, other legumes
Catechins	Apple, tea, grape, wine, lentils
Anthocyanidins	Cherry, grape, bilberry, cherry, cranberry, peach, plum, hawthorn, loganberry, cocoa.

Extraction of Flavonoids from Plants

The pharmacological activities of medicinal plants are closely related to types of natural compounds those are present in bioactive plant material. Each of natural chemical compounds may have preferred effective method of extraction which facilitates getting the chemicals compounds out of the plants and into the herbal remedy that is being prepared. For extraction of flavonoids from plant material, freeze-dried plant sample mixed with 70% HPLC grade methanol and shake for 15 min at room temperature. After centrifugation (3,000 rpm, 5 min), the supernatant is filter on 90 mm filter paper. The pellet is then re-extracted with 70% methanol and finally rinsed with 100% methanol. All three supernatants are pooled together before removal of the methanol under vacuum with a rota-evaporator at 70°C. When the methanol has evaporated, the extract is concentrated and purified using an activated Sep-Pack C18 column (Sep-Pak → RC Cartridge, Water) and eluted with HPLC grade methanol before being stored at 4°C prior to analysis (Nicolas et al., 2005).

Pharmacokinetic Study of flavonoids

The single most important group of phenolics is the flavonoids. They are highly diverse, in both their chemical structure and proposed biological functions. Their metabolic pathways are particularly complex with, in many cases, multiple alternative metabolic fates. Profiling of the components of a pathway over time provides a dynamic view of the metabolic events occurring in the plant (Kevin and Michael, 1997). The extent of absorption of flavonoids is an important unsolved problem because of the limited data available about them, particularly in humans. Animal studies show that flavonoids present in foods are to be considered non-absorbable because they are bound to sugars as P-glycosides (with the exception of catechins). In fact, only free flavonoids, without a sugar molecule (so-called aglycones), are thought to be able to pass through the gut wall. The hydrolysis of the glycosidic bonds occurs only in the colon by micro-organisms that at the same time degrade dietary flavonoids. This is because no enzymes capable of splitting the bond are present or secreted into the gut. After absorption, the subsequent metabolism of flavonoids is quite well known from animal studies, while less data for humans are available. The liver is main and primary responsible site for the metabolism of absorbed flavonoids. The intestinal wall and kidney are the secondary sites of the metabolism of the absorbed flavonoids. However, this depends on the flavonoids: those found in citrus fruits are poorly metabolized by the intestinal microflora, quercetin is not absorbed in humans, rutin is poorly absorbed, whereas procyanidolignanes are readily absorbed in mice. Many flavonoids are metabolized by intestinal bacteria and these flavonoids are converted to hormone-like compounds with weak estrogenic and antifecondative activities. The possibility of an enterohepatic cycle has been postulated: micro-organisms in the colon can hydrolyse glucuronides and sulphates, which then presumably enables absorption of the liberated aglycones. Flavonoids, once absorbed, influence many biological functions including protein synthesis, cell proliferation differentiation and angio-

Biosynthesis of Flavonoids

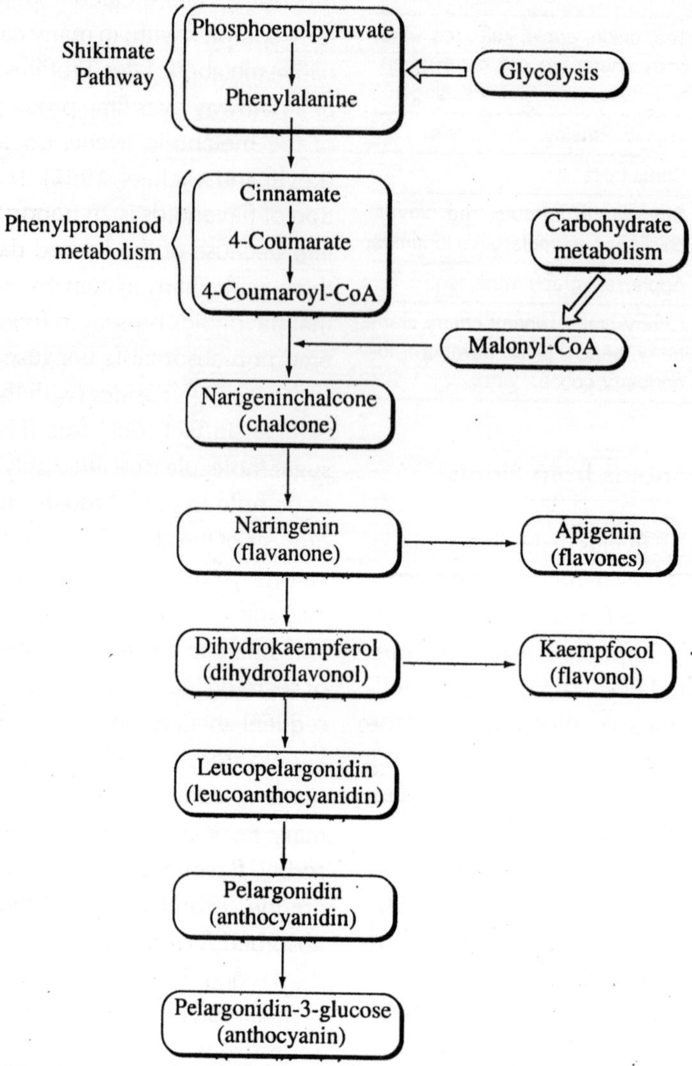

Fig. 23.3: Biosynthetic pathway of various flavonoids

genesis, making them beneficial in a various human disorders (Giulia et al., 1999).

Pharmacological Importance of Flavonoids

The use of flavonoids are in the treatment of disease is to large extent is much older than the science of chemistry. Flavonoids have been used in folk as well as modern medicine around the world. Therefore, it seems that these compounds are important not only for plants, but also for animals including humans (Giulia et al., 1999). The important role of flavonoids in diet and medicine is becoming more and more recognized. From past two decades many researcher has much concentrated on the study of antibacterial, antifungal and antiviral activities of different flavonoids.

Anti fungal activity

Azotobacter vinelandii	Quercetin, Rutin, Epicathenin	Nishino et al., 1987
Alternacia tennisima	Apigenin, Echinacin	Pathak et al., 1991
Cladosporium herbarum	Phaseolinisoflavan	Marchelli et al.,1973
Candida albicans	Chloroflavonin	Pham et al., 1993
Candida tropicalis	Quercetin	Sato et al., 1996
Fusarium solani, Botrytis cinerea, Verticillium dahliae	Chrysoeriol	Sanabria et al., 1991

Antibacterial activity

Organism	Flavonoids	References
Clostridium perfingens	Hydroxyethylrutoside	Ratsimamanga et al., 1994
Klebsiella pneumonia	Rutin	Singh et al. 2008.,
Pseudomonas aeruginosa	Rutin, Naringin, Baicalin, Hydroxyethylrutosine	Ng et al., 1996 Singh et al. 2008
Streptococcus pyogenes	Apigenin	Amoros et al., 1992
Streptococcus viridians	Apigenin	Bamard et al., 1993
Streptococcus jaccalis	Chrysin	Mahmood et al., 1993
Streptococcus baris	Chrysin	Naghski et al., 1947
Streptococcus pneumonia	Chrysin	Tereschuk et al., 1997
Staphylococcus aureus	Quercetin, Baicalin, Quercetogetin, Fisetin, iso-liquiritigenin, Naringin+rutin, Naringin+ Hespertin, Hespertin,	Kujumgier et al., 1999
Staphylococcus albus	Fisetin	Weidenboemer and Jha,1993
Escherichia coli, Bacillus subtilis	Quercetin	Ran et al., 1992
Bacillus anthracis	Rutin	Bashir et al.,1994
Proteus vulgaris	Datisetin	Ishii et al., 1995
Shigella boydii	Hespertin,Naringin+Rutin, Naringenin+Hespertin	Gabor and Eperjessy, 1966

Antiviral activity

Rabies virus	Quercetin, Quercetrin, Rutin	Ghazal et al., 1992
Herpes Virus	Quercetin	Kell et al., 1987
Para influenza virus	Quercetin, Rutin	Deca, et al., 1987
Herpes simplex virus type 1	Apigenin, Chrysin	Tahara et al., 1987
Herpes simplex virus type 1	Galangin, Quercetin, Kempferol	Singh et al., 1988
Potato virus	Morin, Rutin+Quercetin	Tripathi and Rastogi, 1981
Influenza virus	Rutin+Quercetin	Tripathi and Rastogi, 1981
Herpes simplex virus type 2	Quercetin	Bakay et al., 1968
Respiratory syncytial virus	Quercetin, Naringin	Bakay et al., 1968
Immuno-deficiency virus infection	Apigenin	Tsuchiva et al., 1985
Polio virus, Mengo virus, Pseudorabies virus	Quercetin	Hayashi et al., 1993

Flavonoids in heart disease

In order to study the role of dietary flavonoids in coronary heart disease prevention; qucertin, kaempaferol, myricetin, luteolin, apigenin are major phytonutrient which help in prevention of heart disease (Itoigawa et al.,1999). Flavonoids have high propensity to transfer electrons, chelate ferrous ions, and scavenge reactive oxygen species (Kandaswami et al.,1994). Because of these properties, and also been considered as potential protectors against chronic cardiotoxicity caused by the cytostatic drug doxorubicin. Doxorubicin is a very effective antitumor agent but its clinical use is limited by the occurrence of a cumulative dose-related cardiotoxicity, resulting in, for example, congestive heart failure (negative inotropic effect). In a recent report, the cardiotoxicity of doxorubicin on the mouse left atrium has been inhibited by flavonoids, 7-monohydroxyethylrutoside and 7′, 3′, 4′-trihydroxyethylrutoside (Lackeman et al., 1986; Huesken et al., 1995; Bast et al., 2007).

Flavonoids in Antioxidant activity

Plant polyphenolics, such as flavonoids are described as scavengers of reactive oxygen species (ROS), via inhibition of oxido-reductases (Rawat et al. 2008). Flavonoids inhibit LPO in vitro at the initiation stage by acting as scavengers of superoxide anions and hydroxyl radicals. It has been proposed that flavonoids terminate chain radical reactions by donating hydrogen atoms to the peroxy radical forming a flavonoid radical; this flavonoid radical reacts with free radicals terminate the propagation chain reaction (Torel et al.,1986; Afanas'ev et al.,1989; Robak, 1988). In addition to their antioxidative properties, some flavonoids act as metalchelating agents and inhibit the superoxide-driven Fenton reaction, which is an important source of active oxygen radicals (Bravo, 1994). The flavones and catechins seem to be the most powerful flavonoids for protecting the body against reactive oxygen species (ROS). Body cells and tissues are continuously threatened by the damage caused by free radicals and ROS which are produced during normal oxygen metabolism or are induced by exogeneous damage (Groot, 1994, Wegener and Fintelmann, 1999). Free radicals and ROS have been implicated in a large number of human diseases (Ares and Outt, 1998). Quercetin, kaempferol, morin, myricetin and rutin, by acting as antioxidants, exhibited beneficial effects such as anti-inflammatory, antiallergic, antiviral, as well as anticancer activity. They have also been suggested to play a protective role in liver diseases, cataracts, and cardiovascular diseases. Quercetin and silybin, acting as free radical scavengers, were shown to exert a protective effect in liver reperfusion ischemic tissue damage (Hillwell, 1994; Fraga et al., 1987). The scavenging activity of flavonoids has been reported in some research papers to be in the order: Myrcetin > quercetin > rhamnetin > morin > diosmetin > naringenin > apigenin > catechin > 5,7-dihydroxy-3′,4′,5′-trimethoxy- flavone > robinin > kaempferol > flavones (Ratty, 1988). Morin, myricetin, kaempferol and quercetin have also been suggested as stabilizers for fish oil as an alternative to synthetic antioxidants (Husain, 1987).

Flavonoids in Lipid lowering activity and Heart disease

Many of plant flavonoids are responsible for the antilipidemic activity; the lipid lowering studies have observed in *in vitro* and *in vivo*. Oxidative modification of low-density lipoproteins (LDL) by free radicals is an early event in the pathogenesis of atherosclerosis. The rapid uptake of oxidatively modified LDL *via* scavenger receptor leads to the formation of foam cells. Oxidized LDL also has a number of other atherogenic properties. A number of mechanisms are likely to contribute to inhibition of LDL oxidation by flavonoids. Flavonoids may directly scavenge some radical species by acting as chainbreaking antioxidants (Whalley et al., 1990). In addition, they may recycle other chain-breaking antioxidants such as á-tocopherol by donating a hydrogen atom to the tocopheryl radical (Francel, 1993). Transition metals such as iron and copper are important pro-oxidants, and some flavonoids can chelate divalent metal ions, hence preventing free radical formation. The ability of quercetin, and the quercetin glycosides, to protect LDL against oxidative modification has shown a significant protective effect (Igarashi et.al., 1995; Fuhrman et al., 1995; Anlis et al., 1997). Influence of flavonoids on blood coagulation has been studied, the anticoagulant action of heparin was antagonized by *T. hircanicum* extracted. The ability of different flanovoids to inhibit the procoagulant activity of adherent human monocyties has been studied recently and hinokiflavone, a bioflavonoid has been found to be very effective in inhibiting the interleukin-1â induced expression of tissue factor on human monocytes (Raj and Shalinikapoor, 1999). The ability of (+)-catechin to inhibit LDL oxidation induced by copper and several cell lines including mouse macrophages, human monocyte-derived macrophages, and vascular endothelial cells isolated from human umbilical cords have been investigated (Mangiapane et al., 1992). As expected, LDL modified by cells or copper-induced oxidation was endocytosed and degraded by human macrophages more quickly than native LDL. However, in the presence of (+)-catechin, the rate of endocytosis and degradation by macrophages was similar to that of native LDL (Mangiapane et al., 1992).

Effects of flavonoids in blood vessels

Flavonoids quercetin and rutin are used in capillary fragility and phlebosclerosis and displayed pharmaceutical importance. The activities of certain flavonoids in inhibiting capillary permeability and Arthus phenomenon were found to be in the following order, hesperitin > rutin > quercetin > naringenin > kaempferol > isoquercitol. It has been suggested that flavonoids, which contain free hydroxyl groups at 3, 3' and 4' positions exert beneficial physiological effects on capillaries (Narayana et al., 2001). Tangeratin, hesperidin, quercetin, and rutin have been found to reduce aggregation of horse erythrocytes; the decrease in blood cell aggregation produced by most of the flavonoids may explain the reported valuable effects of these compounds on abnormal capillary permeability and fragility, the reduction of disease symptoms and their protection against various traumas and stresses (Osman et al.,1998). The flavonoids O-(â- hydroxyethyl) rutoside, (+) catechol, trihydroxyethylrutoside increased the negative charge density of the blood vessel wall *in vitro* and were markedly antithrombogenic (Gryglewski et al., 1987). Quercetin also has been reported to inhibit aggregation of human platelets by several authors. Other antiaggregatory flavonoids reported were 3-methyl quercetin, toxerutin, fisetin, dihydroquercetin and flavone. Nobeletin and sinensetin decreased erythrocyte aggregation and sedimentation *in vitro* and might be useful in dietary control of high blood viscosity syndrome; Patuletin reduced the capillary permeability and was also reported to have antispasmodic and hypotensive effects. (Narayana et al., 2001). Orally administered flavonoids weakly inhibit the vascular permeability and prevent pulmonary haemorrhage. Acacetin at 25-100 mg/kg oral dose to mice reduced capillary fragility and at 50-100 mg/kg it reduced vascular permeability (Alcaraz et al., 1987; Kandaswami et al., 1994).

Flavonoids in antithrombotic activity

Several flavonoids are responsible for the antithrombotic activity; platelet aggregation plays a pivotal role in the physiology of thrombotic disesases. Activated platelets adhering to vascular endothelium generate lipid peroxides and oxygen free radicals which inhibit the endothelial formation of prostacyclin and nitrous oxide. It was shown in the 1960s that tea pigment can reduce blood coagulability, increase fibrinolysis, and prevent platlet adhesion and aggregation (Lou et al.,1989). Selected flavonoids such as quercetin, kaempferol and myricetin were shown to be effective inhibitors of platelet aggregation in dogs and monkeys (Osman et al., 1998). Flavonols are particularly antithrombotic because they directly scavenge free radicals, thereby maintaining proper concentration of endothelial prostacyclin and nitric oxide (Gryglewski et al., 1987). Few study showed that flavonoids are powerful antithrombotic agents *in vitro* and *in vivo* because of their inhibition of the activity of cyclooxegenase and lipoxigenase pathways (Alcaraz and Ferrandiz, 1987).

Flavonoids in antidiabetic activity

Flavonoid, quercetin plays significant role in administration of insulin secretion, and shows antidiabetic activity. Vessel and coworkers reported that quercetin brings about the regeneration of pancreatic islets and proprably increases insulin release in strptozotocin-induced diabetic rats (Vessal et al., 2003). In another study, quercetin stimulate insulin release and enhanced Ca^{2+} uptake from isolated islets cell which suggest a place for flavonoids in noninsulin-dependent diabetes (Hif and Howell, 1984; Hif and Howell 1985).

Flavonoids in antineoplastic activity

Various flavonoids have exhibited antineoplastic activity and detailed studies have revealed that quercetin exerted a dose-dependent inhibition of growth and colony formation (Kontruck et al., 1986; Izzo et al. 1991; Murakami et al., 1992). The flavonoids, kaempferol, catechin, toxifolin and fisetin, also suppress the cell growth (Kim et al., 1993; Gill et al., 1994). On screening the antileukaemic efficacy of naturally occurring and synthetic flavonoids on human promyelocytic leukaemic HL-60 cells, genistein, an isoflavone was found to have strong effect (Hirano et al., 1994; Wei et al., 1990). Cirrus flavonoids (tangeretin) also exhibit antiinvasive activity, but appear to act by a different mechanism. They show a poor affinity for the extracellular matrix and do not bind enzymes to laminin. *In vitro* studies have been made on the antiproliferative effect of citrus flavonoids quercetin, taxifolin, nobletin and tangeretin on human squamous cell carcinoma. Flavonoids extracted from *Scutelluria baicalensis* (baicalein, baicalin and woogonin) exerted *in vitro* a concentration-dependent inhibition of the proliferative response of cultured rabbit vascular smooth muscle cells upon exposure to 5% calf serum. Aside from quercetin and baicalein, epigallocatechin gallate and green tea extract were also reported to inhibit tumor growth by inhibiting mitosis. Some flavonoids (quercetin, epigallocatechin) and green tea extract inhibit tumor growth both by inhibiting some phase of the cell cycle and by blocking or competing for hormone receptor sites. Rutin, on the contrary, does not bind to estrogen binding sites and does not inhibit the growth of hormone-depending tumors (Giulia et al., 1999). Quercetin, but not rutin, was also reported to be effective in inhibiting of *in vitro* bromodeoxyuridine incorporation by cells from transitional cell carcinoma of the bladder. The flavonoids tricin and kaempferol-3-0-P-D-glucopyranoside derived from the traditional Chinese medicinal plant *Wikstroemia Mica,* demonstrated antileukaemic activity in the P-388 leukemic mice. Furthermore, epidemiological studies indicated that diets containing linseed and soy (rich in isoflavonoids and lignans) may protect against colon, breast and prostatic cancer (Giulia et al., 1999).

Flavonoids in osteoclastogenesis

Flavonoids are found to have an inhibitory effect on osteoclastic bone resoption *in vitro*. Flavonoid quercertin was found to increase calcium content in the diaphyseal tissues of rat femoral culture system in vitro, although such an effect was not seen with culture of myricetin, kaempferol, isorhamnetin, curcumin, hesperidin, or astaxanthin. Among various flavonoids, quercetin had unique effect on bone calcification, although the effect of flavonoids on osteoblastic cells remains a matter of some controversy (Masayoshi et al., 2007). Quercetin has been shown to increase osteogenic differentiation of human adipose tissue-derived stromal cells; reverse transcription-polymerase chain reaction (RT-PCR) and real time PCR analysis show that quercetin treatment induces an increase in the gene expression of osteopontin, bone morphogenic protein 2, alkaline phosphatase and Runx 2, which are a marker protein of osteoblastic cells . (Kim et al., 2006). Meanwhile, quercetin has been reported to accelerate the tumor necrosis factor-alphainduced growth inhibition and apoptosis in osteoblastic MC3T3-E1 cells (Son et al., 2006).

Flavonoids as anti-inflammatory agent

Most of the flavonoids shown anti-inflammatory properties and these have been studied both *in vitro* and *in vivo*. Flavone/flavonol glycosides as well as flavonoid aglycons have been reported to Flavones/flavonols kaempferol, quercetin, myricetin, fisetin were reported to possess LO and COX inhibitory activities (Kim et al., 1998; Jachak, 2001). Hesperidin, a citrus flavonoid possesses significant antiinflammatory and analgesic effects (Shahidi et al., 1998). Recently, apigenin, luteolin and quercetin have been reported to exhibit anti-inflammatory activity. Quercetin, gallic acid ethyl ester and some as yet unidentified flavonoids might account for the antinociceptive action reported for the hydroalcoholic extract of *Phyllanthus caroliniensis* (Morino et al.,1997; Alcaraz et al.,1987). Nepetin, a flavonoid obtained from *Nepeta hindostana*, was investigated in both acute and chronic models of inflammation in rats and found to possess significant activity in both proliferative and exudative phases of inflammation. Apigenin and luteolin from *Chamomilla recutita* were found to significantly inhibit the oedema caused by croton oil. This activity may have been due to a direct inhibition of arachidonic acid metabolism or to other mechanisms such as inhibition of histamine release or promotion of scavenging activity. Studies on the *in vivo* anti-inflammatory activity of the flavonoids, particularly hypolaetin-8-P-D-glucoside, sidertoflavone (isolated from the Spanish *Sideritis mugronensis*) and the flavonol glycosides gossypin and hibifolin (isolated from traditional Indian medicinal plants), showed a dose-dependent inhibition of both paw oedema and leucocyte accumulation in the peritoneum in the carrageenan-induced models of oedema and peritonitis. Other studies were carried out on the anti-inflammatory activities of quercetin and quercitrin (Giulia et al., 1999).In an ex *vivo* system utilizing the carrageenan-induced pleurisy model in rats, quercetin reduced in a doserelated manner the induced contractions of both prostaglandin E, and leukotriene B, and leukocyte migration in the exudate. Quercetin also reduced LTB_4, synthesis in cells stimulated with ionophore A23 both *ex-vivo* and *in vitro*. Quercitrin exhibited similar but less activity than quercetin, recently it was reported that quercitrin decreased colonic damage and the incidence of diarrhea and normalized colonic fluid transport in rats with chronic experimental colitis. Other *in vivo* studies have been carried out on the anti-inflammatory and analgesic activities of flavonoids, such as those extracted from *Citrus aurantium* (hesperidin), *Machaerium villosum* (duartin) and from *Cyclolobium clausseni* (clausse-quinone) (Giulia et al., 1999).

Flavonoids in hepatoprotective activity

A large number of flavonoids have also been found to possess hepato-protective activity; in a study carried out to investigate silymarin, apigenin, quercetin and naringenin as putative therapeutic agents against microcrystin LR- induced hepatotoxicity, silymarin was found to be the most effective natural compound for hepatic protection (Carlo et al., 1993). Rutin and venorutin showed regenerative and hepato-protective effects in experimental cirrhosis (Lorenz et al., 1973). The results of several clinical investigations showed the efficacy and safety of flavonoids in the treatment of hepatobiliary dysfunction and digestive complaints, such as sensation of fullness, loss of appetite, nausea and abdominal pain. Silymarin normalizes cell phospholipid synthesis without showing any demonstrable effect on undamaged cells where by counteracting fatty liver. Moreover, earlier findings on a hepato-protective effect and the prevention of NSAIDs-induced gastropathy may be confirmed (Ruiyc, 1991; Scevola et al., 1984).

Effect of flavonoids on hormones

Flavonoids plays important role in regulatory activity of hormones, by binding to 17 beta-hydroxy steroid dehydrogenases, which regulates estrogen and androgen levels in humans and to 3 beta-hydroxy steroid dehydrogenase, which regulates progestin and androgen levels in males and females respectively (Noro et al., 1983). Quercetin, myricetin, rutin, kaempferol affect the transport, metabolism and action of thyroid hormones. Quercetin myricetin, rutin, kaempferol, galangin, spirenoside and robinin are potent non-toxic ITH deiodinase inhibitors in microsomal membranes, and intact rat hepatocytes. Myricetin, rutin, kaempferol are specific high affinity competitors for L- T_4-binding to human TBPA, weaker antagonists in the T3-5′-deiodinase reaction, and very poor inhibitors of T_3 binding to the nuclear T_3 receptor. Further investigation needs the role of ITH deiodination for tissue specific expression of thyroid hormone action as well advance the knowledge of specific interaction of flavonoids with antithyroidal agent with extra-thyroidal mechanism of action in the process of T_4 bioactivation to the thyromimetically active T_3 (Petkov et.al.,1981).

Effect of flavonoids on enzymes

The biochemical activities of flavonoids and their metabolites depend on their chemical structure and the relative orientation of various moieties on the molecule. Flavonoids display a remarkable array of the effect of enzymes and inhibit a number of enzymes such as aldose reductase(Jager et al., 1998), xanthine oxidase (Koch et al., 1992), phosphodiesterase (Alcaraz et al., 1987), Ca^{2+} ATPase (Narayana et al., 2001), lipo-oxygenase (Baumann et al., 1980) and cyclooxygenase (Varma et al.,1976). Flavonols like quercetin, myricetin and kaempferol inhibit the activity of the adenosine deaminase of endothelial cells, while flavones are inactive (Nagai et al.,1992). Quercetin, morin, myricetin and kaempferol are effective in antagonizing bradykinin responses which is vasodilator compound (Bamard et al., 1993). Effects of luteolin and quercetin on inhibition of tyrosine kinase on cell growth and metastasis; they have inhibitory properties on the 5'-nucleotidase (5'-ribonucleotide phosphohydrolase) activity (Hur et al., 1994; Beladi et al., 1987). Flavonoids can inhibit intracellular Ca^{2+} elevation by reducing phospholipase-C activity (Musci et al., 1985) and they possess potent inhibitory effects on several enzyme systems such as protein kinase-C, protein tyrosine kinase, phospholipase A2 and others (Melzig et.al., 1996). Silymarin acts a strong antioxidant by virtue of its ability to act as an acceptor of O_2 or CCl_3 radicals; by trapping O_2 related free radicals silymarin hinders their interaction with polyunsaturated fatty acid and abolishes the enhancement of lipid peroxidation (Huang et al.,1999 ; Kavutru et.al. 1999). Apigenin inhibits phosphodiesterase (PDE) and the effect was greater on cAMP-PDE than cGMP-PDE levels by 40% and cGMP level remained unchanged. Some flavonoids are predominant inhibitors of either cyclo-oxygenase or lipoxygenase, others are equally effective against both enzymes. Numerous reports of a high standard have appeared on the inhibition by flavonoids of a perplexing number and variety of enzymes, e.g. hydrolases (such as aglucuronidase), hyaluronidase, alkaline phosphatase, arylsulphatase, H^+-ATPases of lysosomal and granular membranes, Na^+/K^+-ATPase of the plasma membrane, a-galactosidase, c-AMP phosphodiesterase, lipases, lyases (such as DOPA-decarboxylase), transferases (like catechol-O-methyltransferase), hydroxylases (like aryl hydroxylase), oxidoreductases (like aldose reductase) and kiriases (e.g. hexokinase) (Narayana et al., 2001).

CONCLUSION

From billions of year natural products have proven to be a great source of various biologically active compounds. Thus, in an effort to discover a new pharmacologically active compounds; many research group in field of biology and chemistry successfully screening the plant extracts to detect secondary metabolites with significant biological activities that could be used as templates for the development of new drugs. Flavonoids are a large group of polyphenolic compounds that have been known for a long time to exert diverse pharmacological and biochemical effects and used as a nutraceuticals. In this review we presented many evidences of their pharmacological and biochemical activities. In that respect, flavonoids represent an enormous source of natural dietary antioxidant, antilipidemic, antimicrobial, antineoplastic, antidiabetic, antithrombotic drug for human welfare. However, due to their low bioavailability in natural sources indicates that the need for further investigations with accuracy in each and every step; including isolation, purification, pharmacokinetic study to clinical trials for development of new drug discovery.

REFERENCE

Afanas'ev IB, Dorozhko AI, Brodskii AV, Kostyuk VA, and Potapovitch AI. Chelating and free radical scavenging mechanisms of inhibitory action of rutin and quercetin in lipid peroxidation. *Biochem. Pharmacol.* 38, 1763-1769, (1989).

Alcaraz MJ, Ferrandiz ML. Modification of arachidonic metaboilism by flavonoids. *J Ethnopharmacol.* 21, 209-229, (1987).

Amoros M, Simoes CMO, Girre L, Sauvanger F, Cormier M. Inhibition of HIV infection by Baicalin- A flavonoid compound purified from chinese herbal medicine. *J Nat Prod* 55, 1732-1739, (1992).

Anlis GT Mc, Enany JMc, Pearce J, Young IY. The effect of various dietary flavonoids on the susceptibility of low-density lipoproteins to oxidation in vitro using both metallic and nonmetallic oxidising agents. *Biochem Soc Trans*, 25, 142-148, (1997).

Ares JJ, Outt PE. Gastroprotective agents for the prevention of NSAID induced gastropathy. *Curr Pharm Des.* 4, 7-36, (1998).

Bakay M, Mucsi I, beladi I, Gabor MM. Antiviral flavonoids from Alkena orientalis. *Acta Microbiol* 15, 223-32, (1968).

Bamard DL, Smee DF, Huffman JH, Meyerson CR, Sidwell RW. Review of Quercetin and related bioflavonoids. *Chemotherapy.* 39, 203-211, (1993).

Bashir AK, Abdulla AA, Wasti IA, Wassan ES, Amiri MH, Crabb TA. New bioactive flavonoids incube resin insecticide. *Int J Pharmcogn*, 34, 366-372, (1994).

Bast A, Kaiserov H, den Hartog GJM, Haenen GRMM, van der Vijgh WJF. Protectors against doxorubicin-induced cardiotoxicity: Flavonoids. *Cell Biol Toxicol*, 23, 39-47, (2007).

Baumann J, Von Brucchau, Sen F, Wurm G. Flavonoids and related compounds as inhibition of arachidonic acid peroxidation. *Prostaglandin*, 20, 627-639, (1980).

Beladi I, Musci I, Pusztai R, Bakay M, Rosztoczy I, Gabor M. Bioactivity of flavonoids. *Stud Org Chem*, 1, p. 443, (1987).

Beretz A, Anton R, Stoclet JC. Flavonoid compounds are potent inhibitors of cyclic AMP phosphodiesterase. *Experimentia*, 34, 1045-1055, (1977).

Brahmachari G, Gorai D. Recent development in the research on naturally occurring flavonoids: An overview. In: G. Brahmachari (ed). *Chemistry of Natural Products:Recent Trends & Developments*, Research Signpost, Kerala, India, pp. 61-159, (2006).

Bravo L, Abia R, Eastwood MA, Saura-Calixto, F. Degradation of polyphenols (catechin and tannic acid) in the rat intestinal tract. Effect on colonic fermentation and faecal output. *Brit. J. Nutr*, 71, 933-946, (1994).

Carlo GD, Autore G, IZZOAA, Moiolino P, Mascolo N, Viola P, Diurno MV, Capawa F. Inhibition of intestinal motility and secretion by flavonoids in mice and rats; structure-activity relatiohships. *J Pham Pharmacol*, 45, 1045-1059, (1993).

Cody V. Crystal and molecular structure of flavonoids. In Plant Flavonoids in Biology and Medicine II: Biochemical, Celhdar, and Medicinal Properties, p. 29-44, Alan R. Liss, New York, NYUSA, (1988).

Coultate TP. Food: The Chemistry of its Components, 2nd ed. The Royal Society of Chemistry, pp. 137-149, (1990).

Cook NC, Samman S, Flavonoids-Chemistry, metabolism, cardioprotective effects, and dietary sources. *Nutritional Biochemistry* 7, 66-76, (1996).

Deca RT, Gouzalez IJ, Mactinez TMV, Moreno J, Romo SCA. Soil Biol. In vitro antifungal activity of some flavonoids and their metabolites. *Biochem*, 19, 223-231, (1987).

Dieter Treutter. Significance of flavonoids in plant resistance: a review. *Environ Chem Lett*. 4, 147-157, (2006).

Duarte J, Vizcaino FP, Utrilla P, Jimenez J, Tamargo J, and Zarzuelo A. Vasodilatory effects of flavonoids in rat aortic smooth muscle. Structure activity relationships. *Biochem. Pharmacol*, 24, 857-862, (1993).

Fahad Ullah Mohd, Wasim Khan Md. Food as Medicine: Potential Therapeutic Tendencies of Plant Derived Polyphenolic Compounds. Asian Pacific Journal of Cancer Prevention, Vol 9, 187-196, (2008).

Fotie Jean. The Antiprotozoan Potential of Flavonoids. Pharmacognosy Reviews, Vol 2, Issue 3, 1-19, (2008).

Fraga CG, Mactino US, Ferraro GE, Coussio JF, Boveris A. Flavonoids as antioxidants evaluated by in vitro and in situ liver chemiluminescence. *Biochem Med Metabol Biol*, 36, 717-720, (1987).

Francel EN, Kanner J, German JB, Packs E, Kinsella JE. Inhibition of oxidation of human low-density lipoprotein by phenolis substances in red wine. *Lancet*, 341, 454-457, (1993).

Fuhrman B, Lavy A, Aviram M. Consumption of red wine with meals reduces the susceptibility of human plasma and low-density lipoproteins to lipid peroxidation. *Am Soc Clin Nutr*, 61, 549-554, (1995).

Gabor M, Eperjessy E. Antimicrobial activity of flavonoids from leaves of chinese herb. *Nature*, 212, 1273-1279, (1966).

Geissman TA. Flavonoid compounds, tannins and related compounds, In: Florkin M. and Stotz, EH, (Ed), Pyrrole Pigments, Isoprenoid Compounds and Phenolic Plant Constituents. Elsevier, New York pp. 265, (1963).

Ghazal SA, Abuzarqua M, Mahansneh AM. Effect of plant flavonoids on immune and inflammatory cell function. *Phytother Res,* 6; 265-271, (1992).

Gill B, Sanz MJ, Terencio MC, Ferrandiz ML, Bustos G, Paya M. The flavonoids. *Life Sci,* 54, 333-339, (1994).

Giulia Di Carlo, Nicola Mascolo, Angelo A. Izzo, and Francesco Capasso. Flavonoids: old and new aspects of a class of natural therapeutic drugs. *Life Sciences*, 65(4), 337-353, (1999).

Grace PA. Ischaemia-reperfusion injury, *Br J Surg*, 81, 637-647, (1994).

Gryglewski RJ, Korbut R, Robak J, Swips J. On the mechanism of anti thrombotic action of flavonoids. *Biochem Pharmacol,* 36, 317-322, (1987).

Groot De, H. Reactive oxygen species in tissue injury. *Hepatogastroenterology*, 41, 328-332, (1994).

Hanasaki Y, Ogawa S, and Fnkui S. The correlation between active oxygens scavenging and antioxidative effects of flavonoids. *Free Radical Biol. Med,* 16, 845-850, (1994).

Harsteen B. Flavonoids A class of natural products of high pharmacological potency. *Biachem Pharmacol,* 32, 1141-1148, (1983).

Hayashi K, Hayashi T, Arisawa M, Morita N. *In vitro* inhibition of viral disease by flavonoids. *Antiviral Chem Chemother*, 4, 49-58, (1993).

Hertog MGL; Hollman PCH; Katan MB; Kromhout D. Intake of potentially anticarcinogenic flavonoids and their determinants in adults in the Netherlands. *Nutrition and Cancer,* 20, 21-29, (1993).

Hertog MGL. Epidemiological evidence on potential health properties of flavonoids. *Proceedings of the Nutrition society,* 55, 385-397, (1996).

Hif CS, Howell SL, Effects of epicatechin on rat islets of langerhans. *Diabetes,* 33, 291-296, (1984).

Hif CS, Howell SL. Effects of flavonoids on insulin secretion and Ca^{+2} handling in rat islets of langerhans. *J Endocrinol*, 107, 1-8, (1985).

Hillwell B. Free radicals, antioxidants and human disease: Curiosity, cause or constipation? *Lancet*, 344, 721-724, (1994).

Hirano T, Gotoh M, Oak K. Natural flavonoids and lignans are plant cytostatic agents against.

Human Leukemic HL-60 cells. *Life Sci*, 55, 1061-1069, (1994).

Hope WC, Welton AF, Fielder-Nagy C, Batula-Bernardo C, Coffey JW. In vitro inhibition of the biosynthesis of slow reacting substances of anaphylaxis (SRS-A) and lipoxygenase activity of quercetin. *Biochem. Pharmacol,* 32, 367-371, (1983).

Holden JM, Schubert A, Wolf WR, Beecher GR. A system for evaluating the quality of published nutrient data:selenium, a test case. *Food Nutr, Bull.,* 9 (Suppl.), 177-193, (1987).

Hollman PCH; Bijsman MNCP; van Gameren Y; Cnossen EPJ; De Vries JHM; and Katan MB. The sugar moiety is a major determinant of the absorption of dietary flavonoid glycosides in man. *Free Rad. Res.,* 31, 569-573, (1999).

Hollman PCH, Katan MB. Absorption, metabolism and health effects of dietary flavonoids in man. *Biomed and Pharmacother*, 51, 305-310, (1997).

Huang Y, Hwang J, Lee P, Ke F, Huang J, Huang C, Kanda Swamic, Jr BM, Lee M. Effects of Luteolin and Quercetin inhibitors of tyrosine kinasa on cell growth and metastasis-associated properties in A43 Al cells over expressing epidermal growth factor receptors. *Br J Pharmaco,* 128, 999-1010 (1999).

Huesken BCP, Dejong J, Beekman B, Onderwater RCA. Flavonoids as cardioprotective agents. *Cancer Chemotheapy Pharmacol*, 37, 55-62, (1995).

Hur CQ, Chen K, Shi Q, Kilkuskie RE, Cheng YC, Lee KH. Apoptosis of HIV infected cell following treatment with Shosoikorso. *J Nat Prod*, 57, 42-50, (1994).

Husain SR, Cillard J, Cillard P. Hydroxy radical scavenging activity of flavonoids. *Phytochemistry,* 26, 2489-2492, (1987).

Igarashi K, Ohmuna M. Effect of Isoharnneti, Rhamnetin and Quercetin on the concentrations of cholesterol and lipoperoxide in the serum and liver and on the blood and liver antioxidative enzyme activities in rats. *Biosci Biotech Biochem*, 59, 595-601, (1995).

Ishii E, Odate J, Ogma T, Myata T. Flavonoids: New aspects of a class of natural therapeutic drugs. *Chem Abste*, 122, 1969544, (1995).

Itoigawa M, Takeya K, Ito C, Furu Kawa H. Structure activity relationship of cardiotonic flavonoids in guinea pig papillary muscle. *J Ethnopharmacol*, 65, 267-272, (1999).

Izzo AA, Dicarlo G, mascolo N, Capasso F, Autore G. Antiulcer effects of flavonoids. Role of endogenous PAF. *Phytotherapy Res*, 8,179-181 (1991).

Jachak SM. Natural products: Potential source of COX inhibitors., 2(1), 12-15, CRIPS (2001).

Jager W, Zembsch B, Wolschann P, Pittenauer E, Senderavicz AM. Metabolism of the anticancer drug flavopiridol, a new inhibitor of cyclin dependent kinases in rat liver. *Life Sci*, 62, 1861-1873, (1998).

Justesen U, Knuthsen P, Leth T. Determination of plant polyphenols in Danish foodstuffs by HPLC-UV and LC-MS detection. *Cancer Letters,* 114, 165-167, (1997).

Kandaswami C, Middleton E. Free radical scavenging and antioxidant activity of plant flavonoids. In: Armstrong D ed. Free radicals in diagnostic medicine. Ed 2. New York: Plenum Press; 351-376, (1994).

Kavutru M, Melzig MF. *In vitro* effects of selected flavonoids on the 5'- nucleotidase activity. *Pharmazine*, 54, 457-459, (1999).

Kell KP, Manadi AM, Adiyasora ZF, Kunaera RM, IZV. Akad.Naun. Kaz. SSR. Bioflavonoids and health effects in man. *Chem Abst* 107, 36667, (1987).

Kevin Robards, Michael Antolovich. Analytical Chemistry of Fruit Bioflavonoids A Review. *Analyst,* Vol. 122, 11R–34R, (1997).

Kim HK, Namgoong SY, Kim HP. Biological actions of flavonoids-I. *Arch Pharmacol Res*, 16, 18-27, (1993).

Kim HP, Mani I, Iversen L, Ziboh VA. Effects of naturally occurring flavonoids and bioflavonoidson epidermal cycloxygenase and lipoxygenase from guinea pigs. *Prostag Leukot Essent Fatty acids,* 58, 17-24 (1998).

Kim YJ, Bae YC, Suh KT, Jung JS Quercetin, a flavonoid, inhibits proliferation and increases osteogenic differentiation in human adipose stromal cells. *Biochem Pharmacol*, 72, 1268-1278, (2006).

Kontruck SJ, Radecki T, Brozozowski T, Antiulcer and gastroprotective effects of solon, a synthetic flavonoid derivative of sophorandin. Role of endogenous prostaglandins. *Bur J Pharmac*, 125,185-192, (1986).

Koch HP, Jager W, Groh U, Plank G. *In vitro* inhibition of adenosine deaminase by flavonoids and related compounds. New insight into the mechanism of action of plant phenolics. *Methods Find Exp Clin Pharmacol*, 14, 413-417, (1992).

Konstantinos Katsenis. Micronized Purified Flavonoid Fraction (MPFF): A Review of its Pharmacological Effects, Therapeutic Efficacy and Benefits in the Management of Chronic Venous Insufficiency. *Current Vascular Pharmacology*, 3, 1-9, (2005).

Kühnau J. The flavonoids: a class of semi-essential food components: their role in human nutrition. *World Review of Nutrition,* 24, 117-120, (1976).

Kujumgier A, Tsvetkova J, Serkedjieva Y, Bankova V,christov R, Popov S. Antibacterial, antifungal and antiviral activity of propolis of different geographic origin. *J Ethno Pharmacol* 64, 235-240, (1999).

Lackeman GM, Claeys M, Rwanagabo PC, Herman AG, Vlietinck A. Chronotropic effect of quercetin on guinea pig right atrium. *J Planta Med,* 52, 433-439, (1986).

Lou FQ, Zhang MF, Zhang XG, Liu JM, Yuan WL. A study on tea pigment in prevention of antherosclerosis. *Chin Med J (Engl),* 102, 579-583 (1989).

Lorenz W, Kusche J, Barth H, Mathias CH. Action of several flavonoids on enzyme of histidine metabolism *in vitro.* In Histamine (Ed. Cz. Maslinski) Dowden, Hutchinson and Ross. Stroudsberg. Pennsylvania, pp. 265-269, (1973).

Mahmood N, Pizza C, Aquino R, De Tammasi N, Piacente S, Colman S, Bruke A, Hay AJ. Inhibition of HIV infection by flavonoids. *Antiviral Res,* 22, 189-197, (1993).

Mangels AR; Holden JM; Beecher GR; Forman MR; Lanza, E. Carotenoid content of fruits and vegetables: An evaluation of analytical data. *J. Am. Diet. Assoc,* 93, 284-296, (1993).

Mangiapane H, Thomson J, Salter A, Brown S, Bell GD, and White DA. The inhibition of the oxidation of low density lipoprotein by (+)-catechin, a naturally occurring flavonoid. *Biochem. Pharmacol,* 43, 445-450, (1992).

Marchand Lee L; Murphy SP; Hankin JH; Wilkens LR; Kolonel LN. Intake of flavonoids and lung cancer. *J. Nat. Can.Inst.,* 92(2), 154-160, (2000).

Marchelli R, Vining LC. Recent advances in the discovery and development of flavonoids and their antiviral activity. *JCS Chem Comm,* 555, (1973).

Masayoshi Y, Reiko H, Satoshi U, Kaori I. Effects of flavonoid on calcium content in femoral tissue culture and parathyroid hormone-stimulated osteoclastogenesis in bone marrow culture in vitro. *Mol Cell Biochem,* 303, 83-88, (2007).

Melzig MF. Inhibition of adinosine deaminase activity of aortic endothelial cells by selected flavonoids. *Planta Med,* 62, 1-20, (1996).

Middleton E, Jr. and Kandaswami C. (1993) The impact of plant flavonoids on mammalian biology: Implications for immunity, inflammation and cancer. In *The Flavonoids: Advances in ResearchSince.* (J.B. Harborne, ed.), Chapman and Hall, London, UK, pp. 619-652, (1986).

Middleton E. The flavonoids. *Trends Pharmacol Sci,* 5, 335-338, (1984).

Monbrison F. de, Maitrejean M, Latour C, Bugnazet F, Peyron F, Barron D. and Picot S. In vitro antimalarial activity of flavonoid derivatives dehydrosilybin and 8-(1;1)-DMA-kaempferide. *Acta Tropica,* 97(1), 102-107, (2006).

Morino M, Tsuzuki T, Ishikawa Y, Shirakami T, Yoshimura M, Kiyosuke Y, Matsunaga K, Yoshikumi C, Saijo N. Specific regulation of HSPS in human tumour cell lines by flavonoids. *In vivo,* 11, 265-270, (1997).

Murakami S, Muramatsu M, Otomo S. Gastric H+/K+ ATPase inhibition by catechins. *J Pharm Pharmacol,* 44, 926-928, (1992).

Musci I, Pragathi M. The nutritional significance of flavonoids, some physiological consideration. *Experientia,* 41, 930, (1985).

Naghski J, Copley MJ, Couch JF. Antifungal activity of plant polyphenols. *Science,* 105, 125-131, (1947).

Nagai T, Miyaichi Y, Tomimori T, Suzuki Y, Yamaha H. Antiviral activity of two flavonoids from Tanacetum microphyllum. *Antiviral* Res, 19, 207-216, (1992).

Narayana K Raj, Sripal Reddy M, Chaluvadi MR, Krishna DR. Bioflavonoids classification, pharmacological, biochemical effects and therapeutic potential. *Indian Journal of Pharmacology,* 33, 2-16, (2001).

Ng TB, Ling JML, Wang ZT, Cai JN, Xu GJ. Examination of coumarins, flavonoids and poly saccharopeptides for anti fungal activity. *Gen Pharmacol*, 27, 1237-1242, (1996).

Nicolas R, Phillips M, Judith W. Phenolic Compounds: Extraction and Analysis. In: A.J. Marquez (ed) Lotus japonicas Handbook, pp. 349-355, (2005).

Nishino C, Enoki N, Tawata S, Mori A, Kobayashi K, Fukushima M. Tea flavonids and microbial disease: A review. *Agric Biol Chem* 51,139-145, (1987).

Noro T, Oda Y, Miyasa, Ueno A, Fukushim S. Inhibition of adinosine deaminase activity of aortic endothelial cells by selected flavonoids. *Chem Pharm Bull*, 31, 3984-3991, (1983).

Osman HE, Maalej N, Shanmuganayagam D, Folts JD. Grape juice but not orange or grapefruit juice inhibits plate activity in dogs and monkey's. *J. Nutr*; 128, 2307-2312, (1998).

Pathak D, Pathak K, Singla AK. Flavonoids as medicinal agents- Recent evidences. *Fitoterapia*; I XII (5), 371-389, (1991).

Petkov E, Nickdor N, Uzunov P. Inhibitory effects of flavonoids on xanthine oxidase. *Planta Med,* 43,183-87, (1981).

Pham TK, Vinh PT, Nong HD, Nguyen DK. Flavonoids as antimicrobial agents. *Tap chi Duoc Hoc*, 6, 14-21 (1993).

Ran SS, Lee CK, Kim YS, Characteristics and accurrance of plant polyphenols. *Yak Hak Hoechi*, 36, 407-414 (1992).

Raj KJ, Shalinikapoor. Flavonoids- A review of biological activities. *Indian Drugs*, 36, 668-678, (1999).

Ratsimamanga VS, Rasoanaivo P, Rafemanantsoa C, Ratsimamanga AR, frappier F. Effect of Quercetin on Staphylococcus aureus *in vitro. Fitoterapia*, 65, 551-558, (1994).

Ratty AK. Effects of flavonoids on nonenzymatic lipid peroxidation: structure activity relationship. *Biochem Med Metabol Biol*, 39, 67-79, (1988).

Rawat, AKS, Govindarajan R, Singh DP. High-performance liquid chromatographic method for the quantification of phenolics in 'Chyavanprash' a potent Ayurvedic drug. *Journal of Pharmaceutical and Biomedical Analysis*, 43, 527-532, (2007).

Rawat AKS, R. Govindarajan, Dhirendra P Singh. Validated RP–LC Method for Standardization of Ashokarishta: A Polyherbal Formulation. *Chromatographia*, November No. 9/10, 68, 873-876, (2008).

Robak J. and Gryglewski, RJ. Flavonoids are scavengers of superoxide anions. *Biochem. Pharmacol.* 37, 837-841, (1988).

Ruiyc. Advances in pharmacological studies of silymarin. *Mem Inst Oswaldo Cruz.* 86, 79-85, (1991).

Sato M, Fujiwara S, Tsuchiya H, Fujii T, Linuma M, Tosa H, Ohkawa Y. Role of flavonoids in microbial diseases. *J. Ethnopharmacol*, 54, 171-178, (1996).

Sanabria GA, Ospina SA, Ceron JA, Raman MJ. Quercetin and related bioflavonoids: A review. *Rev Colomb Cienc Quim Farm*, 19,44-51, (1991).

Scevola D, Bacbacini G, Grosso A, Bona S, Perissoud D. Flavonoids and hepatic cyclic monophasphates in liver injury. *Boll Ins Sieroter Milan*, 63, 77-82, (1984).

Shahidi F, Yang Z, Saleemi ZO. Natural flavonoids as stabilizers. *J Food Lipids*, 1, 69-75, (1998).

Singh U P, Pandey VB, Singh KN, Singh RON. Structural and biogenic relationships of isoflavonoids. *Can J Bot*, 166, 1901-1910, (1988).

Singh M, Govindarajan R, Rawat AKS, Khare PB. Antimicrobial Flavonoid Rutin from *Pteris Vittata* L. Against Pathogenic Gastrointestinal Microflora. *American Fern Journal*, 98(2), 98-103,(2008).

Son YO, Kook SH, Choi KC, Jang YS, Jeon YM, Kim JG, Lee KY, Kim J, Chung MS, Chung GH,

Lee JC. Quercetin, a bioflavonoid, accelerates TNF-alpha-induced growth inhibition and apoptosis in MC3T3-E1 osteoblastic cells. *Eur J Pharmacol*, 529, 24-32, (2006).

Tapas, A R Sakarkar DM, and Kakde RB. Flavonoids as Nutraceuticals: A Review. *Tropical Journal of Pharmaceutical Research*, September 7 (3), 1089-1099, (2008).

Tahara S, Hashidoka Y, Mizutani J. Flavonoids as medicines. *Agri Biol Chem*, 51, 1039-1045, (1987).

Tereschuk ML, Riera MVQ, Casteo GR, Afdala LR. Antimicrobial activity of flavonoids from leaves of Tagetes minuta. *J Ethnopharmacol*, 56, 227-236, (1997).

Tsuchiva Y, Shimizu, Hiyama Y, Itoh K, Hashimoto Y, Nakarama M, Horie T, Morita N. Inhibitory effect of flavonoids on fungal diseases. *Chem Pharm Bull,* 33, 3881-3890, (1985).

Tripathi VD, Rastogi RP. *In vitro* anti-HIV activity of flavonoids isolated from Garcinia multifolia. *J Sci Indian Res*, 40, 116-121, (1981).

Torel J, Cillard J, and Cillard P. Antioxidant activity of flavonoids and reactivity with peroxy radical. *Phytochemistry*, 25, 383-385, (1986).

Varma SD, Kinoshita JH. Inhibitory effects of plant polyphenols on rat liver glutathione-S-transferase. *Biochem Pharmacol*, 25, 2505-2510, (1976).

Vessal M, Hemmati M, Vasei M. Antidiabetic effects of quercetin in streptozocin induced diabetic rats. *Comp Biochem Physiol C*, 135, 357-364, (2003).

Wegener T, Fintelmann V. Flavonoids and bioactivity. *Wein Med Wochem Schr*, 149, 241-247, (1999).

Weidenboemer M, Jha H.C. Inhibition of fungal infections of flavonoids. *Pestic Sci*, 38, 347-353, (1993).

Wei H, Tye L, Bresnick E, Birt DF. Inhibitory effect of Apigenin, a plant flavonoids on epidermal ornithine decarboxylase skin tumor promotion in mice. *Cancer Res*, 50, 499-502, (1990).

Whalley De C, Rankin SM, Houct JRS, Jessup W, Leake DS. Flavonoids inhibit the oxidative modification of low density lipoproteins by macrophages. *Biochem Pharmacol,* 39, 1743-1750, (1990).

Wollenweber E. Occurrence of flavonoid aglycones in medicinal plants. *Prog Clin Biol Res*, 280, 45-55, (1988).

chapter 24

Bioactive Triterpenoid Saponins from Medicinal Plants

Santanu Saha and E. V. S. Subrahmanyam

INTRODUCTION

Natural products have been an exemplary source of medicine since existence of human civilizations and this approach has been in practice over the years for discovering new drug molecules. The secondary metabolites have been played a major role in natural product based drug discovery process for millennia and that has initiated the evolution of present contemporary medicine (Clardy and Walsh, 2004; Young-Won et al., 2006). Saponins (triterpenoid and steroid) are such secondary metabolites which can be found widely in nature.

Saponins name derived from Latin word 'sapo', which means soap, because of their ability to form soap- like foam in aqueous solution. Saponins contain sugar moieties, which are linked glycosidically to hydrophobic aglycone part that may be triterpenoids or steroids. Based on this aglycone part saponins are classified as triterpenoid saponins and steroidal saponins. It has also seen that some other classes of saponins are also present in nature like glycosteroidalkaloids. The aglycones (both, triterpenoid and steroid) are synthesized from 2, 3 oxidosqualene by enzymatic cyclization, and then followed by glycosylation to produce respective saponins. The difference between triterpenoid and steroid saponins are attributed to number of carbon atoms of aglycone skeleton. The triterpenoids are having 30 carbon atoms, where steroids contain 27.

Triterpenoid saponins are distributed only in higher plants, unlike steroidal saponins, which are produced by plants, lower marine animals and also by some bacteria (Yoshiki et al., 1998; Minale et al., 1996). The structural diversity of triterpenoid saponins has been seen due to presence of various classes of triterpenoid skeletons, which also found to be responsible for their diverse biological action. Till date many research works have been carried out to find biologically active triterpenoid saponins from plants. In this section, we have collated the information about the bioactive triterpenoid saponins from various plants. Before reviewing bioactive triterpenoid saponins, we describe the biosynthesis of this compound to understand their structural diversity.

Biosynthesis of Triterpenoid Saponins

The biosynthesis of triterpenoid saponins are initiated from mevalonic acid and further proceed via isoprenoid pathway. In Isoprenoid pathway, at first 3 isoprene units of 5 carbon atoms are producing15 carbon atom molecule farnesyl pyrophosphate through geranyl pyro - phosphate. Two molecules of this farnesyl pyro-phosphate linked in a tail-to-tail manner to form squalene of 30 carbon atoms. This squalene oxidized to 2, 3 oxidosqualene and followed by enzymatic cyclisation to produce various skeletons of triterpenoid and sterols (Fig. 1) as aglycone parts of saponins (Abe et al., 1993; Haralampidis et al., 2002). The enzymatic cyclization process is regulated by diverse type of 2, 3 oxidosqualene cyclases (OSCs) like lanosterol synthase, cycloartenol synthase, dammarenediol synthase, β-amyrin synthase (Abe et al., 1993; Wendt et al., 2000; Haralampidis et al., 2002; Wendt, 2005).

The biosynthesis of triterpenoid or sterol follows Ruzicka deduced "biogenetic rule of isoprene", which is governed by cation activated oxidosqualene cyclization of "chair-chair-chair" or "chair-boat-chair" conformation, rearrangement and deprotonation reaction (Ruzicka et al., 1953; Eschenmoser et al., 1955; Ruzicka, 1959, 1963; Xu et al., 2004). 2, 3- oxidosqualene cyclization of the "chair-chair-chair" conformation results in tetracyclic dammarenyl cation and that may be converted to dammarene-like triterpenoids by the dammarenediol synthase (DS) (Baek et al., 1997; Haralampidis et al., 2002; Wendt, 2005). The tetracyclic dammarenyl cation may undergo to further rearrangements to form tetracyclic C17 baccharenyl carbocation and can be followed by reaction to produce pentacyclic C25 lupenyl carbocation. The lupeol synthase (LuS) catalyzes the conversion of pentacyclic C25 lupenyl carbocation to lupane triterpenoid (Yook et al., 2002; Wendt et al., 2000; Haralampidis et al., 2002; Wendt, 2005). Further, the rearrangement of lupenyl carbocation lead to produce oleanane type or β-amyrin triterpenoids and ursane type or α-amyrin triterpenoids, which is mediated by β-amyrin synthase (βAS) and α-amyrin synthase(αAS) respectively (Wandji et al.,2003; Haralampidis et al., 2002; Vincken et al., 2007).

On the other hand, enzymatic cyclisation of "chair-boat-chair"conformation of 2,3-oxidosqualene produces tetracyclic protosteryl C-20 carbocation, which is then converted to sterols like cycloartenol (in plant) and lanosterol(in animals and fungi) by cycloartenol synthase (CS) and lanosterol synthase (LS), respectively(Abe et al., 1993; Kennelly et al., 1996; Radwan et al., 2004; Haralampidis et al., 2002; Xu et al., 2004; Vincken et al., 2007).

In the final step of saponin biosynthesis, all sapogenins (triterpenoid and sterols) go through the various chemical decorations (oxidation, substitution, acylation, glycosylation, benzoylation, and so on) mediated by cytochrome P450-dependent monooxygenases, glycosyltransferases, acyltransferases, benzoyltransferases, and other enzymes. But the detail mechanisms of these reactions are still unknown (Zhong and Yue, 2005). Various sugar moieties like glucose, galactose, rhamnose, glucouronic acid will be attached to carbon skeletons by glycosylation reaction. In case of triterpenoid saponins, sapogenins attach to chain of sugar and/or uronic acid units at C3 position, unlike steroidal saponins. Whereas oxidation reaction causes the attachment of functional groups (hydroxyl groups, carbonyl groups and carboxylic acids) at various positions of carbon skeletons.

Chemistry of Triterpenoid Saponins

Saponins are surface active glycosides that are widely available in nature. Chemically saponins are composed of aglycone and sugar moieties which are produced by hydrolysis of saponins. The structure of saponins are varied depend on variety of aglycone or sapogenins are attached. Commonly triterpenoid and steroids are served as aglycones which lead to name saponins as triterpenoid saponins and steroidal saponins, respectively. Triterpenoid saponins are generally occur in higher plant kingdom where as steroidal saponins are common in wide range of plant species and in some bacteria. The diverse chemical class of saponins also include steroidal glycoalkaloids, which consists of glycosidically linked steroidal alkaloid with monosaccharide moieties (Haralampidis et al., 2002; Vincken et al., 2007).

The non polar aglycone part of triterpenoid saponins include diverse skeletons of triterpenoids and that is attached to one or more polar sugar moieties (Oleszek, 2002). In last the few decades, several works have been carried out on biosynthesis, isolation and characterization of naturally occurring triterpenoid saponins, gave an extensive knowledge about the various classes of triterpenoids which boost up the further classification process for this class of saponins. Therefore, based on triterpenoid carbon skeletons which produced in biosynthetic pathway (see biosynthesis of triterpenoid saponins); triterpenoid saponins are classified in various classes like dammarene, lupanes, oleananes and ursanes. These classes of saponins are distributed in various medicinal plants.

The sugar moieties which are attached to these carbon skeletons, are found to be monosaccharides (e.g. glucose, xylose, arabinose, pyranose, rhamnose, etc.) only, but differ in number. Based on the number of sugar chains attached, triterpenoid saponins are also classified, like, monodesmoside (containing single sugar chain), bidesmoside (containing two sugar chains), tridesmoside (containing three sugar chains). It has seen that 18 monosaccharide residues can be attached through sugar chains to oleanane skeleton. During biosynthesis several substituents such as -OH, -COOH, -CHO, $-CH_2OH$ and $-CH_3$ are also introduced to different position of aglycone skeleton.

Bioactive Triterpenoid Saponins from Medicinal Plants

Triterpenoid saponins are distributed in dicotyledon plants such as alliums, ginseng, liquorice, quillaja, horse chestnut, spinach and so on. These diverse classes of triterpenoid saponins have been observed in many dicotyledonous families such as Sapindaceae, Caryophyllaceae, Linaceae, Rutaceae, Myrtaceae. Triterpenoid saponins are also reported to be seen in various legumes, like soyabeans, beans, peas, etc. The triterpenoid saponins, Soyasaponin- I, Soyasaponins I-III, and Dehydrosoyasaponin-I were isolated from peas and soyabean (Taylor et al., 2004). The most bioactive triterpenoid saponins have been reported as ginsenosides from Panax *ginseng* and *Panax notoginseng*. Chemically Ginsenosides contain dammarane as well as oleanane type of triterpenoid skeletons. Ginsenosides like ginsenoside Rb1, Rg1 and 20(S) protopanaxadiol have been isolated from Ginseng plant species, were found to be responsible for immunomodulation, cytotoxicity and antitumor, antiviral, antibacterial activities (Ng et al., 2006; Liu et al., 2009; Christensen, 2009). The triterpenoid saponins from *Quillaja saponaria* Molina have been reported for immunomodulatory and adjuvant activity. The purified quillaja saponins found to be as QS-7, QS-17, QS-18, and QS-21 from this plant species (Nord and Kenne, 2000; Guo et al., 2000). Symplocososides and Escins from *Symplocos chinensis* (Fu et al., 2005; Li et al., 2005), Avicins from *Acacia victoriae* (Li et al., 2005), Madecassoside and Asiaticoside from *Centella asiatica* (Sampson et al. 2001), are few examples of triterpenoid saponins which have been isolated and also reported for their various biological activities. Few structures of isolated triterpenoid saponins illustrated in Fig. 2.

Here, we attempt to discuss about triterpenoid saponins from various plants with their biological actions and the mechanism for respective activities.

Immunological Activity by Triterpenoid Saponins

Botanicals alter immune functions in mode of modulating cytokine secretion, immunoglobulin secretion, cellular co-receptor expressions, lymphocyte expressions and phagocytosis, to exhibit immunomodulatory activity (Patwardhan and Gautam, 2005; Plaeger, 2003). Many saponins from natural sources have been included in this list of botanical immunomodulators (Kensil, 1996). Triterpenoid saponins from *Quillaja saponaria* Molina and *Panax ginseng* C.A. Meyer, lead this list for its profound action on immune systems. *In vitro* study reported the increase of immune cell proliferation by Quillaja and other saponins either as crude extract or as pure compound (Chavali et al., 1987; Plohmann et al., 1997; Lacaille-Dubois et al., 1999). In another study Quillaja saponins QH-A and QH-C in various formulations showed an *in vitro* and *in vivo* induction of IL-6 (Behboudi et al., 1997). The purified saponins QS-7, QS-17, QS-18, and QS-21 from quillaja bark increase the antibody levels by 100 fold or more in Ag BSA and beef liver cytochrome b5 immunized mouse. The same study also confirmed the toxicity of QS-18 unlike QS-7 and QS-21 (Kensil et al., 1991). The action of Quil A (quillaja saponins) on Th1/ Th2 immune response and the production of cytotoxic T-lymphocytes (CTLs) have promoted it as vaccine adjuvant (Sjölander et al., 1997; So et al., 1997; Coulter et al., 1998). Further this, saponin led to form immune-stimulating complex (ISCOM), in combination with cholesterol, phospholipid, amphiphatic proteins. The adjuvant activity of ISCOM or quillaja saponins alone have been in interest for vaccine based research, since early 80's. The *in vivo* study on ICR mice reported significant increase of IgG1 level along with adjuvant effect on antigen specific IgG2a, IgG2b and IgG3 of QS-21 in combination with three type O-side-chain polysaccharide containing vaccine, compare to immunogenicity of vaccines alone (Coughlin et al., 1995). In another study ISCOMs induced antibody response and/or protective immunity were evaluated in many experimental mammalian animals (Mowat et al., 1999). Pham et al. (Pham et al., 2006) reported the isolation of QS-7, QS-17, QS-18, and QS-21 by fractionation of Quil A and out of which only QS-7 was able to form prominent structures and a minor amount of ISCOMs in combination with lipid. The immunomodulatory activity of ginsenoside Rg1 from *Panax ginseng* was evaluated by stimulating humoral immune responses of sheep red blood cells immunized mice. Ginsenoside Rg1 also increased the number of T-helper cells and production of IL-1 by macrophages (Kenarova et al., 1990). Further study reported the Th2 specific immune response of Ginsenoside Rg1 by enhancing CD4(+) T cells and Th2 cytokine IL-4 (Lee et al., 2004). A crude ginseng extract (GS) and the purified ginsenoside R(b1) (R(b1)) were evaluated for their adjuvant effects in dairy cattle at immunisation with ovalbumin (OVA) and/or a Staphylococcus aureus bacterin. Both GS and R(b1) were safe adjuvants, and R(b1) had the strongest adjuvant effects, when used for immunisation against S. aureus in dairy cattle (Hu et al., 2003). Ginseng-fraction Rb1 containing Porcine parvovirus (PPV) vaccines induced IL-4 and IL-10 in pre-boost animals and IFN-gamma, IL-2, IL-4, IL-10 and TNF-alpha in post-boost mice along with similar antibody titres in pre and post-boost mice, concluded the balanced Th1 and Th2 immune response of Rb1 fraction as vaccine adjuvant (Rivera et al., 2005). Protopanaxadiol saponins (Rg3, Rd, Rc, Rb1 and Rb2) and protopanaxatriol saponins (Rg1, Re and Rg2) from the root of *Panax ginseng* were evaluated for their adjuvant effects in ovalbumin (OVA) immunized mice by increasing antibody responses and cytokine production. The study showed Rg1, Re, Rg2, Rg3 and Rb1 have more potent adjuvant properties than the others, indicating that they are the major constituents contributing to the adjuvant activities of total ginseng saponins (Sun et al., 2007). Saponins extracted from ginseng stems and leaves (GSLS) and GSLS with oil emulsion showed potent adjuvant effects by modulating cellular and humoral immune responses and by promoting both Th1 and Th2 immune responses of mice to vaccination against foot-and-mouth disease virus (FMDV) serotype Asia 1 (Song et al., 2009). Triterpenoid saponins from *Glycyrrhiza uralensis* showed humoral and cellular immune response similar to Quil A in Ovalalbumin immunized ICR mice by stimulating splenocyte proliferation and enhancing OVA-specific IgG, IgG1, and IgG2b antibody responses (Sun and Pan, 2006). Platycodin D2 (PD2), triterpenoid saponin from *Platycodon grandiflorum* showed potent immunomodulatory activity in Ovalalbumin immunized ICR mice by stimulating splenocyte proliferation and enhancing OVA-specific IgG, IgG1, and IgG2b antibody responses, which concluded the balanced Th1 and Th2 directing immune response by the saponins (Xie et al., 2008; Xie et al., 2008). A novel triterpenoidal saponin, called pulcherrimasaponin (CP05) from the leaves of *Calliandra pulcherrima* Benth showed vaccine adjuvant activity similar to QS21 saponin (*Quillaja saponaria* Molina) with fucose-mannose ligand (FML) antigen of *Leishmania donovani* by enhancing FML specific antibody responses and delayed type hypersensitivity against leishmanial antigen (Silva et al., 2005). Another study specified the vaccine adjuvant activity by monoterpene deprived fraction of CP05 in comparison with QS21 saponin with same FML vaccines. Where intact saponins CP05, which lacks the C4 aldehyde group was unable to augment anti-FML antibody, CD4(+) and CD8(+) Leishmania specific lymphocytes and IFN-gamma splenocyte secretion (Nico et al., 2005). Eight pure triterpenoid saponins from *Polygala senega* L. have been reported for potent immunomodulatory activity against OVA immunized mice and enhancement of IL-2 levels in *in vitro* study of spleen cell culture from immunized mice (Katselis et al., 2007). Triterpenoid saponins from *Acacia victoriae*, have been reported for its modification of NF-êâ molecule to prevent stimulation of genes involved in immune and inflammatory pathways in response to stress signal (Haridas et al., 2001).

Cytotoxicity and antitumor activity by triterpenoid saponins

Triterpenoid saponins from plant species reported for antitumor activity for allogeneic sarcoma 180 and syngeneic DBA/2-MC.SC-1 fibrosarcoma tumor models, which presumed to be driven by immunomodulation effect by augmentation of TNF-alpha release (Plohmann et al., 1997). Asterlingulatoside C and D, triterpenoid saponins from *Aster lingulatus,* showed good inhibitory activity against DNA synthesis in human leukemia HL-60 cells with IC50 values of 8.8 and 6.1 microM, respectively (Shao et al., 1997). Novel triterpenoid saponins, capilliposide A-C from *Lysimachia capillipes* evaluated for cytotoxic activity, where only capilliposide B showed significant cytotoxicity against human A-2780 cells (Tian et al., 2006). *Albizia adianthifolia* (Mimosaceae) triterpenoid saponins reported for induction of apoptosis on human leukemia cells. The result showed cytotoxic and/or lymphoproliferative effect of adianthifoliosides A, B, and D (AdA, AdB, and AdD) and prosapogenins (Pro1 and Pro2) on human leukemia T-cells (Jurkat cells), where only lymphoproliferative effect found on splenocytes. The study suggested the apoptosis as an alternative mechanism for cytotoxic activity other than membrane permeabilization formation (Haddad et al., 2004). Study on triterpenoid saponins form Chinese horse chestnut seeds showed vacuolization, apoptotic nuclei fragmentation and apoptotic body formation in human leukaemia cells as signs of apoptosis, which could be established the mechanism of action for cytotoxic effect. Where as, antiproliferative activity of saponins on the same cell lines were caused by cell cycle arrest at G1-S phase (Niu et al., 2008). Ginsenoside Rg3 exhibited the antiproliferative activity by seems to be same mechanism. The apoptosis induction in human cancer and other cell lines by saponins irrespective of triterpenoid or steroid can be caused by stimulating cytochrome c—caspase 9—caspase 3 pathway (Lee et al., 2000; Liu et al., 2000;

Haridas et al., 2001; Cai et al., 2002). The property was followed for cytotoxic activity showed by triterpenoid saponins from *Securidaca inappendiculata* (Yui et al., 2001). Symplocososides Ġ-K, triterpenoid saponins from root of *Symplocos chinensis*, showed significant cytotoxicity against cancer cell lines KB, HCT-8, Bel-7402, BGC-823 and A549 with IC (50) values ranging from 0.82 muM to 5.09 muM, except for symplocososide I against cancer cell lines KB, BGC-823, A549 and symplocososide K against cancer cell line BGC-823 with IC (50) values >10.00 muM (Fu et al., 2005).

However, the diverse groups of saponins from variety of plant species have shown cytotoxic activity in different manner. As in recent work, apoptosis based mechanism for cytotoxicity of triterpenoid saponins was challenged by avicin D. This triterpenoid saponins were able to cause the death for apoptosis inhibitor (benzyloxycarbonyl-valyl-alanyl-aspartic acid (O-methyl)-fluoro-methylketone) treated and apoptosis-resistant cells. This non-apoptotic cell death claimed to be mediated by different mechanism, autophagy, which can be regulated by set of events like, decreasing cellular ATP levels, stimulating the activation of AMP-activated protein kinase (AMPK), and inhibiting mammalian target of rapamycin (mTOR) and S6 kinase activity. The autophagy cell death was found to be decreased by inhibiting the events from AMPK to mTOR, which put a further support to hold autophagy as a mechanism for cell death (Xu et al., 2007). Soyasaponins from soyabean also showed the cytotoxicity for human colon cancer cells by induction of macroautophagy (Ellington et al., 2005). The triterpenoid saponins-initiated tumor-specific cytotoxicity seems to be structure related and sugar moieties were found to be responsible for this action (Hosny and Rosazza, 2002). The finding further supported by a work on enzymatic hydrolysis of virgaureasaponin 1 (triterpenoid saponins), where sugar moieties showed the cytotoxic activity (Bader et al., 1998). The study on cytotoxic activity of hederagenin also supported the structural activity relationship (Chwalek et al., 2006).

Anti-inflammatory activity by triterpenoid saponins

Six triterpenoid saponins from the roots of *Codonopsis lanceolata*, were investigated for anti-inflammatory activity. The isolated new compound named codonolaside III, showed promising inhibitory effect for xylene-induced mouse ear edema compare to other triterpenoid saponins (Xu et al., 2008). A new triterpenoid saponin from *Carthamus tinctorius* linn., showed anti-inflammatory activity in experimental model (Yadava and Chakravarti, 2008). A comparative study of anti-inflammatory activity in mice model between isolated triterpenoid saponins and total saponins extract of *Aesculus chinensis*, showed a potent activity by isolated compound than total extract (Wei et al., 2004). Inhibition of carrageenan induced rat paw oedema was showed by triterpenoid saponins from *Polygala japonica*. The saponins were found to inhibit the production of inflammatory mediators–nitric oxide (NO) in LPS-stimulated RAW264.7 macrophages, advocated the anti-inflammatory activity by compounds (Wang et al., 2008). Anti-rheumatic effect of triterpenoid glycoside niga-ichigoside F1 (NIF1) and its aglycone 23-hydroxytormentic acid (23-HTA) from *Rubus coreanus* (Rosaceae) were investigated in Freund's complete adjuvant-induced rheumatism in rats. The saponins were significantly decreasing rheumatoid arthritis (RA) factor and C-reactive protein (CRP) factor, which was found to be reason for anti-rheumatic effect of compounds (Nam et al., 2006). The triterpenoid saponins (Avicin) showed anti-inflammatory activity by suppressing proinflammatory components of the innate immune system in human cells by redox regulation (Haridas et al., 2004). Triterpenoid saponins, clematichinenosides AR and AR (2) from *Clematis chinensis* Osbeck, also showed anti-inflammatory activity by the same mechanism (Liu et al., 2009). In structure-activity relationship study for anti-inflammatory activity of tubeimosides showed the key role of C-16 hydroxyl group for the effect. In the study Tubeimosides I, II, and III form *Bolbostemma paniculatum* (Maxim) Franquet (Cucurbitaceae) were investigated for anti-inflammatory activity, where C-16 hydroxyl group containing tubeimosides II only showed potent effect (Yu et al., 2001).

Antiviral activity by triterpenoid saponins

Diverse group of triterpenoid saponins have been reported for antiviral activity against various viruses and their mechanism of action also found to be erratic. Tubeimoside-1 (Tub), the triterpenoid saponin from *Bolbostemma paniculatum* (Maxim) Franquet, showed anti-HIV activity by mechanism of inhibiting HIV core protein p24 production and HIV mediated cytopathogenesis HTLV-IIIB and also by neutralizing the infection of 2 other isolates, HTLV-IIIRF and HTLV-IIIMN (Yu et al., 1994). Triterpenoid saponins (zingibroside R1) were also reported for anti-HIV activity mediated by cytotoxicity (Hasegawa et al., 1994). Gleditsia saponin C and gymnocladus saponin G from *Gleditsia japonica* and *Gymnocladus chinensis*, respectively, were shown anti-HIV activity by following the same principles (Konoshima et al., 1995). *Ardisia japonica* triterpenoid saponins showed anti-HIV activity in *in vitro* experiment (Piacente et al., 1996). Where as, triterpenoid saponins from natural sources showed antiviral activity against herpes simplex virus type 1 either by inhibiting viral DNA synthesis (by oleanolic group) or by inhibiting viral capsid protein synthesis (by ursane group) but never shown any cytotoxic activity (Simões et al., 1999). Antiviral activity of Quillaja extracts against six viruses: vaccinia virus, herpes simplex virus type 1, varicella zoster virus, human immunodeficiency viruses 1 and 2 (HIV-1, HIV-2) and reovirus were also supported the mechanism based upon direct virucidal activity other than cell cytotoxicity (Roner et al., 2007). Oleanolic acid glycosides from *Calendula arvensis* were reported for antiviral effects by inhibition of vesicular stomatitis virus (VSV) and rhinovirus (HRV) infection in cell cultures (De Tommasi et al., 1991). The study on synthetic triterpenoid saponins revealed the responsibility of sugar linkage for antiviral activity (Takechi et al., 2003). In other study acylated triterpenoid saponins from *Maesa lanceolata* showed antiviral activity which was related to the diacylation of compounds (Apers et al., 2001). Some triterpenoid saponins were also found to be effective against type A influenza virus by their structure modification (Flekhter et al., 2007). Six triterpenoid saponins (oblonganoside A-F) from *Ilex oblonga* were reported for their activity against Tobacco mosaic virus (TMV) by inhibiting TMV replication (Wu et al., 2007). In a recent study, astragaloside IV, a triterpenoid saponin from Chinese herb radix Astragali (huangqi) showed potent anti-hepatitis B virus (HBV) activity in duck hepatitis B virus (DHBV)-infected ducklings (Wang et al., 2009), which also supported the previous anti-HBV activity showed by whole extract of same plant.

Other Activities of Triterpenoid Saponins

Saponins are found to have hemolytic activity, irrespective of their aglycone structure. The triterpenoid saponins form *Symplocos glomerata* King showed 50% haemolysis of a 10% suspension of sheep erythrocytes (Waffo-Teguo et al., 2004). Acylated triterpenoid saponins from *Harpullia austro-caledonica* also caused 100% haemolysis of a 10% suspension of sheep erythrocytes (Voutquenne et al., 2005). In another study, Maesasaponin mixture B from *Maesa lanceolata* hemolyzed 50% of human erythrocytes (1% suspension) at concentration of 1.6 microg/mL (Sindambiwe et al., 1998). However the mechanism for hemolytic activity is not fully understood. In that context Lin and Wang reported that triterpenoid saponins (dioscin) possibly caused the destabilization of membrane by penetrating the membrane lipid bilayer and consequent membrane curvature, which may eventually result in the hemolysis of red cells (Lin and Wang, 2009). Soyasaponinsl and III, and dehydrosoyasaponin I caused membrane hyperpolarization by opening large Ca-dependent K conductance channels, which relaxed smooth muscle (McManus et al., 1993). Glycosides Rb1, Rg1, 20(S) protopanaxadiol also showed the effect on lipid bilayer (DPPC) for phase transition (Akoev et al., 1997). The ability of acylated triterpenoid saponins from ginseng to integrate transiently into membrane and to form pore like structure, were suggested that the hemolytic activity directly dependent on the numbers of polar groups in aglycone moiety (Namba et al., 1973). It was also observed that triterpenoid saponins with a single sugar chain (monodesmosides) showed more hemolytic potential than those with a two sugar chains (bidesmosides) (Fukuda et al., 1985; Woldemichael and Wink, 2001).

Besides, cell membrane permeabilization and hemolytic activity triterpenoid saponins like hederagenin or oleanolic acid also showed antifungal activity on Yeast as well as Dermatophyte species and *Candida glabrata* (Favel et al., 1994). Triterpenoid saponins from *Pithecellobium racemosum* (M.) were found to have moderate antifungal activity against T. mentogrophytes, C. albicans and S. cerevisiae with MIC values of 6.25, 12.5 and 12.5 micrograms/ml respectively (Khan et al., 1997). Glycosides of polygalacic acid were evaluated for antifungal activity in micro-dilution assay by using various funguses: *Candida albicans, C. glabrata, C. krusei* and *C. tropicalis* (Bader et al., 2000). The molluscicidal activity was also found in glycosides of oleanolic acid of *Dialium guineense* (Houghton et al., 1997). Platycodin A, from *Platycodi radix* exhibited significant neuroprotective activities against glutamate-induced toxicity, exhibiting cell viability of about 50%, at concentrations ranging from 0.1 microM to 10 microM (Son et al., 2007). Sixteen triterpenoid saponins from *Polygala tenuifolia* Willd., showed protective action on neurotoxicity induced by glutamate and serum deficiency in PC12 cells at the concentration of 10 (-5) mol/L (Li et al., 2008). Sapinmusaponins Q and R of *Sapindus mukorossi* demonstrated potent anti-platelet aggregation activity than aspirin (Huang et al., 2007). The triterpenoid saponins were also showed anti-sweetning activity (Yoshikawa et al., 1997; Yoshikawa et al., 2000).

Clinical trial studies of natural triterpenoid saponins

In context of drug discovery research, clinical trial studies proclaimed medicinal efficacy of triterpenoid saponins. ISCOMATRIX adjuvant and HPV16E6E7 fusion protein comprised HPV16. Immunotherapeutic successfully developed HPV16 E6E7 specific cell mediated immunity in immunized patients compare to placebo recipients, in a phase I clinical trial, which proved the safe and increasing immunity property of immunotherapy in presence of ISCOMATRIX adjuvant and HPV16E6E7 fusion protein (Frazer et al., 2004). The immunoadjuvant property of Quillaja saponin containing ISCOMATRIX has been evaluated along with recombinant NY-ESO-1 protein ("cancer-testis" antigen) in human by inducing high-titer antibody responses, strong delayed-type hypersensitivity reactions, and NY-ESO-1 epitopes- specific circulating CD8(+) and CD4(+) T cells (Davis et al., 2004). The adjuvant effect of QS-21 was also observed along with MPL in vaccine formulation, which was able to induce strong and persistent humoral and T cell responses against hepatitis B surface antigen (Vandepapelière et al., 2008). Ginseng saponins in the form of Shengxueling (SXL), a Chinese medicinal preparation showed immediate effect in treating of refractory idiopathic thrombocytopenic purpura (ITP) in human with less adverse effect (Shao et al., 2007).

The immunity related anti-rheumatoid arthritis effect of *Panax notoginseng* saponins (PNS) has been observed by changing indexes including platelet counts, immnuoglobulins (IgG, IgA, IgM), complement (C)3, rheumatoid factor (RF), C-reactive protein (CRP), ceruloplasmin (CER), haptoglobin (HPT), and alpha1-acid glycoprotein (AAG) in 43 patients (Zhang et al., 2007). Ginsenoside-Rd showed selective competitive Ca^{2+} receptor antagonist in a phase II randomized double-blind clinical study with patients, which proved its effect on acute ischemic stroke (Liu et al., 2009). Ginsenoside Rg3 (Shenyi Capsule) treatment in combination with chemotherapy showed improvement of the postoperative life span of patients with non-small cell lung cancer (NSCLC) in comparison to chemotherapy alone. It has seen that ginsenoside Rg3 (Shenyi Capsule) treatment increased NK cells and ratio of CD4/CD8 was maintained normal in capsule treated or combined treated patients, unlike only chemotherapy treatment patients (Lu et al., 2008). The effect of *Panax quinquefolius* saponin (PQS) on blood lipid and insulin sensitivity was approved by clinical study on patients of coronary heart disease (CHD) with blood glucose abnormality (BGA). The treatment of PQS in combination with conventional drug decreased fasting plasma glucose (FPG), total cholesterol (TC), low-density lipoprotein cholesterol (LDL-C) where as it increased Homa-beta values to show effects on blood lipid and insulin sensitivity, respectively (Zhang et al., 2007). Another triterpenoid saponin, escin shortened the time to recovery of gastrointestinal motility significantly in cancer patients after colorectal surgery (Xie et al., 2009).

Here, in **Table 1**, we have listed out the reported triterpenoid saponins with their sources and biological activities.

CONCLUSION

Triterpenoid saponins are produced by many different plant species, primarily dicots. These classes of saponins are synthesized from mevalonic acid via isoprenoid pathway, which lead to develop diverse classes of triterpenoid skeletons. Aglyclone skeletons then undergo glycosylated with various monosaccharides. Due to their complex structures, various functions have been observed, like hemolysis, immunomodulation, adjuvant effect, antiviral, antifugal, antitumor. The mechanism for immunomodulatory activity of triterpenoid saponins were found to be the effect on T-helper cells , Th1/Th2 specific cytokines (IL-2, IL-4, IFN-γ, TNF-α) and cytotoxic T-lymphocytes, which also helped to develop it as a potent adjuvant for various vaccine preparations. Effect of triterpenoid saponins on pro-inflammatroy cytokines are also responsible for its anti-inflammatory activity. The cell-membrane permeabilization and antiproliferative activity of saponins has been reported as mechanism for its cytotoxic and antitumor activity. Due to cell- membrane permeabilization property triterpenoid saponins are also found to have hemolytic activity. The neuroprotective activity of triterpenoid saponins has been observed in *in vivo* studies against glutamate induced cell toxicity. Triterpenoid saponins showed antiviral activity either by inhibiting viral DNA synthesis or by inhibiting viral capsid protein synthesis, and it also showed direct virucidal activity. Several clinical studies of natural triterpenoid saponins have proved its claimed biological activities.

Structure-activity relationship studies showed that aglycone and sugar moieties are responsible for various activities. Aglycones are claimed to have cell-membrane permeabilization and antiviral potential. Whereas sugar moieties are found to be responsible for immunomodulation or adjuvant activity, antitumor activity by cell cycle arrest and anti-inflammatory activity. It has been observed that same class of saponins able to show various activities. The cause of these findings have not been clearly understood yet. This requires further extensive studies on isolated compounds to find out their proper mechanism of actions for various activities.

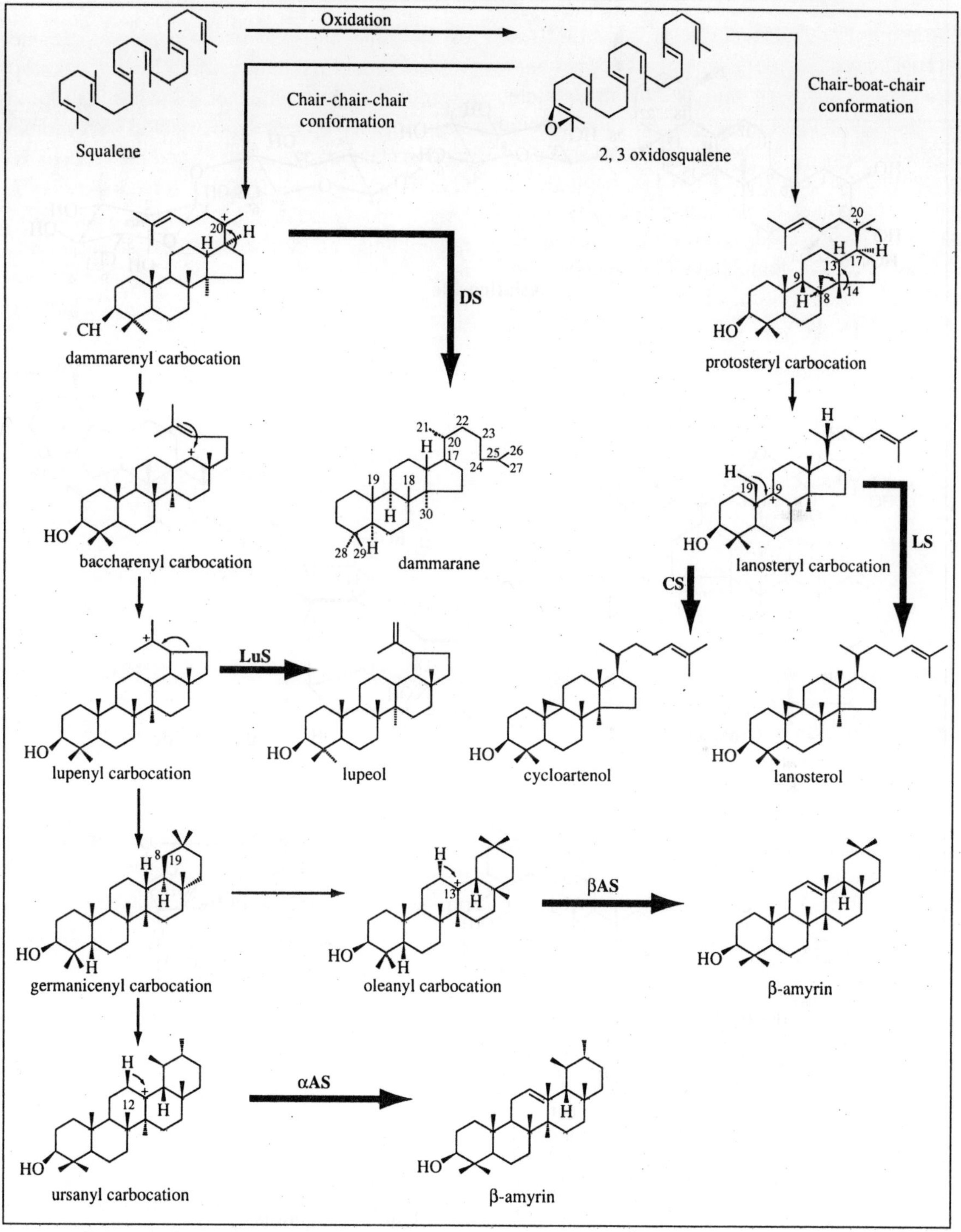

Fig. 24.1: Cyclization of 2, 3- oxidosqualene to produce various steroid and triterpenoid skeletons by the help of different oxidosqualene cyclase enzymes: DS- dammarenediol synthase, CS- cycloartenol synthase, LS- lanosterol synthase, LuS- lupeol synthase, αAS- β-amyrin synthase, αAS- α-amyrin synthase

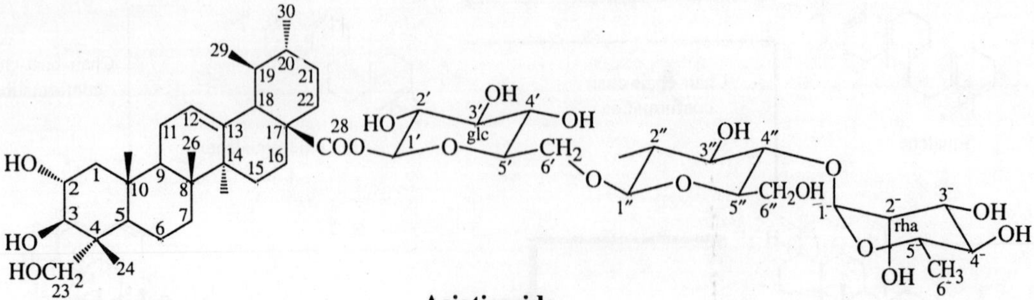

Asiaticoside

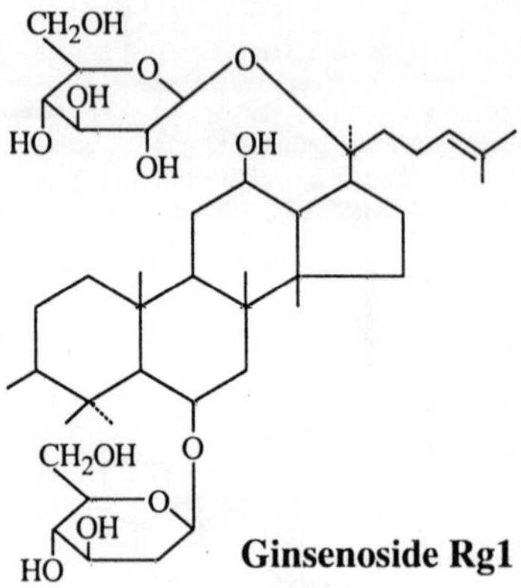

Ginsenoside Rg1

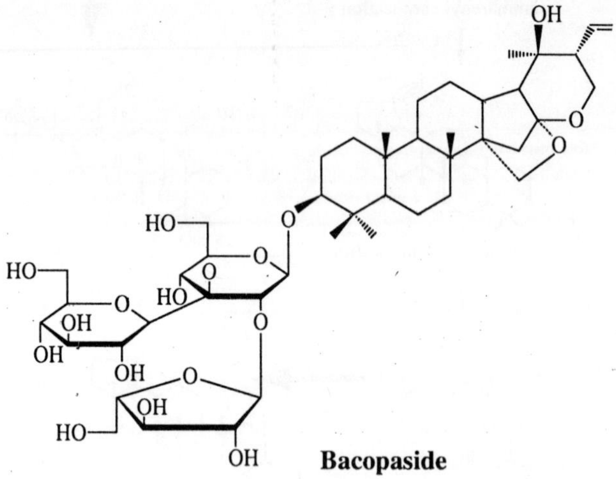

Bacopaside

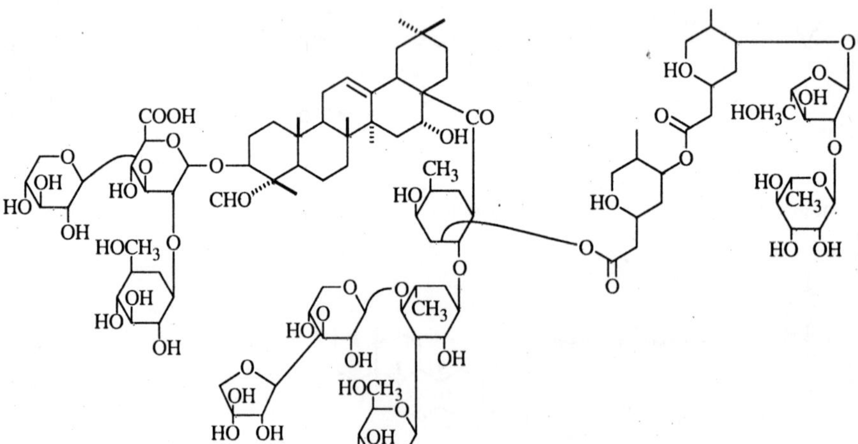

Quillaja saponins

Contd. to next page.

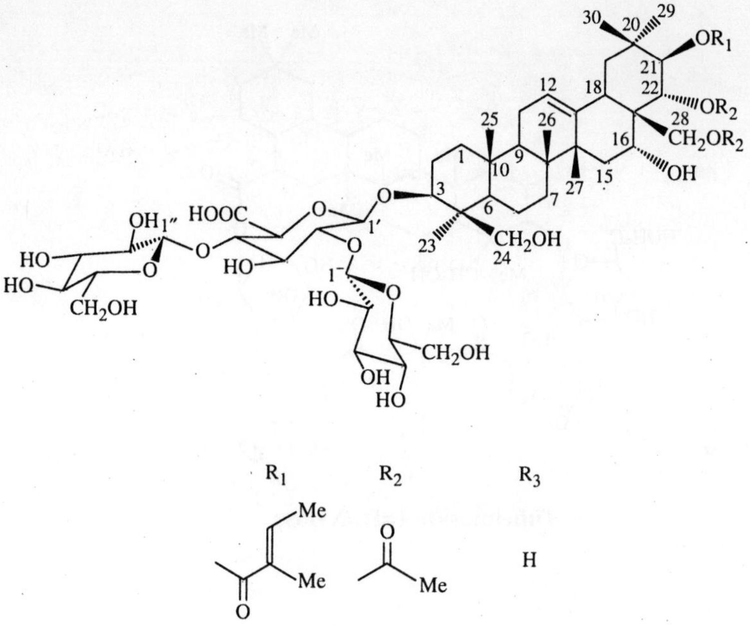

Escin I a

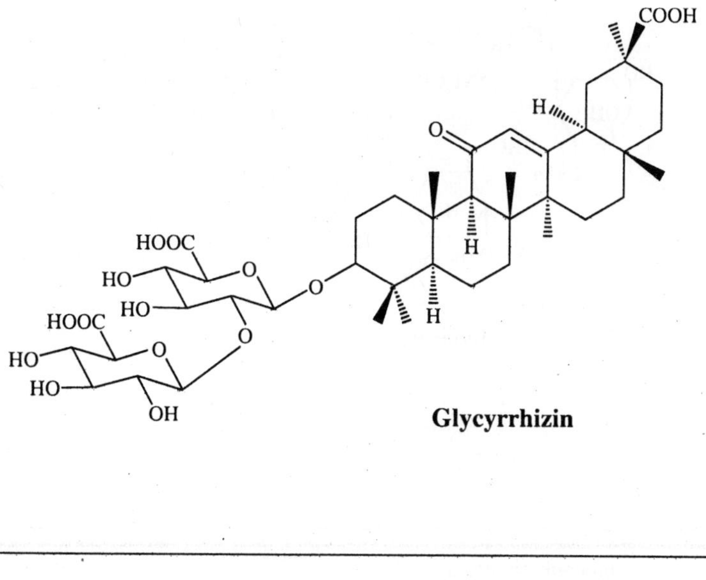

Glycyrrhizin

Contd. to next page.

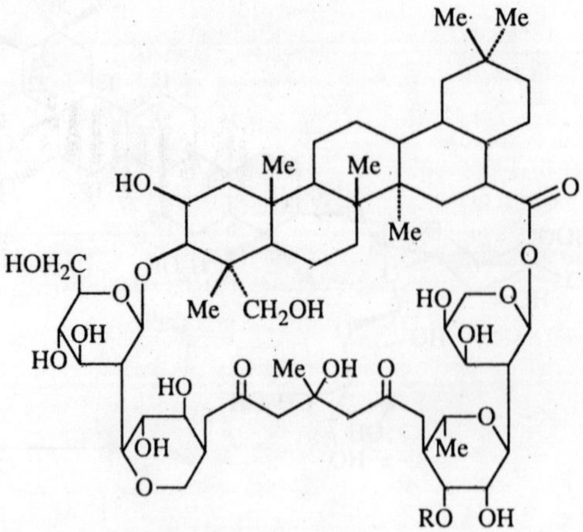

Tubeimoside 1=R=Xylose

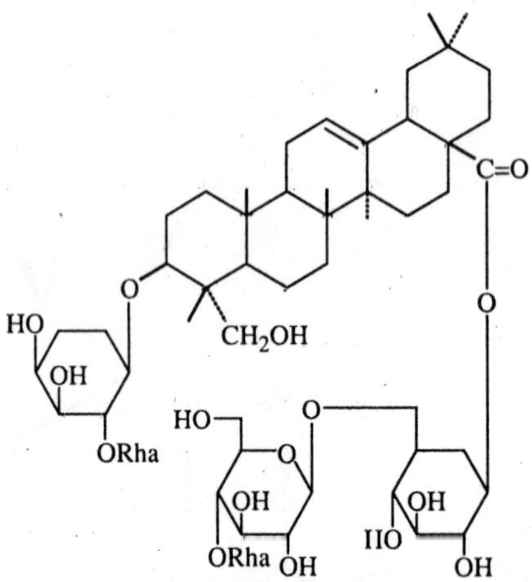

Hederasaponin

Fig. 24.2: Structures of isolated triterpenoid saponins

Table 24.1: List of isolated triterpenoid saponins along with their sources and biological actions

Source	*Name of compound*	*Biological activity*	*Reference*
Acacia victoriae	Avicins	Anticancer	Haridas et al., 2001
Acanthopanax senticosus	Acanthopanaxoside E	Pancreatic lipase-inhibition activity	Li et al., 2007
Aesculus chinensis	Escin Ia, Ib, IVc–f, Isoescin Ia and Ib	Anti-HIV activity by inhibiting HIV-1 protease	Yang et al., 1999
Albizia grandibracteata	Grandibracteosides A-C	Antitumor activity against KB and MCF7 tumoral cell	Krief et al., 2005
Ardisia crenata Sims.	Ardisicrenoside K and L	Antifungal	Liu et al., 2007
Aster sedifolius	Astersedifolioside A-C	Antiproliferative effect in KiMol, a transformed Thyroid cell line	Corea et al., 2004
Bacopa monniera	Bacopasides IX-XI, bacopaside I and II, bacopasaponsin C and D	Memory impairment activity	Zhou et al., 2009
Bohadschia vitiensis	Bivittoside D	Spermicidal activity	Lakshmi et al., 2008
Bredemeyera floribunda	Bredemeyeroside B	Antidote activity for *Snake venom*	Daros et al., 1996
Bupleurum falcatum	Saikosaponin-A(SSA)	Inhibition of allergic asthma	Park et al., 2002
Cimicifuga racemosa	Actein	Anti-HIV activity	Sakurai et al., 2004
Cynara cardunculus L.	Cynarasaponins 1-3	Antimutagenic	Krizkova et al., 2004
Dianthus superbus var. Longicalycinus herbs	Dianosides	Analgesic and Antihepatotoxic actions	Hikino et al., 1984
Dianthus versicolor	Dianversicosides A-G	Cytotoxic activity	Ma et al., 2009
Glinus oppositifolius	Glinosides A and B	Antiplasmodial activity	Traore et al., 2000
Glochidion eriocarpum	Glochieriosides A and B, and Glochidone	Cytotoxic activity againsthuman cancer cell lines	Kiem et al., 2009
Grindelia robusta Nutt and *G. lanceolata Nutt.*	Grindeliasapogenin D	Haemolytic activity	Kreutzer et al., 1990
Gynostemma pentaphyllum	Gypenosides	Vasorelaxation activity	Tanner et al., 1999
Gypsophila oldhamiana	Gypsosaponins A-C	Pancreatic lipase-inhibition activity	Zheng et al., 2007
Hedera colchica Koch	Hederacolchiside-A (HCol-A1)	Immunomodulatory activity	Barthomeuf et al., 2004
Hedera helix	Alpha-hederin	Cytotoxic activity	Danloy et al., 1994
Ixeris sonchifolia	Ixeris saponins A-C	Cytotoxicity against cancer cell lines	Feng et al., 2003

Contd. to next page.

Lonicera japonica	Loniceroside C	Anti-inflammatory activity	Kwak et al., 2003
Maesa balansae	Maesabalides I-VI	Anti-leishmanial activity	Germonprez et al., 2005
Mitragyna inermis	Quinovic acid glycosides	Anti-tumor activity	Cheng et al., 2002
Pentaclethra macroloba	Macrolobin-A and B	Antidote for Bothrops snake venome	da Silva et al., 2007
Phytolacca tetramera	Phytolaccosides B, E and F	Antifungal activity	Escalante et al., 2002
Scabiosa tschiliensis	Scabiosaponins A-K, and Hookerosides A and B	Pancreatic lipase inhibition activity	Zheng et al., 2004
Swartzia langsdorffii Raddi.	Oleanane type triterpenoid saponins- A2, B2, C and D	Molluscicidal activity	Magalhaes et al., 2003
Symphytum officinale	Symphytoxide A	Hypotensive activity	Ahmad et al., 1993
Symplocos chinensis	Symplocososide A- F	Cytotoxic Activity	Tang et al., 2004
Trevesia palmata	Bisdesmosidic saponins 1-6	Antiproliferative activity	De Tommasi et al., 2000
Vaccaria segetalis	Segetoside B	Inhibition of Luteal cell activity	Sang et al., 2002
Viola hondoensis	Acutoside A	Metalloproteinase (MMP)-1 inhibitory activity	Moon et al., 2004
Wistaria brachybotrys	Wistariasaponins D and G	Antitumor activity	Konoshima and Kozuka, 1991
Zygophyllum fabago L.	Zygophylosides O and P	Nitric Oxide (NO) inhibitory activity	Feng et al., 2008

REFERENCES

Abe I, Rohmer M, Prestwich GC. Enzymatic cyclization of squalene and oxidosqualene to sterols and triterpenes. *Chem Rev*, 93, 2189-2206, (1993).

Ahmad VU, Noorwala M, Mohammad FV, Sener B, Gilani AH, Aftab K. Symphytoxide A, a triterpenoid saponin from the roots of *Symphytum officinale. Phytochemistry*, 32(4), 1003-1006, (1993).

Akoev VR, Elemesov RE, Abdrasilov BS, Kim Y. A, Park HJ. Effects of triterpenoid glycosides of the dammaran series and their aglycons on phase transitions of dipalmitoylphosphatidylcholine. *Membr Cell Biol*, 10 (6), 657-663, (1997).

Apers S, Baronikova S, Sindambiwe JB, Witvrouw M, De Clercq E, Vanden Berghe D, Van Marck E, Vlietinck A, Pieters L. Antiviral, haemolytic and molluscicidal activities of triterpenoid saponins from *Maesa lanceolata*: establishment of structure-activity relationships. *Planta Med*, 67(6), 528-532, (2001).

Bader G, Seibold M, Tintelnot K, Hiller K. Cytotoxicity of triterpenoid saponins. Part 2: Relationships between the structures of glycosides of polygalacic acid and their activities against pathogenic Candida species. *Pharmazie*, 55(1), 72-74, (2000).

Bader G, Wray V, Just U, Hiller K. Enzymatic hydrolysis of the cytotoxic triterpenoid glycoside virgaureasaponin 1. *Phytochemistry*, 49 (1), 153-156, (1998).

Baek NI, Kim JM, Park JH, Ryu JH, Kim DS, Lee Y. H, Park JD, Kim SI. Ginsenoside Rs(3), a genuine dammarane-glycoside from Korean red ginseng. *Arch Pharm Res*, 20(3), 280-282, (1997).

Barthomeuf C, Boivin D, Beliveau R. Inhibition of HUVEC tubulogenesis by hederacolchiside-A1 is associated with plasma membrane cholesterol sequestration and activation of the Ha-Ras/MEK/ERK cascade. *Cancer Chemother Pharmacol*, 54(5), 432-440. (2004).

Behboudi S, Morein B, Villacres-Eriksson M. *In vivo* and *in vitro* induction of IL-6 by *Quillaja saponaria* Molina triterpenoid formulations. *Cytokine*, 9(9), 682-687, (1997).

Cai J, Liu M, Wang Z, Ju Y. Apoptosis induced by dioscin in Hela cells. *Biol Pharm Bull*, 25(2), 193-196, (2002).

Chavali SR, Francis T, Campbell JB. An in vitro study of immunomodulatory effects of some saponins. *Int J Immunopharmacol*, 9(6), 675-683, (1987).

Cheng ZH, Yu BY, Yang XW, Zhang J. Triterpenoid saponins from bark *Mitragyna inermis*. *Zhongguo Zhong Yao Za Zhi*, 27(4), 274-277, (2002).

Christensen LP. Ginsenosides chemistry, biosynthesis, analysis, and potential health effects. *Adv Food Nutr Res*, 55, 1-99, (2009).

Chwalek M, Lalun N, Bobichon H, Plé K, Voutquenne-Nazabadioko, L. Structure-activity relationships of some hederagenin diglycosides: haemolysis, cytotoxicity and apoptosis induction. *Biochim Biophys Acta*, 1760 (9), 1418-1427, (2006).

Clardy J, Walsh C. Lessons from natural molecules. *Nature*, 432, 829-837, (2004).

Corea G, Iorizzi M, Lanzotti V, Cammareri M, Conicella C, Laezza C, Bifulco M. Astersedifolioside A-C, three new oleane-type saponins with antiproliferative activity. *Bioorg Med Chem*, 12(18), 4909-4915, (2004).

Coughlin RT, Fattom A, Chu C, White AC, Winston S. Adjuvant activity of QS-21 for experimental E. coli 018 polysaccharide vaccines. *Vaccine*, 13(1), 17-21, (1995).

Coulter A, Wong TY, Drane D, Bates J, Macfarlan R, Cox J. Studies on experimental adjuvanted influenza vaccines: comparison of immune stimulating complexes (Iscoms) and oil-in-water vaccines. *Vaccine*, 16(11-12), 1243-1253, (1998).

da Silva JO, Fernandes RS, Ticli FK, Oliveira CZ, Mazzi MV, Franco JJ, Giuliatti S, Pereira PS, Soares AM, Sampaio SV. Triterpenoid saponins, new metalloprotease snake venom inhibitors isolated from *Pentaclethra macroloba*. *Toxicon*, 50(2), 283-291, (2007).

Danloy S, Quetin-Leclercq J, Coucke P, De Pauw-Gillet MC, Elias R, Balansard G, Angenot L, Bassleer R. Effects of alpha-hederin, a saponin extracted from *Hedera helix*, on cells cultured in vitro. *Planta Med*, 60(1), 45-49, (1994).

Daros Mdo D, Matos FJ, Parente JP. A new triterpenoid saponin, bredemeyeroside B from the roots of *Bredemeyera floribunda*. *Planta Med*, 62(6), 523-527, (1996).

Davis ID, Chen W, Jackson H, Parente P, Shackleton M, Hopkins W, Chen Q, Dimopoulos N, Luke T, Murphy R, Scott AM, Maraskovsky E, McArthur G, MacGregor D, Sturrock S, Tai TY, Green S, Cuthbertson A, Maher D, Miloradovic L, Mitchell SV, Ritter G, Jungbluth AA, Chen YT, Gnjatic S, Hoffman EW, Old LJ, Cebon JS. Recombinant NY-ESO-1 protein with ISCOMATRIX adjuvant induces broad integrated antibody and CD4(+) and CD8(+) T cell responses in humans. *Proc Natl Acad Sci USA*, 101(29), 10697-10702, (2004). Erratum in: *Proc Natl Acad Sci U S A*, 102(27), 9734 (2005).

De Tommasi N, Autore G, Bellino A, Pinto A, Pizza C, Sorrentino R, Venturella P. Antiproliferative triterpene saponins from *Trevesia palmate*. *J Nat Prod*, 63(3), 308-314, (2000).

De Tommasi N, Conti C, Stein ML, Pizza C. Structure and in vitro antiviral activity of triterpenoid saponins from *Calendula arvensis*. *Planta Med*, 57(3), 250-253, (1991).

Ellington AA, Berhow M, Singletary KW. Induction of macroautophagy in human colon cancer cells by soybean B-group triterpenoid saponins. *Carcinogenesis*, 26 (1), 159-167, (2005).

Escalante AM, Santecchia CB, Lopez SN, Gattuso MA, Gutierrez Ravelo A, Delle Monache F, Gonzalez Sierra M, Zacchino SA. Isolation of antifungal saponins from *Phytolacca tetramera*, an Argentinean species in critic risk. *J Ethnopharmacol*, 82(1), 29-34, (2002).

Eschenmoser A, Ruzicka L, Jeger O, Arigoni D. Zur Kenntnis der Triterpene. *Helv Chim Acta,* 38, 1890–1904, (1955).

Favel A, Steinmetz MD, Regli P, Vidal-Ollivier E, Elias R, Balansard G. In vitro antifungal activity of triterpenoid saponins. *Planta Med*, 60(1), 50-53, (1994).

Feng XZ, Dong M, Gao ZJ, Xu SX. Three new triterpenoid saponins from *Ixeris sonchifolia* and their cytotoxic activity. *Planta Med*, 69(11), 1036-1040, (2003).

Feng YL, Wu B, Li HR, Li YQ, Xu LZ, Yang SL, Kitanaka S. Triterpenoidal saponins from the barks of *Zygophyllum fabago* L. *Chem Pharm Bull (Tokyo)*, 56(6), 858-60, (2008).

Flekhter OB, Medvedeva NI, Kukovinets OS, Spirikhin LV, Galkin EG, Galin FZ, Golovanov DG, Pavlova NI, Savinova OV, Boreko EI, Tolstikov GA. Synthesis and antiviral activity of lupane triterpenoids with modified cycle E. *Bioorg Khim*, 33(6), 629-634, (2007).

Frazer IH, Quinn M, Nicklin JL, Tan J, Perrin LC, Ng P, O'Connor VM, White O, Wendt N, Martin J, Crowley JM, Edwards SJ, McKenzie AW, Mitchell SV, Maher DW, Pearse MJ, Basser RL. Phase 1 study of HPV16 specific immunotherapy with E6E7 fusion protein and ISCOMATRIX adjuvant in women with cervical intraepithelial neoplasia. *Vaccine*, 23(2), 172-181, (2004).

Fu GM, Wang YH, Gao S, Tang MJ, Yu SS. Five New Cytotoxic Triterpenoid Saponins from the Roots of *Symplocos chinensis*. *Planta Med*, 71(7), 666-672, (2005).

Fukuda K, Utsumi H, Shoji J, Hamada A. Saponins can cause the agglutination of phospholipid vesicles. *Biochemica et Biophysica Acta*, 820, 199-206, (1985).

Germonprez N, Maes L, Van Puyvelde L, Van Tri M, Tuan DA, De Kimpe N. In vitro and in vivo antileishmanial activity of triterpenoid saponins isolated from *Maesa balansae* and some chemical derivatives. *J Med Chem*, 48(1), 32-37, (2005).

Guo S, Falk E, Kenne L, Ronnberg B, Sundquist BG. Triterpenoid saponins containing an acetylated branched D-fucosyl residue from *Quillaja saponaria* Molina. *Phytochemistry*, 53(8), 861-868, (2000).

Haddad M, Laurens V, Lacaille-Dubois MA. Induction of apoptosis in a leukemia cell line by triterpene saponins from *Albizia adianthifolia*. *Bioorg Med Chem*, 12(17), 4725-4734, (2004).

Haralampidis K, Trojanowska M, Osbourn AE. Biosynthesis of triterpenoid saponins in plants. *Adv Biochem Eng,* 75, 31-49, (2002).

Haridas V, Arntzen CJ, Gutterman JU. Avicins, a family of triterpenoid saponins from *Acacia victoriae* (Bentham), inhibit activation of nuclear factor-kappaB by inhibiting both its nuclear localization and ability to bind DNA. *Proc Natl Acad Sci USA*, 98(20), 11557-1162, (2001). Comment in: *Proc Natl Acad Sci USA*, 98(20), 10986-10988, (2001).

Haridas V, Hanausek M, Nishimura G, Soehnge H, Gaikwad A, Narog M, Spears E, Zoltaszek R, Walaszek Z, Gutterman JU. Triterpenoid electrophiles (avicins) activate the innate stress response by redox regulation of a gene battery. *J Clin Invest*, 113(1), 65-73, (2004).

Haridas V, Higuchi M, Jayatilake GS, Bailey D, Mujoo K, Blake ME, Arntzen CJ, Gutterman JU. Avicins: triterpenoid saponins from *Acacia victoriae* (Bentham) induce apoptosis by mitochondrial perturbation. *Proc Natl Acad Sci USA*, 98(10), 5821-5826, (2001).

Hasegawa H, Matsumiya S, Uchiyama M, Kurokawa T, Inouye Y, Kasai R, Ishibashi S, Yamasaki

K. Inhibitory effect of some triterpenoid saponins on glucose transport in tumor cells and its application to *in vitro* cytotoxic and antiviral activities. *Planta Med*, 60(3), 240-243, (1994).

Hikino H, Ohsawa T, Kiso Y, Oshima Y. Analgesic and antihepatotoxic actions of dianosides, triterpenoid saponins of *Dianthus superbus* var. longicalycinus herbs. *Planta Med*, 50(4), 353-355, (1984).

Hosny M, Rosazza JP. New isoflavone and triterpene glycosides from soybeans. *J Nat Prod*, 65(6), 805-813, (2002).

Houghton PJ, Odukoya OA, Adelusi A, Omogbai EK, Sanderson L, Whitfield PJ. Control of water-borne parasitic diseases with natural products: the potential of *Dialium guineense* as a molluscicide. *Trop Doct*, 27 (Suppl 1), 26-29, (1997).

Hu S, Concha C, Lin F, Persson Waller K. Adjuvant effect of ginseng extracts on the immune responses to immunisation against *Staphylococcus aureus* in dairy cattle. *Vet Immunol Immunopathol*, 91(1), 29-37, (2003).

Huang HC, Tsai WJ, Liaw CC, Wu SH, Wu YC, Kuo YH. Anti-platelet aggregation triterpene saponins from the galls of *Sapindus mukorossi*. *Chem Pharm Bull (Tokyo)*, 55(9), 1412-1415, (2007).

Katselis GS, Estrada A, Gorecki DK, Barl B. Adjuvant activities of saponins from the root of *Polygala senega* L. *Can J Physiol Pharmacol*, 85(11), 1184-1194, (2007).

Kenarova B, Neychev H, Hadjiivanova C, Petkov VD. Immunomodulating activity of ginsenoside Rg1 from *Panax ginseng*. *Jpn J Pharmacol*, 54(4), 447-454, (1990).

Kennelly EJ, Cai L, Kim NC, Kinghorn AD. Abrusoside E, a further sweet-tasting cycloartane glycosides from the leaves of *Abrus precatorius*. *Phytochemistry*, 41, 1381–1383, (1996).

Kensil CR. Saponins as vaccine adjuvants. *Crit Rev Ther Drug Carrier Syst*, 13(1-2), 1-55, (1996).

Kensil CR, Patel U, Lennick M, Marciani D. Separation and characterization of saponins with adjuvant activity from *Quillaja saponaria* Molina cortex. *J Immunol*, 146(2), 431-437, (1991).

Khan IA, Clark AM, McChesney JD. Antifungal activity of a new triterpenoid glycoside from *Pithecellobium racemosum* (M.). *Pharm Res*, 14(3), 358-361, (1997).

Kiem PV, Thu VK, Yen PH, Nhiem NX, Tung NH, Cuong NX, Minh CV, Huong HT, Hyun JH, Kang HK, Kim YH. New triterpenoid saponins from *Glochidion eriocarpum* and their cytotoxic activity. *Chem Pharm Bull (Tokyo)*, 57(1), 102-105, (2009).

Konoshima T, Kozuka M. Constituents of leguminous plants, XIII. New triterpenoid saponins from *Wistaria brachybotrys*. *J Nat Prod*, 54(3), 830-836, (1991).

Konoshima T, Yasuda I, Kashiwada Y, Cosentino LM, Lee KH. Anti-AIDS agents, 21. Triterpenoid saponins as anti-HIV principles from fruits of *Gleditsia japonica* and *Gymnocladus chinensis*, and a structure-activity correlation. *J Nat Prod*, 58(9), 1372-1377, (1995).

Kreutzer S, Schimmer O, Waibel R. Triterpenoid sapogenins in the genus Grindelia. *Planta Med*, 56(4), 392-394, (1990).

Krief S, Thoison O, Sevenet T, Wrangham RW, Lavaud C. Triterpenoid saponin anthranilates from *Albizia grandibracteata* leaves ingested by primates in Uganda. *J Nat Prod*, 68(6), 897-903, (2005).

Krizkova L, Mucaji P, Nagy M, Krajcovic J. Triterpenoid cynarasaponins from *Cynara cardunculus* L. reduce chemically induced mutagenesis in vitro. *Phytomedicine*, 11(7-8), 673-678, (2004).

Kwak WJ, Han CK, Chang HW, Kim HP, Kang SS, Son KH. Loniceroside C, an antiinflammatory saponin from *Lonicera japonica*. *Chem Pharm Bull (Tokyo)*, 51(3), 333-335, (2003).

Lacaille-Dubois MA, Hanquet B, Cui ZH, Lou ZC, Wagner H. A new biologically active acylated triterpene saponin from *Silene fortunei*. *J Nat Prod*, 62(2), 404, (1999).

Lakshmi V, Saxena A, Mishra SK, Raghubir R, Srivastava MN, Jain RK, Maikhuri JP, Gupta G. Spermicidal activity of bivittoside D from *Bohadschia vitiensis*. *Arch Med Res*, 39(7), 631-638, (2008).

Lee EJ, Ko E, Lee J, Rho S, Ko S, Shin MK, Min BI, Hong MC, Kim SY, Bae H. Ginsenoside Rg1 enhances CD4(+) T-cell activities and modulates Th1/Th2 differentiation. *Int Immunopharmacol*, 4(2), 235-244, (2004).

Lee SJ, Ko WG, Kim JH, Sung JH, Moon CK, Lee BH. Induction of apoptosis by a novel intestinal metabolite of ginseng saponin via cytochrome c-mediated activation of caspase-3 protease. *Biochem Pharmacol*, 60(5), 677-685, (2000).

Li B, Abliz Z, Fu G, Tang M, Yu S. Characteristic fragmentation behavior of some glucuronide-type triterpenoid saponins using electrospray ionization tandem mass spectrometry. *Rapid Commun Mass Spectrom*, 19(3), 381-390, (2005).

Li C, Yang J, Yu S, Chen N, Xue W, Hu J, Zhang D. Triterpenoid saponins with neuroprotective effects from the roots of *Polygala tenuifolia*. *Planta Med*, 74(2), 133-141, (2008).

Li F, Li W, Fu H, Zhang Q, Koike K. Pancreatic lipase-inhibiting triterpenoid saponins from fruits of *Acanthopanax senticosus*. *Chem Pharm Bull (Tokyo)*, 55(7), 1087-1089, (2007).

Li XX, Davis B, Haridas V, Gutterman JU, Colombini M. Proapoptotic triterpene electrophiles (avicins) form channels in membranes: cholesterol dependence. *Biophys J*, 88(4), 2577-2584, (2005).

Lin F, Wang R. Hemolytic mechanism of dioscin proposed by molecular dynamics simulations. *J Mol Model*, (2009) (In Press).

Liu DL, Wang NL, Zhang X, Gao H, Yao XS. Two new triterpenoid saponins from *Ardisia crenata*. *J Asian Nat Prod Res*, 9(2), 119-127, (2007).

Liu LF, Ma XL, Wang YX, Li FW, Li YM, Wan ZQ, Tang QL. Triterpenoid saponins from the roots of *Clematis chinensis* Osbeck. *J Asian Nat Prod Res*, 11 (5), 389-396, (2009).

Liu WK, Xu SX, Che CT. Anti-proliferative effect of ginseng saponins on human prostate cancer cell line. *Life Sci*, 67(11), 1297-1306, (2000).

Liu X, Xia J, Wang L, Song Y, Yang J, Yan Y, Ren H, Zhao G. Efficacy and safety of ginsenoside-Rd for acute ischaemic stroke: a randomized, double-blind, placebo-controlled, phase II multicenter trial. *Eur J Neurol*, 16(5), 569-575, (2009).

Liu Y, Li J, He J, Abliz Z, Qu J, Yu S, Ma S, Liu J, Du D. Identification of new trace triterpenoid saponins from the roots of *Panax notoginseng* by high-performance liquid chromatography coupled with electrospray ionization tandem mass spectrometry. *Rapid Commun Mass Spectrom*, 23(5), 667-679, (2009). Erratum in: *Rapid Commun Mass Spectrom*, 23(7), 1095-1096, (2009).

Lu P, Su W, Miao ZH, Niu HR, Liu J, Hua QL. Effect and mechanism of ginsenoside Rg3 on postoperative life span of patients with non-small cell lung cancer. *Chin J Integr Med*, 14(1), 33-36, (2008).

Ma L, Gu YC, Luo JG, Wang JS, Huang XF, Kong LY. Triterpenoid saponins from *Dianthus versicolor*. *J Nat Prod*, 72(4), 640-644, (2009).

Magalhaes AF, Tozzi AM, Santos CC, Serrano DR, Zanotti-Magalhaes EM, Magalhaes EG, Magalhaes LA. Saponins from *Swartzia langsdorffii*: biological activities. *Mem Inst Oswaldo Cruz*, 98(5), 713-718, (2003).

McManus OB, Harris GH, Giangiacomo KM, Feigenbaum P, Reuben JP, Addy ME, Burka JF, Kaczorowski GJ, Garcia ML. An activator of calcium-dependent potassium channels isolated from a medicinal herb. *Biochemistry*, 32(24), 6128-6133, (1993).

Minale L, Iorizzi M, Palagiano E, Riccio R. Steroid and triterpenoid oligoglycosides of marine origin. *Adv Exp Med Biol*, 404, 335-356, (1996).

Moon HI, Chung JH, Lee JK, Zee OP. Triterpenoid saponin from *Viola hondoensis* W. Becker et H Boss. and their effect on MMP-1 and type I procollagen expression. *Arch Pharm Res*, 27(7), 730-733, (2004).

Mowat AM, Smith RE, Donachie AM, Furrie E, Grdic D, Lycke N. Oral vaccination with immune stimulating complexes. *Immunol Lett*, 65(1-2), 133-140, (1999).

Nam JH, Jung HJ, Choi J, Lee KT, Park HJ. The antigastropathic and anti-rheumatic effect of nigaichigoside F1 and 23-hydroxytormentic acid isolated from the unripe fruits of *Rubus coreanus* in a rat model. *Biol Pharm Bull*, 29(5), 967-970, (2006).

Namba T, Yoshizaki M, Tominori T, Kobashi K, Mitsui K. Hemolytic and its protective activity of ginseng saponins. *Chem Pharm Bull (Tokyo)*, 21(2), 459-461, (1973).

Ng KM, Che CM, Wo SK, Tam PK, Lau AS. Analytical application of acetate anion in negative electrospray ionization mass spectrometry for the analysis of triterpenoid saponins—ginsenosides. *Rapid Commun Mass Spectrom*, 20(10), 1545-1550, (2006).

Nico D, Santos FN, Borja-Cabrera GP, Palatnik M, Palatnik de Sousa CB. Assessment of the monoterpene, glycidic and triterpene-moieties' contributions to the adjuvant function of the CP05 saponin of *Calliandra pulcherrima* Benth during vaccination against experimental visceral leishmaniasis. *Vaccine*, 25(4), 649-658, (2007).

Niu YP, Wu LM, Jiang YL, Wang WX, Li LD. Beta-escin, a natural triterpenoid saponin from Chinese horse chestnut seeds, depresses HL-60 human leukaemia cell proliferation and induces apoptosis. *J Pharm Pharmacol*, 60(9), 1213-1220, (2008).

Nord LI, Kenne L. Novel acetylated triterpenoid saponins in a chromatographic fraction from *Quillaja saponaria* Molina. *Carbohydr Res*, 329(4), 817-829, (2000).

Oleszek WA. Chromatographic determination of plant saponins. *J Chromatogr*, 967, 147-162, (2002).

Park KH, Park J, Koh D, Lim Y. Effect of saikosaponin-A, a triterpenoid glycoside, isolated from *Bupleurum falcatum* on experimental allergic asthma. *Phytother Res*, 16(4), 359-363, (2002).

Patwardhan B, Gautam M. Botanical immunodrugs: scope and opportunities. *Drug Discov Today*, 10(7), 495-502, (2005).

Pham HL, Ross BP, McGeary RP, Shaw PN, Hewavitharana AK, Davies NM. Saponins from *Quillaja saponaria* Molina: isolation, characterization and ability to form immuno stimulatory complexes (ISCOMs). *Curr Drug Deliv*, 3(4), 389-397, (2006).

Piacente S, Pizza C, De Tommasi N, Mahmood N. Constituents of *Ardisia japonica* and their *in vitro* anti-HIV activity. *J Nat Prod*, 59(6), 565-569, (1996).

Plaeger SF. Clinical immunology and traditional herbal medicines. *Clin Diagn Lab Immunol*, 10(3), 337-338, (2003).

Plohmann B, Bader G, Hiller K, Franz G. Immunomodulatory and antitumoral effects of triterpenoid saponins. *Pharmazie*, 52(12), 953-957, (1997).

Plohmann B, Bader G, Hiller K, Franz G. Immunomodulatory and antitumoral effects of triterpenoid saponins. *Pharmazie*, 52 (12), 953-957, (1997).

Radwan MM, El-Sebakhy NA, Asaad AM, Toaima SM, Kingston DGI. Kahiricosides II–V, cycloartane glycosides from an Egyptian collection of

Astragalus kahiricus. *Phytochemistry*, 65, 2909-2913, (2004).

Rivera E, Ekholm Pettersson F, Inganäs M, Paulie S, Grönvik KO. The Rb1 fraction of ginseng elicits a balanced Th1 and Th2 immune response. *Vaccine*, 23(46-47), 5411-5419, (2005).

Roner MR, Sprayberry J, Spinks M, Dhanji S. Antiviral activity obtained from aqueous extracts of the Chilean soapbark tree (*Quillaja saponaria* Molina). *J Gen Virol*, 88(1), 275-285, (2007).

Ruzicka L. History of the isoprene rule: Faraday lecture. *Proc Chem Soc*, 341–360, (1959).

Ruzicka L. Perspectives of the biogenesis and chemistry of terpenes. *Pure Appl Chem*, 6, 493-522, (1963).

Ruzicka L, Eschenmoser A, Heusser H. The isoprene rule and the biogenesis of terpenic compounds. *Experientia*, 357-367, (1953).

Sakurai N, Wu JH, Sashida Y, Mimaki Y, Nikaido T, Koike K, Itokawa H, Lee KH. Anti-AIDS agents. Part 57: Actein, an anti-HIV principle from the rhizome of *Cimicifuga racemosa* (black cohosh), and the anti-HIV activity of related saponins. *Bioorg Med Chem Lett*, 14(5), 1329-32, (2004).

Sampson JH, Raman A, Karlsen G, Navsaria H, Leigh IM. In vitro keratinocyte antiproliferant effect of *Centella asiatica* extract and triterpenoid saponins. *Phytomedicine*, 8(3), 230-5, (2001).

Sang SM, Lao AN, Leng Y, Cao L, Chen ZL, Uzawa J, Shigeo Y, Fujimoto Y. A new triterpenoid saponin with inhibition of luteal cell from the seeds of *Vaccaria segetalis*. *J Asian Nat Prod Res*, 4(4), 297-301, (2002).

Shao KD, Zhou YH, Shen YP, Ye BD, Gao RL, Zhang Y. Treatment of 37 patients with refractory idiopathic thrombocytopenic purpura by shengxueling. *Chin J Integr Med*, 13(1), 33-36, (2007).

Shao Y, Ho CT, Chin CK, Poobrasert O, Yang SW, Cordell GA. Asterlingulatosides C and D, cytotoxic triterpenoid saponins from *Aster lingulatus*. *J Nat Prod*, 60(7), 743-746, (1997).

Silva BP, Soares JB, Souza EP, Palatnik M, Sousa CB, Parente JP. Pulcherrimasaponin, from the leaves of *Calliandra pulcherrima*, as adjuvant for immunization in the murine model of visceral leishmaniasis. *Vaccine*, 23(8), 1061-1071, (2005).

Simões CM, Amoros M, Girre L. Mechanism of antiviral activity of triterpenoid saponins. *Phytother Res*, 13(4), 323-328, (1999).

Sindambiwe JB, Calomme M, Geerts S, Pieters L, Vlietinck AJ, Vanden Berghe DA. Evaluation of biological activities of triterpenoid saponins from *Maesa lanceolata*. *J Nat Prod*, 61(5), 585-590, (1998).

Sjölander A, van't Land B, Lövgren Bengtsson K. Iscoms containing purified Quillaja saponins upregulate both Th1-like and Th2-like immune responses. *Cell Immunol*, 177(1), 69-76, (1997).

So HS, Yoon HS, Choi DY, Kwon YS, Sung JH, Lee TG, Park ES, Cho HS, Lee BM, Cho JM, Ryu WS. Effect of a novel saponin adjuvant derived from *Quillaja saponaria* on the immune response to recombinant hepatitis B surface antigen. *Mol Cells*, 7(2), 178-186, (1997).

Son IH, Park YH, Lee SI, Yang HD, Moon HI. Neuroprotective activity of triterpenoid saponins from *Platycodi radix* against glutamate-induced toxicity in primary cultured rat cortical cells. *Molecules*, 12(5), 1147-1152, (2007).

Song X, Bao S, Wu L, Hu S. Ginseng stem-leaf saponins (GSLS) and mineral oil act synergistically to enhance the immune responses to vaccination against foot-and-mouth disease in mice. *Vaccine*, 27(1), 51-55, (2009).

Sun HX, Pan HJ. Immunological adjuvant effect of *Glycyrrhiza uralensis* saponins on the immune responses to ovalbumin in mice. *Vaccine*, 24(11), 1914-1920, (2006).

Sun J, Hu S, Song X. Adjuvant effects of protopanaxadiol and protopanaxatriol saponins from ginseng roots on the immune responses to ovalbumin in mice. *Vaccine*, 25(6), 1114-1120, (2007).

Takechi M, Doi K, Wakayama Y. Biological activities of synthetic saponins and cardiac glycosides. *Phytother Res*, 17(1), 83-85, (2003).

Tang M, Shen D, Hu Y, Gao S, Yu S. Cytotoxic triterpenoid saponins from *Symplocos chinensis*. *J Nat Prod*, 67(12), 1969-1974, (2004).

Tanner MA, Bu X, Steimle JA, Myers PR. The direct release of nitric oxide by gypenosides derived from the herb *Gynostemma pentaphyllum*. *Nitric Oxide*, 3(5), 359-365, (1999).

Taylor WG, Fields PG, Sutherland DH. Insecticidal components from field pea extracts: soyasaponins and lysolecithins. *J Agric Food Chem*, 52(25), 7484-90, (2004).

Tian JK, Xu LZ, Zou ZM, Yang SL. Three novel triterpenoid saponins from *Lysimachia capillipes* and their cytotoxic activities. *Chem Pharm Bull (Tokyo)*, 54(4), 567-569, (2006).

Traore F, Faure R, Ollivier E, Gasquet M, Azas N, Debrauwer L, Keita A, Timon-David P, Balansard G. Structure and antiprotozoal activity of triterpenoid saponins from *Glinus oppositifolius*. *Planta Med*, 66(4), 368-371, (2000).

Vandepapelière P, Horsmans Y, Mori P, Van Mechelen M, Janssens M, Koutsoukos M, Van Belle P, Clement F, Hanon E, Wettendorff M, Garçon N, Leroux-Roels G. Vaccine adjuvant systems containing monophosphoryl lipid A and QS21 induce strong and persistent humoral and T cell responses against hepatitis B surface antigen in healthy adult volunteers. *Vaccine*, 26(10), 1375-1386, (2008).

Vincken JP, Heng L, de Groot A, Gruppen H. Saponins, classification and occurrence in the plant kingdom. *Phytochemistry*, 68(3), 275-297, (2007).

Voutquenne L, Guinot P, Froissard C, Thoison O, Litaudon M, Lavaud C. Haemolytic acylated triterpenoid saponins from *Harpullia austro-caledonica*. *Phytochemistry*, 66(7), 825-835, (2005).

Waffo-Teguo P, Voutquenne L, Thoison O, Dumontet V, Nguyen VH, Lavaud C. Acetylated glucuronide triterpene bidesmosidic saponins from *Symplocos glomerata*. *Phytochemistry*, 65(6), 741-750, (2004).

Wandji J, Tillequin F, Mulholland DA, Chi Shirri J, Tsabang N, Seguin E, Verite P, Libot F, Fomum ZT. Pentacyclic triterpenoid and saponins from *Gambeya boukokoensis*. *Phytochemistry*, 64, 845-849, (2003).

Wang H, Gao J, Kou J, Zhu D, Yu B. Anti-inflammatory activities of triterpenoid saponins from *Polygala japonica*. *Phytomedicine*, 15(5), 321-326, (2008).

Wang S, Li J, Huang H, Gao W, Zhuang C, Li B, Zhou P, Kong D. Anti-hepatitis B virus activities of astragaloside IV isolated from radix. Astragali. *Biol Pharm Bull*, 32(1), 132-135, (2009).

Wei F, Ma LY, Jin WT, Ma SC, Han GZ, Khan IA, Lin RC. Antiinflammatory triterpenoid saponins from the seeds of *Aesculus chinensis*. *Chem Pharm Bull (Tokyo)*, 52(10), 1246-1248, (2004).

Wendt KU. Enzyme mechanisms for triterpene cyclization: new pieces of the puzzle. *Angew Chem*, 44, 3966-3971, (2005).

Wendt KU, Schulz GE, Corey EJ, Liu DR. Enzyme mechanisms for polycyclic triterpene formation. *Angew Chem*, 39, 2812-2833, (2000).

Woldemichael GM, Wink M. Identification and biological activities of triterpenoid saponins from *Chenopodium quinoa*. *J Agricul and Food Chem*, 49, 2327-2332, (2001).

Wu ZJ, Ouyang MA, Wang CZ, Zhang ZK. Six new triterpenoid saponins from the leaves of *Ilex oblonga* and their inhibitory activities against TMV replication. *Chem Pharm Bull (Tokyo)*, 55(3), 422-427, (2007).

Xie Q, Zong X, Ge B, Wang S, Ji J, Ye Y, Pan L. Pilot postoperative ileus study of escin in cancer patients after colorectal surgery. *World J Surg*, 33(2), 348-354, (2009).

Xie Y, Deng W, Sun H, Li D. Platycodin D2 is a potential less hemolytic saponin adjuvant eliciting Th1 and Th2 immune responses. *Int Immunopharmacol*, 8(8), 1143-1150, (2008).

Xie Y, Pan H, Sun H, Li D. A promising balanced Th1 and Th2 directing immunological adjuvant, saponins from the root of *Platycodon grandiflorum. Vaccine*, 26(31), 3937-3945, (2008).

Xu LP, Wang H, Yuan Z. Triterpenoid saponins with anti-inflammatory activity from *Codonopsis lanceolata. Planta Med*, 74(11), 1412-1415, (2008).

Xu R, Fazio GC, Matsuda PT. On the origins of triterpenoid skeletal diversity. *Phytochemistry*, 65, 261–291, (2004).

Xu ZX, Liang J, Haridas V, Gaikwad A, Connolly FP, Mills GB, Gutterman JU. A plant triterpenoid, avicin D, induces autophagy by activation of AMP-activated protein kinase. *Cell Death Differ*, 14 (11), 1948-1957, (2007).

Yadava RN, Chakravarti N. Anti-inflammatory activity of a new triterpenoid saponin from *Carthamus tinctorius* linn. *J Enzyme Inhib Med Chem*, 23(4), 543-548, (2008).

Yang XW, Zhao J, Cui YX, Liu XH, Ma CM, Hattori M, Zhang LH. Anti-HIV-1 protease triterpenoid saponins from the seeds of *Aesculus chinensis. J Nat Prod*, 62(11), 1510-1513, (1999).

Yook CS, Liu XQ, Chang SY, Park SY, Nohara T. Lupane-type glycosides from the leaves of *Acanthopanax gracilistylus. Chem. Pharm. Bull*, 50, 1383-1385, (2002).

Yoshikawa K, Hirai H, Tanaka M, Arihara S. Antisweet natural products. XV. Structures of Jegosaponins A-D from *Styrax japonica* Sieb. et Zucc. *Chem Pharm Bull (Tokyo)*, 48(7), 1093-1096, (2000).

Yoshikawa K, Mizutani A, Kan Y, Arihara S. Antisweet natural products. XII. Structures of sitakisosides XI-XX from *Stephanotis lutchuensis* Koidz. var. japonica. *Chem Pharm Bull (Tokyo)*, 45(1), 62-67, (1997).

Yoshiki Y, Kudou S, Okubo K. Relationship between chemical structures and biological activities of triterpenoid saponins from soybean. *Biosci Biotechnol Biochem*, 62(12), 2291-2299, (1998).

Young-Won C, Marcy JB, Hee BC, Kinghorn AD. Drug Discovery from Natural Sources. *The AAPS Journal*, 8 (2), 239-253, (2006).

Yu LJ, Ma RD, Jiang SB. Effects of tubeimoside-1 on HIV core protein p24 and cytopathogenesis *in vitro. Zhongguo Yao Li Xue Bao*, 15(2), 103-106, (1994).

Yu TX, Ma RD, Yu LJ. Structure-activity relationship of tubeimosides in anti-inflammatory, antitumor, and antitumor-promoting effects. *Acta Pharmacol Sin*, 22(5), 463-468, (2001).

Yui S, Ubukata K, Hodono K, Kitahara M, Mimaki Y, Kuroda M, Sashida Y, Yamazaki M. Macrophage-oriented cytotoxic activity of novel triterpene saponins extracted from roots of *Securidaca inappendiculata. Int Immunopharmacol*, 1(11), 1989-2000, (2001).

Zhang JH, Wang JP, Wang HJ. Clinical study on effect of total panax notoginseng saponins on immune related inner environment imbalance in rheumatoid arthritis patients. *Zhongguo Zhong Xi Yi Jie He Za Zhi*, 27(7), 589-592, (2007).

Zhang Y, Lu S, Liu YY. Effect of panax quinquefolius saponin on insulin sensitivity in patients of coronary heart disease with blood glucose abnormality. *Zhongguo Zhong Xi Yi Jie He Za Zhi*, 27(12), 1066-1069, (2007).

Zheng Q, Koike K, Han LK, Okuda H, Nikaido T. New biologically active triterpenoid saponins from *Scabiosa tschiliensis. J Nat Prod*, 67(4), 604-613, (2004).

Zheng Q, Li W, Han L, Koike K. Pancreatic lipase-inhibiting triterpenoid saponins from *Gypsophila oldhamiana. Chem Pharm Bull (Tokyo)*, 55(4), 646-650, (2007).

Zhong JJ, Yue CJ. Plant cells: secondary metabolite heterogeneity and its manipulation. *Adv Biochem Eng Biotechnol*, 100, 53-88, (2005).

Zhou Y, Peng L, Zhang WD, Kong DY. Effect of Triterpenoid Saponins from *Bacopa monniera* on Scopolamine-Induced Memory Impairment in Mice. *Planta Med*, (2009) (In Press).

chapter 25

Quality Control, Standardisation, Efficacy and Safety of Herbal Medicines

Pharkphoom Panichayupakaranant

INTRODUCTION

The use of traditional medicine (TM) and complementary alternative medicine (CAM) has evolved over centuries in various cultures. TM and CAM have been used throughout the history of mankind, with varying degrees of success, for the treatment or prevention of diseases. TM and CAM can involve the use of medicinal substances (from medicinal plants, minerals or materials from animals), or involve non-medication (e.g. acupuncture, chiropractic). These alternative approaches to therapy are increasingly gaining in popularity, even in the western society. The use of herbal medicines (phytotherapy) in particular has grown exponentially over the last few decades in the West (Eisenberg et al., 1998; Smith, 1998; Defelice, 1995; Zundorf and Dingermann, 1997; Brevoort, 1998; World Health Organization, 2004).

Herbal medicines, or phytomedicines, are plant-derived medicines that contain one or more plants, and one or more active chemical compounds, or more usually a complex mixture of chemical compounds that act individually or in synergistic combination in the body to treat, prevent or manage various diseases. The world-wide market for various categories of 'botanical therapeutics' probably run into 100s of billion of US dollars, especially if we include registered plant drugs (new chemical entities, NCEs), botanical drugs (herbal or phytomedicines), dietary supplements (nutraceuticals) and functional or medicinal foods that are all derived from plants (Raskin et al., 2002). If we add to this the use of herbs in aromatherapy, cosmetics and toiletries, one begins to appreciate the vast increase in the use of herbs in recent times. Indeed the line between 'medicines', 'supplements' or 'cosmetics' are truly blurring, since successful use in all these categories depends on some 'active' plant ingredient(s). In many developing Asian and African countries, herbal medicines and traditional medicinal practitioners have always been popular. Even in Japan, the most developed Asian country, herbal medicine usage has always been very high when compared to modern or western medicine. Although modern medicines are available in developing countries (albeit at high cost), herbal medicines have often maintained popularity for historical and cultural reason. Concurrently, many people in developed countries have begun to turn to alternative or complementary therapies, including use of phytomedicines, dietary supplements and functional or medicinal foods. This resurgence in interest in plant-derived medicines is partly due to (a) growing dissatisfaction with modern orthodox medicines, (b) perception that such medicines are natural and therefore pure and without side-effects, (c) progress in production of higher quality herbal medicines, and (d) in some cases proven clinical efficacy and safety.

The traditional preparations for medical and cosmetic use, until recently, included dried bulk herbs (used as infusions, or teas), tinctures, decoctions, fluid extracts and dermal preparations (poultices, lotions, ointments, salves, balms, liniments and creams). The use of these was largely based on tradition, and few if any were properly tested for stability, safety and efficacy. In the last 20 years, various multinational pharmaceutical, and specialized nutraceutical companies, have begun to offer better quality herbal medicines in modern formulations (tablets, capsules, creams etc), but mostly in an *unregulated manner*. Whereas the herbal medicine industry has expanded rapidly, governmental legislation has not kept pace with this development (see section 3.5 and 3.6). Quality control and development of standardised herbal medicines with consistent safety and efficacy should be key issues, and need to be prioritized from the earliest stages of the development process (Canigueral et al., 2008).

The assurance of safety, quality and efficacy of herbal medicines has now become a key issue for health authorities, the herbal medicine industry, and the public. The increased use of such medicines in self-medication products has brought with it demands from the public and physicians for clinical testing to give scientific validity to claims made by the manufacturers of these products. This presents a problem, since a large number of herbal medicines on the market are not standardised and use of these by uninformed clinicians in controlled clinical trials have often resulted in contradictory results (see section 3.5). Very few of the regulatory authorities around the world strictly regulate herbal medicines and supplements (see section 3.6). Therefore these are often (a) insufficient dosage data on the product label for the customer, (b) spurious claims made by manufacturers, and (c) variable content of active ingredients in the products, making it is difficult to assess the purity and safety of these marketed products.

This situation has improved in the last decade, mostly due to the work of research scientists, national and international health authorities/organization, and a few ethical manufacturers. Methods for quality assurance and the standardisation of many herbal medicines have now been developed. Some of these standardised commercial products have also recently been re-examined in controlled clinical trials with some success. In this chapter, the author discusses the issues relating to un-standardised products, factors causing variability and consequences of using clinically unproven products (section 3). The following section (section 4) describes the process and analytical methods required for achieving quality assurance and standardised products, and presents eight detailed examples of this in section 5. The final section 6 describes the recent interest in preparation of standardised constituent-rich herbal extracts which four detailed examples.

WHY QUALITY CONTROL AND STANDARDISATION OF HERBAL MEDICINES IS IMPORTANT

Quality Control and Standardisation

Quality control involves processes that maintain the quality of a manufactured product. A high quality herbal medicine will contain the correct plant material, or mixture of plant materials, or their extracts, exactly as stated on the product label, free from contamination with other undeclared plant materials, and free from pesticides, radioactive particles, heavy metals, microbes and mycotoxins (World Health Organization, 2007a). This WHO publication outlines potential hazardous contaminants and residues in herbal medicines, provides general principles for assessing the safety of herbal medicines, and recommends methods for determining the level of these contaminants in plant materials. It stresses that there is a lack of research data and that the accepted limits suggested in the guidelines are referenced and extrapolated from work carried out in the food area.

Apart from 'quality', the other main issue in the production and use of herbal medicines is 'standardisation'. Until recently very few manufacturers supplied products containing standardised extracts. Standardisation is a method of assuring minimum (and maximum) level of active ingredients in the extract or the final product. This process is becoming increasingly important, along with 'quality control/assurance', as a means of ensuring a consistent supply of high-quality herbal medicines. Standardisation can be defined as the establishment of reproducible pharmaceutical quality by comparing a product with established reference substances, and by defining minimum and maximum amount of one or more compounds, or groups of compounds that are necessary in the product for efficacy and safety. In the field of phytomedicines, standardisation may apply to the herbal raw materials, or to extracts prepared from raw materials. Many national and international agencies have prepared pharmacopoeial monographs of the most commonly used phytomedicines, and these monographs provide information on standards of active ingredients to be used in establishing the quality of herbal medicines (U.S. department of Health Human Services Food and Drug Administration Center for Drug Evaluation and Research, 2009).

Problems caused by poor quality unstandardised herbal medicines

Although herbal medicines are generally perceived by the public as 'natural' products, and therefore safe, there is voluminous evidence in the scientific literature that their use is not entirely risk-free. The risk is multiplied many fold if the products marketed are of poor quality, and do not contain 'standardised' levels of active compounds. The problems are further compounded by the fact that there are literally 1000s of companies world-wide offering various bands of the more commonly used herbal medicines that are of variable quality, with variable levels of the active ingredients. As self-medication by the public with these unregulated products has increased in recent years, there has been a concomitant increase in reported adverse effects, and hospital admission attributable to use of herbal preparation (Drew and Mayers, 1997; Rates, 2001). These side-effects and other toxicities from herbal medicines occurred primarily because until recently the vast majority of such herbs and supplements had not been thoroughly investigated for safety and efficacy, and it was not appreciated that their concomitant use with other herbs or orthodox medicines would result in serious drug-drug interactions.

Drew and Mayers (1997) classify adverse effects of herbal medicines as those occurring due to (a) intrinsic properties of the herb, and (b) extrinsic factors, such as failure of good manufacturing practice. All drugs, whether synthetic or plant-derived, may cause toxicity if taken at inappropriate dose levels, particularly if their potential for dose related toxicity, drug-drug interaction, and idiosyncratic reaction is not carefully ascertained prior to marketing. With herbal medicines there have been, at least in the past, problems caused by (a) misidentification, (b) lack of standardisation, (c) contamination, (d) substitution, (e) deliberate adulteration, (f) incorrect preparation and/or dosage, and (g) inappropriate or incomplete labelling and/or advertising. Thankfully the situation is improving at present, particularly because various international agencies are cooperating on the development of guidelines for the herbal industry. For a historical perspective of the many serious toxicological problems caused in the past by poor quality unstandardised herbal medicines, the reader is referred to Drew and Mayers

(1997), Chan et al. (1992), Perharic et al. (1994), De Smet (1995), Capasso et al. (2000), Rates (2001), Valli and Giardina (2002), Chan (2003), Flaster and Lassiter (2004), Wirth et al. (2005) and Teng et al. (2008). Even in the year 2010, important herbal medicines continue to be marketed by manufacturers, which contain wrong or ineffective levels of the herb. For example a recent metabolomic quality control study of claimed antimalarial *Artemisia afra* clearly illustrates this point (Van der Kooy et al., 2008). However, the adverse effects of most herbal drug are relatively less frequent when the drugs are used properly compared with synthetic drugs, but well controlled clinical trials now confirm that they really exist (Bagheri et al., 1998; Drew and Mayers, 1997; De Smet, 1995; D'Arcy, 1993; Brown, 1992).

Factors affecting quality and phytochemical content of herbal medicines

The quality of herbal medicines is a major challenge because the content of active constituents in plants varies according to a large number of factors, and therefore generally the plants used in phytomedicine have a complex and inconstant chemical composition. The factors include the choice of the highest yielding plant species/variety, genetic composition of the plant, growth conditions (e.g. soil composition), geographical origin (climatic variation), age, and the specific parts of the plants harvested for processing. These factors are *intrinsic* to the plant i.e. plant genetics, growth conditions and similar variables will result in differences in levels of the active constituents in different biological variations of the plant(s). Two *extrinsic* factors can result in further variability in the level of active compounds in the harvested plants. Firstly, the harvesting season and conditions, and storage of the fresh and dried plant material can all result in changes in levels of the active constituents. Secondly, the subsequent processing (e.g. pre-chopping/mincing, drying, grinding, extraction procedures) can also affect the levels of active compounds, and may ultimately result in variability and loss of 'quality'.

Plant Selection and Harvesting

(a) Plant Collection and Cultivation

The quality assurance of a phytomedicine should start at the very beginning of the production process i.e. at the stage of selection of the plant or plants that afford the highest yield of the required phytochemical(s). The manufacturers of the herbal medicines in the past have not always been in control of this process, since they often purchased bulk plant material from the commodities market. If dried whole plant parts are purchased (e.g. seed, roots, leaves etc), at least there is a chance for some identification and authentication step by the manufacturer. Very often, the supply of plant material is in bulk powdered form, or even in liquid or dry extract, and this is problematic in terms of quality control tests.

Some of the herbal plant materials are derived from plants that are not cultivated, but gathered from the wild in their natural habitat. Such plant material is said to be 'wild-crafted'. There is a greater chance with wild-crafting of misidentification and adulteration with other unwanted plant or plant parts, since very often un-skilled or untrained labour is used in such plant collection from remote locations. There is also the added ethical problem of aggressive harvesting leading to the plant species becoming extinct. Therefore, ideally herbal plants should be cultivated, which allows the production of homogenous material, thus guaranteeing chemical homogeneity (Labadie, 1986). Cultivation will also provide a chance to produce 'organic herbal products', since plants can be grown, if at all possible, without the use of man-made fertilizers, herbicides and pesticides. This in turn will lower the levels of the potential hazardous contaminants in the final product (see section 3.1, and WHO guidelines, 2007a). To have some guarantee of authenticity and quality of plant materials, the manufacturers should ideally cultivate and harvest their own plants, or at least supervise this process if purchasing from a supplier of herbal plants. There are now numerous companies around the world that specialize in cultivating herbal plants strictly according to Good Agriculture Practice (GAP), and who also use Good Manufacturing Practice (GMP) for production and quality control of plant materials and their extracts.

(b) Plant Authentication and Quality Control

Once the plant material has been selected, or harvested (in the correct season), or purchased from a bulk-supplier, the first step undertaken by the manufacturer of the phytomedicine should be proper botany identification, even if the supplier have provided some certificates of analysis as part of the purchase contract. Proper botanical authentication should ideally involve independent botanical experts, and voucher specimens should be lodged with a herbarium (or in-house) for *each batch* of harvested or purchased plant material. This authentication should be followed by checks on 'quality' of the plant material, and testing for contaminants according to guidelines (e.g. the WHO guidelines, 2007a). The final stage (see section 3.3.2) is of course a detailed and qualitative and quantitative phytochemical screening, and preparation of 'standardised extract', using appropriate chemical, biological or botanical reference standards, prior to formulation and marketing of the phytomedicine.

Inadequate quality control as outline above, using macroscopic, microscopic, chemical and spectroscopic/chromatographic techniques has often in the past resulted in serious consequences through mis-identification. Flaster and Lassiter (2004) have recently highlighted this issue of authentication. They present an argument for an in-house herbarium, and cite numerous examples of incorrect identification e.g. adulteration of Eastern European comfrey leaf (*Symphytum officinale* L., Boraginaceae) with deadly night shade leaf (*Atropa belladonna* L., Solanaceae), presence of toxic castor bean seed (*Ricinus communis* L., Euphorbiaceae) and precatory bean seeds (*Abrus precatorius* L., Fabaceae) in cultivated and wild-harvested materials. It has been reported that 50% of the Echinacea sold in the USA from 1908 through 1991 was actually *Parthenium integrifolium* (Foster, 1985). Both these herbs have the common name of 'Missouri Snakeroot'; this suggests that herbs intended for use in phytotherapy should always be referred to by their scientific name and subjected to proper authentication process. This particular mis-identication of Echinacea is not confined to the herbal industry, but has also occurred in a reputable academic department (e.g. Bauer et al., 1985) and the subsequent retraction after this error was recognized in a further publication (Bauer et al., 1987).

Plant processing

(a) Fresh plant material and drying

Whereas some botanical training is recommended for personnel involved in plant collection and harvesting of wild or cultivated plants, *plant processing* should ideally only be carried out by well trained professional staff. After the plant material (leaves, roots, rhizomes, barks, flowers, pods, etc) has been freshly harvested, there is an initial visual inspection conveyer belt to remove any unwanted parts, or parts of other plants, followed by thorough multiple rinsing with distilled water to remove any particulate adulterants (dust, soil, insect etc). The plant material is then usually "tumble" dried in a stream of cool air to remove traces of the rinsing water. The resulting 'fresh' plant material should immediately be sampled randomly (several samples from different parts of the batch), and subjected to (a) authentication by professional botanists, and 'voucher specimens' prepared and lodged as appropriate for future reference, (b) tests to determine the exact moisture content (~ 60-80%) (c) quality control tests according to the WHO guidelines (2007a), and (d) detailed phytochemical determination, both qualitative and quantitative. This should ideally be the starting point for any further scientific studies (Fig. 25.1A). Very few of the scientific papers in fact report on the phytochemical determination of freshly collected plant materials; most proceed to dry the plant material, process it further to a powder, and report yields of 'active' constituents in the crude solvent extracts of these dried plant materials.

Most freshly collected plant materials have a high water content (~ 80%) and if not stored correctly will undergo rapid deterioration through enzymatic processes and/or microbial growth. If the chemical constituents in the plant material are known to be heat labile, it may be necessary to store the fresh material in cold storage (5°C), and the fresh material subjected as quickly as possible to careful processing without an intermediate drying step. Most plant materials are in fact dried prior to further processing since this stabilizes the content of the chemicals in the plant material. The exact procedure used for drying is dependent on the nature of the specific plant material. The drying can be carried out in a shady place at ambient temperature if the plant constituents are known to be heat labile, or in an oven at low temperatures with controlled air flow. When the stability of the chemical constituents in the plant material is unknown, or if they are known to be unstable, the fresh plant material should undergo a stabilization process consisting of freezing, lyophilisation, use of alcohol vapor etc (Williamson et al., 1996). If the correct drying process is used for any specific plant or plant material, the moisture content should drop to about 15% or below and there should be no significant loss of any of the chemical constituents. The obtained dried plant material at this stage should ideally be subjected to the same quality control and chemical screening as described above for the 'freshly' collected samples, so that any loss of constituents can be assessed and quantified, taking into account the water content of the fresh and dried samples (Fig. 25.1B).

(b) Size reduction and extraction

The dried herbal plant material is then subjected to mincing or chopping to reduce the plant material into a much smaller size suitable for feeding into a grinder to further reduce it to a powder. This powder is often sieved to define the particle size ranges in the obtained powder. This powdered plant material should again be subjected to the same quality control and chemical screening as described before for fresh plant material. If this powdered plant material is to be stored for several weeks or months, it is prudent to sample it at weekly intervals to check the stability of the chemical constituents under the storage conditions (Fig. 25.1C). The storage of the dried plant material, or of the fine powder obtained after grinding, also requires care to avoid loss of chemical constituents. When the stability of these materials is unknown, it is best to store them in moisture resistant and air-tight containers that exclude light, at low temperatures (below 20°C) until required for further processing into plant extracts.

Powdered plant material is still often used in herbal formulations around the world, but more often now the powder is subjected to a suitable extraction process (see section 4.2.1) to provide ultimately a crude extract. This crude extract can also be subjected to further enrichment, to provide

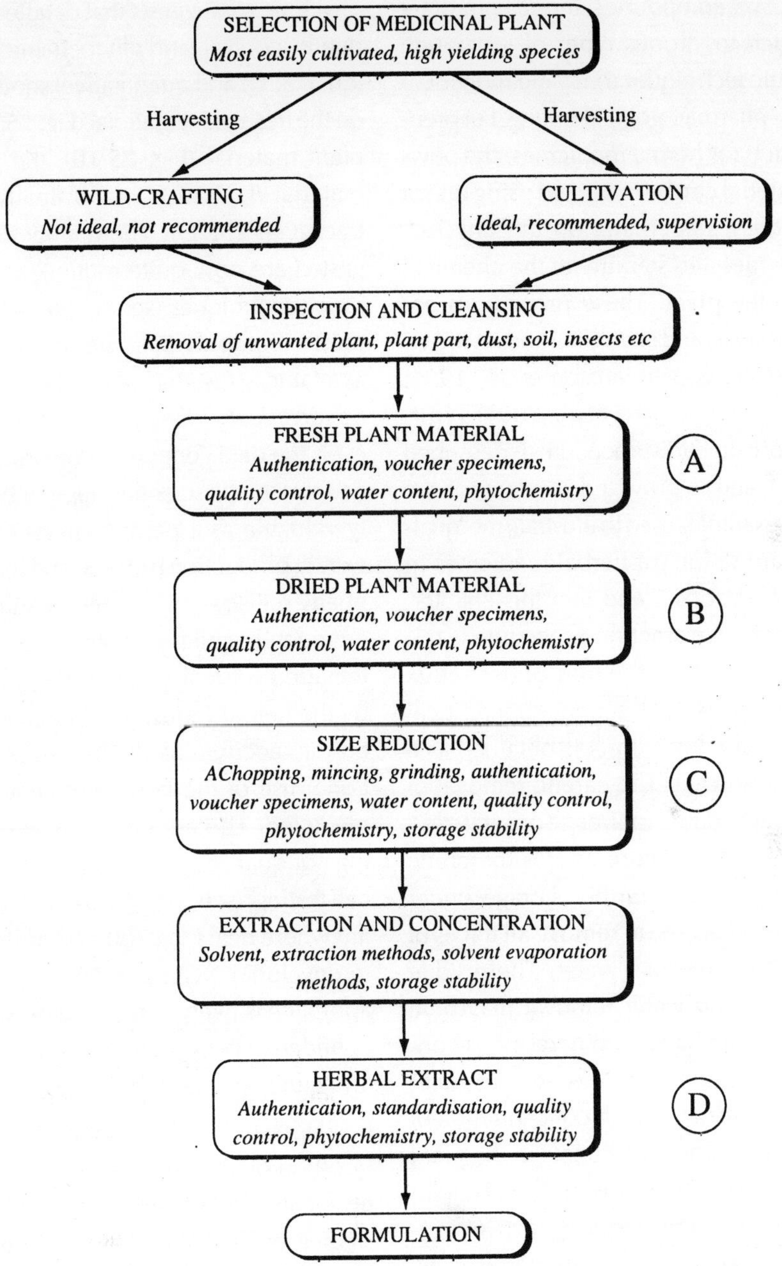

Fig. 25.1. Schematic diagram illustrating the various steps that should ideally be involved in the production of herbal extract prior to formulation. *A - D are steps where ideally quality control, authentication and full phytochemical screening (qualitative and quantitative) should be undertaken. For some herbs, the drying step is not used; the fresh plant material is processed directly. This figure was kindly developed & designed by Professor L A Damani, visiting Professor at the Prince of Songkla University.*

'active constituent-rich extract' (see section 6). Of course if the aim is to identify one or more components as the 'active' compounds, the crude extract can be subjected to various types of separation chromatographic techniques to isolate individual components for pharmacological testing. For preparation of extracts for herbal medicines, the powdered plant material can be extracted using one of several techniques, depending on the physicochemical properties and stability of the chemical constituents in the plant. These procedures are detailed in many texts, and in original and reviewed scientific publications (Williamson et al., 1996; Huie, 2002; Ong, 2004; Liang et al., 2004). A further discussion of extraction procedures is described in section 4.2.1 and is provided in many of the individual herb examples used to illustrate the 'quality' and 'standardisation' of herbal medicines in various parts of sections 5 and 6 of this chapter. Irrespective of which extraction procedure is utilized (e.g. maceration, extraction under reflux conditions, solid-phase extraction, supercritical fluid extraction, etc), the extract is obtained as a solution in some solvent. The careful removal of this solvent under vacuum (or freeze or spray drying) at the lowest temperature affords the crude extract. This may require further storage under vacuum for a period of time to remove all traces of the solvent and any residual water. The residue after trace solvent and water removal may be a solid powder, or may have an oily resinous consistency. The concentrate step (i.e. solvent/water removal) also may result in high concentration of acidic or phenolic plant constituents in the plant extract. It is prudent to check how these will chemically affect the levels of the required 'active' constituent. Extracts need to be carefully stored in airtight, moisture-resistant containers in the dark at low temperatures, and long term stability assessed under storage conditions (Fig. 25.1D).

Figure 25.1 is a diagrammatic representation of the various steps that should ideally be involved in the production of herbal extracts prior to the formulation of the herbal medicine for marketing. This scheme suggests that detailed authentication, quality control, and phytochemical determination (qualitative and quantitative) should be carried out on the fresh plant material (Fig. 25.1A), on the dried plant material (Fig. 25.1B), the powdered plant material (Fig. 25.1C), and finally on the dry extract (Fig. 25.1D). The quality control tests suggested are now quite routine, and the standardisation techniques (see section 4, 5 and 6) for the most commonly used herbs are beginning to be available. *This kind of testing need not therefore be technically difficult, or cost-prohibitive.* However, the data generated from this type of detailed and systematic scientific approach can be extremely valuable as a permanent record of the herbal extract production process, and indeed can be part of any registration dossier for submission to governmental regulatory authorities. This type of systematic protocol has not always been followed by the herbal industry, which have relied mostly on the 'accumulated knowledge' from the traditional use of the herb over centuries in folklore medicine. The additional expenditure for carrying out quality control/standardisation, and clinical testing (see section 3.5), is not likely to be anywhere nears the 300-400 million US $ it costs to develop a NCE. But the reward of a scientific approach is likely to be increased acceptance and confidence in the marketed product by the public and clinicians, and therefore increased sales.

Figure 25.1 does not address the important question of any safety evaluation in animal models for specific diseases, or acute/chronic toxicity studies, or clinical evaluation since at present most herbal medicines are not regulated. However, if good standardised herbal extracts or formulated products become the norm, then these can then readily be used in scientific investigations, or in clinical trials with some confidence (see section 3.5).

Examples to illustrate factors affecting quality and phytochemical content of herbal extracts

The effects of plant part, harvesting period, drying and storage on anthraquinone glycoside content in the leaves of *Sennna alata* L. have been demonstrated (Panichayupakaranant and Intaraksa, 2003). Determination of anthraquinone glycoside content in the dried leaves of *S. alata* from Songkhla province, Thailand, collected from different positions of the plant and at different time period, indicated that anthraquinone glycosides markedly accumulated in the leaves collected from the upper positions of the plant (young and mature leaves) (Table 25.1). The anthraquinone glycoside content was lower for the leaves collected from the lower positions of the plant (older leaves). As regards the effect of harvesting period, it was found that the young leaves harvested in March and September, and the mature leaves harvested in June, gave higher amounts of anthraquinone glycosides. *S. alata* begins to blossom in November and fruits in December (Table 25.1). In December, the anthraquinone glycosides were found to accumulate more in the flowers and pods than in the leaves. The effects of the drying method were also been demonstrated. The temperature and the method of drying both play an important role in the quality of *S. alata* raw material preparation. The leaves that had been dried by using a hot air oven at 50°C contained a higher anthraquinone glycoside content [1.43% w/w dry weight (DW)] than those either using the hot air oven at 80°C (0.44% w/w DW), or those that had been dried in the sun for three days (0.95% w/w DW). This indicates that the anthraquinone glycosides are not stable at the high temperatures.

Table 25.1. Anthraquinone glycoside content in leaves (collected at different leaf-positions), flowers and pods of *S. alata*, harvested in different months (from Panichayupakaranant and Intaraksa, 2003).

Leaf-positions or plant part	Anthraquinone glycoside content (% w/w DW; Mean SE)			
	March	June	September	December
1 - 3	1.8 0.02*	1.2 0.12	1.6 0.06*	1.1 0.10
4 - 6	1.4 0.02*	1.6 0.07	1.1 0.08	1.3 0.13
7 - 9	1.0 0.01	1.2 0.12	0.9 0.08	1.2 0.12
10 - 12	1.0 0.01	1.2 0.04	0.9 0.06	n.s.
13 - 15	n.s.	0.8 0.05*	n.s.	n.s.
Flower	n.s.	n.s.	n.s.	2.2 0.11*
Pod	n.s.	n.s.	n.s.	1.8 0.08*

The plants were harvested from Songkhla province, Southern Thailand, and divided into six groups according to the positions of the leaves on the plant counted from the top, that is, leaf-positions 1-3, 4-6, 7-9, 10-12, 13-15, respectively. The plant leaves were dried by using a hot air oven at 50°C for 24 hours. n = 3 individual experiments. * Significantly different from the others when compared within the column, $p < .05$. n.s. no sample.

A study on the stability of anthraquinone glycosides in *S. alata* leaf powders, kept in air tight containers at room temperature, revealed that after nine months, the content of the anthraquinone glycosides in the leaf powder did not decrease significantly (initial level 1.6 ± 0.01% w/w DW, 9 months 1.6 ± 0.02% w/w DW), but it decreased by approximately 25% when stored for one year (1.2 ± 0.01% w/w DW) (Panichayupakaranant and Intaraksa, 2003).

Studies on the factors affecting the quality of *Rhinacanthus nasutus* (also see sections 5.7 and 6.2) raw materials, including distribution of rhinacanthins in plant parts and period of plant harvesting, have also been reported (Panichayupakaranant et al., 2006). Determination of total rhinacanthin content in the dried leaves, stems and roots of *R. nasutus*, which were collected at different time periods, has demonstrated that rhinacanthins markedly accumulated in the roots and leaves, but less so in the stems of the plant (Table 25.2). These results are in agreement with the part of *R. nasutus* that is recommended for use in traditional and primary health care systems (Farnsworth and Bunyapraphatsara, 1992). The leaves and roots harvested in July were found to yield higher amounts of rhinacanthins. In July, *R. nasutus* is not yet in bloom. Thus, *R. nasutus* leaves and roots should be harvested before the plant goes into flower. Although the leaves and roots harvested in other periods gave a lower content of total rhinacanthins, they still passed the lower limit of the total rhinacanthins (not less than 1% w/w DW) as set by Panichayupakaranant et al. (2006). The other examples of factors (e.g. plant part, plant cultivar, geographic origin, drying, extraction, etc) that affect the content of the active constituents of herbal plants are shown in Table 25.3.

Table 25.2. Total rhinacanthins in the dried leaves, stems and roots of *Rhinacanthus nasutus* harvested in different times (from Panichayupakaranant et al., 2006)

Period of harvesting	Total rhinacanthins (% w/w DW; Mean SE)		
	Leaves	Stems	Roots
April 2003	3.6 0.1*	2.1 0.0*	4.3 0.3*
July 2003	5.6 0.0*	1.0 0.0*	5.7 0.1*
October 2003	4.4 0.1*	0.6 0.0*	4.7 0.0*
January 2004	3.3 0.0*	0.8 0.0*	4.2 0.0*

The plants were harvested from Songkhla province, southern Thailand, and dried by using a hot air oven at 50°C for 24 hours.
*The data was analysed by one way analysis of variance (ANOVA; complete factorial design). The level of statistical significance was taken at $p< 0.05$ when compared to the data within the same column.

Table 25.3. Examples of factors affecting the content of active constituents of herbal plants

Factors	Herbal plants	Active constituents	References
Plant part	*Centella asiatica* (L.) Urban(Umbelliferae)	asiaticoside, madecasoside, asiatic acids	Zainol et al., 2008
	Echinacea purpurea (L.) Moench (Asteraceae)	alkylamides and cichoric acid	Wills and Stuart, 1999b
	Lonicera japonica thunb. (Caprifoliaceae)	sweroside	Kwak et al., 2008
Plant cultivar	*Beta vulgaris* Subspecies *cycla* (Chenopodiaceae)	flavonoid	Gil et al., 1998
	Impatiens balsamina L. (Balsaminaceae)	lawsone, bllawsone and lawsone methyl ether	Sakunphueak and Panichayupakaranant , 2010
Geographic origin	*Centella asiatica* (L) Urban (Umbellifereae)	asiaticoside	Randriamampionona et al., 2007
	Coriandrum sativum L. (Umbellifereae)	essential oil	Pasquale et al., 1995
	Glycyrrhiza glabra L. (Leguminosae)	glycyrrhizic acid and isoliquiritigenin	Statti et al., 2004
	Hypericum brasiliense Choisy (Guttiferae)	betulinic acid and phenolic compounds	Abreu and Mazzafera, 2005

Contd. to next page.

Drying method	*Filipendula ulmaria* L. (Rosaceae) and *Salix alba* L. (Salicaceae)	phenolic compounds (total phenols, salicylates, quercetin)	Harbourne et al., 2009
Packing and storage	*Beta vulgaris* Subspecies *cycla* (Chenopodiaceae)	flavonoid and vitamin C	Gil et al., 1998
	Spinacia oleracea L. (Chenopodiaceae)	flavonoid and vitamin C	Gil et al., 1999
Extraction conditions	*Senna alata* L. (Leguminosae)	anthraqinone	Panichayupakaranant et al., 2009a
	Zingiber cassumunar Roxb.(Zingiberaceae)	phenylbutanoid derivatives	Kaewchoothong et al., 2008

Variation of active contents in herbal medicines on the market

Herbal medicine available world-wide are generally of poor quality and the content of any putative 'active' ingredient (or mixture of ingredients) can vary considerably in products marketed by different manufactures, and even ' batch to batch' variation in products from the same company can occur (Osowski et al., 2000; Kressmann et al., 2002). The effectiveness of any herbal product depends on its ability to deliver an effective dose of active compounds. It is obvious that adulteration, or inclusion of the wrong species of plant in the herbal medicine, will result in decreased effectiveness of the product. Even if the correct plant species is selected, the final products from different manufacturers may contain variable amounts of the active contents. This may be due to different procedures used in processing of the harvested plants (e.g. drying temperature, extraction conditions, etc), or simply a total breakdown of good manufacturing practice standards. For example, Echinaceae species are very commonly used worldwide, including in most European contries (particularly Germany) and the USA, but products on the market have variable levels of active ingredients due to adulteration (Bauer and Wagner, 1987), or use of different species of Echinacea (Bauer et al., 1989). Wills and Stuart (1998) have also reported that about 20% of retail Echinacea products in Australia contained near-zero levels of caffeoyl phenols and alkylamides, two of several active compounds in Echinacea. In laboratory experiments these authors showed that use of high temperatures in the drying process results in substantial loss of the various active compounds in Echinacea (Wills and Stuart, 1999a). They subsequently carried out a survey of sixty-two dried Echinacea samples traded in Australia (Wills and Stuart, 1999b).. The survey revealed that low levels of the active constituents in commercial samples were consistent with the use of high temperatures during the drying of the fresh plant material. Wills et al., (2000) have also drawn attention to problems with quality of traded Valerian samples in Europe. For example, of the thirty one products (tinctures, tablets, capsules) available in the Netherlands at that time, the content of valerenic acid varied widely (< 1 to 25 mg/ml) (Bos et al., 1996). These types of inconsistence supports the systematic scientific approach suggested in Fig. 25.1 (section 3.3.2), i.e. full chemical determination of fresh plant material, and again at each of the subsequent processing stages in production of the herbal medicines.

There are numerous other studies of marketed herbal medicines that illustrate the inconsistencies exemplified by Echinacea and Valerian products above. For examples, of the fifty four marketed products of St. John's Wort, only two were found to contain hypericin and pseudohypericin contents within 10% of that stated on the product label (Draves and Walker, 2003). Garrard et al., (2003) have carried out an interesting survey of a total of 880 herbal products available to the public for the ten most commonly purchased herbs sold in 1998 in the United States. They did not make an attempt to analyze all these products to determine the levels of active constituents. They collected benchmark information about ingredients of these ten herbs and daily dosage recommendations (RDD) from a then recent text book (Fetrow and Avila, 2001), and compared this information with that given in the label of each of the 880 products they had purchased. Their survey revealed that only 43% were consistent with a benchmark in ingredients and RDD, 20% in ingredients only, and 37% were either not consistent or label information was insufficient.

These examples clearly suggest that worldwide there is a wide variation in herbal products on the market, and supports a case for some mandatory requirements set by regulatory authorities to ensure that herbal products on sale at the very least contain the correct ingredients at levels consistent with recommended daily dosage (RDD).

Consequences of the use of poor quality, unstandardised herbal medicines

The first obvious consequence of poor quality herbal medicines is that they will have no efficacy or variable efficacy, and in some cases toxicity (see section 3.2). This will result in loss of confidence in these products by the public and loss of sales. As has been stated before, there is now a strong feeling that some clinical testing of the most widely used herbal medicines should be carried out to provide scientific support for their use. Indeed clinical trials have been conducted over the last few decades, but unfortunately the results have often been contradictory. One reason for this is the fact that the products often used in these trials were of poor quality, with unstandardised levels of active constituents. For example, Ginger (*Zingiber officinale*) is widely used as a spice, but also as an herbal medicine for treating pregnancy-related nausea and vomiting (Boone and Shields, 2005; Borrelli et al., 2005; Willetts et al., 2003; Keating and Chez, 2002; Vutyavanich et al., 2001). A recent systematic review of six double-blind, randomized controlled trials has shown that ginger may be effective in treating pregnancy-related nausea and vomiting (Borrelli *et al.*, 2005). However, other studies have shown that ginger is not effective in the treatment of postoperative nausea, motion sickness, or nausea of other etiology (Chrubasik *et al.*, 2005). The factors contributing to the variability in clinical response to ginger are not known, but could be due to differences in the quality of the ginger products used, or to differences in the composition of the ginger powders and ginger extracts used in the studies. If ginger is to be used successfully as an herbal medicine, the composition of its major components will have to be determined and standardised. None of the ginger powders or extracts used in previous clinical studies was analysed prior to use and this represents a major limitation of the studies.

Wolsko et al., (2005) have recently carried out a systematic and detailed assessment of the extent to which published randomized controlled trials of herbal medicines between the years 2000 - 2004 had characterised and verified the levels of active constituents of the herbal medicine under study. They selected published English language randomised controlled trials evaluating single herb preparations of Echinacea, Gingko, Saw palmetto and St. John'a wort. Of the 81 randomized trials they carefully examined, only 15% (12) reported performing tests to quantify actual contents, and 4% (3) provided adequate data to compare actual with expected content values of at least one chemical constituent. Numerous studies have demonstrated that marketed herbal medicines are very often of poor quality, with variable levels of active constituents (see section 3.4). The use of such products in clinical trials has, not surprisingly, led to irreproducible and contradictory results.

However, nowadays more and more emphasis is being put on the use of standardised materials in clinical trials. For example, a systematic review of *Andrographis paniculata* for the treatment of upper respiratory infection (URI) by the Natural Standard Research Collaboration (2006) found that the majority of these clinical trials were carried out using the product standardised to contain 5.25 mg andrographolide and deoxyandrographolide per tablet. The results of these trials collectively suggest that this herb is effective in reducing symptom severity and duration in URI, both in children and adults, provided that the treatment is started within 36 to 48 hours of the onset of symptoms (Kligler et al., 2006).

Standardised extract should also always be used in laboratory investigations for any particular pharmacological activity, so that data between different laboratories can be compared. For example a recent investigation of the antioxidant activity of the leaves of *Mangifera indica*, utilizing standardised extracts, has resulted in the identification of very potent antioxidant activity in this plant. The standardised ethanolic and aqueous extracts of *M. indica* leaf prepared to contain mangiferin concentration of 73 ± 0.17 mg/g of dry weight of the extract had free radical scavenging activity (IC_{50}) of 0.17 ± 0.02 mg/ml, and total phenolic content of 590 ± 48 mg/g of extract. The protection exhibited by these extracts against lipid peroxidation was superior to butylated hydroxytoluene and commercial grape seed extract (Ling et al., 2009).

Methods for good quality control and standardisation are now available for many of the most commonly used herbs, and it is hoped that future studies are carried out on these standardised extracts or formulated products. Scientific journals are becoming strict on publication of basic investigations and clinical trials that have used unstandardised or poor quality herbal products (Gagnier et al., 2006; Verhagen et al., 2003).

Regulatory issues on herbal medicines

Some plants contain extremely potent pharmacological substances, and these obviously are controlled in most countries. For example digitalis, rauwolfia, belladonna, poppy, coca etc are all strictly controlled by national agencies similar to the Food and Drug Administration (FDA) in the USA. Similarly, other national agencies have lists and tight control on growing, purchasing, holding or marketing of plants that have highly toxic constituents e.g. nux vomica beans (which contains strychnine). Apart from these classes of plants, generally most herbal medicines are not subjected to legislative control and have been freely available as 'over-the- counter' herbal supplements for centuries. It is only in recent years that scientists have begun to carry out detailed phytochemical, pharmacological, safety, efficacy, and clinical studies on some of the more commonly used herbal medicines.

There are numerous problems in the enactment of laws controlling the use of herbal medicines. Firstly, it is claimed that these herbs have long history of safety, since they have been used in traditional folklore medicine over many millennia. The counter argument is that folk medicines have moved a long way from its original use in family groups or small villages to herbal shops in urban areas. Now modern, often more concentrated preparations are marketed by herbal industries. The traditionally used herbal preparations (e.g. infusions) were probably of low potency, but contained a finely balanced mixture of plant constituents acting in synergy to cure or manage minor ailments. Secondly, the herbal companies are marketing more concentrated semi-purified extracts, and some claim that such 'refinements' may be removing some of the beneficial plant constituents in the extraction process. It therefore seems prudent to carry out some phytomedical efficacy and safety testing on these modern 'herbal extracts', since it is clear now that the use of herbal medicines is not entirely risk-free (see sections 3.2 and 3.5). However, legislative control of such multi-component mixtures is difficult, particularly if more than one of the plant constituents are active, or if all these constituents act in synergy. Requiring herbal industries to carry out the detailed testing that is now necessary for newly developed single-component modern synthetic drugs would be too cost-prohibitive. In a recent review, Canigueral et al., (2008) makes the point that, quote *"we should not disregard the legacy of traditional wisdom because ethnopharmacology and knowledge provided by existing clinical trials (be they open, observational studies or small, double-blind investigations) is a source of invaluable insight into the safety and efficacy of herbal medicines"*, unquote.

Despite this view (Canigueral et al., 2008), most scientists (including Çanigueral et al., 2008) now believe that the production of herbal medicines nowadays has reached a level of sophistication where quality and standardised products are available, and such products can be subjected to some of the rules regulating clinical research of synthetic drugs. At the very least, national regulatory agencies need to provide some detailed guidelines for the herbal industries, since the safety and efficacy of the modern quality standardised herbal medicines are readily evaluable by methods of modern clinical pharmacology (Calapai and Caputi, 2007). At present most of the phytochemical, safety and efficacy research is carried out by academic researchers. If the associations of the herbal industries were to fund more of this type of academic research, the data generated on every aspect of the production of herbal medicines, from plant selection, processing, extraction, standardisation, formulation (Fig. 25.1), right up to some safety and efficacy studies, would be extremely useful in providing scientific backing to the use of traditional herbal medicines.

The actual regulations of herbal medicines vary from country to country. In some countries where herbs have a widespread use (e.g. China and India), national agencies have compiled detailed monographs, which set out limits of active constituent(s), and provide information on quality control and standardisation procedures, and therefore information on dosage (RDD, recommended daily dosage) can be obtained from such databases. Most herbal medicines in Europe are under strict guidelines of individual member countries of the European bloc countries (CPMP/QWP/2820100), and European guideline should be looked upon as a model for production of good quality standardised herbal medicines. In the United States, herbal medicines are marketed as 'dietary supplements', and it is left largely to the manufacturers to ensure that such supplements are safe and labelled appropriately. Thus US FDA can only take action to restrict the use of an herbal product after it has been shown to be unsafe (http://vm.cfsan.fda.gov/%7Edms/supplemnt.html). The US FDA has proposed guidelines for current good manufacturing practice rules for dietary supplements (http://www.cfsan.fda.gov/~lrd/fr030313.html), but no strict regulations have yet been enacted. It is disheartening to read a report in the year 2008 entitled "Why the United States Still Needs Improved Dietary Supplement Regulation and Oversight" (Morrow, 2008).

Numerous publications have in recent years reviewed the current regulation of herbal medicines in different countries (Benzi and Ceci, 1997; Kumar et al., 2007; Calixto, 2000; Morrow, 2008), but it is the detailed WHO guidelines (World Health Organization, 2007a; 2007b) that hopefully will ultimately lead to some global harmonisation of the regulations on herbal medicine production and use, as well as rules for some form of risk-monitoring system.

STANDARDISATION OF HERBAL MEDICINES

General Considerations

Apart from the enormous analytical and technical problems in standardisation of herbal medicines, standards for ingredients and recommended daily doses (RDDs) have not been clearly established by any of the regulatory authorities in the world. In some Asian countries where herbal medicines are widely used (e.g. China, India, Thailand), and in some European countries (e.g. Germany), monographs of the more commonly used herbal products have appeared in national pharmacopoeias and similar botanical data bases. These monographs can be a source of information to estimate RDDs. Furthermore, a text book by Fetrow and Avila (2001) provides a benchmark for ingredients and dosage levels for a large number of plants used in complementary and alternative medicines.

At the international level, the World Health Organization (WHO) (World Health Organization, 2004) has developed a strategy to review traditional medicines and included within this review is a program to develop monographs for herbal ingredients. In European countries, the European Scientific Cooperative on Phytotherapy (ESCOP) was established to advance the scientific status of phytomedicine and to assist with the harmonisation of their regulatory status. Additionally, the Association of South East Asian Nations (ASEAN) has established a committee to assure the quality of herbal medicines, particularly those most widely and commonly used by the people in the ASEAN countries, as well as to promote their utilisation in primary health care.

A Pharmacopoeia is a collection of quality standards for medicines and their components. In order to obtain marketing authorization for a medical product, the ingredients or the medicinal product must generally comply with a pharmacopoeial standard. Thus, pharmacopoeial standards may provide guidance on acceptable purity criteria for that ingredient.

An important aspect of the quality control of herbal extracts is the need to use consistent quality herbal extracts. Standardised extracts arise out of the need to create a uniform product, with batch-to-batch consistency. An herbal extract should be standardised for content of the active constituents to the limits that are set in its monograph. The extract, for which the active constituents (single or groups) are known, can be standardised so that it contains a known amount of the active ingredients in a clearly defined amount of an herbal extract. For example, pomegranate fruit peel extract, which is used in antioxidant preparations, should be standardised to contain ellagic acid content not less than 13% w/w (Panichayupakaranant et al., 2010a). Similarly, *Senna alata* leaf extract that is used in antifungal preparations should be standardised to contain total anthraquinone content not less than 16% w/w (Sakunpak *et al.*, 2009). However, where possible, it is better to define a 'fingerprint' of the herbal extract.

There are two types of standardisations. One is based on identifying and quantifying an extract to a pure compound e.g. curcumin, capsaicin, allicin, etc. The second identifies and concentrates one or more as active constituents, making it as a concentrated active constituent extract. This means that other naturally occurring constituents in the extract are displaced. The examples of the latter are rhinacanthin-rich *Rhinacanthus nasutus* extract (Panichayupakaranant et al., 2009b), madecassoside and asiaticoside-rich *Centella asiatica* extract (Jia and Lu, 2008), and anthraquinone-rich *Senna alata* extract (Sakunpak *et al.*, 2009).

By definition, a standardised herbal extract involves pre-determining one or a number of biochemical constituents as either active, or as marker, compounds, and this result in three very distinct types of herbal extracts.

1. The active constituent extracts

The active constituent extracts may be only a partial representation of the herb's normally occurring constituents. This limits the broad range of known traditionally properties and uses of the herb in favor of a single use. For example, curcumin, capsaicin, asiaticoside, etc.

2. The active constituent-enriched extracts

The high degree of concentration necessary to produce this type of extract causes a corresponding displacement and lack of other constituents, which in a few cases have subsequently been shown to be even more effective than the originally presumed active constituent. For example, the antifungal activity of rhinacanthin-rich *Rhinacanthus nasutus* extract againt *Trichrophyton rubrum* (MIC 7.5 μg/ml) is higher than that of its main active constituent, rhinacanthin-C (MIC 15.1 μg/ml) (Panichayupakaranant et al., 2009b). The antifungal activity of anthraquinone (aloe-emodin and emodin) rich *Senna alata* extract against *T. mentagrophytes* and *Microsporum gyseum* (MICs 62 and 250 μg/ml, respectively) is higher than that of its main active constituents, aloe-emodin (inactive) and emodin (MICs 125 and 1000 μg/ml, respectively (Sakunpak *et al.*, 2009).

3. Marker extract

This type of the extracts establishes that a specified amount of a marker compound is present in the extract. It must be noted that a marker does not represent the active constituent, but is selected as a biochemical constituent characteristic of the plant. The marker extracts are used for positive identification, or to create a higher degree of uniform potency, but not proven as active constituents. For the latter, it remains to be proven whether this is consistent with the potency of the whole herb.

Procedures and analytical methods used for achieving "standard" herbal medicines

Currently, quality-related problems (lack of consistency, safety, and efficacy) seem to be overshadowing the potential genuine health benefits of various herbal preparations. A major cause of these problems seems to be related to the lack of simple and reliable analytical methods for the chemical analysis of herbal materials.

The active constituent is responsible for the intended pharmacological activity or therapeutic effects of a botanical raw material, or herbal preparation. However, a marker compound is a chemical constituent that is also used for identification and/or standardisation processes, especially when the active constituents are not known or identified. Chemical standardisation often involves chemical identification by spectroscopic or chromatographic fingerprint techniques, and quantitative analysis for active constituents or marker compounds if available.

The key challenges in the development of analytical methods for botanicals and herbal preparations are: (a) analysis of active compounds or markers in a complex or crude extract, (b) lack of standard reference substances, (c) target analytes may be thermally labile, (d) selection of extraction and separation methods, and (e) batch-to-batch variation of the composition of the plant material obtained. The analytical methods developed should be validated. With the chemical fingerprint, the method should be able to perform composition analysis and monitor the batch-to-batch variation of the plant materials obtained for use. Methods that are simple, rapid and environmentally friendly are attractive options for the user. For the analysis of botanicals and herbal preparations, a holistic solution involving the combination of the methods of extraction, separation and analytical techniques are required.

Extraction Techniques

Sample preparation is the crucial first step in the analysis of botanicals or herbal preparations, because it is necessary to extract the desired chemical components from the herbal materials for further separation and characterisation. A brief summary of the experimental conditions for some methods of extraction are shown in Table 25.4 (Ong, 2004).

(a) *Liquid–liquid extraction*

Liquid–liquid extraction (LLE) transfers target analytes from a liquid matrix into another immiscible liquid-phase according to solubility differences. Most classical extractions are performed in separating funnels to extract analytes from an aqueous biological or environmental solution into a non-polar or less polar organic solvent. Classical LLE operates manually, requiring repetitive coalescence and phase separation, which can be very slow when emulsions form, and in turn this technique produces a large volume of organic solvent waste. Some alternative techniques include membrane-separated liquid extraction (MSLE) (Jonsson and Mathiasson, 2000), countercurrent chromatography (CCC), single drop microextraction (SDME) (Xu et al., 2007), and laminar flow techniques (Wang et al., 2002).

Table 25.4. Summary of the experimental conditions for various extraction methods for herbal materials (from Ong, 2004)

Methods	*Common solvent used*	*Temperature* (°C)	*Pressure applied*	*Time required*	*Volume of solvent required* (*ml*)
Sonication	Alcohol or mixture of alcohol and water	Can be heated	N/A	1 h	50-100
Soxhet extraction	Alcohol or mixture of alcohol and water	Depending on solvent used	N/A	3-18 h	150-200
Microwave assisted extraction	Alcohol or mixture of alcohol and water	80-150	Depending on if it is closed or open vessel extraction	10-40 min	20-50
Supercritical Fluid extraction	Carbon dioxide or Carbon dioxide with modifiers, such as methanol	40-100	250-450 atm	30-100 min	N/A
Pressurized liquid extraction (PLE)	Methanol	80-200	10-20 bar	20-40 min	20-30
Pressurized hot water extraction (PHWE)	Water or water with 10-30% ethanol	80-300	10-50 bar	40-50 min	40-45
Surfactant assisted PHWE	Water with surfactants, such as Triton X100 or SDS	80-200	10-20 bar	40-50 min	40-45

(b) *Ultrasonic extraction*

Although the use of ultrasonic energy to aid the extraction of medicinal compounds from plant materials can be found in the literature as early as the 1950s, mechanistic aspects of the usefulness of ultrasonically assisted extraction are worth noting. Fundamentally, the effects of ultrasound on the cell walls of plants can be described as follows (Vinatoru, 2001):

(1) Some plant cells occur in the form of glands (external or internal) filled with essential oil. A characteristic of external glands is that their skin is very thin and can be easily destroyed by sonication, thus facilitating release of essential oil contents into the extraction solvent.

(2) Ultrasound can also facilitate the swelling and hydration of plant materials to cause enlargement of the pores of the cell wall. Better swelling will improve the rate of mass transfer and, occasionally, break the cell walls, thus resulting in increased extraction efficiency and/or reduced extraction time.

As a novel approach to extraction and sample preparation for herbs, Huie and co-workers (Fang et al., 2000) have recently employed ultrasound to assist the surfactant-mediated extraction of ginsenosides from American ginseng. In this approach the surfactant-mediated extraction process can be divided into two parts: (1) solubilisation of active ingredients from the solid herbal material into the extraction solvent (aqueous surfactant solution); and (2) the cloud-point phase separation of the aqueous surfactant solution containing the active ingredients into a bulk aqueous phase and a smaller volume surfactant-rich phase (analyte concentration). In ultrasonically assisted extraction the use of aqueous surfactant solution containing 10% Triton X-100 as the extraction solvent was found to result in faster extraction kinetics and higher recovery compared to methanol and water.

Recently, trends in analytical extraction have been a movement toward less (organic) solvent consumption, faster extraction time, improved quantification (i.e., higher recoveries, better reproducibility, and a drive towards ever lower detection limits), and extraction selectivity (Raynie, 2004). The conventional methods e.g. heat-reflux extraction is time-consuming and labourious, and involves lengthy operation techniques, bulk amount of solvents and ultimately thermal decomposition of the target molecules at continuous high temperature (Zhou and Liu, 2006). Thus, development of 'modern' extraction techniques with significant advantages over conventional methods (e.g. reduce in organic solvent consumption and in sample degradation, elimination of additional sample clean-up and concentration steps before analysis, improvement in extraction efficiency, selectivity, etc.) for the extraction and analysis of herbal materials is likely to play an important role in the overall effort of ensuring and providing high-quality herbal products to consumers worldwide. In order to reduce the use of organic solvents and improve the extraction processes, newer sample preparation methods, such as microwave assisted extraction (MAE), supercritical fluid extraction (SFE) and pressurized liquid extraction (PLE) have been introduced for the extraction of analytes present in plant materials (Ong, 2004).

(c) *Microwave-assisted extraction*

In contrast with conventional liquid–solid extraction methods (e.g. Soxhlet extraction) in which a relatively long extraction time (typically 3-48 h) is required, microwave-assisted extraction (MAE) uses microwave energy for solution heating, which results in significant reduction of the extraction time (usually less than 30 min). This is because the microwaves heat the solvent directly, thus accelerating the speed of heating. For example, it has been demonstrated that the percentage extraction of tashinones from the root of *Salvia miltiorrhiza* by MAE was the same or even higher than conventional extraction methods. However, MAE only needed 2 minutes, but extraction at the room temperature, extraction under heat reflux conditions, ultrasonic extraction and Soxhlet extraction needed 24h, 45 min, 75 min and 90 min, respectively (Pan et al., 2002). Besides the advantage of high extraction speed, MAE also enables a significant reduction in the consumption of organic solvent (typically less than 40 ml, compared with the 100–500 ml required in Soxhlet extraction) (Zygmunt and Namiesnik, 2003; Huie, 2002; Camel, 2000; Eskilsson and Björklund, 2000). Recent applications of MAE in medicinal plant analysis are shown in Table 25.5.

Among the conditions commonly studied for optimization of MAE process, the effects of solvent composition, solvent volume, extraction temperature, and matrix characteristics seem to be most important for plant materials. For example, Hao et al., (2002) recently performed a kinetic study of the effects of these conditions on the MAE of artemisinin from *Artemisia annua* L. Their results indicated that the optimal conditions of MAE of artemisinin from *A. annua* were as follows: No. 6 extraction solvent oil is the best solvent, solvent to raw material ratio greater than 11.3, microwave radiation for 12 min, raw materials size less than 0.125 mm in diameter. The extraction rate of artemisinin was increased with the increase of grinding degree, solvent to material ratio and dielectric constant of solvent mixture containing hexane and cyclohexane.

Table 25.5 Recent applications of microwave-assisted extraction in medicinal plant analysis

Analytes	*Medicinal plants*	*Microwave conditions*	*References*
Artemisinin	*Artemisia annua* dried leaves	60 s power on and the cool to room temperature and repeated until the duration of microwave radiation is 12 min	Hao et al., 2002
Coumarin, *o*-coumaric and melilotic acids	*Melilotus officinalis*	two successive irradiations of 5 min each at 50 °C	Martino et al., 2006
Glycyrrhizic acid	Licorice root	15 s power on, 15 s power off for three times, 85–90°C and then 3 s power on for heating and 15 s power off for cooling	Pan et al., 2000
Phenolic compounds	*Rosmarinus officinalis* *Origanum dictamnus* *Origanum majorana* *Teucrium polium Vitex agnus-cactus* *Styrax officinalis*	45 s power on (750 W), 30 s power off and then 15 s power on, allow to cool after each irradiation repeated until the duration of microwave radiation is 4 min	Proestos and Komaitis, 2008
Solanesol,	Tobacco leaves	45 s power on to reach 60°C and then 3 s power on for heating (700 W) and 9 s power off for cooling	Zhou and Liu, 2006
Tanshinones (tanshinone IIA, cryptotanshinone and tanshinone I	*Salvia miltiorrhiza* dried root	25 s power on to reach 80°C and then 3 s power on for heating and 10 s power off for cooling	Pan et al., 2001; Pan et al., 2002
Tea phenol	Black tea	120s power on (600W) and 1 min power off for cooling	Spigno and de Faveri, 2009

(d) *Supercritical fluid Extraction*

An environment friendly method of sample preparation mainly means the use of environment friendly solvents such as water, supercritical fluids, etc. Supercritical fluid extraction (SFE) is a typical environment friendly method. Supercritical fluids, the intervening physical state between gas and liquids, possess unique properties. In particular, their viscosity is lower than that of liquids, allowing faster diffusion and more efficient extractions. Using such fluids, SFE acquires ability to perform selective extractions by adjusting the fluid properties by regulating pressure, temperature and the content of modifiers. Carbon dioxide is currently the solvent of choice. Non-polar supercritical CO_2 produces high extraction efficiency for compounds from non-polar to low polarity. Co-solvent systems combining CO_2 with one or more small amounts of modifiers (d"15%) extend the utility of CO_2 to polar and even ionic compounds. The numerous adjustable parameters have not only made SFE flexible but also tedious in optimisation and difficult in use. Important points in favour of SFE are its relatively short extraction time, mild pressures and temperatures used, which minimise the risks of losing activity to preserve the integrity of functional compounds of food and natural products, and to extract labile compounds from environmental samples (Sun et al., 2006; Wang et al., 2004; Stashenko et al., 2004). Recent applications of SFE in medicinal plant analysis are shown in Table 25.6.

Table 25.6 Recent applications of supercritical fluid extraction in medicinal plant analysis

Analytes	*Medicinal plants*	*Extraction conditions*	*References*
Essential oil	Chamomile (*Matricaria chamomilla*) flower	CO_2; 250 bar; 40 °C; flow rate 13 kg/h; 90 min	Kotnik et al., 2007
Essential oil	Portuguese-grown rose geranium (*Pelargonium* sp.)	CO_2; 90–100 bar, 40 °C; flow rate 1.6 kg/h; 15-30 min	Gomes et al., 2007
Diterpene, triterpene and casticin	*Vitex agnus castus* fruit	CO_2; 450 bar; 45 °C; flow rate 7 kg/h; 4-7 h	Cossuta et al., 2008
Bioactive compounds	*Helianthus annuus*	CO_2 and 5% water as a modifier; 100–500 bar; 35-50 °C	Casas et al., 2007
Lignans and cinnamic acid	*Schisandra chinensis*	CO_2; 27 MPa; 50 °C, flow rate 0.4 or 0.8 g/min; 2-7 h	Sovova et al., 2007
Essential oil	*Piper nigrum*	CO_2; 100 bar; 40 °C; flow rate 3 kg/h	Perakis et al., 2005
Ginsenosides	North American ginseng (*Panax quinquefolius*)	CO_2 and MeOH or DMSO as modifiers; 20.7, 34.5 and 48.3 MPa; 110 °C	Wood et al., 2006

(e) *Pressurized-liquid Extraction*

Pressurized-liquid extraction (PLE) emerged in the mid-1990s and Benthin et al., (1999) were the first to conduct a comprehensive study on the feasibility of applying PLE to medicinal herbs. The sample in a stainless-steel cell was extracted with an organic solvent at a temperature ranging up to 200 °C under a relatively high pressure, typically 4-20MPa. Under these conditions, the solubility of the analytes and the mass transfer are increased, and the viscosity and the surface tension of the solvents are decreased, which can improve the contact of the analytes with the solvent and thus enhance the extraction (Ramos et al., 2002). PLE has been developed in order to reduce the use of solvents and time in the methods of extraction. The technique uses organic solvents at elevated temperature and pressure, which drastically improves the speed of the extraction process. The parameters that have a significant effect on the extraction efficiencies of marker compounds in botanicals and herbal preparations by PLE are the time for extraction/volume of solvent, applied temperature and the nature of solvent used. The time for extraction was set at 20 min as it was found that a significant portion of the target analytes would be extracted. The pressure was observed to have little effect on the extraction efficiency as it was applied to keep the solvent in the liquid phase. It has been reported that the extraction efficiency of marker compounds in botanicals and herbal preparations by PLE was comparable or higher than Soxhlet extraction (Ong, 2004). The enhanced performance when using PLE over Soxhlet extraction and other conventional methods of extraction are the higher solubility of analytes in solvent and higher diffusion rate as a result of higher temperature. At higher temperature, the strong solute-matrix interaction caused by van der Waals forces, hydrogen bonding and dipole attractions between solute molecules and active sites on the matrix were disrupted. The used of pressurized solvent extraction of anti-diabetic compound, charantin, from fruits of *Momordica charantia* (bitter melon) has been reported (Pitipanapong et al., 2007). Compared with Soxhlet extraction, PLE could achieve similar yields but with lower extraction time and solvent volume usage, suggesting that it is an attractive new method for fast extraction of charantin.

Separation Techniques

Separation procedures are dependent mainly on some physicochemical properties of the compounds. It is relatively easy to separate compounds that have different physical properties by simple techniques such as solvent extraction. If the various compounds are similar to each other in their polarity, any slight difference in any one of their physical properties, e.g. molecular size, is exploited to achieve separation. The separation of plant constituents for herbal product analysis is mainly carried out using chromatographic techniques e.g. thin layer chromatography (TLC), gas liquid chromatography (GC), high performance liquid chromatography (HPLC). One further technique, which has fairly wide application in herbal product analysis, is capillary electrophoresis.

(a) *Thin layer chromatography* (TLC)

TLC is an adsorption chromatography in which samples are separated based on the interaction between a thin layer of adsorbent and a selected solvent. A thin layer of an adsorbent attached on a plate is used as stationary phase, while the selected solvent is the mobile phase. TLC was the common method of choice for herbal analysis before instrumental chromatography methods such as GC and HPLC were established. Even nowadays, TLC is still frequently used for the analysis of herbal medicines since various pharmacopoeias still use TLC to provide the first characteristic fingerprints of herbal extracts. TLC is mainly used as a simple method for initial screening, with semi-quantitative evaluation together with other chromatographic techniques.

TLC has the advantage of many-fold possibilities of detection in analysing herbal medicines. In addition, TLC is rather simple and can be employed for multiple sample analysis. For each plate (20 × 20 cm), more than 30 spots of samples can be studied simultaneously. Thus, the use of TLC to analyse herbal medicines is still popular. With the help of the CAMAG video store system (CAMAG, Switerland) and TLCQA-UV methods (Chau et al., 1998) it is possible to get useful qualitative and quantitative information from the developed TLC plate. Moreover, with the help of image analysis and digitised technique developed in computer science, the evaluation of similarity between different samples is also possible. TLC is a convenient method of determining the quality and possible adulteration of herbal products. For further details about TLC the readers could consult the book by Wagner et al. (1996).

(b) *Gas chromatography* (GC)

GC is a method for separating components of mixtures of volatile compounds. In this technique, species distribute between a mobile gas and a stationary liquid phase. Thus, when sample molecules are in the liquid phase they are stationary. The rate of migration for a chemical species is determined by how much of it distributes into the gas phase. The higher the percentage of material in the gas phase, the faster it will migrate. For example, a species that distributes itself 100% into the gas phase will migrate at the same rate as the flowing gas. On the other hand, a species that distributes 100% into the stationary phase will not migrate at all. Species that distribute themselves partly in both phases will migrate at an intermediate rate (Burchfield and Storrs, 1962).

It is well-known that many pharmacologically active components in herbal medicines are volatile chemical compounds. Thus, the analysis of volatile compounds by GC is very important in the analysis of herbal medicines. The GC analysis of the volatile oils has a number of advantages. Firstly, the GC of the volatile oil gives a reasonable "fingerprint" which can be used to identify the plant. The composition and relative concentration of the compounds in the volatile oil are characteristic of the particular plant and the presence of impurities in the volatile oil can be readily detected. Secondly, the extraction of the volatile oil is relatively straight forward and can be standardised and the components can be readily identified using GC–MS analysis. The relative quantities of the components can be used to monitor or assess certain characteristics of the herbal medicines. Changes in composition of the volatile oil may also be used as indicators of oxidation, enzymatic changes or microbial fermentation (Liang et al., 2004).

The advantages of GC clearly lie in its high sensitivity of detection for almost all the volatile chemical compounds. This is especially true for the usual FID detection and GC–MS. Furthermore, the high selectivity of capillary columns enables separation of many volatile compounds simultaneously within very short times. Thus, over the past decades, GC is a popular and useful analytical tool in the research field of herbal medicines (Uekusa et al., 2009; Ma et al., 2008; Ruan and Li, 2007; Hu et al., 2006; Lu et al., 2006; Shen et al., 2004, Lee et al., 2004; Guo et al., 2004). With the use of GC–MS, reliable information on the identity of the compounds is available as well. However, the most serious disadvantage of GC is that it is not convenient for analysis of polar and non-volatile compounds. For this, it is necessary to use tedious sample work-up which may include derivatisation. Therefore, the HPLC become another necessary tool for the comprehensive analysis of the herbal medicines.

(c) *High-performance liquid chromatography* (HPLC)

HPLC is a popular method for the analysis of herbal medicines because it is easy to learn and use, and is not limited by the volatility or stability of the samples. In a liquid chromatographic process, a liquid permeates through a porous solid stationary phase and elutes the solutes into a flow-through detector. The stationary phase is usually in the form of small-diameter (5-10 mm) uniform particles, packed into a cylindrical column. The typical column is constructed from a rigid material (such as stainless steel or plastic) and generally 5-30 cm long and the internal diameter is in the range of 1-9 mm.

In general, HPLC can be used to analyse almost all the compounds in the herbal medicines, and it has therefore received the most extensive application in recent years in the analysis of herbal medicinal preparations (Tan et al., 2008; Xie et al., 2007; Chan et al., 2007; Xie et al., 2005; Ohtake et al., 2004). Reversed-phase (RP) columns are probably the most popular columns used for the analysis of herbal medicines. It is noteworthy that the optimal separation conditions for the HPLC involves many factors; compositions and pH of the mobile phases, flow rate, mode of elution, sample preparation method, detection system, etc. Thus, experimental suitable protocols should be designed for the optimal separation of each mixture of compounds (Xie et al., 2007; Xie et al., 2005). In order to obtain better separation, some new techniques have been recently developed in the research field of liquid chromatography. These are micellar electrokinetic capillary chromatography (MECC) (Wang et al., 2007; Zhu et al., 2007), high-speed counter-current chromatography (HSCCC) (Chen et al., 2009; Deng et al., 2009), reversed-phase ion-pairing HPLC (RP-IPC-HPLC) (Wybraniec, 2006), and strong anion-exchange HPLC (SAX-HPLC) (Müller et al., 2009). These newer techniques will provide new opportunities for more effective separation for certain specific extracts of some herbal medicines.

HPLC coupled to a photodiode array detector (HPLC-PDA) has been widely used for the analysis of crude plant extracts. The UV spectra of natural products obtained on-line by HPLC-PDA give useful information on the type of constituents and in the case of certain classes of compound (Hostettmann et al., 1984). HPLC-PDA has become a common technique in most analytical laboratories in the world now. With the additional UV spectral information, the qualitative analysis of complex samples in herbal medicines turns out to be much easier than before. For instance, checking peak purity and comparing with the available standard spectrum of the known compound to the one in the investigated sample. With the introduction of electrospray mass spectrometry, the coupling of liquid chromatography and mass spectrometry (LC–MS) has opened a new way for the wide and routine application of this technique to the analysis of herbal medicines. Several valuable review articles dealing with LC–MS and its applications have been published (Chen and Pramanik, 2009; Xu et al., 2007; Oleszek and Bialy, 2006; Hayen and Karst, 2003).

(d) *Capillary electrophoresis* (CE)

CE was introduced in early 1980s as a powerful analytical and separation technique (Jorgensen and Lukacs, 1981) and has since been extensively developed. It allows an efficient way to acquire data on the purity and complexity of a sample, and can handle virtually every kind of charged sample component ranging from simple inorganic ions to DNA. There has been an obvious increase in use of electrophoretic methods, especially capillary electrophoresis, in the analysis of herbal medicines (Cianchino et al., 2008; Zhou et al., 2008; Hsieh et al., 2006; Molnár-Perl and Füzfai, 2005; Sun et al., 2002) in last decade. CE is a promising technique for the separation and analysis of active ingredients in herbal medicines since it needs only small amounts of standards, and can analyse samples rapidly with very good separation ability. It is also a good tool for producing the chemical fingerprints of the herbal medicines, since it has similar technical characteristics of liquid chromatography.

Qualitative and quantitative analysis of herbs, herbal extractions and herbal medicine fomulations

For qualitative and quantitative analysis of phytochemicals, chromatography can be used. In general, one or two markers, or pharmacologically active components, in herbs are currently employed for evaluating the quality and authenticity of herbs or herbal extractions, for the identification of a single herb or herbal medicine preparation, and for assessing the quantitative herbal composition of an herbal formulated product. This kind of determination, however, does not give a complete picture of an herbal product, because multiple constituents are usually responsible for its therapeutic effects. These multiple constituents may work synergistically and not all are necessarily present in the extract. Moreover, the chemical constituents in component herbs in the herbal medicines may vary depending on harvest seasons, plant origins, drying processes and other factors (see section 3.3 and 3.4). Thus, it seems to be necessary to determine most of the phytochemicals of herbal products in order to ensure the reliability and repeatability of pharmacological and clinical research, to understand their bioactivities, and possible side effects of active compounds, and to enhance product quality control.

In recent years, significant efforts have been made to devise methods for the quality control of herbal materials as well as herbal preparations by utilizing quantitative methods and/or qualitative fingerprinting technologies (Lin et al., 2001; Yang et al., 2005). Both methods have advantages and disadvantages. Quantitative analysis aims to separate and identify the marker compounds from herbs or herbal preparations and then use them as indicators, or standards, to assess quality. Determining the effective or principal chemical constituents and the toxic compounds is crucial to the quality control of herbs and herbal preparations. Much attention has been drawn to the development of chromatographic methods in this field, and a great number of such papers have been published. But for quality control of complex systems, the determination of only a few compounds cannot give a comprehensive and accurate assessment of all active constituents in herbal medicinal products. This approach is therefore inherently inadequate for quality control and stability evaluation of herbal medicinal products (Xie et al., 2007). Several chromatographic techniques, such as HPLC, GC, CE and TLC, can be applied for this kind of documentation. In this way, the full herbal product can be regarded as the active 'compound'. The concept of phytoequivalence was developed in Germany in order to ensure consistency of herbal products (Tyler, 1999). According to this concept, a chemical profile, such as a chromatographic fingerprint, for an herbal product should be constructed and compared with the profile of a clinically proven reference product.

By definition, a chromatographic fingerprint of an herbal product is, in practice, a chromatographic pattern of the extract of some common chemical components of pharmacologically active and/or chemical characteristic (Ong, 2002). This chromatographic profile should be featured by the fundamental attributions of "sameness" and "differences" so as to chemically represent the herbal product investigated (Welsh, 1996). It is suggested that with the help of chromatographic fingerprints obtained, the authentication and identification of herbal medicines can be accurately conducted ("sameness"), even if the amount and/or concentration of the chemical characteristic constituents are not exactly the same for different samples of this herbal preparation (hence, "differences") (Valentao et al., 1999). We should globally consider multiple constituents in the herbal product extracts, and not consider only one and/or two marker components for evaluating the quality of the herbal products.

In any herbal product and its extract, there are hundreds of unknown components and many of them are in low amounts. Moreover, there usually exists variability within the same herbal material. Consequently, to obtain reliable chromatographic fingerprints that represent pharmacologically active and chemical characteristic components is not an easy task. Fortunately, chromatography offers very powerful separation ability, such that the complex chemical components in herbal product extracts can be separated into many relatively simple sub-fractions. Furthermore, the recent approaches of applying 'hyphenated' chromatography and spectrometry, such as HPLC-PDA, GC-MS, HPLC-MS and HPLC-NMR, could provide the additional spectral information which will be very helpful for the qualitative analysis, and even for on-line structural elucidation. With the help of the spectral information the 'hyphenated' instruments show greatly improved performances in terms of the elimination of instrumental interferences, retention time shift correction, selectivity, chromatographic separation abilities, measurement precision (Gong et al., 2001a; 2001b; 2001c) A chemical fingerprint obtained by 'hyphenated' chromatography, will without question, remain the primary tool for quality control of herbal medicines for many decades.

EXAMPLES TO ILLUSTRATE PROCEDURES AND TECHNIQUES FOR STANDARDISATION OF HERBAL MEDICINES

General considerations

This section provides eight detailed examples where one or more of the procedures (e.g. extraction, concentration, separation, and analytical methods) described in section 4 have been utilized to achieve quality control and 'standard' herbal extracts.

Centella asiatica (L.) Urban

Centella asiatica (L.) Urban is an ethnomedical plant used in different continents by diverse ancient cultures and tribal groups. The areal part of *C. asiatica* is claimed to possess a wide range of pharmacological effects, and is used for wound healing (Suguna et al., 1996), mental disorders (Apparao et al., 1973), atherosclerosis, fungal and bacterial infections (Oyedeji et al., 2005; Zaidan et al., 2005), as an antioxidant and anticancer drug (Jayashree et al., 2003; Babu et al., 1995). *C. asiatica* has also been reported to be useful in the treatment of inflammations, diarrhoea, asthma, tuberculosis, and various skin lesions and ailments like leprosy, lupus, psoriasis and keloid. In addition, numerous clinical reports verify the ulcer-preventive and anti-depressive sedative effects of *C. asiatica* preparations, as well as their ability to improve venous insufficiency and microangiopathy. These properties have been ascribed to the pentacyclic triterpenes: asiatic acid (I), madecassic acid (II), asiaticoside (III) and madecassoside (IV) (Fig. 25.2) (Zheng and Qin, 2007).

The estimation of the terpene acids (I, II) and the glycosides (III, IV) of *C. asiatica*, was until recently carried by a titrimetric method (Castellani et al., 1981). This method determines only content of total terpene acids. For the determination of glycosides, the extract must first be hydrolyzed to convert the glycosides to acids, and then the total terpene acids are chemically estimated. Hence this method is non-selective, non-specific and lacks precision and accuracy of modern chromatographic methods. A reversed-phase gradient HPLC method has recently been developed to assay the four constituents (I-IV) in crude plant extracts (Inamdar et al., 1996). Chromatographic separation was performed with a μ-Bondapak, C_{18} 10 μm, 30 × 0.39 cm, S.S. column (Waters) and a water-acetonitrile mobile phase, with UV detection at 220 nm. The initial solvent was water: acetonitrile at 80 : 20% v/v, changed to 45 : 55% v/

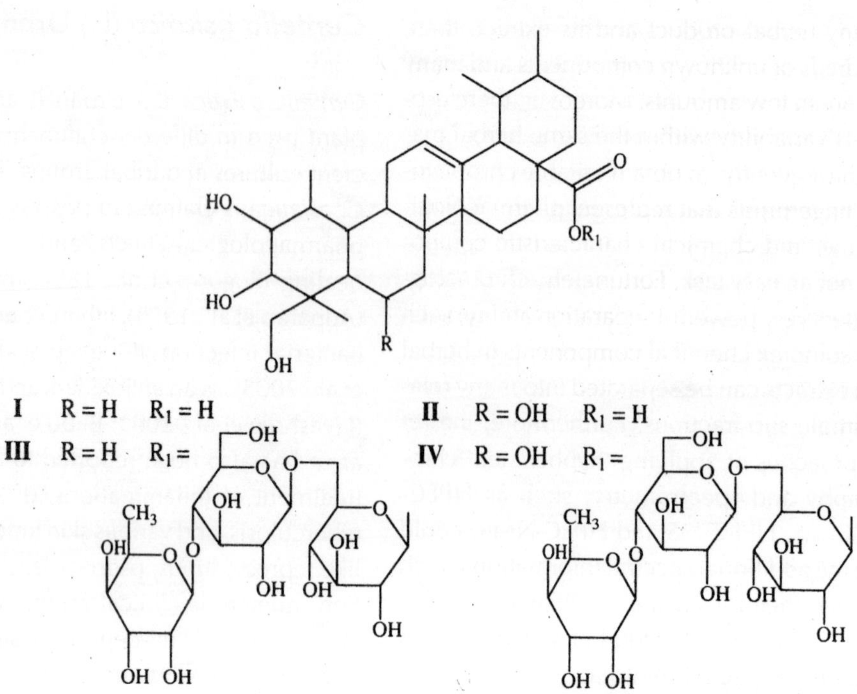

Fig. 25.2. Structures of asiatic acid (I), madecassic acid (II), asiaticoside (III), madecassoside (IV).

v at 30 mins and re-set to 80 : 20% v/v at 45 mins. A 20μl volume of sample was injected onto the column. All the four compounds (I-IV) could be separated in a single run. Optimum separation was obtained by using a linear gradient of acetonitrile in water from 20 to 55% in 30 mins. This HPLC method of analysis is precise, accurate and rapid. The method was used to assay the active components I-IV in the plant extracts and pharmaceutical preparations containing *C. asiatica* extracts.

Zingiber officinale Roscoe

Ginger (*Zingiber officinale* Roscoe) is widely used as a spice, but also as a dietary supplement for treating nausea (Kawai, 1994), postoperative nausea and vomiting (Chaiyakunapruk et al., 2006), motion sickness (Chrubasik et al., 2005) and pregnancy-related nausea (Willetts et al., 2003; Vutyavanich et al., 2001). 6-Gingerol, 6-shogaol, 8-gingerol, and 10-gingerol (Fig. 25.3) have been identified as the principal pungent components of ginger powder (Chrubasik et al., 2005; Yoshikawa et al., 1993; Harvey, 1981). They have been shown to have anti-platelet and anti-inflammatory (Nurtjahja-Tjendraputra et al., 2003; Srivastava, 1986), antioxidative (Ippoushi et al., 2003), antitumorigenic and immunomodulatory (Bode et al., 2001; Keum et al., 2002; Kim et al., 2002a; Lee and Surh, 1998), anti-*Helicobacter pylori* (Mahady et al., 2003), and antifungal (Ficker et al., 2003) properties.

A high-performance liquid chromatographic method that is suitable for the analysis of 6-gingerol, 6-shogaol, 8-gingerol, and 10-gingerol in a wide variety of ginger-containing dietary supplements, spices, teas, mints, and beverages has been described (Schwertner and Rios, 2007). 6-Gingerol, 6-shogaol, 8-gingerol, and 10-gingerol were extracted from various ginger-containing products with ethyl acetate and analysed by HPLC on a C-8 reversed phase column with methanol-water (65 : 35% v/v) as a mobile phase. The quantitation wavelength was set at 282 nm. The recoveries of 6-, 8-, and 10-gingerol, and 6-shogaol from the ginger dietary supplements and ginger-containing products were 94.7, 93.6, 94.9 and 97.1% w/w, respectively. The within-day coefficients of variation for 6-gingerol, 6-shogaol, 8-gingerol, and 10-gingerol standards (at 50 μg/ml) were 2.54, 2.38, 2.55, and 2.31%, respectively. The lower limit of quantitation was 25 ng injected. The standard curves for 6-, 8-, and 10-gingerol and 6-shogaol were linear from 10.0 to 1000 μg/ml (correlation coefficient e" 0.996). On the basis of the HPLC analysis, ginger powder contained 0.25, 0.127, 0.047, and 0.036% of 6-gingerol, 6-shogaol, 8-gingerol, and 10-gingerol, respectively. The 6-gingerol concentration in the different ginger dietary supplements was found to be higher than that of the 8- or 10-gingerol concentration, but not always higher than that of 6-shogaol.

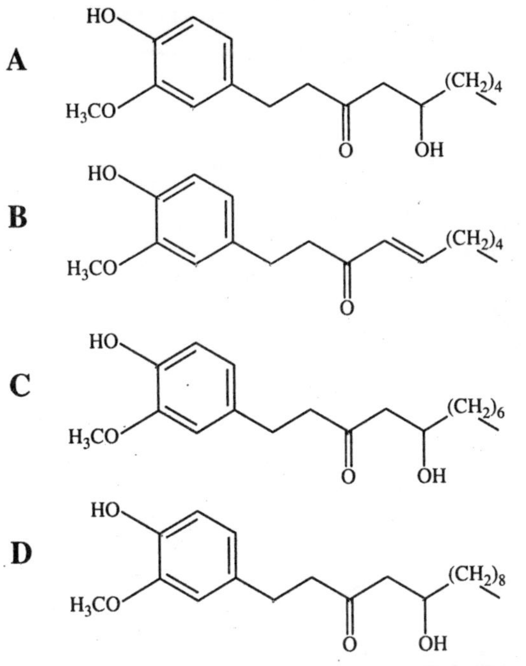

Fig. 25.3. Chemical structures of 6-gingerol (A), 6-shogaol (B), 8-gingerol (C), and 10-gingerol (D).

Ginkgo biloba L.

Ginkgo biloba L. is one of the most popular herb nutrition supplements, with terpene lactones (ginkgolides and bilobalide) and flavonoids being the two major groups of active components. Ginkgo flavonoids have been associated with reduced lipid peroxidation in vascular walls and nerve cells. Ginkgolides are well known to be antagonists of platelet-activating factor. The enriched ginkgo extracts used for the preparation of ginkgo products are usually standardised to contain 24% w/w flavonoids and 6% w/w terpene lactones. There is a report on quantitative analysis of the total content of flavonoids and terpene lactones of Ginkgo products using high performance liquid chromatography with ultraviolet (UV) and evaporative light scattering detection (ELSD) (Li and Fitzloff, 2002). The reported methods are reliable and sensitive with detection limits of 2 ng for flavonoids on column, with HPLC-UV and 20-35 ng for terpene lactones on column with HPLC-ELSD.

A fingerprint profile method was developed using a capillary HPLC/MS method which can identify more than 70 components from the *G. biloba* product (Ding *et al.*, 2008). The full scan of MS base peak of the reference sample of *G. biloba* extract, which was proven to be of the best quality, has resulted in the identification of more than 70 peaks. The method allows the flavonoids and terpene lactones to be detected simultaneously and information of both the parent ion and its fragmentation can be obtained in just one HPLC/MS run. This method could be viewed as complementary to specific quantitative analysis of some bioactive components of the herb.

Garcinia mangostana L.

The rind of the mangosteen (*Garcinia mangostana* L.) has been used for hundreds of years in Southeast Asia as a medicine for skin infections, wounds, dysentery and diarrhoea. The rind contains high amounts of xanthones, which have several biological activities, including antioxidant (Moongkarndi et al., 2004; Williams et al., 1995), antibacterial (Chomnawang, 2005; Iinuma et al., 1996), antifungal (Gopalakrishnan et al., 1997), anti-inflammatory (Nakatani et al., 2002), antitumor (Matsumoto et al., 2005), antiplatelet aggregation (Rajtar et al., 1999; Lin et al., 1996), vasorelaxant activities (Cheng and Kang, 1997), histamine and serotonin receptor blockers (Chairungsrilerd et al., 1996) and HIV-1 protease inhibition (Chen et al., 1996). A simple HPLC-PDA has been reported which quantitatively analyses six xanthones, including 3-isomangostin, 8-desoxygartanin, gartanin, α-mangostin, 9-hydroxycalabaxanthone and β-mangostin (Fig. 25.4) (Ji *et al.*, 2007). Separation was performed on a Phenomenex Luna C18 (150 mm × 3.00 mm, 5 μm) column. The mobile phase consisted of water with 0.1% trifluoroacetic acid (A), methanol with 0.1% trifluoroacetic acid (B) and isopropanol (C), which were applied in the following gradient elution: 50% A/30% B/20% C (v/v/v) to 10% A/70% B/20% C (v/v/v) in 45 minutes; finally in the next 2 minutes to 80% A/20% C (v/v) and held at that composition for another 5 minutes. The xanthones were identified by retention time, ultraviolet spectra and quantified at 320 nm. The precision of the method was confirmed by the relative standard deviation (R.S.D.), which was d" 4.6%. The recovery was in the range from 96.6% to 113.4%. A good linear relationship was established in over two orders of magnitude range. The limits of detection (LOD) for six xanthone compounds were 0.248 μg/ml. The developed methods were applied to the determination of six xanthones in *G. mangostana* products. The satisfactory results showed that the methods are effective for the analysis of real samples.

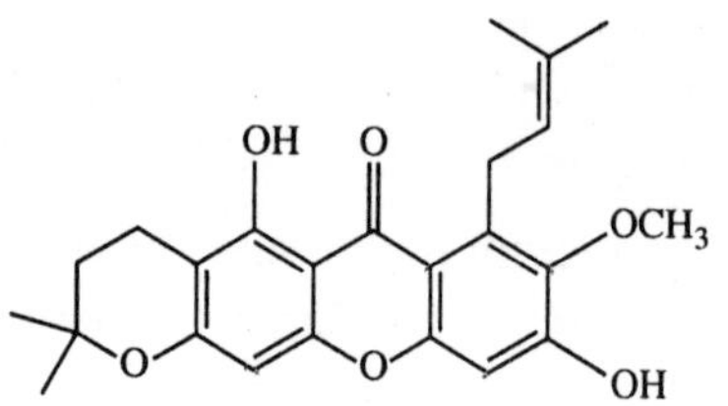
(1)

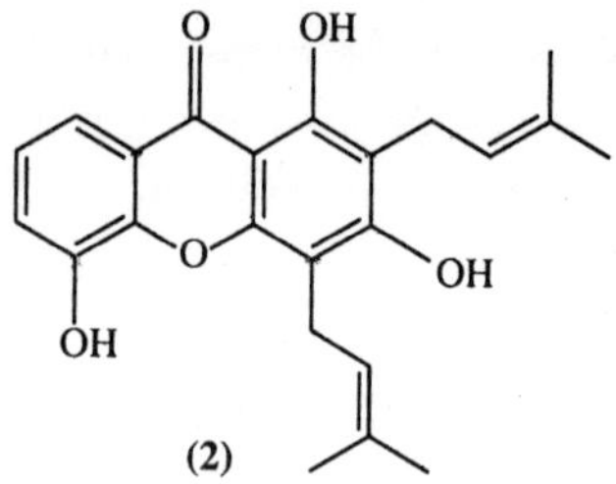
(2)

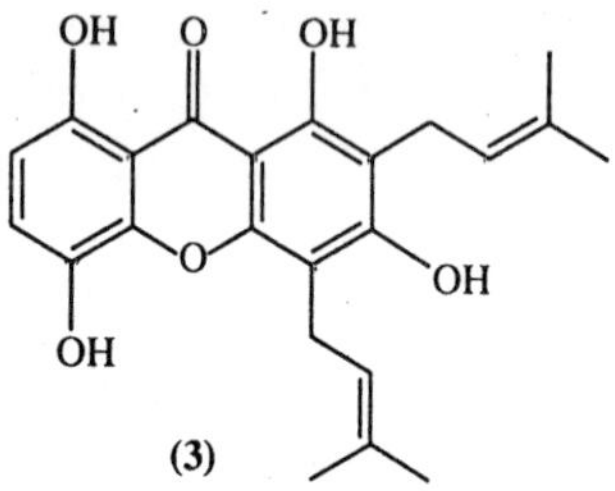
(3)

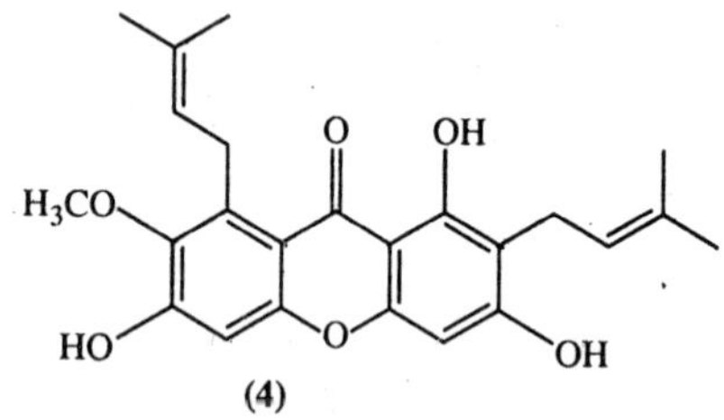
(4)

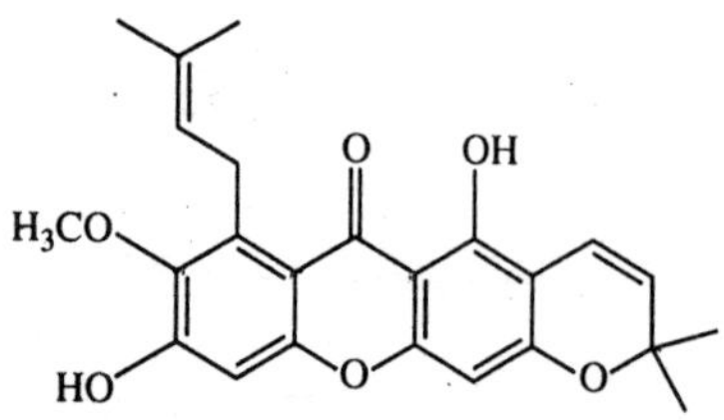
(5)

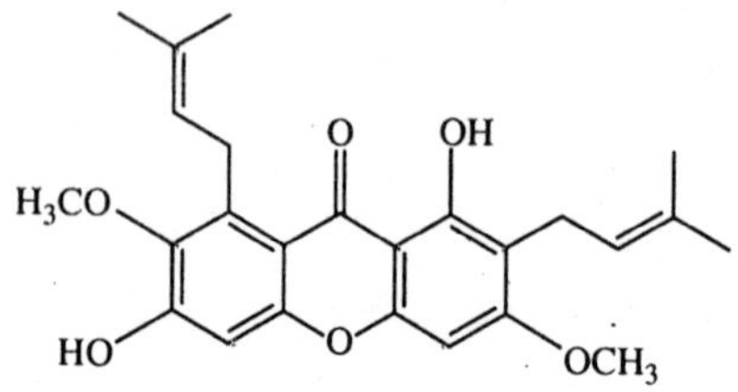
(6)

Fig. 25.4. Structures of xanthones: (1) 3-isomangostin; (2) 8-desoxygartanin; (3) gartanin; (4) a-mangostin; (5) 9-hydroxycalabaxanthone; (6) β-mangostin.

Punica granatum L.

Pomegranate (*Punica granatum* L.) fruits are widely consumed fresh and in commercial products as juice, jam and wine. Pomegranate fruit husk/peel is a rich source of hydrolysable tannin belonging to ellagitannins. In the commercial promegranate juice industry, these ellagitannins are extracted from the husk in significant quantities into the juice due to their hydrophilic properties. Promegranate fruit peel, a by-product of the pomegranate juice industry, is therefore an inexpensive and abundant source of ellagitannins. Pomegranate extracts are also being investigated for their potential use as natural food preservatives and nutraceuticals (Negi et al., 2003). It has been reported that the methanol extracts of the fruit peel contain 192 mg of total phenolics per gram, and exhibit antioxidant activity with Trolox equivalent antioxidant capacity (TEAC) values of 394.66 and 316.29 mmol/100 g dry weight, as evaluated by 1,1-diphenyl-2-picrylhydrazyl (DPPH) and 2,2′-azinobis (3-ethylbenzothiazoline-6-sulphonic acid (ABTS) assay, respectively (Surveswaran et al., 2007). The major types of phenolic compounds were reported as hydrolysable tannin (punicalin, punicalagin, gallagic acid, ellagic acid) and gallic acid. In addition, the antioxidant compounds found in pomegranate fruit peel extract were phenolic compounds; ellagic acid and flavonol; quercetin and kaempferol (Lansky and Newman, 2007). On the basis of DPPH radical scavenging assay-guided purification, ellagic acid (Fig. 25.5) was isolated from the methanol extract of pomegranate fruit peel. On the basis of DPPH radical scavenging assay and β-carotene bleaching test, ellagic acid exhibited stronger antioxidant activity than standard quercetin with EC_{50} values of 2.1 ± 0.02 and 4.3 ± 1.21 μM, respectively, while those of the standard quercetin were 8.3 ± 0.23 and 4.4 ± 0.77 μM, respectively (Panichayupakaranant *et al.*, 2010b).

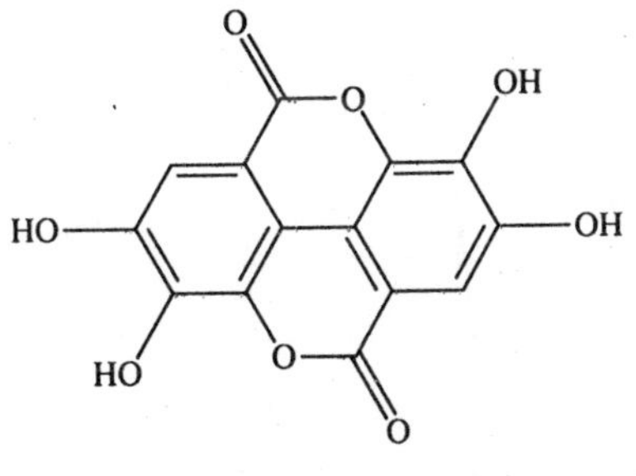

Fig. 25.5. Structure of ellagic acid

A reversed-phase HPLC for simultaneous quantitative determination of ellagic acid, quercetin and kaempferol in the fruit peel extract using a solvent gradient has been established (Panichayupakaranant *et al.*, 2010b). The method involved the use of a TSK-gel ODS-80Tm column with a mixture of 2% aqueous acetic acid and methanol (gradient elution mode: 0-15 min, 40-60% v/v methanol and 15-20 min, 60% v/v methanol) as the mobile phase and detection by UV at 254 nm. On the basis of the HPLC analysis, only ellagic acid was found as the major constituent in the methanol extract of pomegranate fruit peel (Fig 25.6). Neither quercetin nor kaempferol were found. The parameters of linearity, repeatability, reproducibility, accuracy and specificity of the method were evaluated. The recovery of the method was 98.5% and linearity (correlation coefficient > 0.9995) was obtained for ellagic acid. A high degree of repeatability and reproducibility (R.S.D. values less than 5%) were also achieved. Specificity of the method was evaluated using UV-absorption spectra produced by PDA detector. The lower limits of detection and quantification were 1.00 and 2.50 μg/ml, respectively.

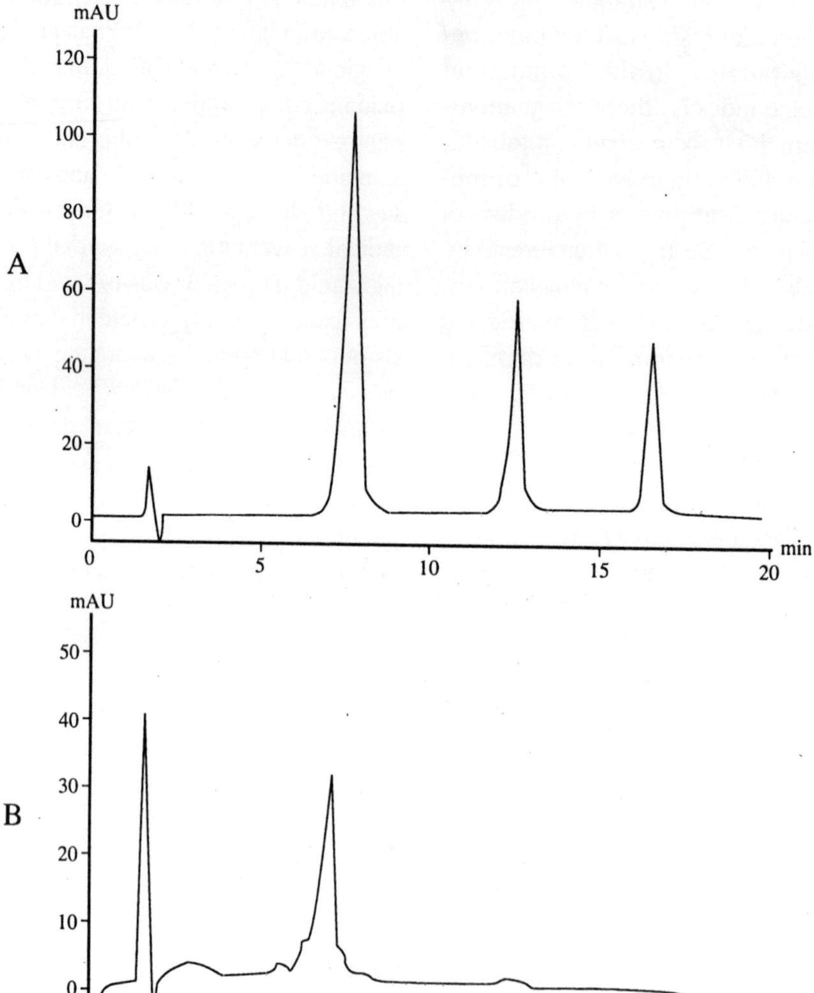

Fig. 25.6. HPLC-chromatograms of (A) authentics: ellagic acid (1), quercetin (2) and kaempferol (3); (B) methanol extract of pomegranate fruit peel. (from Panichayupakaranant et al., 2010b)

Rhinacanthus nasutus (L.) Kurz

Rhinacanthus nasutus (L.) Kurz, a small shrub of Acanthaceae family, has long been used in Thai traditional medicine for treatment of tinea versicolor, ringworm, pruritic rash, abscess pain, and skin diseases (Farnsworth and Bunyapraphatsara, 1992). It has been reported that rhinacanthin-C, rhinacanthin-D and rhinacanthin-N (Fig. 25.7) isolated from *R. nasutus* possesses antifungal (Pan-

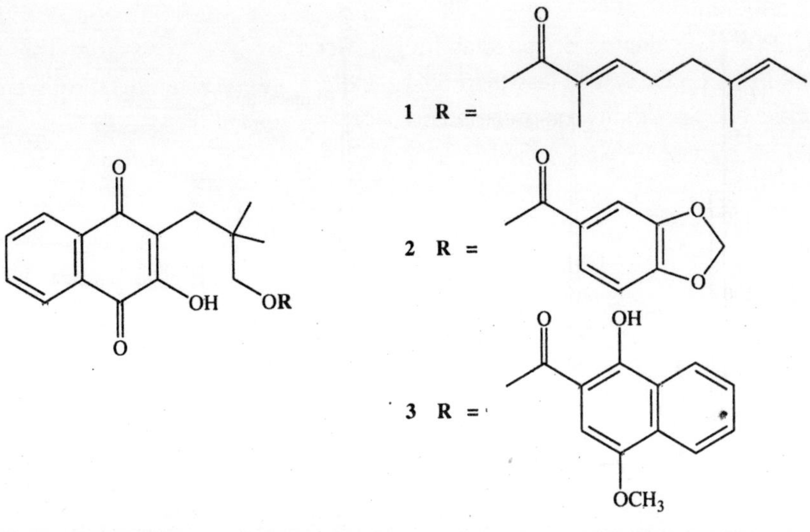

Fig. 25.7. Structures of rhinacanthin-C (1), -D (2) and -N (3).

ichayupakaranant et al., 2009b), cytotoxic (Gotoh et al., 2004; Wu et al., 1998) and antiviral (Sendl et al., 1996) activities.

A reversed-phase HPLC has been established for the simultaneous determination of rhinacanthin-C, rhinacanthin-D and rhinacanthin-N in *R. nasutus* leaves (Panichayupakaranant et al., 2009b). The method involves the use of a TSK-gel ODS-80Ts column (5 μm, 4.6 x 150 mm) with the mixture of methanol and 5% aqueous acetic acid (80:20, v/v) as the mobile phase. All three compounds were eluted within 20 minutes with satisfactory resolution (Fig. 25.8). The parameters of linearity, repeatability, accuracy and specificity of the method were evaluated. The recovery of the method was 94.3-100.9% and good linearity (correlation coefficient ≥ 0.9999) was obtained for all rhinacanthins. A high degree of specificity as well as repeatability and reproducibility (R.S.D. values less than 5%) were also achieved. The limit of detection and quantification of all rhinacanthins were 0.75 and 3.0 μg/ml, respectively. On the basis of the HPLC analysis, rhinacanthin-C was a major rhinacanthin, the content of which was 1.9% w/w, while rhinacanthin-D (0.16% w/w) and rhinacanthin-N (0.07% w/w) were minor constituents.

Senna alata (L.) Roxb.

Senna alata (L.) Roxb. (*Cassia alata* L.) is a plant belonging to the family Leguminosae. In Thailand *S. alata* leaves have long been traditionally used for the treatment of constipation and dermatophyte infections (Farnsworth and Bunyapraphatsara, 1992). Anthraquinone glycosides were demonstrated as the active constituents for the laxative properties (Elujoba et al., 1989), while the aglycones including aloe-emodin, rhein, emodin and chrysophanol (Fig. 25.9) exhibited antifungal activity (Manojlovic et al., 2002; Agarwal et al., 2000).

A reversed-phase HPLC has been established for the simultaneous determination of four anthraquinones; rhein, aloe-emodin, emodin and chrysophranol in *S. alata* leaves (Panichayupakaranant *et al.*, 2009a). The method involves the use of a TSK-gel ODS-80Tm column (5 μm, 4.6 x 150 mm) with a mixture of methanol and 2% aqueous acetic acid (70:30, v/v) as the mobile phase and UV detection at 254 nm. All four compounds were eluted within 30 minutes with baseline resolution (Fig. 25.10). The parameters of linearity, repeatability, accuracy and specificity of the method were evaluated. The recovery of the method was

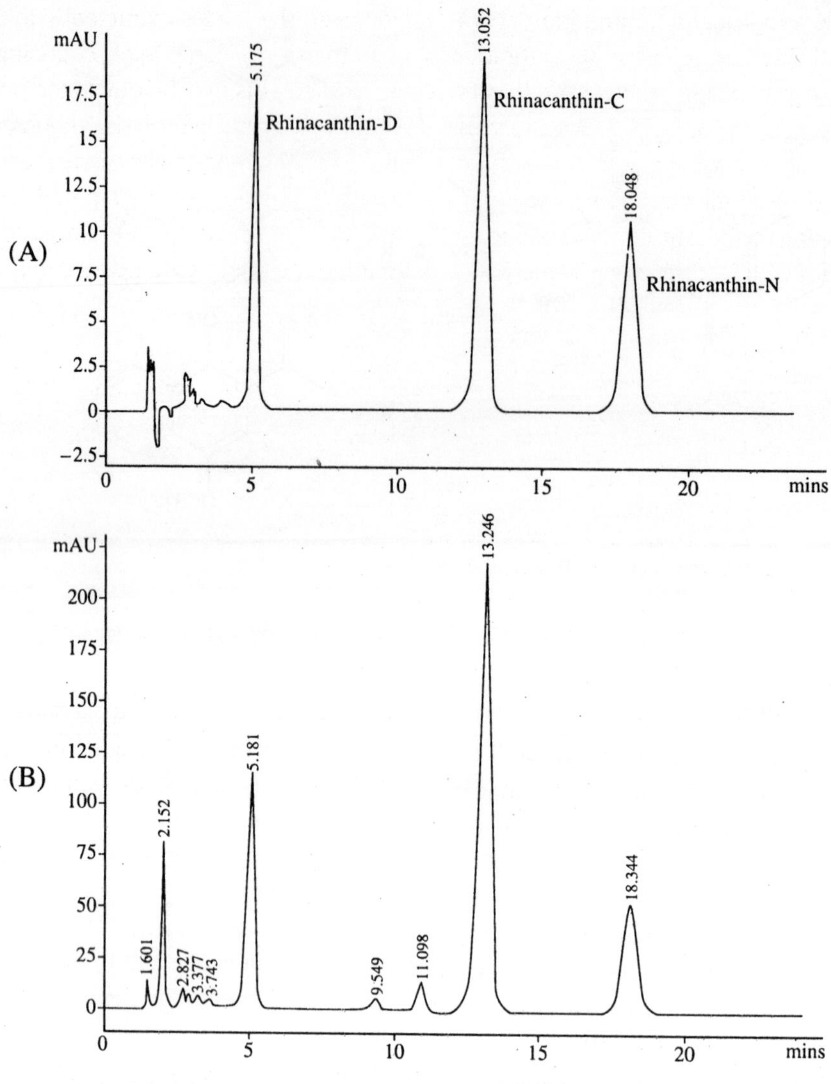

Fig. 25.8. HPLC-chromatograms of (A) the authentic rhinacanthin-C, -D and -N and (B) *R. nasutus* leaf extract. (from Panichayupakaranant et al., 2009b)

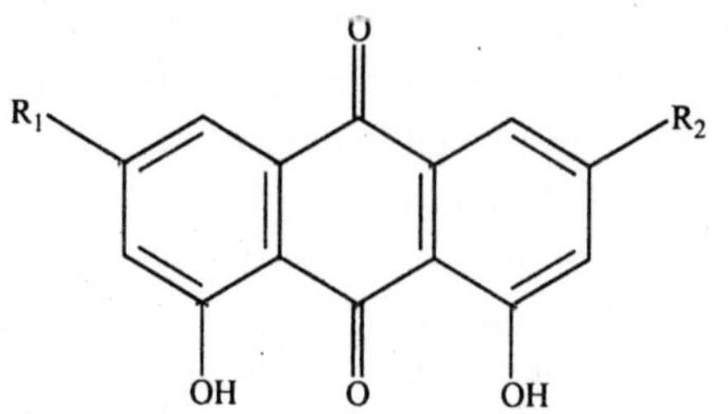

Aloe-emodin : $R_1 = CH_2OH$; $R_2 = H$
Chrysophanol : $R_1 = CH_3$; $R_2 = H$
Emodin : $R_1 = CH_3$; $R_2 = OH$
Rhein : $R_1 = COOH$; $R_2 = H$

Fig. 25.9. Chemical structures of anthraquinones found in *Senna alata*.

100.3 - 100.5% and linearity (correlation coefficient > 0.9998) was obtained for all anthraquinones. A high degree of specificity as well as repeatability and reproducibility (R.S.D. values less than 5%) were also achieved. On the basis of HPLC analysis, only rhein and aloe-emodin are the major aglycone of anthraquinone found in the methanol extract of *S. alata* leaves (Table 25.7). However, the leaves extracted with 5% v/v HCl in methanol are capable of producing emodin in the extract. This may be due to the occurrence of emodin glycoside hydrolysis. Although, chrysophanol has been reported as a constituent in *S. alata* leaves, it was not detected in both extracts. This may be due to very small amounts of this anthraquinone being accumulated in *S. alata* leave.

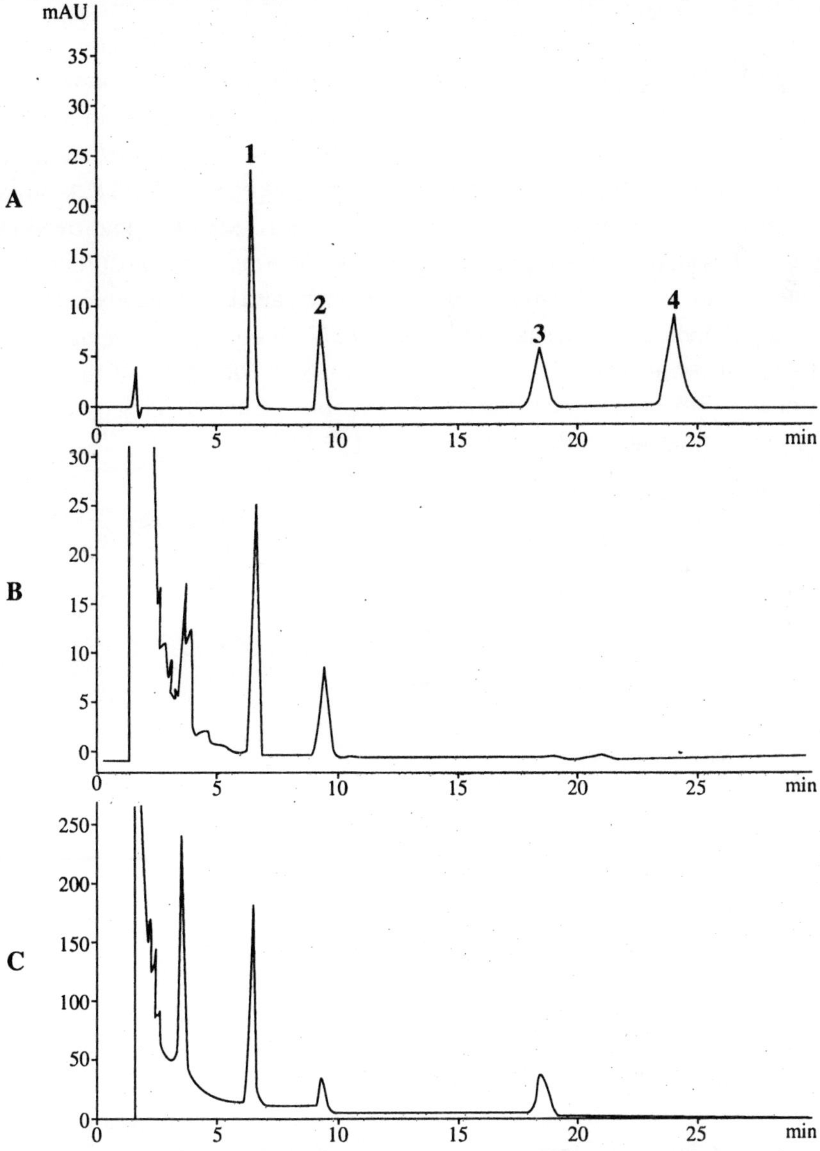

Fig. 25.10. HPLC-chromatograms of (A) authentics: aloe-emodin (1), rhein (2), emodin (3) and chrysophanol (4); (B) methanol extract and (C) 5% HCl in methanol extract of *S. alata* leaves. (from Panichayupakaranant et al., 2009a)

Table 25.7. Anthraquinone content of dried *S. alata* leaf extracted with methanol and 5% HCl in methanol analyzed by HPLC (from Panichayupakaranant et al., 2009a)

Compounds	Anthraquinone content (% w/w) Mean S.D.	
	Methanol extract	5% v/v HCl in methanol extract
Rhein	0.02 0.002	0.15 0.009
Aloe-emodin	0.03 0.008	0.04 0.011
Emodin	n.d.	0.13 0.008
Chrysophanol	n.d.	n.d.

n.d. not detected

Curcuma longa L.

Turmeric (*Curcuma longa* L.) is a rich source of phenolic compounds, curcuminoids. It is widely used as a dietary spice and coloring agent in food and herbal medicine. It is valuable for its pharmacological activities, such as anti-inflammatory, anti-microbial, anti-oxidant, anti-parasitic, anti-mutagenic and anti-cancer affects (Ahsan et al., 1999; Çýkrýkçý et al., 2008; Péret-Almeida et al., 2005). The turmeric extract generally contains three different diaryl heptanoids, which are curcumin, demethoxycurcumin and bisdemethoxycurcumin (Fig. 25.11) (Péret-Almeida et al., 2005; Jayaprakasha et al., 2002 G.K. Jayaprakasha, L.J.M. Rao and K.K. Sakariah, Improved HPLC method for the determination of Curcumin, Demethoxycurcumin, and bisdemethoxycurcumin, *Journal of Agricultural and Food Chemistry* **50** (2002), pp. 3668–3672. **Full Text** via CrossRef | View Record in Scopus | Cited By in Scopus (35)Jayaprakasha *et al.*, 2002).

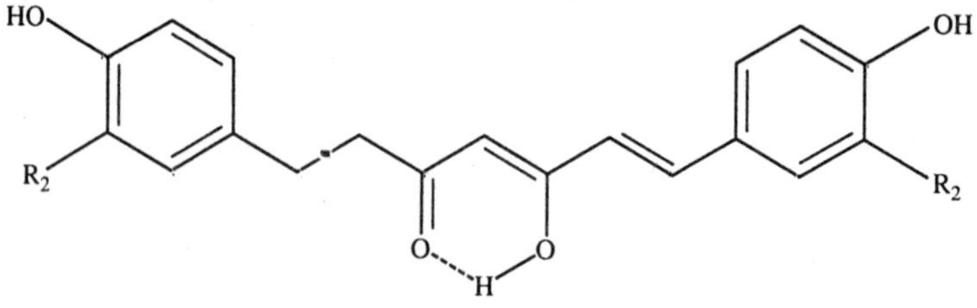

Compounds	R_1	R_2
Curcumin	OCH_3	OCH_3
Demethoxycurcumin	H	OCH_3
Bisdemethoxycurcumin	H	H

Fig. 25.11. Chemical structures of curcuminoids.

Curcuminoids are responsible for the biological activity of *C. longa* and are present to the extent of 2 - 5% w/w (Govindarajan, 1980). Curcuminoids are recognized for their broad spectrum of biological activities and safety in foods or pharmaceuticals. Curcumin is known for its antioxidant, anti-anti-inflammatory, antimicrobial, antiparasitic, antimutagenic, and anticancer properties (Mahattanadul et al., 2006a; Mahattanadul et al., 2006b; Şrimal, 1997). The effect of curcuminoids on the proliferation of MCF-7 human breast tumor cells has been reported. Demethoxycurcumin exhibited the best inhibitory effect on MCF-7 cells, followed by curcumin and bisdemethoxycurcumin (Simon et al., 1998). The antioxidant activity of demethoxycurcumin and bisdemethoxycurcumin was as efficient as the well-known strong antioxidant curcumin (Ahsan et al., 1999). Commercially available curcumin consists of a mixture of three naturally occurring curcuminoids with curcumin as the main (~77% w/w) constituent (Ahsan et al., 1999).

Several methods including HPLC, GC, LC/MS and spectrophotometric methods have been described for the determination of curcumin content in turmeric (Michaleas *et al.*, 2006; Holzgrabe et al., 2005; Péret-Almeida *et al.*, 2005; Jayaprakasha et al., 2002; Subcommittee on the Establishment of the Thai Herbal Pharmacopoeia, 1998). These techniques are time consuming and their specificity, accuracy and precision are not as good as the NMR method, which provides simultaneous identification and quantitation. High-resolution NMR spectroscopy is an effective tool for structure elucidation. For quantitative analysis, the advantages of ^{1}H NMR method are manifold. It is rapid, noninvasive, and does not require any sample pre-clean steps. Standard compounds are not required for preparing calibration curves, and it detects the components present in herbal preparations simultaneously in a single measurement. It had been observed that quantitative NMR spectroscopy is less time consuming, easy to perform, produces more accurate and precise results and leads to a higher reproducibility, compared with HPLC methods (Holzgrabe *et al.*, 2005; Michaleas *et al.*, 2006). A rapid, sensitive and accurate ^{1}H NMR method has been developed for the quantitation of curcumin isolated from *Curcuma longa* rhizome (turmeric) extract, the results of which were compared with a validated LC-MS/MS method (Gören et al., 2009). The relative standard deviations of the methods were found to be 2.49% and 3.48% for the ^{1}H NMR and LC-MS/MS methods, respectively. The correlation coefficients were 0.998 for ^{1}H NMR and 0.995 for LC-MS/MS assay in the calibration range. The recoveries at 5 mg/ml and 50 ìg/ml concentrations averaged to 99.9-101% for both techniques, respectively.

The uncertainty of the measurement of curcumin via ^{1}H NMR spectroscopy was determined to be 5.80% while in LC-ESI-MS/MS method was 7.38%. The ^{1}H NMR spectroscopic method has the additional advantages to the conventional HPLC-UV, GC and LC/MS methods in that it is fast, selective, accurate and reliable. For the trace analysis of curcumin, LC–MS/MS method would be more suitable, however, in tracing small impurities and/or analogues of curcumin, ^{1}H NMR would be the best spectroscopic technique.

PREPARATION OF ACTIVE CONSTITUENT-RICH EXTRACTS

General considerations

The term of "active principle" refers to the intrinsic chemical substance which induces biological or pharmacological activity. Plants are capable of synthesising a large variety of organic compounds. The active principle may be represented by primary cellular constituents (proteins, lipids, polysaccharides) and by secondary metabolites (alkaloids, glycosides, terpenoids coumarins, flavonoids, saponins, tannins, essential oils, etc.). Pharmacologically active constituents of plants are mostly secondary metabolites generated from the shikimate, acetate-malonate and acetate-mevalonate pathways (Tyler et al., 1988). Secondary metabolites were at one time considered as peripheral to the essential metabolism of the cell (i.e. waste products of metabolism). They are now known to be important in many plant functions, although the full function of most is yet to be fully understood (Williams et al., 1989; Bennett and Wallsgrove, 1994). The role of secondary metabolites includes: (a) protection against predators including insects, animal and marine herbivores, micro-organisms and parasite attack, or protection against the environment, (b) protection against UV radiation, (c) participation in allelopathy (the release of a chemical by an organism into the environment that affects the growth, health, behaviour or population of another organism), and (d) function in over flow storage or in disposal of waste products from primary metabolite or involved in detoxification process (see Wills et al., 2000 for an excellent review).

Many conventional drugs or their precursors are derived from plants. However, there is a difference between administering a pure isolated chemical and the same chemical in a plant matrix. Whether this "chemical complexity" is advantageous, it is still a matter of some debate. Wills et al (2000) are of the view that synergy is an important concept in medicinal plant use. In the context of chemical complexity it applies if the pharmacological effect of a chemical mixture is greater than the arithmetic sum of the effects of individual components. This needs to be taken into account when considering the preparation of active constituent-rich extracts.

The extraction and fractionation processes are important steps for the preparation of an active constituent-enriched extract. Suitable extraction methods, as well as the choice of solvents for extraction, are capable of increasing the yield of active constituent in the extract.

An application of ultrasonic extraction with organic solvents of varying polarity (diethyl ether, hexane and ethyl acetate) has been studied for the extraction of volatile oil in garlic (*Allium sativum*), and the yield and flavor profile of the oil has been studied, in comparison to conventional steam distillation (Kimbaris et al., 2006). There are numerous papers in the literature show that the use of correct temperature is crucial in maintaining the levels of constituents in the essential oil from garlic. The application of ultrasound for the extraction of the essential oil is considered to cause less damage of thermal-sensitive molecules, thus, providing a better approach for the extraction of compounds primarily responsible for the characteristic odour and taste of freshly chopped garlic. It was found that the ultrasound-assisted extraction diminished the danger of thermal degradation of sensitive aroma compounds from garlic.

A few different extracting solvents (methanol, acetone, acetonitrile and ethyl acetate) were evaluated for extraction of xanthones from *Garcinia mangostana* fruit rind using ultrasonic extraction. It was found that acetone was the most appropriate solvent for extracting this plant material, affording the highest yield of xanthones (Ji *et al.*, 2007).

In subsequent sections (6.2-6.5) methods for preparation of some active constituent-rich extracts are described.

Rhinacanthin-rich *Rhinacanthus nasutus* extract

Rhinacanthus nasutus (also see sections 3.3.3 and 5.7), a small shrub of Acanthaceae family, has long been used in Thai traditional medicine for treatment of tinea versicolor, ringworm, pruritic rash, abscess pain, and skin diseases. It has been reported that rhinacanthin-C, rhinacanthin-D and rhinacanthin-N isolated from *R. nasutus* possessed antifungal, cytotoxic and antiviral activities.

A few different extraction solvents were tried to maximise the rhinacanthin content in *R. nasutus* leaf extract. Among the solvents that were used for extraction, methanol gave the highest yield of the crude extract (Table 25.8). The obtained extract using methanol gives a rather low total content of rhinacanthins, despite giving the highest yield of crude extract (18.4% w/w of dried leaves). In contrast, ethyl acetate gave the lowest yield of crude extract, but with the highest content of total rhinacanthins (Panichayupakaranant et al., 2009b). This indicates that ethyl acetate is a suitable extraction solvent.

Table 25.8 Yield and total rhinacanthin content in dried *R. nasutus* leaf extracts (from Panichayupakaranant et al., 2009b)

Solvents	Yield (%w/w S.D.)	Total rhinacanthin content (%w/w S.D.)
Dichloromethane	3.7 0.12	11.7 0.25
Chloroform	4.9 0.22	14.3 0.14
Ethyl acetate	4.8 0.16	33.0 0.16
Ethanol	11.5 0.28	5.4 0.24
Methanol	18.4 0.43	6 7 0.31

Ion exchange chromatographic methods have been developed to improve rhinacanthin concentration in the extract, as well as to diminish the interference from other compounds in the extract. Anion exchange resin is widely used for separation or pre-purification of many compounds. For example, separation of lactic acid has been achieved using a strong basic anion exchange resin, Amberlite IRA-400 (Cao et al., 2002) and weak anion exchanger, Amberlite IRA-92 (Tong et al., 2004). Rhinacanthins are anionic compounds that can be enriched by anion exchange resins. It was found that Amberlite IRA-67 column was capable of improving the rhinacanthin content in the obtained semi-purified extract. The content of total rhinacanthins in the rhinacanthin rich *R. nasutus* extract was increased to 77.5% w/w compared to 37.4% w/w in the crude extract from ethyl acetate extraction (Table 25.9). The interfering compounds, including chlorophyll and other pigments, were also markedly excluded. The weakly basic anion exchanger, Amberlite IRA-67 is therefore suitable for preparation of *R. nasutus* leaf extract (Panichayupakaranant et al., 2009b)

Table 25.9 Total rhinacanthin content in the ethyl acetate extract and rhinacanthin-rich extract of *R. nasutus* leaves (from Panichayupakaranant et al., 2009b)

Compounds	Rhinacanthin content (% w/w; Mean R.S.D.)	
	Ethyl acetate extract	Rhinacanthin-rich extract
Rhinacanthin-C	34.5 1.0	66.4 13.05
Rhinacanthin-D	1.8 4.4	7.5 1.37
Rhinacanthin-N	1.1 0.5	3.6 0.57
Total rhinacanthin	37.4	77.5

The antifungal activity of the rhinacanthin-rich *R. nasutus* extract against *Trichrophyton rubrum, T. mentagrophytes* and *Microsporum gypseum* was evaluated and compared with those of the ethyl acetate crude extract and pure standard rhinacanthins (Panichayupakaranant et al., 2009b). The results showed that antifungal activity of the rhinacanthin-rich *R. nasutus* extract was better than that of the ethyl acetate crude extract (Table 25.10). The antifungal activity of the rhinacanthin-rich *R. nasutus* extract was equal to that of rhinacanthin-C. This may be due to a synergistic effect of all the three rhinacanthins on antifungal activity. Thus, the prepared rhinacanthin-rich *R. nasutus* extract is suitable for the development of a suitable topical application antifungal cream.

Table 25.10 Antifungal activity of rhinacanthins, ethyl acetate extract and rhinacanthin-rich *R. nasutus* extract (from Panichayupakaranant et al., 2009b)

Extracts/Compounds	MIC (g/mL)		
	T. rubrum	*T. mentagrophytes*	*M. gypseum*
Ethyl acetate crude extract	31.2	62.5	500.0
Rhinacanthin-rich extract	7.5	31.2	125.0
Rhinacanthin-C	15.1	31.2	125.0
Rhinacanthin-D	31.2	31.2	125.0
Rhinacanthin-N	62.5	250.0	250.0
Ketoconazole*	0.5	8.0	8.0

* positive control

Anthraquinone-rich *Senna alata* extract

Senna alata (L.) Roxb has been traditionally used for the treatment of dermatophyte infections (also see sections 3.3.3 and 5.8). The anthraquinones, including aloe-emodin, rhein, emodin and chrysophanol have been demonstrated as the antifungal active constituents. Recently, the poor quality of *S. alata* leaves, containing a lower level of anthraquinones than the standard value in the monograph of Thai Herbal Pharmacopoeia (1998), has been a major problem in the production of the herbal medicine from *S. alata*. Although an efficient extraction method for dried *S. alata* leaves was established, extracts with low anthraquinone content (1.67% w/w) were still obtained (Panichayupakaranant et al., 2009a). To improve the potency of the antifungal activity of *S. alata* leaf extracts, the anthraquinone content of the extract need to be increased, and the interfering compounds in the extracts (such as chlorophyll) need to be excluded from the extracts, in particular to improve the physical appearance and stability of the extracts.

A few different extraction solvents were tried to maximise the anthraquinone content in *S. alata* leaf extracts. Dried *S. alata* leaves were extracted under reflux conditions using a mixture of HCl, $FeCl_3$ and water in methanol as the solvent. Water was used for extraction of anthraquinone glycoside, while HCl and $FeCl_3$ were used for hydrolysis and oxidation of anthraquinone glycoside to the aglycone moeity. The concentrations of each component in methanol were varied in order to get a high yielding anthraquinone extract. The results showed that emodin was only observed when acidic methanol was used for extraction, and 5% v/v HCl in methanol gave significantly higher total anthraquinone content than those of 0, 3 and 10% v/v HCl in methanol (Table 25.11). Variations of $FeCl_3$ concentration in methanol with 5% v/v HCl were then examined as the extraction solvents. It was found that only aloe-emodin and emodin were observed in the extract after oxidization with $FeCl_3$. However, the content of total anthraquinones was increased when the concentration of $FeCl_3$ was increase to 5% w/v (Table 12). Therefore, 5% w/v $FeCl_3$ in methanol with 5% v/v HCl was selected for use as the extraction solvent for the extraction of anthraquinones from dried *S. alata* leaves. Naturally occurring anthraquinones in *S. alata* leaves are in both glycoside and aglycone forms (Smith and Sadaquat, 1979). This suggests that oxidization and hydrolysis of anthraquinone glycoside are required in the extraction process in order to increase anthraquinone content in *S. alata* extract (Panichayupakaranant et al., 2009a).

Table 25.11 Anthraquinone content in dried *S. alata* leaf extracts extracted under reflux with various concentrations of HCl in methanol (from Panichayupakaranant et al., 2009a)

HCl concentration (% v/v)	Anthraquinone content (% w/w) Mean S.D.			
	Aloe-emodin	Emodin	Rhein	Total
0	0.03 0.002	n.d.	0.02 0.002	0.05 0.004
3	0.14 0.008	0.11 0.012	0.05 0.009	0.30 0.011
5	0.15 0.009	0.13 0.008	0.04 0.011	0.32 0.007
10	0.14 0.010	0.13 0.002	0.03 0.003	0.30 0.013

n.d. = not detected

Table 25.12 Anthraquinone content in dried *S. alata* leaf extracts extracted under reflux with various concentrations of ferric chloride in 5% v/v HCl in methanol (from Panichayupakaranant et al., 2009a)

$FeCl_3$ concentration (% w/v)	Anthraquinone content (% w/w) Mean S.D.			
	Aloe-emodin	Emodin	Rhein	Total
0	0.15 0.009	0.13 0.008	0.04 0.011	0.32 0.007
2.5	0.54 0.044	0.33 0.070	n.d.	0.87 0.103
5	0.99 0.094	0.47 0.011	n.d.	1.46 0.146
10	1.08 0.095	0.51 0.014	n.d.	1.59 0.093

n.d. = not detected

Since glycosides are usually soluble in water, adequate water may be required to increase the anthraquinone glycoside extraction. An optimization study for water content in the extraction solvent showed that the highest extract anthraquinone levels are obtained when employing 15% v/v water (Table 25.13). Thus, the suitable solvent for anthraquinone extraction from dried *S. alata* leaves should comprise 5% v/v hydrochloric acid, 5% w/v ferric chloride and 15% v/v water in methanol.

Table 25.13 Anthraquinone content in dried *S. alata* leaf extracts extracted under reflux with various concentrations of water in 5% v/v hydrochloric acid and 5% w/v ferric chloride in methanol (from Panichayupakaranant et al., 2009a)

Water concentration (% v/v)	Anthraquinone content (% w/w) Mean S.D.		
	Aloe-emodin	Emodin	Total
0	0.42 0.026	0.71 0.001	1.13 0.025
5	0.64 0.166	0.66 0.014	1.30 0.025
10	0.78 0.056	0.58 0.007	1.36 0.029
15	1.11 0.085	0.56 0.004	1.67 0.016
20	0.87 0.023	0.34 0.027	1.21 0.005

Chromatographic methods were used to concentrate the anthraquinone in the crude leaf extracts of *S. alata*, as well as to greatly reduce the levels of other interfering compounds. Two chromatographic methods, an anion exchange and silica gel vacuum chromatography, were examined to improve the anthraquinone content in the leaf extract (Sakunpak *et al.*, 2009). Both methods were capable of increasing total anthraquinone content in the extracts. However, the extract that was isolated by silica gel vacuum chromatography gave higher content of total anthraquinones than that isolated by anion exchange chromatography (Table 25.14). The silica gel vacuum chromatographic method increased total content of anthraquinones in the extract up to 15-fold compared to level in the crude extract. In addition, isolation by silica gel vacuum chromatography was less time consuming than isolation by anion exchange chromatography. This indicates that silica gel vacuum chromatography is a preferable method for improving the anthraquinone content in *S. alata* leaf extracts. The yield of the anthraquinone-rich *S. alata* extract was 0.73% w/w compared to the weight of dried leaf powder. The total anthraquinone content in the extracts was 16.22% w/w (Table 25.15).

Table 25.14 Anthraquinone content in dried *S. alata* leaf extracts isolated by difference methods (from Sakunpak et al., 2009)

Leaf extracts	Anthraquinone content (% w/w; Mean S.D.)		
	Aloe-emodin	Emodin	Total
Crude extract [a]	0.42 0.03	0.71 0.01	1.13 0.02
Isolated by anion exchange chromatography [b]	3.77 0.07	5.81 0.26	9.58 0.33
Isolated by silica gel vacuum chromatography [b]	10.10 1.13	6.60 0.46	16.70 1.59

[a] Extracted with methanol containing 5% v/v HCl, 5% w/v $FeCl_3$ and 15% v/v water

[b] Data is for processing of crude extract by these method

Table 25.15 Anthraquinone content of the anthraquinone-rich *S. alata* extracts (from Sakunpak et al., 2009)

Lot no.	Yield of the extracts (% w/w)	Anthraquinone content (% w/w; Mean S.D.)		
		Aloe-emodin	Emodin	Total
1	0.7	10.8 1.13	6.6 0.47	17.4 0.61
2	0.9	10.5 0.51	4.7 0.30	15.2 0.93
3	0.8	11.1 1.54	5.9 0.95	17.0 1.68
4	0.7	11.1 0.94	6.7 1.01	17.8 0.93
5	0.7	10.4 0.91	5.9 0.86	16.2 0.64
6	0.7	9.2 0.02	5.8 0.65	15.0 0.79
7	0.7	9.2 0.11	5.8 0.78	15.0 1.04
Mean S.D.	0.7 0.09	10.3 0.75	5.9 0.61	16.2 1.12

Evaluation of antifungal activities of the anthraquinone-rich *S. alata* extract and the standard anthraquinones, aloe-emodin, rhein, emodin, chrysophanol against *Trichophyton rubrum, T. mentagrophytes* and *Microsporum gypseum* found that the anthraquinone-rich extract possessed antifungal activity against all tested dermatophytes with MIC values between 15.62 - 250 μg/ml. This enriched extract showed the highest antifungal activity against *T. rubrum*, with an MIC value of 15.62 μg/ml. All tested dermatophytes were also completely inhibited by emodin and rhein at concentration between 1.95 - 1000 and 31.25 - 1000 μg/ml, respectively. Although chrysophanol has been reported as one of the antifungal active compounds (Ibrahim and Osman, 1995), the antifungal activity of this compound against all tested dermatophytes was not observed at concentrations up to 1,000 μg/ml. Among the tested compounds, aloe-emodin exhibited the strongest antifungal activity against *T. rubrum* with MIC value of 0.98 μg/ml, but was not active against *T. mentagrophytes* and *M. gypseum* at the concentration up to 1,000 μg/ml. Although the antifungal activity of the anthraquinone-rich extract against *T. rubrum* was lower than that of aloe-emodin and emodin, its antifungal activities against *T. mentagrophytes* and *M. gypseum* were markedly higher than those of aloe-emodin and emodin. This is probably due to the synergistic effect of these two active compounds. The results of these studies confirm the potential of the anthraquinone-rich *S. alata* leaf extracts as an effective antifungal preparation, suitable for developing formulations for treatment of fungal infections. The extracts used in future studies should be standardised to the total anthraquinone content not less than 16% w/w (Sakunpak *et al.*, 2009).

Ellagic acid-rich pomegranate fruit peel extract

Pomegranate fruit peel, a by-product of the pomegranate juice industry, is a rich source of hydrolysable tannin belonging to ellagitannins (also see section 5.6). It is therefore an inexpensive and abundant source of ellagitannins. A wide range of clinical applications of pomegranate fruit peel extract for the treatment and prevention of cancer, as well as other diseases, where chronic inflammation is believed to play an essential etiologic role, is suggested (Lansky & Newman, 2007). The reports have revealed that pomegranate fruit peel extract is a potential antioxidant agent for nutraceutical and cosmetic applications (Aguilar *et al.*, 2008). Ellagic acid is considered as an indicative marker for standardisation of the fruit peel extract (Zhou *et al.*, 2008), and as a biomarker for human bioavailability studies involving consumption of ellagitannins from food sources (Seeram *et al.*, 2004). In addition, ellagic acid also has other benefits; it has anti-inflammatory (Ogawa *et al.*, 2002), anti-allergy (Rogerio *et al.*, 2008), anti-cancer properties (Larrosa *et al.*, 2006; Mertens-Talcott & Percival, 2005), it reduces microbial growth (Zambuchini *et al.*, 2008), it inhibits many toxic effects caused by phospholipase A_2 (Da Silva *et al.*, 2008), and it protects against testicular toxicity (Turk *et al.*, 2008). Thus, a method for ellagic acid enrichment in pomegranate fruit peel extract is needed.

Different extraction solvents were examined to maximise ellagic acid content in pomegranate fruit peel crude extract (Panichayupakaranant et al., 2010b). Considering the polarity of ellagic acid, combinations of water and methanol were examined as the extraction solvents. The results showed that 10% v/v water in methanol gave significantly higher ellagic acid content than other extraction solvents (Table 25.16). The crude extract was further purified by partitioning between water and a few organic solvents, including ethyl acetate, *n*-butanol and a mixture of *n*-butanol and ethyl acetate (1:1). It was found that the ethyl acetate fraction showed the highest ellagic acid content, as well as the highest antioxidant activity (Table 25.17). Increasing ellagic acid content resulted in an increase in the antioxidant activity of the extract. Partitioning between water and ethyl acetate was therefore an appropriate method for the preparation of the high antioxidant potency extract of pomegranate fruit peel (Panichayupakaranant et al., 2010b).

Table 25.16 Ellagic acid content in pomegranate fruit peel extracts extracted under reflux with various concentration of water in methanol (from Panichayupakaranant et al., 2010b)

Water concentration (% v/v)	Ellagic acid content Mean (% w/w)	S.D.
0	5.84	0.03
5	7.11	0.17
10	7.66	0.01
15	6.82	0.38
20	6.18	0.62

Table 25.17 Ellagic acid content and antioxidant activity in pomegranate fruit peel extracts, which were partitioned between water and various organic solvents (from Panichayupakaranant et al., 2010b)

Extract/fraction	Ellagic acid content Mean (% w/w)	S.D.	Antioxidant activity† EC_{50} (g/ml)	
Methanol extract	7.06	0.02	38.21	0.14
Ethyl acetate fraction	9.48	0.06	15.17	0.40
n-Butanol fraction	8.16	0.01	22.16	0.51
Ethyl acetate and *n*-butanol fraction	8.57	0.06	18.11	0.50

†Evaluated by DPPH radical scavenging assay

After fractionation of the pomegranate fruit peel extract using liquid-liquid extraction between ethyl acetate and 2% aqueous acetic acid, ellagic acid-rich extract was obtained from the ethyl acetate fraction with a yield of 16.6% w/w compared to the weight of dried fruit peel powder (Table 25.18). The appearance of the crude extract changed from a dark brown semi-solid to a brown powder for the ellagic acid-rich extract. On the basis of HPLC analysis, only ellagic acid was found as the major compound in the ellagic acid-rich extract. This method was capable of increasing the ellagic acid content in the extracts from 7.1% w/w to 13.6% w/w as well as the antioxidant activity (Table 25.18). Preliminary studies on fractionation of the pomegranate fruit peel extract found that liquid-liquid extraction between ethyl acetate and water was an appropriate method for a preparation of the high antioxidant potency extract of pomegranate fruit peel. However, the result from this study indicated that the use of 2% aqueous acetic acid, instead of water, in the liquid-liquid extraction process produced an extract with a higher ellagic acid content and antioxidant activity (Table 25.19). This is due to a suppression of ionization of ellagic acid in aqueous acidic condition that was capable of decreasing water solubility of ellagic acid. Hence it is more soluble in ethyl acetate. According to the satisfactory antioxidant activity of the ellagic acid rich pomegranate, the extracts used in further studies were standardised to the ellagic acid content not less than 13% w/w (Panichayupakaranant et al., 2010a).

Table 25.18 Extraction yield, ellagic acid content and antioxidant activity of the ellagic acid-rich pomegranate fruit peel extract (from Panichayupakaranant et al., 2010a)

Extracts/compounds	Extraction yield (% w/w*)	Ellagic acid content (% w/w**)	Antioxidant activity† ED_{50} (μg/L)
Crude extract	32.5 2.14	7.1 0.02	38.2 0.14
Ellagic acid rich extract	16.6 1.13	13.6 0.89	14.9 0.24
Standard quercetin	-	-	3.6 0.64
Standard ellagic acid	-	-	3.1 0.35

* Compared to the weight of dried powder

** Compared to the weight of the extract

†Evaluated by DPPH radical scavenging assay

Table 25.19 Ellagic acid content and antioxidant activity of the ethyl acetate fractions obtained from liquid-liquid extractions (from Panichayupakaranant et al., 2010a)

Solvents for liquid-liquid extraction	Ellagic acid content (% w/w; Mean S.D.)	Antioxidant activity†, ED_{50}(g/L; Mean S.D.)
Ethyl acetate and water	9.2 0.51	16.3 0.72
Ethyl acetate and 2% aq. acetic acid	13.6 0.89	14.9 0.24

†Evaluated by DPPH radical scavenging assay

Madecassoside and asiaticoside-rich *Centella asiatica* extract

Centella asiatica (L.) Urban is a traditional herbal medicine used in Asiatic countries for hundreds of years. It contains pentacyclic triterpenes, mainly asiaticoside, madecassoside, asiatic acid and madecossic acid (Inamdar *et al.*, 1996), and they have been claimed to possess various pharmacological effects. Reports have revealed that triterpene saponins from *C. asiatica* showed a promising wound healing property (Kimura et al., 2008; Shukla et al., 1999). They apparently also have the benefits of memory improvement, anti-inflammatory, anticancer, antioxidation, and anxiolytic activities (Gnanapragasam et al., 2007; Chen et al., 2006; Gnanapragasam et al., 2004; Kumar et al., 2002; Babu et al., 1995). Thus, an efficient method for the separation of madecassoside and asiaticoside from *C. asiatica* is needed.

The conventional separation method of saponins is normally carried out from the extracts by means of solid–liquid extraction from natural resources, then liquid–liquid extraction is conducted by using different solvents, and then followed by a column chromatography with gradient solvent system (Dinan et al., 2001). Liquid–liquid separation method has been investigated to get mixtures of asiaticoside and madecassoside from extracts of *C. asiatica* (Kim et al., 2002b). However, this separation method is an inefficient process, consuming longer time and more solvent, and results in lower recovery of the products. Alternatively, the adsorption–desorption process, in general, is an efficient separation method with a moderate purification effect and can be used economically for recovering and concentrating targeted phytochemicals in industrial practices.

Recently, there is a growing interest in employing macroporous resins to separate bioactive components from crude extracts of herbal raw materials because of their unique adsorption properties. Other advantages include ideal pore structure and various available surface functional groups, low operation expense, less solvent consumption and easy regeneration. Macroporous resins have also been used to separate bioactive components from the crude extract of *C. asiatica* (Jia and Lu, 2008). The adsorption and desorption identities of five different macroporous resins including HPD100, HPD300, X-5, AB-8 and D101 were investigated by static adsorption and desorption of madecassoside and asiaticoside, and the separation process of these from crude *C. asiatica* extracts with the selected resin was tested by dynamic adsorption and desorption experiments. HPD100 exhibited higher adsorption and desorption capacities and higher adsorption speed for asiaticoside and madecassoside than other resins. Columns packed with HPD100 resin were used to perform dynamic adsorption and desorption tests to optimise the separation process of asiaticoside and madecassoside from crude *C. asiatica* extracts. After gradient elution on HPD100 resin, the content of madecassoside in the product increased from 3.9 to 39.7%, and the recovery yield was 70.4%; for asiaticoside the content increased from 2.0 to 21.5%, and the recovery yield was 72.0%. Thus, HPD100 resin possesses a good ability to separate madecassoside and asiaticoside, and the method can be referenced for the separation of other triterpene saponins from crude extract of herbal raw materials (Jia and Lu, 2008).

CONCLUDING REMARKS

Many people use herbal supplements because they believe natural means safer and fewer side effects. In reality, many herbs can be dangerous intrinsically, or can interact with prescription and over-the-counter drugs. The public needs to be educated that"natural" does not mean necessarily "safe." In addition, the public should be aware that the advertising and literature surrounding herbal products often contains untested and spurious claims. Ideally, only standardised products should be purchased; products with the scientific name and quantity of the botanical clearly identified on the label, and the name and address of the manufacturer, batch number, and expiration date.

Over the last 2 – 3 decades, worldwide interest in herbal medicines has increased, both in developed and developing countries. The surge in growth of the herbal market has attracted much interest from the pharmaceutical companies, which has in turn stimulated the appearance of pre-clinical pharmacological studies and of well-controlled and randomised clinical trials to prove the safety and efficacy of herbal products. The number of scientific papers published on herbal plants has grown exponentially in recent years. In spite of this, so far insufficient data exist to provide an accurate assessment of the quality, efficacy and safety of most herbal medicines on the market.

Chemical analysis of extracts from plant material will play a central role in the development and modernisation of botanicals and herbal preparations. The methods used should be able to identify the active or marker compounds, and/or provide a fingerprint of the phytochemical present in the herb. For the chemical standardisation of botanicals and herbal preparations, the methods involved include, sample preparation procedures (e.g. extraction techniques) and analytical methods (e.g. separation and identification techniques). However, due to the complexity of the plant materials obtained, the use of different methods of extraction, separation and identification may be needed. It is certain that methods that are simple, rapid and environmentally friendly will be preferred, and are likely to play an important role in the effort of providing high quality products to consumers worldwide. Just as for pharmaceutical products, a well-validated method will help in monitoring the stability of the botanicals and herbal preparations over a period of time. It is likely that the combination of chemical standardisation with biological assay will provide further knowledge about therapeutic effects of the medicinal plant. The use of validated methods in the chemical standardisation of botanicals and herbal preparations will enhance the quality of the products, assist in pharmacological studies, performance of credible clinical trials and propel the move towards evidence based medicine.

ACKNOWLEDGEMENTS

I wish to express my deepest and grateful thanks to Professor Dr. L. A. Damani for his kindness in help with the preparation of this manuscript, and for his critical comments. My sincere thanks are also expressed to the researchers, including, Assistant Professor Dr. Anusak Sirikatitham, Dr. Wei Wang, Mr. Tossaton Charoonratana, Mr. Apirak Sakunpak, Mr. Athip Sakunphueak, Miss Atcharaporn Issuriya and Mrs. Niwan Intaraksa, who have contributed to work referenced in this book chapter.

REFERENCES

Abreu IN, Mazzafera P. Effect of water and temperature stress on the content of active constituents of *Hypericum brasiliense* Choisy. *Plant Physiol Biochem*, 43, 241-248, (2005).

Agarwal SK, Singh SS, Verma S, Kumar S. Antifungal activity of anthraquinone derivatives from *Rheum emodi*. *J Ethnopharmacol*, 72, 43-46, (2000).

Aguilar CN, Aguilera-Carbo A, Robledo A, Ventura J, Belmares R, Martinez D, Rodríguez-Herrera R, Contreras J. Production of antioxidant nutraceuticals by solid-state cultures of pomegranate (*Punica granatum*) peel and creosote bush (*Larrea tridentata*) leaves. *Food Technol Biotechnol*, 46, 218-222, (2008).

Ahsan H, Parween N, Khan NU, Hadi SM. Pro-oxidant, anti-oxidant, and cleavage activities on DNA of curcumin and its derivatives demethoxycurcumin and bisdemethoxycurcumin. *Chem Biol Interact*, 121, 161-175, (1999).

Apparao MVR, Srinivasan K, Rao K, The effect of mandookparni (*Centella asiatica*) on the general mental ability (Medhya) of mentally retarded children. *J Res Indian Med*, 8, 9-16, (1973).

Babu TD, Kuttan G, Padikkala J. Cytotoxic and antitumor properties of certain taxa of Umbelliferae with special reference to *Centella asiatica* (L.) Urban. *J Ethnopharmacol*, 48, 53-57, (1995).

Bagheri H, Broué P; Lacroix I, Larrey D, Olives JP, Vaysse PH, Ghisolfi J, Montastru JL. Fulminant hepatic failure after herbal medicine ingestion in children. *Térapie*, 53, 77-83, (1998).

Bauer R, Khan IA, Wagner H. Echinacea Nachweis einer Verfälschung von *Echinacea purpurea* (L.) Moench mit *Parthenium integrifolium* L. (Detection of *Parthenium integrifolium* L. adulteration of *Echinacea purpurea* (L.) Moench), *Dtsch Apoth Ztg*, 127, 1325-1330, (1987).

Bauer R, Khan I, Lotter H, Wagner H, Wray V. Structure and stereochemistry of new sesquiterpene esters from *Echinacea purpurea* (L.) Moench. *Helv Chim Acta*., 68, 2355-2358, (1985).

Bauer R, Reminger P, Wagner H. Alkamides from the roots of *Echinacea angustifolia*. *Phytochemistry* 28, 505-508, (1989).

Bauer R, Wagner H. Neue ergebnisse zur analytik von Echinacea wurzeln. *Sci Pharm*., 55, 159-161, (1987).

Bennett RN, Wallsgrove RM. Tansley review no. 72. Secondary metabolites in plant defense mechanisms. *New Physiologist*, 127, 617-633, (1994).

Benthin B, Danz H, Hamburger M. Pressurized liquid extraction of medicinal plants. *J Chromatogr A*, 837, 211-219, (1999).

Benzi G, Ceci A. Herbal medicines in European regulation. *Pharmacol Res*, 35, 355-362, (1997).

Bode AM, Ma WY, Surh YJ, Dong Z. Inhibition of epidermal growth factor-induced cell transformation and activator protein 1 activation by 6-ginerol. *Cancer Res*, 61, 850-853, (2001).

Boone SA, Shields KM. Treating Pregnancy-related nausea and vomiting with Ginger. *Ann Pharmacother*, 39, 1710-1713, (2005).

Borrelli F. Capasso R. Aviello G. Pittler MH, Izzo AA. Effectiveness and safety of ginger in the treatment of pregnancy-induced nausea and vomiting. *Obstet Gynecol*, 105, 849-856, (2005).

Bos R, Woerdenbag HJ, Hendriks H, Zwaving JH, De Smet PAGM, Tittel G, Wikstrom HV, Scheffer JJC. Analytical aspect of phytotherapeutic valerian preparations. *Phytochem Anal* 7, 143-151, (1996).

Brevoort P. The booming US botanical market: a new overview. *Herbalgram*, 44, 33-48, (1998).

Brown RG. Toxicity of Chinese herbal remedies. *Lancet*, 340, 673, (1992).

Burchfield HP, Storrs E, E. Biochemical applications of gas chromatography. Academic Press, New York, (1962).

Calapai G, Caputi AP. Herbal medicines: Can we do without pharmacologist?. *eCAM*, 4(S1), 41-43, (2007).

Calixto JB. Efficacy, safety, quality control, marketing and regulatory guidelines for herbal medicines (phytotherapeutic agents). *Braz J Med Biol Res*, 33, 179-189, (2000).

Camel V. Microwave-assisted solvent extraction of environmental samples. *Trends Anal Chem*, 19, 229-248, (2000).

Canigueral S, Tschopp R, Ambrosetti L, Vignutelli A, Scaglione F, Petrini O. The development of herbal medicine products: Quality, safety and efficacy as key factor. *Pharm Med*, 22, 107-118, (2008).

Cao X, Yun HS, Koo YM. Recovery of L-(+)-lactic acid by anion exchange resin Amberlite IRA-400. *Biochem Eng J*, 11, 189-196, (2002).

Capasso R, Izzo AA, Pinto L, Bifulco T, Vitobello C, Mascolo N. Phytotherapy and quality of herbal medicines. *Fitoterapia*, 71, S58-S65, (2000).

Casas L, Mantell C, Rodríguez M, Torres A, Macías FA, Martínez de la Ossa E. Effect of the addition of cosolvent on the supercritical fluid extraction of bioactive compounds from *Helianthus annuus* L. *J Supercrit Fluids*, 41, 43-49, (2007).

Castellani C, Marai A, Vacchi E. The *Centella asiatica* Boll. *Chim Farm*, 120, 570-605, (1981).

Chairungsrilerd N, Furukawa K, Ohta T, Nozoe S, Ohizumi Y. Histaminergic and serotonergic receptor blocking substances from the medicinal plant *Garcinia mangostana*. *Planta Med*, 62, 471-472, (1996).

Chaiyakunapruk N, Kitikannakorn N, Nathisuwan S, Leeprakobboon K, Leelasettagool C. The efficacy of ginger for the prevention of postoperative nausea and vomiting: A meta-analysis. *Am J Obstet Gynecol*, 194, 95-99, (2006).

Chan K. Some aspects of toxic contaminants in herbal medicines. *Chemosphere*, 52, 1361-1371, (2003).

Chan TYK, Chan AYW, Critchley JAJH. Hospital admission due to adverse reactions to Chinese herbal medicines, *J Trop Med Hyg*, 95, 296-298, (1992).

Chan W, Lee K, Liu N, Cai Z. A sensitivity enhanced high-performance liquid chromatography fluorescence method for the detection of nephrotoxic and carcinogenic aristolochic acid in herbal medicines. *J Chromatogr A*, 1164, 113-119, (2007).

Chau FT, Chan TP, Wang J. TLCQA: quantitative study of thin-layer chromatography. *Bioinformatics,* 14, 540-541, (1998).

Chen G, Pramanik BN. Application of LC/MS to proteomics studies: current status and future prospects. *Drug Discovery Today*, 14, 465-471 (2009).

Chen Q, Yao S, Huang X, Luo J, Wang J, Kong K. Supercritical fluid extraction of *Coriandrum sativum* and subsequent separation of isocoumarins by high-speed counter-current chromatography. *Food Chem*, 117, 504-508, (2009).

Chen SW, Wang WJ, Li WJ, Wang R, Li YL, Huang YN, Liang X. Anxiolytic-like effect of asiaticoside in mice. *Pharmacol Biochem Behav*, 85 339, (2006).

Chen SX. Wan M, Loh BN. Active constituents against HIV-1 protease from *Garcinia mangostana. Planta Med*, 62, 381-382, (1996).

Cheng YW, Kang JJ. Mechanism of vasorelaxation of thoracic aorta caused by xanthone. *Eur J Pharmacol*, 336, 23-28, (1997).

Chomnawang MT. Surassmo S. Nukoolkarn VS, Gritsanapan W. Antimicrobial effects of Thai medicinal plants against acne-inducing bacteria. *J Ethnopharmacol*, 101, 330-333, (2005).

Chrubasik S, Pittler MII, Roufogalis BD. *Zingiberis rhizoma*: A comprehensive review on the ginger effect and efficacy profiles. *Phytomedicine*, 12, 684-701, (2005).

Cianchino V, Acosta G, Ortega C, Martínez LD, Gomez MR. Analysis of potential adulteration in herbal medicines and dietary supplements for the weight control by capillary electrophoresis. *Food Chem*, 108, 1075-1081, (2008).

Çýkrýkçý S, Mozioðlu E, Yýlmaz H. Biological activity of curcuminoids isolated from *Curcuma longa. Rec Nat Prod*, 2, 19-24, (2008).

Cossuta D, Simandi B, Vagi E, Hohmann J, Prechl A, Lemberkovics E, Kery A, Keve T. Supercritical fluid extraction of *Vitex agnus castus* fruit. *J Supercrit Fluids*, 47, 188-194, (2008).

CPMP/QWP/2820/00 (EMEA/CVMP/815/00), Note for guidance on specifications: test procedures and acceptance criteria for herbal drugs, herbal drug preparation and herbal medicinal products, *EMEA*, (2001).

D'Arcy PF. Adverse reactions and interactions with herbal medicines. 2. Drug interactions. *Adverse Drug React Toxicol Rev*, 12, 147-162, (1993).

Da Silva SL, Calgarotto AK, Chaar JS, Marangoni S. Isolation and characterization of ellagic acid derivatives isolated from *Casearia sylvestris* SW aqueous extract with anti-PLA2 activity. *Toxicon*, 52, 655-666, (2008).

De Smet PAGM. Health risk of herbal remedies. *Drug Saf*, 13, 81-93, (1995).

Defelice SL. The nutraceutical revolution-its impact on food industry R and D. *Trends Food Sci Technol*, 6, 59-61, (1995).

Deng S, Deng Z, Fan Y, Peng Y, Li J, Xiong D, Liu R. Isolation and purification of three flavonoid glycosides from the leaves of *Nelumbo nucifera* (Lotus) by high-speed counter-current chromatography. *J Chromatogr B*, 877, 2487-2492, (2009).

Dinan L, Harmatha J, Lafont R. Chromatographic procedures for the isolation of plant steroids. *J Chromatogr A*, 935, 105, (2001).

Ding S, Dudley E, Plummer S, Tang J, Newton, R. P., Brenton, A. G. Fingerprint profile of *Ginkgo biloba* nutritional supplements by LC/ESI-MS/MS. *Phytochemistry* 69, 1555-1564, (2008).

Draves AH. Walker SE, Analysis of the hypericin and pseudohypericin content of commercially available St. John's wort preparations. *Can J Clin Pharmacol*, 10, 114-118, (2003).

Drew AK. and Mayers SP. Safety issues in herbal medicine: implications for the health professions. *Med J Aust*, 166, 538-541, (1997).

Eisenberg DM, Davis RB, Ettner SL, Appel S, Wilkey S, Van Rompay M, Kessler RC. Trends in alternative medicine use in the United States, 1990-1997: results of a follow-up national survey. *JAMA*, 280, 1569-1575, (1998).

Elujoba AA, Ajulo OO, Iweibo GO. Chemical and biological analyses of Nigerian *Cassia* species for laxative activity. *J Pharmaceut Biomed*, 7, 1453-1457, (1989).

Eskilsson CS, Björklund E. Analytical-scale microwave-assisted extraction. *J Chromatogr A*, 902, 227-250, (2000).

Fang Q, Yeung HW, Leung HW, Huie CW. Micelle-mediated extraction and preconcentration of ginsenosides from Chinese herbal medicine. *J Chromatogr A*, 904, 47-55, (2000).

Farnsworth NR, Bunyapraphatsara N. Thai medicinal plants: Plant recommended for primary health care system, Prachachon, Bangkok, pp 90-217, (1992).

Fetrow CW, Avila JR. Professional's Handbook of Complementary and Alternative Medicines. 2nd ed. Springhouse, Pa, Springhouse Corp., (2001).

Ficker C, Smith ML, Akpagana K, Gbeassor M, Zhang J, Durst T, Assabgui R, Arnason JT. Bioassayguided isolation and identification of antifungal compounds from ginger. *Phytother Res*, 17, 897-902, (2003).

Flaster T, Lassiter J. Quality control in herbal preparations: Using botanical reference standard for proper identification. *HerbalGram*, 63, 32-37, (2004).

Foster S. Herb trades beware. *HerbalGram*, 2, 3, (1985).

Gagnier JJ, Boon H, Rochon P, Moher D, Barnes J, Bombardier C. Reporting randomized, controlled trials of herbal interventions: an elaborated CONSORT statement. *Ann Intern Med*, 144, 364-367, (2006).

Garrard J, Harms S, Eberly LE, Matiak A. Variations in product choices of frequently purchased herbs. *Arch Intern Med*, 2290-2295, (2003).

Gil MI, Ferreres F, Tomas-Barberan FA. Effect of modified atmosphere packaging on the flavonoids and vitamin C content of Minimally Processed Swiss Chard (*Beta vulgaris* Subspecies *cycla*). *J Agric Food Chem*, 46, 2007-2012, (1998).

Gil MI, Ferreres F, Tomas-Barberan F. Effect of post-harvest storage and processing on the antioxidant constituents (flavonoids and vitamin C) of fresh-cut spinach. *J Agric Food Chem*, 47, 2213-2217, (1999).

Gnanapragasam A, Ebenezar KK, Sathish V, Govindaraju P, Devaki T. Protective effect of *Centella asiatica* on antioxidant tissue defense system against adriamycin induced cardiomyopathy in rats. *Life Sci*, 76, 585, (2004).

Gnanapragasam A, Yogeeta S, Subhashini R, Ebenezar KK, Sathish V, Devaki T. Adriamycin induced myocardial failure in rats: Protective role of *Centella asiatica*. *Mol Cell Biochem*, 294, 55, (2007).

Gomes PB, Mata VG, Rodrigues AE. Production of rose geranium oil using supercritical fluid extraction. *J Supercrit Fluids*, 41, 50-60, (2007).

Gong F, Liang YZ, Cui H, Chau FT, Chau BTP. Determination of volatile components in peptic powder by gas chromatography–mass spectrometry and chemometric resolution. *J Chromatogr A*, 909, 237-247, (2001a).

Gong F, Liang YZ, Xu QS, Chau FT, Leung AKM. Gas chromatography–mass spectrometry and chemometric resolution applied to the determination of essential oils in Cortex Cinnamomi. *J Chromatogr A*, 905, 193-205, (2001b).

Gong F, Liang YZ, Xu QS, Chau FT, Ng KM. Evaluation of separation quality in two-dimensional hyphenated chromatography. *Anal Chim Acta*, 450, 99-114, (2001c).

Gopalakrishnan G. Banumathi B, Suresh G. Evaluation of the antifungal activity of natural xanthones from *Garcinia mangostana* and their synthetic derivatives. *J Nat Prod*, 60, 519-524, (1997).

Gören AC, Çýkrýkçý S, Çergel M, Bilsel G. Rapid quantitation of curcumin in turmeric via NMR and LC–tandem mass spectrometry. *Food Chem* 113, 1239-1242, (2009).

Gotoh A, Sakaeda T, Kimura T, Shirakawa T, Wada Y, Wada A, Kimachi T, Takemoto Y, Iida A, Iwakawa S, Hirai M, Tomita H, Okamura N, Nakamura T, Okumura K. Antiproliferative activity of *Rhinacanthus nasutus* (L.) Kurz extracts and the active moiety, rhinacanthin C. *Biol Pharm Bull*, 27, 1070-1074, (2004).

Govindarajan VS. Turmerics chemistry, technology and quality. *CRC Crit Rev Food Sci Nutr*, 12, 199-301, (1980).

Guo F, Liang Y, Xu C, Li X, Huang L. Analyzing of the volatile chemical constituents in Artemisia capillaris herba by GC–MS and correlative chemometric resolution methods. *J Pharm Biomed Anal*, 35, 469-478, (2004).

Hao J, Han W, Huang S, Xue B, Deng X. Microwave-assisted extraction of artemisinin from *Artemisia annua* L. *Sep Purif Technol*, 28, 191-196, (2002).

Harbourne N, Marete E, Jacquier JC, O'Riordan D. Effect of drying methods on the phenolic constituents of meadowsweet (*Filipendula ulmaria*) and willow (*Salix alba*). *LWT - Food Sci Technol*, 42, 1468-1473, (2009).

Harvey DJ. Gas chromatographic and mass spectrometric studies of ginger constituents: Identification of gingerdiones and new hexahydrocurcumin analogues. *J Chromatogr A*, 212, 75-84, (1981).

Hayen H, Karst, U. Strategies for the liquid chromatographic–mass spectrometric analysis of non-polar compounds. *J Chromatogr A*, 1000, 549-565, (2003).

Holzgrabe U. Deubner R. Schollmayer C, Waibel B. Quantitative NMR spectroscopy-applications in drug analysis, *J Pharm Biomed Anal* 38, 806-812, (2005).

Hostettmann K, Domon B, Schaufelberger D, Hostettmann M. On-line high-performance liquid chromatography: Ultraviolet-visible spectroscopy of phenolic compounds in plant extracts using post-column derivatization. *J Chromatogr A*, 283, 137-147 (1984).

Hsieh S, Huang M, Lin B, Chang H. Determination of aristolochic acid in Chinese herbal medicine by capillary electrophoresis with laser-induced fluorescence detection. *J Chromatogr A*, 1105, 127-134, (2006).

http://vm.cfsan.fda.gov/%7Edms/supplemnt.html. Cited 4 July, (2009).

http://www.cfsan.fda.gov/~lrd/fr030313.html. Cited 4 July, (2009).

Hu LF, Li SP, Cao H, Liu JJ, Gao JL, Yang FQ, Wang, YT. GC–MS fingerprint of *Pogostemon cablin* in China. *J Pharm Biomed Anal.*, 42, 200-206, (2006).

Huie CW. A review of modern sample-preparation techniques for the extraction and analysis of medicinal plants. *Anal Bioanal Chem*, 373, 23-30, (2002).

Ibrahim D, Osman H. Antimicrobial activity of *Cassia alata* from Malaysia. *J Ethnopharmacol* 45, 151-156, (1995).

Iinuma M, Tosa H, Tanaka T, Asai F, Kobayashi Y, Shimano R, Miyauchi K. Antibacterial activity of xanthones from guttiferaeous plants against methicillin-resistant *Staphylococcus aureus*. *J Pharm Pharmacol* 48, 861-865, (1996).

Inamdar PK, Yeole RD, Ghogare AB, de Souza NJ. Determination of biologically active constituents in *Centella asiatica*. *J Chromatogr A*, 742, 127-130, (1996).

Ippoushi K, Azuma K, Ito H, Horie H, Higashio H, 6-Gingerol inhibits nitric oxide synthesis in activated J774.1 mouse macrophages and prevents peroxynitriteinduced oxidation and nitration reactions. *Life Sci* 73, 3427-3437, (2003).

Jayaprakasha GK, Rao LJM, Sakariah KK. Improved HPLC method for the determination of curcumin, demethoxycurcumin, and bisdemethoxycurcumin, *J Agric Food Chem*, 50, 3668-3672, (2002).

Jayashree G, Kurup MG, Sudarslal VS, Jacob VB. Anti-oxidant activity of *Centella asiatica* on lymphomabearing mice. *Fitoterapia*, 74, 431-434, (2003).

Ji X, Avula B, Khan IA. Quantitative and qualitative determination of six xanthones in *Garcinia mangostana* L. by LC–PDA and LC–ESI-MS. *J Pharm Biomed Anal*, 43, 1270-1276, (2007).

Jia G, Lu X. Enrichment and purification of madecassoside and asiaticoside from *Centella asiatica* extracts with macroporous resins. *J Chromatogr A*, 1193, 136-141, (2008).

Jonsson JA, Mathiasson L. Membrane-based techniques for sample enrichment. *J Chromatogr A*, 902, 205-225, (2000).

Jorgensen JW, Lukacs KD. Zone electrophoresis in open-tubular glass capillaries *Anal Chem*, 53, 1298-1302, (1981).

Kaewchoothong A, Tewtrakul S, Panichayupakaranant P. HPLC Quantitative determination of anti-inflammatory active compounds in *Zingiber cassumuna* extracts. Paper presented at the 8th joint seminar NRCT-JSPS, Bangkok, Thailand, 3-4 February, (2009).

Kawai T, Kinoshita K, Koyama K, Takahashi K. Anti-emetic principles of *Magnolia obovata* Bark and *Zingiber officinale* Rhizome. *Planta Med*, 60, 17-20, (1994).

Keating A, Chez RA. Ginger syrup as an antiemetic in early pregnancy. *Altern Ther Health Med*, 8, 89-91, (2002).

Keum YS, Kim J, Lee KH, Park KK, Surh YJ, Lee JM, Lee SS, Yoon JH, Joo SY, Cha IH, Yook JI. Induction of apoptosis and caspase-3 activation by chemopreventive [6]-paradol and structurally related compounds in KB cells. *Cancer Lett*, 177, 41-47, (2002).

Kim DS, Kim DS, Oppel MN. Shogaols from *Zingiber officinale* protect IMR32 human neuroblastoma and normal human umbilical vein endothelial cells from beta-amyloid (25–35) insult. *Planta Med*, 68, 375-376, (2002a).

Kim K, Lee SY, Seo SK, Hwang BR. Park JK, *US patent* 6, 417, 349, (2002b).

Kimbaris CA. Siatis GN. Daferera JD. Tarantilis AP. Pappar SC, Polission GM. Comparison of distillation and ultrasound-assisted extraction methods for the isolation of sensitive aroma compounds from garlic (*Allium sativum*), *Ultrason Sonochem*, 13, 54-60, (2006).

Kimura Y, Sumiyoshi M, Samukawa K, Satake N, Sakanaka M. Facilitating action of asiaticoside at low doses on burn wound repair and its mechanism. *Eur J Pharmacol*, 584, 415-423, (2008).

Kligler B, Ulbricht C, Basch E, Kirkwood CD, Abrams TR. Miranda M, Khalsa KPS, Giles M, Boon H, Woods J. *Andrographis paniculata* for the treatment of upper respiratory infection: A systematic review by the natural standard research collaboration. *Explore: J Sci Heal*, 2, 25-29 (2006).

Kotnik P, Skerget M, Knez Z. Supercritical fluid extraction of chamomile flower heads: Comparison with conventional extraction, kinetics and scale-up. *J Supercrit Fluids*, 43, 192-198, (2007).

Kressmann S, Müller WE, Blume HH. Pharmaceutical quality of different *Ginkgo biloba* brands. *J Pharm Pharmacol*, 54, 661-669, (2002).

Kumar MHV, Gupta YK. Effect of different extracts of *Centella asiatica* on cognition and markers of oxidative stress in rats. *J Ethnopharmacol*, 79, 253-260, (2002).

Kumar S, Kumar D, Prakash O. Herbal supplements: Regulation and safety aspects. *Pharmacogn Mag*, 3, 65-72, (2007).

Kwak W, Cho Y, Han C, Shin HJ, Ryu KH, Yoo H, Rhee HI. Extraction and purification method of active constituents from stem of *Lonicera japonica* thunb., its usage for anti-inflammatory and analgesic drug. United States Patent 7314644, (2008).

Labadie RP. Problems and possibilities in the use of traditional drugs. *J Ethnopharmacol*, 15, 221-230, (1986).

Lansky EP, Newman RA. *Punica granatum* (pomagranate) and its potential for prevention and treatment of inflammation and cancer. *J Ethnopharmacol*, 109, 177-206, (2007).

Larrosa M, Tomas-Barberan FA, Espin JC. The dietary hydrolysable tannin punicalagin releases ellagic acid that induces apoptosis in human colon adenocarcinoma Caco-2 cells by using the mitochondrial pathway. *J Nutr Biochem*, 17: 611-625, (2006).

Lee E, Surh YJ. Induction of apoptosis in HL-60 cells by pungent vanilloids, [6]-gingerol and [6]-paradol. *Cancer Lett*, 134, 163-168, (1998).

Lee SH, Jung BH, Kim SY, Chung BC. Determination of phytoestrogens in traditional medicinal herbs using gas chromatography–mass spectrometry. *J Nutr Biochem*, 15, 452-460, (2004).

Li W, Fitzloff JF. HPLC determination of flavonoids and terpene lactones in commercial *Ginkgo biloba* products. *J Liq Chromatogr Related Technol*, 25, 2501-2514, (2002).

Liang Y, Xie P, Chan K. Quality control of herbal medicines. *J Chromatogr B*, 812, 53-70, (2004).

Lin CN, Hsieh HK, Liou SJ, Ko HH, Lin HC, Chung MI, Ko FN, Liu HW, Teng CM. Synthesis and antithrombotic effect of xanthone derivatives *J Pharm Pharmacol*, 48, 887-890, (1996).

Lin G, Li P, Li SL, Chan SW. Chromatographic analysis of *Fritillaria isosteroidal* alkaloids, the active ingredients of Beimu, the antitussive traditional Chinese medicinal herb. *J Chromatogr A*, 935, 321-338, (2001).

Ling LT, Yap S, Radhakrishnan AK. Subramaniam T, Cheng HM, Palanisamy UD. Standardised *Mangifera indica* extract is an ideal antioxidant. *Food Chem*, 113, 1154-1159, (2009).

Lu HM, Liang YZ, Chen S. Identification and quality assessment of *Houttuynia cordata* injection using GC–MS fingerprint: A standardization approach. *J Ethnopharmacol*, 105, 436-440, (2006).

Ma C, Wang W, Li B, Hua L, Xing D, Wang Y, Du L. GC-MS based comparative study of the essential oils from YL2000 ethanol decoction. *World Sci Technol*, 10, 78-82, (2008).

Mahady GB, Pendland, SL, Yun GS, Lu ZZ, Stoia A. Ginger (*Zingiber officinale* Roscoe) and the gingerols inhibit the growth of Cag A+ strains of *Helicobacter pylori*. *Anticancer Res* 23, 3699-3702, (2003).

Mahattanadul S, Nisaudah Radenahmad N, Phadoongsombut N, Thitima Chuchom T, Panichayupakaranant P, Yano S, Reanmongkol W. Effect of curcumin on reflux sophagitis in rats. *J Nat Med*, 60, 198-205, (2006a).

Mahattanadul S, Reanmongkol W, Yano S, Panichayupakaranant P, Phadoongsombut N, Tungsinmunkong K. Preventive and curative effects of curcumin on the development of gastric inflammatory diseases in rats. *J Nat Med*, 60, 191-197, (2006b).

Manojlovic NT, Solujic S, Sukdolak S. Antimicrobial activity of extract and anthraquinones from *Caloplaca schaereri*. *Lichenologist*, 34, 83-85, (2002).

Martino E, Ramaiola I, Urbano M, Bracco F, Collina S. Microwave-assisted extraction of coumarin and related compounds from *Melilotus officinalis* (L.) Pallas as an alternative to Soxhlet and ultrasound-assisted extraction. *J Chromatogr A*, 1125, 147-151, (2006).

Matsumoto K, Akao Y, Ohguchi K, Ito T, Tanaka T, Iinuma M, Nozawa Y. Xanthones induce cell-cycle arrest and apoptosis in human colon cancer DLD-1 cells. *Bioorg Med* Chem, 13, 6064-6069, (2005).

Mertens-Talcott SU, Percival SS. Ellagic acid and quercetin interact synergistically with resveratrol in the induction of apoptosis and cause transient cell cycle arrest in human leukemia cells. *Cancer Lett*, 218, 141-151, (2005).

Michaleas S, Antoniadou-Vyza, E. A new approach to quantitative NMR: Fluoroquinolones analysis by evaluating the chemical shift displacements, J of *Pharm Biomed Anal*, 42, 405-410, (2006).

Molnár-Perl I, Füzfai Z. Chromatographic, capillary electrophoretic and capillary electrochromatographic techniques in the analysis of flavonoids. *J Chromatogr A*, 1073, 201-227, (2005).

Moongkarndi P, Kosem N, Kaslungka S, Luanratana, O, Pongpan N, Neungton N. Antiproliferation, antioxidation and induction of apoptosis by *Garcinia mangostana* (mangosteen) on SKBR3 human breast cancer cell line. *J Ethnopharmacol*, 90, 161-166, (2004).

Morrow JD. Why the United States still needs improved dietary supplement regulation and oversight. *Clin Pharmacol Ther*, 83, 391-393, (2008).

Müller K, Daus B, Mattusch J, Stärk H, Wennrich R. Simultaneous determination of inorganic and organic antimony species by using anion exchange phases for HPLC–ICP-MS and their application to plant extracts of *Pteris vittata*. Talanta, 78, 820-826, (2009).

Nakatani K, Atsumi M, Arakawa T, Oosawa K, Shimura S, Nakahata N, Ohizumi Y. Inhibitions of Histamine Release and Prostaglandin E_2 Synthesis by Mangosteen, a Thai Medicinal Plant. *Biol Pharm Bull*, 25, 1137-1141, (2002).

Negi PS, Jayaprakasha GK, Jena BS. Antioxidant and antimutagenic activities of pomegranate peel extracts. *Food Chem*, 80, 393-397, (2003).

Nurtjahja-Tjendraputra E, Ammit AJ, Roufogalis BD, Tran VH, Duke CC, Effective anti-platelet and COX-1 enzyme inhibitors from pungent constituents of ginger. *Thromb Res*, 111, 259-265, (2003).

Ogawa Y, Kanatsu K, Iino T, Kato S, Jeong Y, Shibata N, Takada K, Takeuchi K. Protection against dextran sulfate sodium-induced colitis by microspheres of ellagic acid in rats. *Life Sci* 71, 827-839, (2002).

Ohtake N, Nakai Y, Yamamoto M, Sakakibara I, Takeda S, Amagaya S, Aburada M. Separation and isolation methods for analysis of the active principles of Sho-saiko-to (SST) oriental medicine. *J Chromatogr B*, 812, 135-148, (2004).

Oleszek W, Bialy Z. Chromatographic determination of plant saponins - An update (2002-2005). *J Chromatogr A*, 1112, 78-91, (2006).

Ong ES. Extraction methods and chemical standardization of botanicals and herbal preparations. *J Chromatogr B,* 812, 23-33, (2004).

Ong ES. Chemical assay of glycyrrhizin in medicinal plants by pressurized liquid extraction (PLE) with capillary zone electrophoresis (CZE). *J Sep Sci*, 25, 825-831, (2002).

Osowski S, Rostock M, Bartsch HH, Massing U. Pharmaceutical comparability of different therapeutic Echinacea preperations. *Res Compl Nat Classical Med*, 7, 294-300, (2000).

Oyedeji OA, Afolayan AJ. Chemical composition and antibacterial activity of the essential oil of *Centella asiatica* growing in South Africa. *Pharm Biol*, 43, 249-252, (2005).

Pan XJ, Liu H, Jia G, Shu YY. Microwave-assisted extraction of glycyrrhizic acid from licorice root. *Biochem En. J*, 5, 173-177, (2000).

Pan XJ, Niu GG, Liu H. Comparison of microwave-assisted extraction and conventional extraction techniques for the extraction of tanshinones from *Salvia miltiorrhiza* bunge. *Biochem Eng J*, 12, 71-77, (2002).

Pan X, Niu G, Liu H. Microwave-assisted extraction of tanshinones from *Salvia miltiorrhiza* bunge with analysis by high-performance liquid chromatography. *J Chromatogr A,* 922, 371-375, (2001).

Panichayupakaranant P, Charoonratana T. and Sirikatitham, A. RP-HPLC analysis of rhinacanthins in *Rhinacanthus nasutus*: validation and application to preparation of rhinacanthin high-yielding extract. *J Chromatogr Sci*, 47, 705-708, (2009b).

Panichayupakaranant P, Chatkrapunt U, Supavita T. Pharmacognostic and chemical studies on the leaves of *Rhinacanthus nasutus*. *Nigerian J Nat Prod Med*, 10, 1-5, (2006).

Panichayupakaranant P, Intaraksa N. Distribution of hydroxyanthracene derivatives in *Cassia alata* and the factors affecting the quality of the raw material. *Songklanakarin J Sci Technol*, 25, 497-502, (2003).

Panichayupakaranant P, Issuriya A, Sirikatitham A and Wang W. Antioxidant assay-guided purification and liquid chromatographic determination of ellagic acid in pomegranate peel. *J Chromatogr Sci*, in press, (2010b).

Panichayupakaranant P, Issuriya A, Sirikatitham A. Preparation method and stability of ellagic acid rich pomegranate fruit peel extract. *Pharm Biol*, 48, 201-205 (2010a).

Panichayupakaranant P, Sakunpak A, Sakunphueak A. Quantitative HPLC determination and extraction of anthraquinones in *Senna alata* leaves. *J Chromatogr Sci*, 47, 197-200 (2009a).

Pasquale R, Rapisarda A, Germanò MP, Ragusa S, Kirjavainen S, Galati EM. Effects of cadmium on growth and pharmacologically active constituents of the medicinal plant *Coriandrum sativum* L. *Water Air Soil Pollut*, 84, 147-157, (1995).

Perakis C, Louli V, Magoulas K. Supercritical fluid extraction of black pepper oil. *J Food Eng*, 71, 386-393, (2005).

Péret-Almeida L. Cherubino APF. Alves RJ. Dufossé L, Glória BAM. Separation and determination of the physico-chemical characteristics of curcumin, demethoxycurcumin and bisdemetho-xycurcumin, *Food Res Int* 38, 1039-1044, (2005).

Perharic L, Shaw D. Colbridge M, House I, Leon C, Murray V. Toxicological problems resulting from exposure to traditional remedies and food supplements. *Drug Saf*, 11, 284-294, (1994).

Pitipanapong J, Chitprasert S, Goto M, Jiratchariyakul W, Sasaki M, Shotipruk A. New approach for extraction of charantin from Momordica charantia with pressurized liquid extraction. *Sep Purif Technol*, 52, 416-422, (2007).

Proestos C, Komaitis M. Application of microwave-assisted extraction to the fast extraction of plant phenolic compounds. *LWT-Food Sci Technol*, 41, 652-659, (2008).

Rajtar G, Zolkowska D, Kleinrok Z. Marona H. Antiplatelets activity of some xanthone derivatives. *Acta Pol Pharm*, 56, 319-324, (1999).

Ramos L. Kristenson EM. Th. Brinkman UA. Current use of pressurised liquid extraction and subcritical water extraction in environmental analysis. *J Chromatogr A*, 975, 3-29, (2002).

Randriamampionona D, Diallo B, Rakotoniriana F, Rabemanantsoa C, Cheuk K, Corbisier A, Mahillon J, Ratsimamanga S, Jaziri ME. Comparative analysis of active constituents in *Centella asiatica* samples from Madagascar: Application for ex situ conservation and clonal propagation. *Fitoterapia*, 78, 482-489, (2007).

Raskin I, R.bnicky DM, Komarnytsky S, Ilic N, Poulev A, Borisjuk N, Brinker A, Moreno DA, Ripoll C, Yakoby N, O'Neal JM, Cornwell T, Pastor I, Fridlender B. Plant and human health in the twenty-first century. *Trends Biotechnol*, 20, 522-531, (2002).

Rates SMK. Plants as source of drugs. *Toxicon*, 39, 603-613, (2001).

Raynie DE. Modern extraction techniques. *Anal Chem*, 76, 4659-4664, (2004).

Rogerio AP, Fontanari C, Borducchi E, Keller AC, Russo M, Soares EG, Albuquerque DA, Faccioli LH. Anti-inflammatory effects of *Lafoensia pacari* and ellagic acid in a murine model of asthma. *Eur J Pharmacol*, 580, 262-270, (2008).

Ruan G, Li G. The study on the chromatographic fingerprint of *Fructus xanthii* by microwave assisted extraction coupled with GC–MS. *J Chromatogr B*, 850, 241-248, (2007).

Sakunpak A, Sirikatitham A, Panichayupakaranant P. Preparation of anthraquinone high-yielding *Senna alata* extract and its stability. *Pharm Biol*, 47, 236-241, (2009).

Sakunphueak A, Panichayupakaranant p. Effects of donor plants and plant growth regulators on naphthoquinone production in root cultures of *Impatiens balsamina. Plant Cell Tissue Organ Cult*, in press, (2010).

Schwertner HA, Rios DC. High-performance liquid chromatographic analysis of 6-gingerol, 8-gingerol, 10-gingerol, and 6-shogaol in ginger-containing dietary supplements, spices, teas, and beverages. *J Chromatogr B*, 856, 41-47, (2007).

Seeram NP, Lee R, Heber D. Bioavailability of ellagic acid in human plasma after consumption of ellagitannins from pomegranate (*Punica granatum* L.) juice. *Clin Chim Acta*, 348, 63-68, (2004).

Sendl A, Chen JL, Jolad SD, Stoddart C, Rozhon E, Kernan M. Two new naphthoquinones with antiviral activity from *Rhinacanthus nasutus. J Nat Prod*, 59, 808-811, (1996).

Shen S, Sha Y, Deng C, Zhang X, Fu D, Chen J. Quality assessment of *Flos Chrysanthemi Indici* from different growing areas in China by solid-phase microextraction-gas chromatography-mass spectrometry. *J Chromatogr A*, 1047, 281-287, (2004).

Shukla A, Rasik AM, Jain GK, Shankar R, Kulshrestha DK, Dhawan BN. In vitro and in vivo wound healing activity of asiaticoside isolated from Centella asiatica. *J Ethnopharmacol*, 65, 1-11, (1999).

Simon A, Allais DP, Duroux JL, Basly JP, Durand-Fontanier S, Delage C. Inhibitory effect of curcuminoidss on MCF-7 cell proliferation and structure-activity relationship. *Cancer Lett*, 129, 111-116, (1998).

Smith EA. Nutraceuticals market is $86 billion, say experts. *Drug Topics Archive*, June 15, (1998).

Smith RM, Sadaquat A. Anthraquinones from the leaves of *Cassia alata* from Fiji. *NZJ Sci* 22, 123-126, (1979).

Sovova H, Opletal L, Bartlova M, Sajfrtova M, Krenkova M. Supercritical fluid extraction of lignans and cinnamic acid from *Schisandra chinensis. J Supercrit Fluids*, 42, 88-95, (2007).

Spigno G, de Faveri DM. Microwave-assisted extraction of tea phenols: A phenomenological study. *J Food Eng*, 93, 210-217, (2009).

Srimal RC. Turmeric: a brief review of medicinal properties. *Fitoterapia*, 68, 483-493, (1997).

Srivastava KC. Isolation and effects of some ginger components of platelet aggregation and eicosanoid biosynthesis. *Prostaglandins Leukot Med* 25, 187-198, (1986).

Stashenko EE, Jaramillo BE, Mart´ýnez JR. Analysis of volatile secondary metabolites from Colombian *Xylopia aromatica* (Lamarck) by different extraction and headspace methods and gas chromatography. *J Chromatogr A*, 1025 105-113, (2004).

Statti GA, Tundis S, Sacchetti G, Muzzoli M, Bianchi A, Menichini F. Variability in the content of active constituents and biological activity of *Glycyrrhiza glabra. Fitoterapia*, 75, 371-374, (2004).

Subcommittee on the Establishment of the Thai Herbal Pharmacopoeia. Thai Herbal Pharmacopeia, Prachachon, Bangkok, pp 38-44, (1998).

Suguna L, Sivakumar P, Chandrakasan G. Effects of *Centella asiatica* extract on dermal wound healing in rats. *Indian J Exp Biol*, 34, 1208-1211, (1996).

Sun M, Temelli F. Supercritical carbon dioxide extraction of carotenoids from carrot using canola oil as a continuous co-solvent. *J Supercrit Fluids*, 37, 397-408, (2006).

Sun X, Gao C, Cao W, Yang X, Wang E. Capillary electrophoresis with amperometric detection of curcumin in Chinese herbal medicine pretreated by solid-phase extraction. *J Chromatogr A*, 962, 117-125, (2002).

Surveswaran S, Cai Y, Corke H, Sun M. Systematic evaluation of natural antioxidants from 133 Indian medicinal plants. *Food Chem*, 102, 938-953, (2007).

Tan X, Li Q, Chen X, Wang Z, Shi Z, Bi K, Jia Y. Simultaneous determination of 13 bioactive compounds in Herba *Artemisiae Scopariae* (Yin Chen) from different harvest seasons by HPLC–DAD. *J Pharm Biomed Anal*, 47, 847-853, (2008).

Teng L, Shaw D, Barnes J. Practice of traditional Chinese herbal medicine shops in central London. *Phytochem Lett*, 1, 94-98, (2008).

Tong WY, Fu XY, Lee SM, Yu J, Liu JW, Wei DZ, Koo YM. Purification of L(+)-lactic acid from fermentation broth with paper sludge as a cellulosic feedstock using weak anion exchanger Amberlite IRA-92. *Biochem Eng J*, 18, 89-96, (2004).

Turk G, Ate°°ahin, A., Sonmez M, Çeriba°i AO, Yuce A. Improvement of cisplatin-induced injuries to sperm quality, the oxidant-antioxidant system, and the histologic structure of the rat testis by ellagic acid. *Fertil Steril*, 89, 1474-1481, (2008).

Tyler VE. Phytomedicines: Back to the Future. *J Nat Prod*, 62, 1589-1592, (1999).

Tyler VE, Brady LR, Robbers JE. Pharmacognosy, 9th ed. Philadelphia, PA: Lea and Febiger, (1988).

US department of Health Human Services Food and Drug Administration Center for Drug Evaluation and Research. Guidance for industry botanical drug products. http://www.fda.gov/cder/guidance/1221dft.htm#P131_3293, Cited 1 July, (2009).

Uekusa K, Ono T, Hayashida M, Nihira M, Ohno Y. GC/MS analysis of an herbal dietary supplement containing ephedrine. *Legal Medicine*, 11, S573-S575, (2009).

Valentao P, Andrade PB, Areias F, Ferreres F, Seabra, RM. Analysis of vervain flavonoids by HPLC/diode-array detector. It application to quality control. *J Agric Food Chem.* 47, 4579-4582, (1999).

Valli G, Giardina EV. Benefits, adverse effects and drug interactions of herbal therapies with cardiovascular effects. *JACC*, 39, 1083-1095, (2002).

Van der Kooy F, Verpoorte R, Marion Meyer JJ. Metabolomic quality control of claimed antimalarial *Artemisia afra* herbal remedy and *A. afra* and *A. annua* plant extracts. *S Afr J Bot*, 74, 186-189, (2008).

Verhagen H, Aruoma OI, van Delft JHM, Dragsted LO, Ferguson LR, Knasmuller S, Pool-Zobel BL, Poulsen HE, Williamson G, Yannai S. The 10 basic requirements for a scientific paper reporting antioxidant, antimutagenic or anticarcinogenic potential of test substances in *in vtro* experiments and animal studies *in vivo*. *Food Chem Toxicol*, 41, 603-610, (2003).

Vinatoru M. An overview of the ultrasonically assisted extraction of bioactive principles from herbs. *Ultrason Sonochem*, 8, 303-313, (2001).

Vutyavanich T, Kraisarin T, Ruangsri RA. Ginger for nausea and vomiting in pregnancy: Randomized, double-masked, placebo-controlled trial. *Obstet Gynecol*, 97, 577-582, (2001).

Wagner H. Bladt S, Rickl V. Plant Drug Analysis: A Thin Layer Chromatography Atlas, second ed., Springer-Verlag, New York, (1996).

Wang X, He Y, Qian L. Determination of polyphenol components in herbal medicines by micellar electrokinetic capillary chromatography with Tween 20. *Talanta*, 74, 1-6, (2007).

Wang Y, Yue S, Li D, Jin M, Li C. Kinetics and mechanism of Y(III) extraction with CA-100 using a constant interfacial cell with larminar flow. *Solvent Extr Ion Exc*, 20, 345-358, (2002).

Wang Z, Ashraf-Khorassani M, Taylor LT. On-line coupling of supercritical CO_2 extraction with reversed-phase liquid chromatography for the quantitative analysis of analytes in aqueous matrices. *J Chromatogr* A, 1033, 221-227, (2004).

Welsh WJ, Lin WK, Tersigni SH, Collantes E, Duta R, Carey MS, Zielinski WL, Brower J, Spencer

JA, Layloff TP. Pharmaceutical fingerprinting: Evaluation of neural networks and chemometric techniques for distinguishing among same-product manufacturers. *Anal. Chem.* 68, 3473-3482, (1996).

Willetts KE, Ekangaki A, Eden JA. Effect of a ginger extract on pregnancy-induced nausea: A randomised controlled trial. *Aust N Z J Obstet Gynaecol*, 43, 139-144, (2003).

Williams DH, Stone MJ, Hauck PR, Rahman SK. Why are secondary metabolites (natural products) biosynthesized? *J Nat Prod*, 52, 1189-1208, (1989).

Williams P, Ongsakul M, Proudfoot J, Croft K, Beilin L. Mangostin inhibits the oxidative modification of human low density lipoprotein. *Free Radic Res* 23, 175-184, (1995).

Williamson E, Okpako DT and Evans FJ. Selection, preparation and pharmacological evaluation of plant material, Wiley, Chichester, (1996).

Wills RBH, Bone K, Morgan M. Herbal products: active constituents, mode of action and quality control. *Nutr Res Rev*, 13, 47-77, (2000).

Wills RBH, Stuart DL. Alkylamide and cichoric acid levels in *Echinacea purpurea* grown in Australia. *Food Chem*, 67, 385-388, (1999b).

Wills RBH, Stuart DL. Generation of high quality Australian *Echinacea purpurea* products. Kingston ACT, Australia: Rural Industries Research and Development Corporation, (1999a).

Wills RBH., Stuart DL. Level of active constituents in manufactured echinacea products. *Chem Aust*, 9, 17-19, (1998).

Wirth JH, Hudgins JC, Paice JA. Use of herbal therapies to relieve pain: A review of efficacy and adverse effects. *Pain Manage Nurs*, 6, 145-167, (2005).

Wolsko PM, Solondz DK, Phillips RS, Schachter SC, Eisenberg DM. Lack of herbal supplement characterization in published randomized controlled trials. *Am J Med*, 118, 1087-1093, (2005).

Wood J, A Bernards MA, Wan W, Charpentier PA. Extraction of ginsenosides from North American ginseng using modified supercritical carbon dioxide. *J Supercrit Fluids*, 39, 40-47, (2006).

World Health Organization. WHO guidelines for assessing quality of herbal medicines with reference to contaminants and residues. World Health Organization, Spain, 1-22, (2007a).

World Health Organization. WHO guidelines on developing consumer information on proper use of traditional, complementary and alternative medicine. World Health Organization, Italy, 1-6, (2004).

World Health Organization. WHO Guidelines on good manufacturing Practices (GMP) for Herbal Medicines. World Health Organization, France, 1-72, (2007b).

Wu TS, Hsu HC, Wu, PL, Teng CM, Wu CY. Rhinacanthin Q, A naphthoquinone from *Rhinacanthus nasutus* and its biological activity. *Phytochemistry*, 40, 2001-2003, (1998).

Wybraniec, S. Effect of tetraalkylammonium salts on retention of betacyanins and decarboxylated betacyanins in ion-pair reversed-phase high-performance liquid chromatography. *J Chromatogr A*, 1127, 70-75, (2006).

Xie Y, Jiang ZH, Zhou H, Xu HX, Liu L. Simultaneous determination of six Aconitum alkaloids in proprietary Chinese medicines by high-performance liquid chromatography. *J Chromatogr A*, 1093, 195-203, (2005).

Xie Y, Jiang Z, Zhou H, Cai X, Wong Y, Liu Z, Bian Z, Xu H, Liu L. Combinative method using HPLC quantitative and qualitative analyses for quality consistency assessment of a herbal medicinal preparation. *J Pharm Biomed Anal*, 43, 204-212, (2007).

Xu L, Basheer C, Lee HK. Developments in single-drop microextraction. *J Chromatogr A*, 1152, 184-192, (2007).

Xu RN, Fan L, Rieser MJ, El-Shourbagy TA. Recent advances in high-throughput quantitative bioanalysis by LC–MS/MS. *J Pharm Biomed Anal*, 44, 342-355, (2007).

Yang LW, Wu DH, Tang X, Pang W, Wang XR, Ma Y, Su WW. Fingerprint quality control of Tianjihuang by high-performance liquid chromatography-photodiode array detection. *J Chromatogr A*, 1070, 35-42, (2005).

Yoshikawa M, Hatakeyama S, Chatani N, Nishino Y, Yamahara J. Qualitative and quantitative analysis of bioactive principles in *Zingiberis Rhizoma* by means of high performance liquid chromatography and gas liquid chromatography. On the evaluation of Zingiberis Rhizoma and chemical change of constituents during *Zingiberis Rhizoma* processing. *Yakugaku Zasshi*, 113, 307-315, (1993).

Zaidan MRS, Noor Rain A, Badrul AR, Adlin A, Norazah, A., Zakiah, I. *In vitro* screening of five local medicinal plants for antibacterial activity using disc diffusion method. *Trop Biomed*, 22, 165–170, (2005).

Zainol NA, Voo SC, Sarmidi MR, Aziz RA. Profiling of *Centella asiatica* (L.) Urban extract. *Malay J Anal Sci*, 12, 322-327, (2008).

Zambuchini B, Fiorini D, Verdenelli MC, Orpianesi C, Ballini R. Inhibition of microbiological activity during sole (*Solea solea* L.) chilled storage by applying ellagic and ascorbic acids. *LWT - Food Sci Technol*, 41, 1733-1738, (2008).

Zheng CJ, Qin LP. Chemical components of *Centella asiatica* and their bioactivities. *J Chin Integr Med* 5, 348-351, (2007).

Zhou B, Wu Z, Li X, Zhang J, Hu X. Analysis of ellagic acid in pomegranate rinds by capillary electrophoresis and high-performance liquid chromatography. *Phytochem Anal*, 19, 86-89, (2008).

Zhou H, Liu C. Microwave-assisted extraction of solanesol from tobacco leaves. *J Chromatogr A*, 129,135-139, (2006).

Zhou X, Sun J, Zhu D, Yuan B, You T. Quality analysis of herbal medicine products prepared from herba sarcandrae by capillary electrophoresis with electrochemical detection. *Chem Res Chin Univ*, 24, 148-153, (2008).

Zhu J, Yu K, Chen X, Hu Z. Comparison of two sample preconcentration strategies for the sensitivity enhancement of flavonoids found in Chinese herbal medicine in micellar electrokinetic chromatography with UV detection. *J Chromatogr A*, 116, 191-200, (2007).

Zundorf I, Dingermann T. Quality evolution: evolution of the quality of phytopharmaceuticals, *Dtsch Apoth Ztg*, 137, 61-62, (1997).

Zygmunt BJ. Namiesnik, J. Preparation of samples of plant material for chromatographic analysis. *Chromatogr Sci*, 41, 109-116, (2003).

chapter 26

Toxicity Problems Associated with Herbs

R. A. Dickson, K. Annan and A. Y. Mensah

INTRODUCTION

Human survival has always depended on plants. The natural world once served as the source of all medicinal agents, with higher plants constituting by far the principal source (Farnsworth, 1986). The use of the medicinal herbs for curing disease has been documented in history of all civilizations. Man in the pre-historic era was probably not aware about some of the health hazards that may be encountered during therapy. With the onset of research into medicinal plants, it has been noted that plants contain active principles, which are responsible, for the curative action of the herbs. Some of these principles commonly referred to as secondary metabolites present in plants may be toxic. With introduction of scientific procedures researchers all over the globe have been able to understand about toxic principles present in the green flora.

The success rate of discovering new drugs from natural sources especially from medicinal plants may be based on the implementation of strategies which invariably explore and exploit the untapped potential of these plants. If the potential of herbs as sources of medicinal entities can be maximized and tapped effectively, the problem of toxicity would have to be critically addressed.

The use of herbs has regularly been under much scrutiny due to the toxicity of some of the plants used. In the orthodox world, it is normal practice for the mention of the use of medicinal herbs to be greeted with an almost automatic reference to toxicity related challenges. One key area is issues bothering especially on hepatotoxicity (Brinker, 1983). More often than not, a frequently quoted excuse for dismissing the use of herbs has to do with the problem of toxicity.

It must however be stated clearly that the problem of toxicity and for that matter adverse drug reactions is also common in the orthodox world. Approximately 8% of all hospital admissions in the US. are due to adverse reactions to synthetic drugs. At least 100,000 people a year die from them. That means at least three times as many people are killed in the US. by pharmaceutical drugs as are killed by drunken drivers. Thousands die each year from supposedly safe over-the-counter remedies. Deaths or hospitalizations due to herbs are so rare that they may be hard to find (Treaure, 1995).

Similar figures apply in the UK. In the area of hepatoxicity, where perhaps the strongest case against some herbs lies, the statistics are horrendously clear-over 80% of cases of hepatic failures presenting for liver transplant or which sometimes result in death are due to poisoning by freely available OTC non-prescription NSAIDs, such as paracetamol and aspirin. Interestingly enough not one case was due to ingestion of medicinal herbs (Treasure, 1995).

It is interesting to note that a more general and predominant view has been that herbs are relatively safer due to the fact that it is obtained from natural sources. However, neither of these extreme schools of thought can be viewed as very realistic. A more realistic and acceptable scientific viewpoint may have to be that any substance ingested in excess is potentially harmful. This general principle would include all plant materials and their products over the years. The use of herbs have frequently been promoted as a 'safer' alternative to certain allopathic drugs. This purported view led to the furtherance of herbal medicine in the nineteenth century. The question to ask however is what the situation is today regarding the issue of toxicity. The very fact that herbalists are provided with maximum recommended doses for every herb in the British Herbal Pharmacopoeia acknowledges the fact that herbs cannot be the harmless plants that some people assume them to be. Nor are they all highly dangerous agents, as some schools of thought seem to presume. They are prescribed with the same detailed consideration with respect to biochemical composition and dosage as any drug.

WHO estimates that as much as 80% of the people in developing countries rely on traditional medicine to meet their healthcare needs (WHO, 2007). Since the main components of these traditional treatments more or less are plant based, it presupposes that issues pertaining to their toxicity must be taken seriously. All toxicity claims have to be examined in a balanced and scientific manner irrespective of whether it is herbal or synthetic based.

Definition of Toxicity

The Oxford Advanced Learner's Dictionary defines toxicity as the quality of being poisonous; the extent to which something is poisonous. The definition of the term toxicity or toxic is ultimately a matter of viewpoint. Many ordinary foods contain constituents that could be regarded as poisonous. These may include cyanogenic glycosides in many fruit seeds and cassava, the isothiocyanates found in some vegetables such as the mustards and lectin-containing soya and kidney beans. Nonetheless these foods are generally regarded as safe and consumed without taking any precautionary measures.

Similarly, both water and oxygen, seemingly harmless, can kill in excessive amounts, so quantity is often an important consideration when it comes to the use of these terms. Reports have appeared in medical journals regarding the toxicity and harmful side effects of some herbal preparations. The first point to note is that virtually all the cases documented relate to herbal products purchased over-the-counter, and not to herbal medications prescribed by accredited a practitioners.

The Source of the Problem

With the ever-increasing use of herbal medicines and the global expansion of the herbal medicines market, safety has become a major concern for both health authorities and the public worldwide.

Limited toxicological data are available on medicinal plants. However potential hepatotoxicity associated with herbal medicines has been discussed for some time (Chitturi and Farrell, 2000; Pittler and Ernst, 2003). Hepatotoxicity has been reported with a number of herbal medicines including Black Cohosh, Comfrey, Ephedra and Kava. *Teucrium* species have also been implicated in hepatotoxicity (Ernst, 2003).

Research into problems with the toxicity of herbal medicines reveals four main potential causes:

I) Herbal material that has been adulterated with toxic non-plant materials, e.g. lead

II) Herbal material that has been adulterated with other plants

III) Plant species of proven toxicity

IV) Interactions between the herbal medicines and orthodox drugs or other substances

I) Herbal material that has been adulterated with toxic nonplant materials, e.g. lead

It is well known that there are many contaminants and residues that may cause toxicity problems in consumers of herbal medicines. Many are natural toxic metals or bacteria. Some arise from past or present use of agents or materials that pollute the environment and subsequently medicinal plants, such as emissions from factories or the residues of certain pesticides. The contamination of herbal medicines with heavy metals/toxic elements continues to be a major international problem (WHO, 2007). A comprehensive review in 1992 summarized test results on products and case histories of patients who had experienced toxic effects as a result of the presence of heavy metals in herbal preparations (US-FDA, 2004). Similar findings continue to be reported and the potential impact on public health is significant (De Smet, 2005). In most cases involving synthetic drugs, these are undeclared in the product and only come to light when the user experiences adverse effects which are sufficiently serious to warrant medical intervention. Exposure to the undeclared drug is revealed in the subsequent investigation of clinical cases. Of particular concern is the deliberate addition of closely related derivatives of pharmaceutical drugs, for example the use of nitrosofenfluramine instead of fenfluramine in weight-loss products (De Smet, 2005).

The situation with the heavy metals/toxic elements in herbal products differs in that whilst these ingredients may arise from the plant ingredients themselves or be introduced as trace contaminants during processing, they are also frequently added intentionally and declared as ingredients within some Traditional Chinese Medicine (TCM) and Asian medicine formulations. The Chinese Pharmacopoeia, for example, includes monographs for realgar (arsenic disulfide), calomel (mercurous chloride), cinnabaris (mercuric sulfide) and hydrargyri oxydum rubrum (red mercuric oxide), and includes formulations for nearly 50 products that include one or more of these substances (Chinese Pharmacopoeia, 2005).

Recent research has also demonstrated that herbs may absorb heavy metals during growth. For these reasons, there is currently a potential global danger to the health and well-being of people where these practices are encouraged. This risk can be reduced by ensuring that herbal medicines with harmful contaminants and residues do not reach the public, by assessing the quality of the medicinal plants, herbal materials and finished herbal products before they reach the market.

In all situations, the acceptable daily intake (ADI) of a toxic chemical, heavy metal or element estimated as the maximum amount of an agent, expressed on a body mass basis, to which an individual in a population may be exposed daily over his or her lifetime without appreciable health risk has to be critically investigated during quality control assessment of herbal medicines (WHO, 2007).

II) Herbal material that has been adulterated with other plant

Cases of serious cardiac arrhythmias were reported in the USA in 1997 following the accidental substitution of plantain with *Digitalis lanata* (Slifman, 1998). Subsequent investigation revealed that large quantities of the contaminated plantain had been shipped to more than 150 manufacturers, distributors and retailers over a two-year period (Slifman, 1998).

Fourteen cases of *podophyllum* poisoning have been reported from Hong Kong following the inadvertent use of the roots *Podophyllum hex-*

andrum instead of *Gentiana* and *Clematis* species. It is reported that this accidental substitution arose because of the apparent similarity in morphology of the roots (But *et al.*, 1996).

Cases of cardiotoxicity resulting from the ingestion of *Aconitum* species used in TCM have been reported from Hong Kong (Tai *et al.*, 1992). In TCM, *Aconitum* rootstocks are processed by soaking or boiling them in water in order to hydrolyse the aconite alkaloids into their less toxic aconine derivatives. Toxicity can, however, result when such processes are uncontrolled and unvalidated. In the UK, the internal use of aconite is restricted to prescription only.

The dangers of confusing Chinese (*Illicium verum* Hook.f.) and Japanese star anise (*Illicium anisatum* L.), have been known for many years as the dried fruits cannot be distinguished through visual examination. Japanese star anise is similar to the Chinese variety but has been reported to cause neurologic and gastrointestinal toxicities due to the presence of anisatin (Read, 1926; Biessels *et al.*, 2002).

III) Classification of plant species of proven toxicity

The classification of plants in terms of a hierarchy of toxicity is usually complicated. To simplify this, three working definitions may be set up, making a distinction among the following:

I) Herbs that are known to contain highly poisonous substances, and are therefore toxic when ingested even in very small amounts. Their use as medicines is strictly controlled e.g., *Atropa belladonna* (Deadly nightshade) of family Solanaceae

II) Herbs that contain high amounts of chemical groups known to be toxic if ingested in large amounts. A maximum recommended dose reflects this e.g., *Symphytum officinale* (comfrey) of family Boraginaceae.

III) Herbs that are non-toxic even when ingested in large amounts, but in isolated cases may cause hypersensitivity reactions e.g., *Althaea officinalis* (marshmallow) of family Malvaceae.

IV) Interactions between the herbal medicines and orthodox drugs or other substances

Interactions occurring between prescribed or over the counter and herbal medicines exist. A systematic review conducted in 2001 of published herb-drug interactions found evidence of interactions involving widely used herbs with prescribed drugs such as warfarin and garlic, St John's Wort and oral contraceptives (Izzo and Ernst, 2001). More research has to be be encouraged in this area.

Idiosyncrasies and Safeguards

It is a scientific fact that, within any given population, each individual will show genetic variation. For example an individual may react adversely to the intake of onions which does not seem to affect a lot of people who consume the same onions. That does not mean that the rest of the population should be advised not to eat onions, but rather that the individual concerned is sensitive to a chemical compound in the vegetable, and should therefore be advised to avoid eating it. Similarly, some individuals are allergic to certain detergents and a host of other substances. Once again, these do not become the subject of a widespread ban, but simply represent a problem for those who are especially sensitive to one of the chemicals present.

The way in which we react to such problems recognizes that, with reasonable precautions, these substances can be freely handled by most of the population without serious risk to health. The same type of logic is applied to conventional pharmaceutical preparations. Most of the population will not show an adverse reaction, but in some cases commonly prescribed drugs (such as penicillin) may cause serious problems. The level of acceptance of side effects is set by the statistical results of clinical trials. Once a drug has satisfied these criteria, it is deemed safe when prescribed at the recommended dosage level. It does not mean that nobody will be harmed by it. The story should not be any different when it comes to herbal medicines.

In as much as herbs prescribed by a qualified medical herbalist may be safe; most do not come supported by data from countless clinical trials, but they do come with a long history of highly successful use. Much of modern orthodoxy only recognizes its own measurements of clinical efficacy, such as double-blind trials. There is very little data available for herbs, since medical researchers are very reluctant to include herbs on clinical trials without prior proof of efficacy or at least evidence of safety. Both the latter factors would be brought up in the initial considerations of an ethics committee, and long-standing historical use of a herb counts for very little indeed. Thus, herbal research at the clinical trial level is generally blocked. If full-scale clinical trials of herbs were routinely allowed, it would soon be concluded that most of the species implicated in questions of toxicity are in fact quite safe when used at the recommended dosage levels. Trials would also reveal the true efficacy of herbal medications. It is hardly a good scientific practice to deliberately seek out isolated examples of toxic herbs, and use these reports to call the whole practice of using herbs as unreliable.

It is a fact that, in Britain, paracetamol is the cause of 100-150 deaths annually. It is also the direct cause of 30,000-40,000 referrals to hospital each year (Editorial, Pharmaceutical Journal, 1997). However, the highlighting of only the negative aspects of such a drug would be fairly criticized by the scientific community as being unbalanced because, when used safely, paracetamol is a very effective drug. The same logic should be applied to the use of herbs, but sadly it is not. There is much prejudice against the use of herbs in clinical practice, most of which is based on ignorance. Most of the adverse reactions to herbs recorded in case histories may be considered to be simply hypersensitivity reactions, which will occur from time to time as is the case in orthodox practice.

Few herbalists would disagree that there should be tight controls on the use and sale of herbs. Over-the-counter remedies should always specify the amount of active principle present and maximum dosages. Generally speaking, however, the protection against overdosing is automatic because, for most products, the amount of constituent present is relatively low. This relates to the form that the herb is in *i.e.* the dried herb, rather than other dosage forms.

Types of herbs from a safety point of view

In practice, three groups of herbs can be identified from a safety point of view (Slifman, 1998; But, 1996; Tai, 1992). There are a handful of herbs that contain near pharmaceutical concentrations of poisonous constituents which should on no account be taken internally by unqualified persons except in homeopathic potencies. Examples are *Atropa belladonna, Arnica spp, Aconitum spp, Digitalis spp*. In many countries availability of these herbs is limited by law.

The second group consists of herbs with powerful actions example plants causing nausea or vomiting. They are perfectly safe used under appropriate conditions. Some of these herbs are restricted in some countries but freely available in others. *Lobelia and Eonymus spp* are examples. There is some inconsistency here, for example Ephedra is restricted, perhaps with justification, in the UK, but is freely available in the US.

Finally, there is an idiosyncratic grouping of herbs which have been alleged, with some scientific support, to exhibit specific kinds of toxicity. The best known is the hepatotoxicity of pyrrolizidine-alkaloid-containing plants such as Comfrey (Symphytum). Other examples are Dryopteris (Male Fern), Viscum (Mistletoe) and Corynanthe (Yohimbe).

DISCUSSIONS AND CONCLUSION

The use of herbal medicinal products continues to increase and there is growing evidence that herbal medicines are used widely by all groups of society including children, pregnant and breast-feeding mothers, women, especially during the menopause, and the elderly. Over the last few years the significance of herb–drug interactions has been recognized and with this the realization that healthcare professionals need to be aware that patients do take herbal medicinal products, and need to understand their effects and appreciate their contribution in attaining a total wellbeing.

Herbal medicine use is thriving worldwide (Ernst, 1998) and herbal medicinal products can offer an alternative even in cases where conventional medicines have failed in life-threatening conditions. Care however has to be taken to ensure that they are of adequate quality and safety, and are used in an appropriate manner. A detailed literature survey on the toxicity of herbal medicines shows the continuous recycling of the same small group of case histories, indicative in itself of the small total number of examples to draw upon and the rarity of toxic effects. There are relatively few professional medical herbalists available to review much of the inaccurate portrayal of the use of herbs which frequently relates to issues of toxicity. Thus, much of it escapes unchallenged. In most cases since members of the general public and the medical profession may not have made contact with these specialists, many will fail to recognize these inaccurate and prejudiced views. As a result, much attention is focused on the toxic effects of some of these herbs especially when combined with orthodox drugs, and this is frequently quoted as a reason to avoid taking the latter even though it may be the preferred option. Any substance taken by mouth is available for interaction with drugs, foods and dietary supplements. These molecules share several features, including toxicity at high levels. Herbs are therefore not an exception.

Bearing in mind these facts, many of the comments regarding the potential interaction of drugs with herbs fail to recognize that a number of those interactions could be identified by examining the biochemical composition of herbs in exactly the same manner as if they were food items or dietary supplements. In any case, many of the species used in herbal medicine may be the same as those used as food crops in some instances. However, once these plants are utilized within the framework of herbal medicine they seem to assume a completely different image, deserving dismissal rather than scientific investigation. Although a very common food item, grapefruit juice has been the subject of detailed analysis and has been found to alter the metabolism of a range of different drugs (Kiani and Imam, 2007). In particular, it increases the bioavailability of felodipine by several times when compared with water. The picture is therefore not that gloomy after all. If similar information about the various herbs of substances obtained from plants were disseminated more widely, there would be little or no grounds for some of these unfounded criticisms. Any possible interactions between the various components of herbs and other drugs would then be common knowledge, rather than the subject of speculation, and appropriate preventative steps could be considered. Highlighting the possible dangers associated with the use of herbs is all very well if it is fairly contrasted with the dangers of orthodox preparations. Liver and kidney damage are recognized side effects of many commonly prescribed allopathic drugs, but this obviously does not stop their being used in the treatment of diseases. Their benefits are considered to far outweigh any adverse side effects. The saying 'no effect without a side effect' seems to be true in the case of herbs as is true also in orthodox practice.

A comprehensive survey of the toxicology of British plants was produced by the Ministry of Agriculture Fisheries and Foods in 1984 (Cooper and Johnson, 1984). Their conclusion was that, although many plants are known to be poisonous, few species present a serious risk and cases of severe poisoning are rare. Reviewing the literature reveals a limited amount of toxicological data for medicinal herbs. However, as mentioned above there are certain constituents that are intrinsically toxic. By considering information provided by detailed biochemical analyses, it is possible to predict the potential adverse effects that may occur with some herbs. For example, the relatively high amounts of sesquiterpene lactones found in the Compositae means that some of the members of this plant family could precipitate a hypersensitivity reaction in susceptiable individuals. Species that might be involved include *Tanacetum parthenium* (feverfew) (Cooper and Johnson, 1984).

Interestingly, the assessment makes the observation that 'as a basic rule, documentation of a long period of use should be taken into consideration when safety is being assessed. This means that when there are no detailed toxicological studies, documented experience on long term use without evidence of safety problems should form the basis of risk assessment. If such an open-minded view were taken of herbal medicine in general, much more research would have been allowed. This not withstanding, the issues of toxicity have to be properly dealt with to increase the confidence of its clients.

In the arena of conventional medicine if a drug is to be effective, it will inevitably have side effects. The medical establishment considers herbal medicines as drugs, and as such, they must also have side effects. Paradoxically tens of thousands of people every year turn to use herbs because they regard plant remedies as being free from undesirable side effects. Herbs are considered to be generally safe and effective agents. There are a few plants that are almost "drug like" and whose action approaches that of pharmaceuticals. Digitalis is the classic example. Herbalists use these plants in near allopathic treatment strategies if at all, and in some countries e.g. UK, their availability is restricted by law (Sliman, 1998).

In the developed world, people who use herbs in the treatment of diseases are already involved in pharmaceutical therapies. Herbal remedies may act either as agonists or potentiate some drug therapies, and an understanding of conventional drugs and their own side effects as well as the toxicities of some of these herbs is an essential prerequisite for effective herbal therapeutics.

Medical orthodoxy at best does not understand the use of herbs in the treatment and management of diseases. It sees it as a threat which it attempts to rubbish, regulate or ridicule. Quackery has a fascinating role in the history of medicine and its institutions, but much of the hostility towards the use of herbs comes from its apparently greater proximity to orthodoxy than for example acupuncture or homeopathy. This is the unfortunate political context in which toxicity and safety of herbal medicines are debated.

This not withstanding, the issues of toxicity of herbs should be properly researched into to increase the confidence of its clients in this all embracing practice. This is because whether the practice is condemned or not, this 'green gold' phenomenon and the craze to return to nature for mans healthcare needs have come to stay.

The very fact that herbalists are provided with maximum recommended doses for every herb in the British Herbal Pharmacopoeia acknowledges the fact that herbs cannot be the harmless plants that some people assume them to be. Nor are they all highly dangerous agents, as some schools of thought seem to presume. They are prescribed with the same detailed consideration with respect to biochemical composition and dosage as any drug. It is therefore imperative that more research into herbs and their related toxicity profiles be studied seriously just as is done for conventional drugs.

REFERENCES

Chitturi S, Farrell GC. Herbal hepatotoxicity: an expanding but poorly defined problem. *J Gastroenterology and Hepatology* 15, 1093-1099, (2000).

Cooper GA, Johnson M. Transgenic *Plants* and World *Agriculture.* Reviews of Environmental Contamination and *Toxicology* 127, 23-67, (1984).

De Smet P. Health risks of herbal remedies: An update. *Clinical Pharmacology Therapeutics* 2004; 76, 1-17, (2004).

Editorial, Pharmaceutical Journal, 1997.

Ernst E. Harmless Herbs? A review of the recent literature. *Am J of Med*, 104,170-178,(1998).

Farnsworth NR. New natural products and plant drugs with pharmacological, biological or therapeutical activity; Wagner H; Wolff P, Eds. Springer-Verlag: Berlin, FRG and New York, NY. pp.1-22, (1986).

Food and Drug Administration. FDA announces major initiatives for dietary supplements. 2004. http://www.fda.gov/bbs/topics/news/2004/NEW01130.html.

Izzo AA, Ernst E. Interactions between herbal medicines and prescribed drugs: a systematic review. *Drugs* 2001, 61, 2163-2175, (2001).

Kiani J, Imam SZ. Medicinal importance of grapefruit juice and its interaction with various drugs. Nutr J. 6, 33 (2007).

Pharmacopoeia of the People's Republic of China (English edition). Chemical Industry Press, 2005.

Pittler MH, Ernst E. Systematic review: hepatotoxic events associated with herbal medicinal products. *Aliment Pharmacol Ther.*, 18, 451-471, (2003).

Treasure, J (1995). http://www.herbological.com.

chapter 27

Modern Methods of Herbal Drugs Extraction

Vivekananda Mandal and Subhash C Mandal

INTRODUCTION

Plants are naturally gifted bio-factories for the synthesis of medicinal compounds, which have seen the discovery of new drugs with high therapeutic value. Today when different chromatographic methods can provide high resolution of complex mixtures, with detection limits down to few nanograms or below but still the whole advanced analytical process can be wasted if an unsuitable sample preparation or extraction method has been applied before the sample reaches the chromatograph. With the herbal drug usage gaining worldwide recognition as evident from the 1994 WHO data, which says that 90% of the worlds population uses medicinal plant for curing and 81% have no access to synthetic drugs, establishment of proper quality and safety becomes a challenging issue (Nyiredy, 2004). In all research associated with natural product, extraction forms the key basic step. Unfortunately, even though most of the research in medicinal plants starts with extraction, but still today not much attention has been paid to this crucial step. Extraction or sample preparation forms the crucial first step in the analysis of herbs, because it is necessary to extract the desired chemical components from the herbal materials for further separation and characterization. Although many traditional sample preparation methods are still in use, the trends in recent years have been towards: (a) The ability to use smaller initial sample sizes even for trace analyses. (b) Greater specificity or greater selectivity in extraction, (c) Increased potential for automation or for on-line methods, reducing manual operations. (d) A more environmentally friendly approach (green chemistry) with less waste and the use of small volumes or no organic solvents.

The conventional extraction methods like Soxhlet, maceration and hydrodistillation are error prone, tedious and often large volume of organic solvents are consumed in the extraction process. In addition, each extraction step adds to the risk of sample loss and contamination. The acceptance of new techniques has been slow, despite the good performances of several novel methods, such as supercritical fluid extraction, pressurized liquid extraction, microwave and ultrasound assisted extraction. These new methods are typically much faster and often more selective than conventional methods, and consume lesser volume of organic solvents. In general, they allow more efficient extraction of analytes and increases sample throughput, thus they are likely to play an important role in the overall effort of ensuring and providing high quality herbal products to consumers worldwide.[2] In this article recent developments and applications of modern extraction techniques for the extraction, clean up, and concentration of analytes from medicinal plants or herbal materials are reviewed. These modern techniques include supercritical fluid extraction (SFE), microwave assisted extraction (MAE) and ultrasound assisted extraction (UAE). Emphasis is placed on brief description of the unique capabilities, working principle and current applications of each modern technique.

SUPERCRITICAL FLUID EXTRACTION

During recent years, there has been a surge in the use of supercritical fluids as an extraction medium in the field of environmental science and natural product chemistry. The existing extraction techniques by liquid solvents are of environmental concern and supercritical fluid extraction technology is providing reliable, safe, selective and above all, cost effective technique over that of other conventional extraction techniques. Today, supercritical fluid extraction using carbon dioxide as the supercritical fluid is a well-established method and widely used. SFE is an advanced separating technique based on the enhanced solvating power of certain gasses above their critical point. Above the critical temperature and pressure, the substance becomes a supercritical fluid and possesses the properties of gas as well as liquid. Thus the confined gas-like mass transfer and the liquid like solvating power of supercritical fluid is the main criteria of their use for extraction (Lang and Wain, 2003). If a liquid is heated in a sealed system, the liquid expands and the vapor above the liquid becomes denser due to evaporation. If heating is continued or pressure applied it is possible to reach a point where the vapor phase is as dense as the liquid phase and a supercritical phase is achieved. Supercritical fluids are produced by heating a gas above its critical temperature or compressing a liquid above its critical pressure. So a pure supercritical fluid is any compound at a temperature and pressure above the critical point. Super critical fluid exhibits a pressure tunable dissolving power. They possess a liquid like density, and their gas like transport properties, less viscosity makes them to diffuse more quickly than liquids into the botanical material and can therefore extract plant products more effectively and faster than conventional organic solvents. In supercritical region, solvating strength is a direct function of density, which in turn is dependent on system pressure. By changing the density of the fluid through temperature and pressure, the solvating strength of the supercritical fluid can be altered. At a constant temperature, extraction at lower pressure will favor non-polar analytes, and extraction at higher pressure will favor polar and higher molecular weight analytes. Thus, the extraction can be optimized for a particular analyte by simply changing the pressure. The use of polarity modifiers also enhances extraction efficiency and selectivity to extract biologically important molecules (Lang and Wain, 2003). Ethanol is generally used in this regard, as it is non-toxic. The amount and identity of polarity modifier and supercritical carbon dioxide density can be varied to optimize the extraction process. The modifier can be mixed with carbon dioxide in a separate pressure chamber or it can be incorporated into the sample matrix in the extraction cell prior to extraction by supercritical fluid. The modifier exerts its effect mainly in two basic ways.

- By interacting with the analyte complex to promote rapid desorption into the supercritical fluid
- By enhancing the solubility properties of supercritical carbon dioxide

Advantages

1) SFE is fast. Mass transfer limitations determine the rate at which the extraction can be performed.
2) Supercritical fluids have solute diffusivities in order of magnitude higher and viscosities in order of magnitude lower than liquid solvents, which results in increased extraction efficiency.

3) SFE is generally completely within 20-60 minutes whereas liquid extraction by Soxhlet can range 10-14 hours.
4) Elimination of multiple steps increases accuracy and reproducibility of the extraction.
5) The solvent strength of a supercritical fluid can easily be controlled where the solvent strength of a liquid is constant.
6) Most of the supercritical fluids are gasses at ambient conditions. Concentration steps are greatly simplified by direct coupling of SFE to chromatographic techniques. Extraction by solid-liquid method (Soxhlet) needs to be concentrated prior to analysis.
7) Supercritical fluid extraction generates less waste solvents and offers less exposure of laboratory personnel to toxic solvents.
8) Yields quantitative recovery of target analytes without loss or degradation during extraction.
9) Offers selective extraction. The selective solvent characteristics of high-pressure carbon dioxide and the low temperature at which the extraction is carried out make it a more versatile extractant for the labile aroma. Selective extraction can be achieved by selecting the fluid polarity and density.
10) The technique avoids purification by adsorption chromatography and keeps the other active ingredients intact in the matrix.

Disadvantages

1. high installation cost
2. Needs specialized operator

Off Line and On Line SFE Techniques

Off line SFE technique allows direct collection of the extracted analytes either in a solvent or passing the supercritical fluid through a column packed with chromatography adsorbent or can be collected in a cryogenic vessel for subsequent analysis. On line SFE technique, comprises of extraction and analysis, which has been used by many researchers as an analytical tool for the study of medicinal plants. The extracted components are transferred directly from the SFE cell into the gas chromatography column via an on-column injector. SFE can be directly coupled with HPLC too with appropriate detector depending upon the type of analysis to be carried out.

Off line SFE is simpler to perform and after extraction the extract can be analyzed by an appropriate analytical method. On line SFE requires an understanding of SFE and chromatographic conditions and the sample extract is not available for different analytical methods. However, sampling handling between extraction and chromatographic analysis is eliminated by an on line analysis and also loss of components can be avoided. Whereas in off line SFE, the analytes are collected in a solvent and loss can occur during collection or handling during subsequent analyses. In recent times SFE has proved out to be an effective alternative tool for the extraction of various volatile compounds, essential oil, flavonoids and many steroidal compounds.

ULTRASOUND EXTRACTION

The range of human hearing is from 16 KHz to 18 KHz (Schiner and Salvador, 2004). Ultrasound is the name given to sound waves having frequencies higher than those to which the human ear can respond. Since many natural products are thermally unstable and many degrade during thermal extraction, so recent times have seen the growth of UAE as an efficient alternative to various conventional thermal extraction process (Hromadkova and Valachovic, 1999). Recent studies have shown that UAE enhances the extraction efficiency by increasing the yield and by shortening the time of extraction of secondary metabolites from various plant tissues. Various studies have demonstrated that ultrasound is capable of accelerating the extraction of organic compounds contained within the plant tissues by disrupting the cell walls and enhancing mass transfer of cell contents. The enhancement of extraction efficiency of organic compounds by ultrasound is attributed to the phenomenon called acoustic cavitation (Ruo et al., 1997). As ultrasound passes through a liquid, the expansion cycles exert negative pressure on the liquid, pulling the molecules away from one another. If the ultrasound intensity is sufficient, the expansion cycle can create cavities or micro-bubbles in the liquid. This occurs when the negative pressure exceeds the local tensile strength of the liquid, which varies with the type and purity of the liquid. Once formed, these bubbles will absorb the energy from the sound waves and will grow during the expansion cycles and recompress during the compression cycle. The potential energy of the expanded bubble transforms into kinetic energy in the form a liquid jet that moves through inside the bubble and penetrates the opposite wall of the bubble. Liquid jets driving into the surface have been observed at speeds close to 400 km/h (Luque-Garcia and Luque de Castro, 2003). The impact of the jets on the solid surface is very strong. This can result in serious damage to impact zones and can produce newly exposed, highly reactive surfaces. Scanning electron micrographs (SEM) have provided evidence of the mechanical effects of ultrasound, mainly shown by the destruction of cell walls and release of cell contents. In contrast to conventional extractions, plant extracts diffuse across cell walls due to ultrasound, causing cell rupture over a shorter period, which ultimately increases mass transfer phenomenon (Vinatora and Toma, 1997).

The main advantages of ultrasound-assisted leaching over conventional Soxhlet extraction are as follows.

1. Cavitation increases the polarity of the system, including extractants, analytes and matrix; this increases the extraction efficiency, which can be similar to or greater than that of conventional Soxhlet extraction
2. Ultrasound-assisted leaching allows the addition of a co-extractant to increase further the polarity of the liquid phase
3. It also allows the leaching of thermolabile analytes, which are generally altered under the working conditions of Soxhlet extraction.
4. The operating time is invariably shorter with faster kinetics than when compared to Soxhlet extraction.

There exist several investigation reports regarding the reduced extraction time for UAE. The efficiency of the extraction of soyisoflavones was improved by ultrasound and complete extraction was achieved within 20 min (Mauricio et al., 2003). Similarly better efficiency than conventional approaches was reported for the extraction of chlorogenic acid from *Eucommia ulmodies* (Li et al., 2005). Higher yield of rutin and hesperidin was obtained while employing ultrasound technique, which was attributed to the disruption of cell walls by cavitational effects (Paniwanyk et al., 2001). To achieve the same recovery of anthraquinone as that achieved by UAE, Soxhlet and Maceration took a much longer time (Hemwinol et al., 2006). Many such similar reports also exist for other natural products. The average time of ultrasonic extraction typically ranges from a few to 30 min, although it can be as long as 70 min. The recoveries obtained during this time are comparable to those obtained after a dozen or so hours of Soxhlet extraction, carried out at the same temperature. The extraction conditions can be optimized with respect to time, polarity and amount of solvent, and the mass and kind of sample. The advantage of this technique is the possibility of extraction of many samples at once in an ultrasonic bath. The extraction is carried out at room temperature, which makes it suitable for the extraction of thermally labile analytes. The need for separation of the extract from the sample following the extraction is a disadvantage of this technique.

MICROWAVE ASSISTED EXTRACTION

Microwaves are non-ionizing electromagnetic waves positioned between X-ray and infrared rays in the electromagnetic spectrum (Eskilsson and Bjorklund, 2000). Microwaves are made up of two oscillating perpendicular fields i.e. electric and magnetic field and the former is responsible for heating. Unlike conventional heating which depends on conduction–convection phenomenon with eventually much of the heat energy being lost to the environment (Mandal et al., 2007), in case of MAE, heating occurs in a targeted and selective manner with practically no heat being lost to the environment as the heating occurs in a closed system. MAE offers a rapid delivery of electromagnetic energy, which is efficiently converted to heat energy by polar solvents. As a result, the delivery of energy takes place to the total volume of solvent and solid plant matrix with subsequent heating of the solvent and solid plant matrix. Even though dried plant material is used for extraction in most cases, but still plant cells contain minute microscopic traces of moisture that serves as the target for microwave heating. The moisture when heated up inside the plant cell due to microwave effect, evaporates and generates tremendous pressure on the cell wall due to swelling of the plant cell. The pressure pushes the cell wall from inside, stretching and ultimately rupturing it, which facilitates leaching out of the active constituents from the ruptured cells to the surrounding solvent thus improving the yield of phyto-constituents (Camel, 2001). This phenomenon can even be more intensified if the plant matrix is impregnated with solvents with higher heating efficiency under microwave. Higher temperature attained by microwave radiation can hydrolyze ether linkages of cellulose, which is the main constituent of plant cell wall, and can convert into soluble fractions within 1 to 2 min. The higher temperature attained by the cell wall, during MAE, enhances the dehydration of cellulose and reduces its mechanical strength and this in turn helps solvent to access easily to compounds inside the cell (Latha, 2006). In order to study cell damage during the MAE experiments, tobacco leaf samples were examined by scanning electron microscopy. Scanning electron micrographs of the untreated sample, heat-reflux extraction sample and microwave treated sample revealed that there were no structural difference between heat-reflux extraction and those of untreated samples, except few slight ruptures on the surface of the sample. However, the surface of the sample was found greatly destroyed after MAE (Zhou and Liu, 2006). This observation suggests that microwave treatment affects the structure of the cell due to the sudden temperature rise and internal pressure increase. During the rupture process, a rapid exudation of the chemical substance within the cell into the surrounding solvents takes place. This mechanism of MAE based on exposing the analytes to the solvent through cell rupture is different from that of heat-reflux extraction that depends on a series of permeation and solubilization processes to bring the analytes out of the matrix. Evidence has also been presented that during the extraction of essential oils from plant materials, MAE allows the desorption of compounds of interest out of the plant matrix (Lucchesi et al., 2004). This occurs due to the targeted heating of the free water molecules present in the gland and vascular systems; this leads to localized heating causing dramatic expansion, with subsequent rupture of their walls, allowing essential oil to flow towards the organic solvent. The effect of microwave energy is strongly dependent on the dielectric susceptibility of both the solvent and solid plant matrix. Most of the time, the sample is immersed in a single solvent or mixture of solvents that absorb microwave energy strongly. Temperature increases penetration of the solvent into the matrix and constituents are released into the surrounding hot solvent. However in some cases only selective heating of sample matrix is brought about by immersing the sample in a microwave transparent solvent (hexane, chloroform). This approach is particularly useful for thermolabile components to prevent their degradation.[2] The marked advantage of MAE are reduced extraction time and solvent usage with improved yield. Microwave power, microwave exposure time, solid-solvent loading ratio and solvent polarity are some of the important factors, which must be optimized to get maximum yield (Mandal et al., 2007). Extraction time was found to be drastically reduced from 12 h to few seconds in case of extraction of ginseng saponin using MAE (Shu and Chang, 2003). Using MAE only 30 sec was found to be sufficient for the extraction of cocaine when compared to several hours of conventional heating (Bieri and Ilias, 2006). It took only 2 minutes for complete exhaustive extraction of tanshinones from *Salvia miltiorrhiza*, whereas for the extraction of equivalent quantity of tanshinones it took 90, 75 and 45 minutes by Soxhlet, ultrasonic and heat reflux extraction respectively (Pan et al., 2002). A 12-min MAE could recover 92.1% of artemisinin from *Artemisia annua* L, while several-hour Soxhlet extraction could only achieve about 60% recovery (Hao et al., 2002). A 4–5 min MAE (ethanol–water) of glycyrrhizic acid from licorice root achieved a higher extraction yield than extraction (ethanol–water) at room temperature for 20–24 h. MAE can also reduce solvent consumption as it requires only few ml of the solvent than when compared to large volume of solvents required in conventional extraction process.[2] The basic idea should be that in MAE the plant matrix should be just immersed in the extracting solvent.

CONCLUSION

Chemical analysis of extracts from plant material will play a central role in the development and modernization of herbal medicines. The majority of extraction procedures for the determination of plant metabolites are developed in such a way that the final extract introduced into the GC and HPLC columns contains only the analytes with all interferences removed. This is one area where conventional techniques have spelled utter disaster. However, due to complexity of the plant materials obtained, different methods using different methods of extraction and separation tools may be needed. It is certain that methods that are simple, rapid and environmentally friendly will be preferred and is likely to play an important role in the effort in providing high quality products to consumers worldwide. Just as for pharmaceutical products, a well-validated method will help in monitoring the stability of the botanicals and herbal preparations over a period of time. In this regard SFE, MAE, UAE have shown great hopes through their improved ability for extraction of analytes from complicated plant matrices in a much reduced time and with using very less amount of solvent. Even though such systems may be costly but once installed subsequent production cost will be very less because of their unique abilities as discussed. The need for development of existing methods of separation and introduction of new techniques of high resolution and effectiveness must be seriously felt. In all probability, such developments will give rise to the discovery of new effective compounds from phytopharmaceutical sources. More research is needed to improve the understanding of extraction mechanism, remove technical barriers, improve the design and scale up of the novel extraction systems for their better industrial applications.

REFERENCES

Bieri S. Ilias Y. Focused microwave assisted extraction combined with solid phase microextraction and gas chromatography- mass spectrometry for the selective analysis of cocaine from coca leaves. *J Chromatogr A*, 1112, 127, (2006).

Camel V. Microwave assisted solvent extraction of environmental samples. *Trends Anal Che.*, 19, 229, (2000).

Eskilsson CS, Bjorklund E. Analytical scale microwave assisted extraction. *J Chromatogr A*, 902, 227, (2000).

Hao J, Han W, Huang S, Xwe B, Beng X. Microwave assisted extraction of artemisinin from Artemisia Annua L. *Sep Purif Technol,* 28, 191, (2002).

Hemwinol S, Pavasant P, Shotpruk A. Ultrasound assisted extraction of anthraquinones from roots of *Morinda Citrifolia. Ultrason Sonochem*, 13, 543, (2006).

Hromadkova Z, Valachovic P. Comparison of classical and ultrasound assisted extraction of polysaccharides from *Salvia officinalis* L. *Ultrason* Sonochem., 5, 163, (1999).

Latha C. Microwave assisted extraction of embelin from *embelia ribes. Biotechnol Lett*, 10.1007, 10529, (2006).

Lang Q, Wain MC. Supercritical fluid extraction in herbal and natural product studies-a practical review. *Talanta*, 53, 771, (2001).

Li H, Chen B, Yao S. Application of ultrasonic technique for extracting chlorogenic acid from *Eucommia ulmodies* Oliv. *Ultrason Sonochem,* 12, 295, (2005).

Luque-Garcia JL, Luque de Castro MD. Ultrasound: a powerful tool for leaching. *Trends Anal Chem.*, 22, 41, (2003).

Lucchesi ME, Chemat F, Smadja J. Solvent free microwave extraction of essential oil from aromatic herbs: comparison with conventional hydrodistillation. *J Chromatogr A*, 1043, 323, (2004).

Mandal V, Mohan Y, Hemalatha S. Microwave assisted extraction-an innovative and promising extraction tool for medicinal plant research. *Phcog. Rev*, 1, 7, (2007).

Mandal V, Mohan Y, Hemalatha S. Research Article Optimization of curcumin extraction by microwave assisted *in vitro* plant cell bursting by orthogonal array designed extraction process and HPTLC analysis. *Phcog Rev*, 11, 132, (2007).

Mauricio A, Palma M, Barroso CG. Ultrasound assisted extraction of soy isoflavones. *J Chromatogr A*, 1012, 119, (2003).

Nyiredy S. Separation strategies of plant constituents- current status. *J Chromatogr B*, 812, 35, (2004).

Paniwanyk L, Beaufoy E, Mason TJ. The extraction of rutin from flower buds of *Sophora japonica. Ultrason Sonochem,* 8, 299, (2001).

Pan X, Niu G, Liu H. Comparison of microwave assisted extraction and conventional extraction techniques for the extraction of tanshinones from Salvia miltiorrhiza bunge. *Biochem Engg J.*, 12, 71, (2002).

Ruo F, Yiyun Z, Ciguang B. Sonochemistry in China. *Ultrason Sonochem*, 4, 183, (1997).

Schiner EC, Salvador MJ. Comparison of classical and ultrasound assisted extractions of steroids and triterpenoids from Chesta spp. *Ultrason Sonochem*, 11, 415, (2004).

Shu YY, Chang YS. Microwave assisted extraction of ginsenosides from ginseng root. Microchem. J, 74, 131, (2003).

Vinatora M, Toma M. The use of ultrasound for the extraction of bioactive principles from plant metabolites. *Ultrason Sonochem*, 4, 135, (1997).

Zhou HY, Liu CZ. Microwave assisted extraction of solanesol from tobaccoleaves. *J Chromatogr A*, 1129, 135, (2006).

chapter 28

Hairy Root Culture: An Indispensable Source for Harvesting Plant Secondary Metabolite without Sacrificing Natural Germplasm

Moumita Gangopadhyay and Sabita Bhattacharya

INTRODUCTION

Secondary metabolites are not essential to plant growth and produced in very small amounts which include diverse group of compounds such as alkaloids, anthocyanins, flavonoids, terpinoids, tannins etc. They have high economical and pharmacological importance and industries are deeply interested in large variety of chemical substances being produced by plants. These compounds have very complicated structure and in many cases are not eco-friendly or cost effective for chemical synthesis. Traditional agricultural method is time consuming and affected by different eco-geographical factors. In this situation plant cell culture played important role for obtaining desirable secondary metabolite and act as a form of "living factory" for the further exploitation of the plant kingdom as a chemical resources. The biggest challenge for producing secondary metabolites from plant cell culture is that most of the metabolites are organ specific, as the biosynthetic ability of synthesizing secondary metabolite accumulates in specific plant tissue. A new route for production of secondary metabolite from hairy root culture provided up new areas where microorganism can be exploited for production of industrially valuable root specific pharmaceuticals, flavors, dyes, nutraceuticals and cosmetics. *Agrobacterium rhizogenes*, a gram negative soil grown bacterium is the causative agent of hairy root disease in dicotyledonous plants. The transformation leads to the emergence of roots at the site of infection which are capable of unlimited growth and can be utilized commercially by bio-industries. So, in recent years, hairy root culture has emerged as useful to study the biology and engineering of plant chemical production. The present article deals with the mechanism of plant pathogen interaction, utility and limitations of hairy root culture as well as a glimpse on the different bioreactors suitable for the scale up of hairy root culture.

History of Hairy Root Culture

The term "hairy root" was first coined by Steward et al. (1900). In 1930, Ricker et al., first named the hairy root causing organism *Phytomonas rhizogenes,* which was later renamed *A. rhizogenes.* The first transformation of higher plants using *A. rhizogenes* was done by Ackermann in 1973 (Ackermann, 1977). More than 450 species of many different genera and families of higher plants are known to be susceptible to the infection by *A. rhizogenes* (Hamill and Lidgett, 1977). *A. rhizogenes* is a gram negative, non-sporing, motile, rod shaped bacterium, closely related to rhizobium which, produce nitrogen fixing nodules on leguminous plants.

Taxonomy

Kingdom Bacteria
Order Rhizobiales
Family Rhizobiaceae
Genus *Agrobacterium*
Species *Agrobacterium rhizogenes*

The Genome Structure

The ability of root induction by *A. rhizogenes* lies in its typical genome structure, the molecular biology of which has not been properly understood till date. Virulent strains of *A. rhizogenes*, contains a large megaplasmid (more than 200 kb) which plays a key role in hairy root formation. Most of the genes involved in hairy root formation are not borne on the chromosome, but on this root inducing (Ri) Plasmid. This plasmid carries three genetic components, first is a mobile DNA element, t-DNA which is integrated into the nucleus of infected cells where it is subsequently stable and integrated into the host genome and transcribed causing the formation of proliferative multi-branched adventitious roots at the site of infection; called as hairy root diseases in dicotyledonous plants. The transferred DNA (t-DNA) located on the Ri plasmids are approximately 10 to 30 kbp in size (Barker et al., 1983; Byurne et al., 1983), generally represent less than 10% of the Ri plasmid. The second one is the virulence area (*vir*), which contains several *vir* genes which do not enter the plant cell but, together with the chromosomal DNA, cause the transfer of t-DNA. The third one is, so-called border sequences (25 bp), resides in the *Agrobacterium* chromosome. The Ri-plasmids are grouped into two main classes according to the opines, which are produced as specific food for bacteria (Chilton et al., 1982) synthesized by hairy roots. First, agropine-type strains induce roots to synthesise agropine, second, mannopine-type strains induce roots to produce mannopine. Agropine-type strains are considered to be the most virulent and therefore frequently used in the establishment of hairy root cultures.

The Genes Responsible for Hairy Root Formation

The t-DNA of the agropine-type Ri-plasmid consists of two separate t-DNA region tl-DNA and tr-DNA. The genes encoding auxin synthesis (*tms*1 and *tms*2) and agropine synthesis (*ags*) have been localized on the tr-DNA of the agropine type of Ri-plasmid. While in mannopine type Ri-plasmids contain only one t-DNA that shares considerable DNA sequence homology with tl of the agropine-type plasmids. tl-DNA regions of t-DNA consists of 4 genetic loci, *rolA*, *rolB*, *rolC*, and *rolD*, which affect hairy root induction. The complete nucleotide sequence of the tl-region revealed the presence of 18 open-reading frames (ORFs), 4 of which, ORFs 10, 11, 12 and 15, respectively, correspond to the *rolA*, *rolB*, *rolC*, and *rolD* loci. It was also shown that *rolA*, *rolB*, and *rolC* play the most pivotal role in hairy root induction. *rol*B seems to be the most crucial in the differentiation process of transformed cells, protruding stigmas and reduced length of stamens; while *rolA* is associated with internodes shortening and leaf wrinkling; *rolC* causes internodes shortening and reduced apical dominance and *rolD* provide the accessory functions. Although the tr-DNA is not essential for hairy root formation it has been shown that the *aux*1 gene harbored in this segment provides to the transformed cells with an additional source of auxin. The plasmid vir genes are essential for the formation of the product that controls t-DNA movement. Vir A, B, C, D, E, G and Vir H are organized regions of 30 kbp vir regions. The product of Vir A specifies and inner membrane protein that recognize plant phenolic compounds due to the wound of plant tissue and passes the information to the product of Vir G which then itself act as transcriptional activator which finally leads to t-DNA transfer. Vir H locus encodes a protein which is responsible for bacterial survival during infection process.

Gene Transfer Mechanism from *Agro-bacterium Rhizogenes* to Plant Genome

The vir gene expression, generation of t-DNA copy, formation of T strand protein complex, movement of the T-complex through the bacterial membranes, targeting of the T complex into and within the plant cell, targeting of the T complex into the cell nucleus, it's stabilization, and finally integration of T strand into cell DNA are seven successive steps of transfer of DNA from *Agrobacterium* to plant cell.

Step 1 Bacterial colonization on the wounding site of plant tissue is prerequisite for transformation. The production of phenolic compounds at the wounding site is sensed by one of the Vir A gene product which initiates induction of expression of remaining Vir loci.

Step 2 The product of Vir C and Vir D play pivotal role in this step. Two Vir D specific product Vir D_1 and Vir D_2 are essentially required for synthesis of t-DNA strand. The Vir C locus decodes for two polypeptides Vir C_1 and Vir C_2 that are shown to enhance t-DNA border nicking.

Step 3 The t-DNAstrand is likely to exist as a DNA protein complex. The Vir E, specially Vir E_2 protein is the most abundant protein synthesized in Vir induced *Agrobacterium* cells. The Vir D_2 bounds to the leading end of the T-complex. Thus T-complex is compressed of the t-DNA strand, Vir D_2 and Vir E_2.

Step 4 The product of Vir B locus produces transmembrane channel outside the bacterial cell wall because of its 11 open reading frame known as Vir B_1 to Vir B_{11}, the last one helps to pump the T complex out of the bacterial cell.

Step 5 The uptake of T-complex into the plant cell though yet not understood clearly but assume this mechanism somewhat analogues to bacterial conjugation.

Step 6 The T-complex (T- DNA strand, Vir D_2 and Vir E_2) in this step enters within plant cell nucleus. The N terminal of Vir D_2 has role to nick the T-DNA border while C terminus helps in the nuclear uptake of the T strand. The Vir E_2 help to Vir D_2 to target the T complex to the nuclear pore in a polar direction which facilitates it's linear uptake.

Step 7 Generally t-DNA insertions can occur in any chromosome of the plant genome (Ambros *et al*, 1986) or it may occur randomly. Single strand of plant DNA participates in this process. At the 5′ end of the T strands invades a short nick the plant DNA's short starch of homology, very few nucleotides which partial pairing between both ends followed by repairing of any overhangs of t-DNA end followed by it's legation to the plant DNA ends. As hairy root formation involves the transfer of DNA from the bacterium to the plant nucleus and the response of plant cell to the root inducing plant hormone-auxin. It was noticed that t_l DNA of Ri plasmid appear to sensitize the transformed cell to auxin, which determined the root growth and typical characteristics of hairy roots.

Transformation Protocol

Different scientists in different time proposed many protocols for successful transformation (Rech et al., 1988; Tepfer et al., 1987). Surface sterilization, overnight co culture and direct infection at the wound site of plant tissue with *A. rhizogenes* are commonly used procedure for transformation. However successful infection procedure depends on particular plant species and specific plant tissue.

Hairy root induction and establishment of hairy root culture

To succeed in establishing a hairy root culture system for a certain species, several essential conditions should be taken into consideration. These conditions include the bacterial strain of *A. rhizogenes*, an appropriate explants, a proper antibiotic to eliminate redundant bacteria after infection, and a suitable culture medium. Agropine strains are the most used strains owing to their strongest ability. Most plant materials such as hypocotyls, leaf, stem, stalk, petiole, shoot tip, cotyledon, protoplast, storage root or tuber can be used to induce hairy root (Mugnier, 1988; Han et al., 1993; Giri et al., 2001). The level of tissue differentiation determines the ability to give rise to transformed roots after *A. rhizogenes* inoculation. In this case, successful infection of some species can be achieved by the addition of acetosyringone. Cefotaxime sodium, Carbencilin disodium, vancomycin, ampicilin sodium or streptomycin sulphate ranging in concentration from 100 to 500 μg/ml areused to kill or eliminate bacteria (Spano et al., 1981; Drews et al., 1995; Krollcka et al., 2001). However for different species, the proper explant material, antibiotic treatment, first emergence of hairy root after infection may vary and the age of the material is most critical, with juvenile material being optimal. The decontaminated hairy root can be subcultured on phytohormones free medium. Generally hairy roots are considered to be stable and easy to subculture. Nonetheless, hairy root culture also possess a certain amount of heterogeneity, even if derived from a single root tip, and the repeated selection seems to be important to obtain high scopolamine producing hairy root lines, so selection of appropriate hairy root line are prerequisite for establishing hairy root culture (Yukimune et al., 1994).

The confirmatory test for hairy root culture

a) Morphological characteristics

Palgeotropism is common phenomenon in the roots transformed with *A. rhizogenes* (Tepfer, 1984), have an alter phenotype such as profuse lateral branching, as a result due to increase biomass and consequent increase in the number of elongating tips.

b) Biochemical markers

The opines are effective biochemical marker for identification of transformed roots has been done through paper electrophoresis (Bakkali et al., 1997, Bais et al., 2001). Due to instability of opine genes within transformed roots this process is not popularly used.

c) Genetic marker

t-DNA identification of the host plant genome acts as a reliable genetic marker to confirm transformation. The most widely used procedure is Southern blot hybridization (White et al., 1982). Other procedures include DNA "dot blotting" (Draper and Scott, 1988), localization of t-DNA in plant chromosome by "in situ hybridization" (Ambros et al., 1986) and Polymerase chain reaction (Jaziri et al., 1994).

APPLICATIONS OF HAIRY ROOT CULTURE

Production of secondary metabolite formation

For 25 years, hairy roots have been investigated as a biological system for the production of valuable phytochemicals that are useful as pharmaceuticals, cosmetics and food additives. These roots can also synthesize more than a single metabolite and therefore prove economical for commercial production purposes. Many medicinal plants have been transformed successfully by *A. rhizogenes* and induced a relatively high productivity of secondary metabolites which are potentially important pharmaceutical products. Sevon et al., (2002) has summarized the most important alkaloid produced by hairy root culture including *Atropa belladonna* L., *Catharanthus tricophyllus* L., and *Datura candida* L. A substantial research effort has already been put in for the production of antitumour alkaloids such as campothecin, vinblstine and taxol with this technique. Hairy root culture of Chinese medicinal plant *Trichosanthes kirilowii* have been seen producing trichosanthin, a *riboseme* inactivating proteins, can inhibit multiplication of the Human Immuno Deficiency (HIV) THE AIDS virus. In recent year, hairy root culture has emerged as useful to study the biology and engineering of plant chemical production.

Understanding and manipulating of root specific metabolism

There are several ways in which we can visualize roots are chemical factories, the underground growth habit of roots poses major technical difficulties for their study and has hindered biochemical research in particular. A recent reincarnation of a classic plant organ culture system has extremely useful in reinvigorating research on root metabolism. Hairy root culture provided many insights into root specific metabolism and its regulation. This system has been used to follow the production of bioactive proteins. Hairy root culture provided many insights into root specific metabolism and its regulation. This system has been used to follow the production of bioactive proteins. Hairy roots will have a continuing role as an experimental model in plant metabolic engineering. Plants also have considerable potential for the production of biopharmaceutical proteins and peptides. Applications vary from the production of natural products and foreign proteins to a model for phyto-remediation of organic and metal contaminants. As the demand for biopharmaceuticals is expected to increase, it would be wise to ensure that they will be available in significantly larger amounts on a cost-effective basis.

Production compounds not found in untransformed roots

Transformation may affect the metabolic pathway and produce new compounds that can not be produced normally in untransformed roots. In *Scutellaria baicalensis* Georgi, accumulated glucoside conjugates of flavonoids instead of the glucose conjugates accumulated in untransformed roots (Nishikawa et al., 1997).

Regeneration of whole plants

Most importantly can transfer T-DNA from binary vectors and enables the production of transgenic plants containing the foreign genes carried on a second plasmid. This property has been used to produce transgenic plants (Tepfer et al., 1984; Christey et al., 1987). Regeneration of transformed plants through hairy roots have been reported in medicinal plant species is limited (Lee et al., 2004; Chaudhuri et al., 2006). Evaluation of secondary metabolite from regenerated plants from hairy roots has been started quite recently (Jung and Tepfer, 1987; Tanaka and Matsumoto, 1993; Aoki et al., 1997; Yoshimostu et al., 2003).

Why hairy root culture prefers over other plant tissue culture?

Traditional agricultural methods often require months to years to obtain a crop (Kiren et al., 1997). Furthermore the levels of secondary metabolite production are affected by eco-geographical factors. The transformed roots are highly differentiated and can cause stable and extensive production of secondary metabolites, where as other plant cell cultures have a strong tendency to be genetically and biochemically unstable and often synthesize very low levels of secondary metabolites (Rhodes et al., 1990; Merkil et al., 1997). Normally, root cultures need an exogenous phytohormone supply and grow very slowly, resulting in the very poor or negligible synthesis of secondary metabolites.

These hairy roots can be maintained as organ cultures for a long time and subsequent shoot regeneration can be obtained without any cytological abnormality. Rapid growth of hairy roots on hormone-free medium and high plantlet regeneration frequency allows clonal propagation of elite plants. This property can be utilized by genetic manipulations to increase biosynthetic capacity. The secondary metabolite production of hairy roots is highly linked to cell differentiation. Alkaloid production decreased clearly when roots were induced to form callus, and reappeared when the roots were allowed to re-differentiate. For this reason undifferentiated callus culture sometime loosed biosynthetic ability to accumulate secondary metabolite (Rekem and Goldberg, 1985; Charlwood and Charlwood, 1991).

Production enhancement in hairy root culture

To obtain a high density root culture, the culture conditions should be maintained at the optimum level. The composition of the culture medium; sucrose percentage; supply of exogenous growth hormone, specially auxin sensitivity, nature of nitrogen source; light; temperature and the presence of biotic and abiotic elicitors; even use of heavy metals enhanced secondary metabolite production. Media manipulations have been reported to aid in the release of metabolites.

Use of bioreactors for commercial production of secondary metabolite from hairy root culture

In many industrialized countries, more and more individuals are turning to herbal medicines and plant-derived products to offset the high costs of personal healthcare. Many efforts have been made to commercialize production of the medical plant metabolites from plant-cell culture. Specific yields for several natural products are higher in plant cell and hairy root culture. Currently, the cost of biopharmaceuticals limits their availability. Plant-derived biopharmaceuticals are cheap to produce and store, easy to scale up for mass production, and safer than those derived from animals and microorganisms. Bioreactor is a vessel constructed of glass, polycarbonate or steel in which cell or organ is cultured. Bioreactors must have sufficient mixing and mass transfer ability to provide adequate nutrient supply under operating ($_p$H, temperature, dissolved oxygen etc) conditions.

Scaling up of hairy roots in novel bioreactors can provide the best conditions for optimum growth and secondary metabolite production than in native root culture (Srivastava et al., 2007). Hairy root morphology is quite plastic so the bioreactor design for root culture is a balancing act between plant tissues and surrounding controlled environment (Wyslouzil et al., 2000). Thus exploitation of hairy root culture in commercial scale depends on the development of suitable bioreactor system. Several bioreactor designs have been reported for hairy root culture roughly divided into two types namely Liquid phase; Gas phase and Hybrid reactors that are a combination of both (Kim et al., 2002). Among liquid phase reactors stirred tank; air lift; bubble columns and turbine blade reactor are commonly used. Here roots are submerged in the liquid medium. The major disadvantage of this reactor is the requirement of high energy for large scale operation (Ravishankar and Venkataramon,

1990).

Reactors in which liquid is the depressed phase and gas in the continuous phase appear to offer continuous conditions and roots are exposed to air and liquid nutrients are delivered as mist (Weathers et al., 1999). One of the major advantages of this type is the complete control of the gases in the culture environment. Different types of gas phase reactors have been used in research activities among them trickle bed; radial flow and nutrient mist reactors are important. The disadvantage of this reactor is that there is no way to uniformly distribute the roots in the chamber without manual loading. A hybrid reactor system made up of bubble column and nutrient mist bioreactor was used to study the transient growth characteristics and nutrient utilization rates of *Artemisia annua* hairy roots (Kim et. al., 2003).

Potential problems encountered in hairy root culture

Several decades have passed since the hairy root culture was established, however this system has not been utilized globally in commercial scale. To resolve the bottleneck of this application future research should focus on the establishment of effective and economical scaled up culture systems that can reduce the consumption but obtain the biggest benefits. If such breakthrough is achieved, the application is more likely (Srivastava, et al., 2007).

CONCLUSION

Due to the high level, stable secondary metabolite production, hormone independent growth and suitability for adaptation to bioreactor system, hairy root technology has offered new opportunities for eco friendly in vitro production of plant secondary metabolites. For first world developing countries this technique is an alternative towards a more self reliant and sustainable development while for developed countries this technology plays vital role in developing an alternative source for obtaining secondary metabolite without destroying natural germplasm which directly impacted on biodiversity conservation. So the future of hairy root culture is very bright for their commercially stable, high level synthesis of secondary metabolites.

REFERENCES

Ackermann C. Pflanzen aus *Agrobacterium rhizogenes*-Tumoren an Nicitiana tabecum. *Plan. Sci. Let.* 8, 23-30, (1977).

Ambros PF, Matzke AJM, and Matzke, M.A. Localization of *Agrobacterium rhizogenes* T-DNA in plant chromosomes by insitu hybridization. *Embo J*, 5, 2073-2077, (1986).

Aoki T, Matsumoto H, Asako Y, Matsunaga Y, and Shimomura U. Variation of alkaloid productivity among several clones of hairy roots and regenerated plants of *Atropa belladonna* transformed with *Agrobacterium rhizogenes* 15864. *Plant Cell Rep*, 16, 282-286, (1997).

Bais HP, George J, Ravishankar GA, Sudha G. Influence of exogenous hormones on growth and secondary metabolite production in hairy root cultures of Chicorium intybus L.cv. Lucknow local. *In vitro Cell Dev Biol-Plant*, 37, 293-299, (2001).

Bakkali AT, Jaziri M, Foreis A, Vander Heyden Y, Vanhaelen M. and Home SJ. Lawsone accumulation in normal and transformed cultures of henna, Lawsonia inermis. *Plant Cell Tiss Org Cult*, 51, 83-87, (1997).

Barker RF, Idler KB, Thomson DV, and Kemp JD. Nucleotide sequence of the T-DNA region from the *Agrobacterium tumefaciens* octopine Ti plasmid pTi 15955. *Plant Molecul Bio*, 2, 335-350, (1983).

Byurne MC, Koplow J, David C, Tempe J and Chilton J. Structure of T-DNA in roots transformed by *Agrobacterium rhizogenes*. *J Molecul and Appl Gen*, 2, 201-209, (1983).

Charlwood BV, Charlwood KA. Terpenoid production in plant cell culture. In: Harborne, J.B., Ecological Chemistry and Biochemistry of Plant Terpenoids. Clarendon Press, Oxford, (1991), pp. 95-132.

Chaudhuri KN, Ghosh B, Tepfer D, Jha S. Spontaneous plant regeneration in transformed roots and calli from Tylophora indica: changes in morphological phenotype and tylophorine accumulation associated with transformation by *Agrobacterium rhizogenes*. *Plant Cell Rep*, 11, 223-246, (2006).

Chilton MD, Tepfer DA, Petit A, David C, Casse-Delbart F, and Tempe J. *Agrobacterium rhizogenes* inserts T-DNA into the genomes of the host plant root cells. *Nature*, 295, 432-434, (1982).

Christey MC, and Sinclair BK. Regeneration of transgenic rape (*B. napus*) and turnip (*B. campestris*) plants via *Agrobacterium rhizogenes* mediated transformation. *Plant Sci*, 87, 161-169, (1992).

Draper J, and Scott R. The isolation of plant nuclic acids. In Plant Genetic Transformation and Gene Expression-A Laboratory Manual Draper J, Scott R, Armitage P, and Walden R, Eds. Blackwell Scientific Publications, London. pp 192-236, (1988),

Drews FE, Staden JV. Initiation of Solasodine production in hairy root cultures of *Solanum mauritianum* Scop. *Plant Grow Regula*, 17, 27-31, (1995).

Giri A, Ravindra ST, Dhingra V, and Narasu ML. Influence of different strains of *Agrobacterium rhizogenes* on induction of hairy roots and artimisinin production in Artemisia annua. *Currt Sci*, 81, 378-382, (2001).

Hamill JD, and Lidgett AJ. Hairy root cultures-Oppertunities and key protocols for studies in metabolic engineering. In: Hairy roots: Culture and applications. Doran P, Ed. Harwood Academic Publishers, Amsterdam, pp 1-30, (1977).

Han KH, Keathley DE, Davis JM, and Gordon MP. Regeneration of a transgenic woody legume (*Robinia pseudocacacia* L. black locust) and morphological alterations induced by *Agrobacterium rhizogenes* mediated transformation. *Plant Sci*, 88, 149-157, (1993).

Jaziri M, Yoshimatsue K, Homes J, and Shimorua K. Traits of transgenic *Atropa belladonna* doubly transformed with different *Agrobacterium rhizogenes* strains. *PCTOC*. 38, 257-262, (1994).

Jung G, and Tepfer D. Use of Genetic transformation by Ri T-DNA of *Agrobacterium rhizogenes* to stimulate biomass and tropane alkaloid production *Atropa belladonna* and *Calystagia sepium* roots grown *in vitro*. *Plant Sci*, 50, 145-152, (1987).

Kieran PM, Macloughlin PF, and Malone DM. Plant cell suspension culture: some engineering considerations. *J Biotech*, 59, 39-52, (1997).

Kim YJ, Wyslouzil BE, and Weatrhers PJ. Invited review: Secondary metabolism of hairy roots in liquid and gas phse reactors. *In vitro Cell Dev Biol Plant*, 38, 1-10, (2002).

Krollcka A, Staniszewska I, Blelawski K, Mallnski E, Szafranek J, Lojkowska E. Establishment of hairy root cultures of Ammi majus. *Plant Sci*, 160, 259-264, (2001).

Lee MH, Yoon S, Jeong JH, and Choi YE. *Agrobacterium rhizogenes*- mediated transformation of *Taraxacum platycarpum* and changes of morphological characters. *Plant Cell Rep*, 22, 822-827, (2004).

Merkel A, Christen P, and Kapetanedis I. Production of Diosgenin by hairy root cultures of *Trigonella- foenum graceum* L. *Plant Cell Rep*, 16, 632-636, (1997).

Mugnier J. Establishment of new axenic hairy root lines by inoculation with *Agrobacterium rhizogenes*. *Plant. Cell. Rep.* 7, 9-12, (1988).

Nishikawa K, and Ishimaru K. Flavonoids in root cultures of Scutella baicalensis. *J Plant Physio*, 151, 633-636, (1997).

Ravishankar GA, Venkataramon LV. Food applications of plant cell cultures. *Cur Sci*, 59, 914-920, (1990).

Rech RL, Golds TJ, Hammatt N, Mulligan BJ, and Devey MR. *J Experimen Bota*, 39, 1275-1285, (1988).

Rhodes MJC, Robins RJ, Hamill JD, Parr AJ, Hilton MH, Walton NJ, Properties of transformed root culture. In : Charlwood BV, Rhodes MJC, eds. Proceeding of the Phytochemical society of Europe secondary product of plant tissue culture, Clarendon press Oxford, London, pp. 201-225, (1990).

Ricker AJ, Banfield WM, Wright WH, Keitt GW, and Sangen HE. Studies on infectious hairy root of nursery apple tree. *J Agricul Res*, 41, 507-540, (1930).

Rokem JS, and Goldberg I. Secondary metabolites from plant cell suspension cultures: methods for yield improvement. Advances in biotechnological processes 4. New York: Alan R. Liss, 241-274(1985).

Sevon N, Oksman C, and Krishi M. *Agrobacterium rhizogenes*-mediated transformation: root cultures as a source of alkaloids. *Planta Med*, 68, 859-868, (2002).

Spano L, Mariotti D, Carardarelli M, Branca C, Constantino P. Morphogenesis and auxin sensitivity of transgenic tobacco with different complements of Ri T-DNA. *Plant Physiol*, 87, 479-483, (1988).

Srivastva S, Srivastva A. Hairy root culture for mass-production of High value secondary Metabolite. *Criti Re Biotech*, 27:29-43, 2007.

Steward FC, Rolfs FM, and Hall FHA. fruit disease survey of West Ern NewYork in 1900. Newyork *Agric Exp Sta Bact*,191, 291-331, (1900).

Tanaka N, and Matsumoto T. Regeneration from *Ajuga* hairy roots with high productivity of 20-hydroxyecdysone. *Plant Cell Rep*, 13, 87-90, (1993).

Tepfer D. Genetic transformation of several species of higher plants by *Agrobacterium rhizogenes*: phenotypic consequences and sexual transmission of the transformed genotype and phenotype. *Cell.* 37, 959-967, (1987).

Tepfer D. Genetic transformation of several species of higher plants *Agrobacterium rhizogenes*. Sexual transmission of the transformed genotype and phenotype. *Cell.* 37, 959-967, (1984).

Weathers PJ, Wyslouzil BE, Wobbe KK. The biological response of hairy roots to oxygen level in bioreactors. *Invitro Cell Dev Biol Plant*, 35, 286-289, (1999).

White FF, Ghidossi G, Gordon MP, and Nester EW. Tumor induction by *Agrobacterium rhizogenes* involves the transfer of plasmid DNA to the plant genome. *Proc Nat Acad Sci USA*, 79, 3193-3197, (1982).

Wyslouzil BE, Waterbury RG, and Weathers PJ. The growth of single roots of *Artemisia annua* in nutrient mist reactors. *Biotechn Bioeng*, 72, 143-150, (2000).

Yoshimatsu K, Shimonrura K, Yamazaki M, Saito K, and Kiuchi F. Transformation of Ipecac (*Cephaelis ipecacuanha)* with *Agrobacterium rhizogenes.Planta Med*, 69, 1018-1023, (2003).

Yukimune Y, Hara Y, and Yamada Y. Tropene alkaloid production in root cultures of *Duboisia myoporoides* obtained by repeated selection. *Bioscí Biotechn & Biochem*, 58, 1443-1446, (1994).

chapter 29

Regulatory Requirements for Herbal Medicines in India: Ensuring Quality, Safety and Efficacy

Subhash C. Mandal (Sr.)

INTRODUCTION

Herbal medicines are being used in India since Vedic age and it has been documented in Rigveda. It has been mentioned in Charak Samhita. Initially herbs have been used by the people traditionally from their experience and gradually a group of experts evolves who were called as apothecaries. Herbal medicines are also used since long back in other different countries like China. In India herbal medicines are being used in Ayurveda, Siddha, Unani and Homoeopathic system of medicines. Ayurvedic system is being practiced since 6000 B.C., Chinese herbal medicines is being practiced since 5000 B.C. whereas the modern system of medicines started since 1800 A.D.

This was popular may be because of the experience and abundant availability of plants in India due to its varied agro climatic zones. We are having around 45,000 species of plants in the Indian conditions, out of which 15,000-20,000 plants have proven medicinal value. The traditional system utilizes around 7,000-7,500 species in its formulations. Ayurveda uses 2000, Unani 1000, Siddha 1300, Tibetian 500 and 200 varieties in the modern medicine (Mukherjee and Wahile, 2006).

Interest on herbal products has been increasing since last few decades not only in underdeveloped and developing countries, but also in the developed countries. A large number of big pharma companies started to redirect their business strategy by investing large amount of finance in research and manufacturing of herbal medicines. Some Govt. institutions are also emphasizing on research on herbal medicines.

Herbal medicine has a Global market of US$ 80-100 billion (Gohil and Patel, 2007) and this market is expected to reach US$2500 billion by the year 2010 and US$ 5 trillion by the year 2050 according to the World Bank report. The Indian herbal drug market is about $ 1 billion and the export of herbal crude extract is about $ 80 million. (Mukherjee, 2001). We have about 7800 manufacturing units engaged in manufacturing of herbal drugs in India, which are consuming 200 tons of herbs annually.

Initially there was no regulation for controlling the quality of herbal medicines and the practitioners relied on their experience on proper identification of the plant. Gradually some regulation developed and the first organized regulation on quality is the Drugs and Cosmetics Act 1940 and Drugs and Cosmetic Rules 1945. This act initially prescribed the standards of Ayurvedic, Siddha and Unani medicines and laid down rules and regulation on manufacturing.

Standards of Drugs as per existing legislature of India

Standards of medicines are prescribed in the Drugs and Cosmetic Act 1940 and individual monographs has been prescribed in the respective Pharmacopoeias. Recently the Govt. of India has published 4 volumes of Ayurvedic Pharmacopoeia encompassing standards of 326 drugs, which is grossly inadequate in comparison to the number of herbs used in the Ayurvedic system of medicines. A positive step has been taken in this direction by publishing of the Herbal Pharmacopoeias, having standards of 52 drugs (IDMA, 2002).

Unfortunately neither the herbal products nor the herbal Pharmacopoeias have any statutory standing in our country (Govt. of India, 2005). That there are a large number of herbal products in the market though it is difficult to categorize these products as per the Drugs and Cosmetics Acts and Rules. Some herbal drugs are also marketed as food or nutritional supplements, with medicinal claims.

Keeping this problem in mind, status of herbal products was surveyed through different sources including Pharmacopoeias of different countries (WHO, 1998; WHO 2001; WHO, 2005).

In some countries herbal products are considered as drugs, e.g. China, UK, Canada, Germany, etc. while some countries do not grant herbal products, the status of drugs e.g. USA, Netherlands etc. They consider it as nutritional supplements, and have framed definite legislation for it e.g. USA (Marwick, 1995).

In India there are some gray areas in case of status of herbal drugs (Table 3.1.I) and there exists no definite policies about food supplements. Recently Govt. of India has published Food Safety act to resolve this problem (Govt. of India, 2006). As per the experts this said act has not been implemented and failed to resolve the problem.

Sometimes mere mentioning of a drug in some textbooks is considered sufficient as per existing legislature, whereas the texts are not properly defined (Govt. of India, 2005).

Table 3.1.I: Standards of Herbal Drugs as per Indian legislation.

System of Medicine	*Standard*
Modern Drugs	The second schedule of Drugs and Cosmetics Act.
Homeopathic Drugs	The second schedule of Drugsand Cosmetics Act.
Ayurvedic, Siddha and Unani Drugs	Rule 168 of Drugs & Cosmetics Act.
Herbal	?

3.1. Standards of Ayurvedic Drugs:

Standards required to be complied with in manufacturing for sale or distribution of Ayurvedic, Siddha and Unani Drugs are laid down in Drugs and Cosmetics Rules, which are given in the table below.

Table 3.1.II: Standards of Ayurvedic, Siddha and Unani drugs as per D and C Rules.

Sl. No.	*Class of Drugs*	*Standards to be complied with*
1.	Single drugs included in Ayurvedic Pharmacopoeia	The standards for identity, purity and strength as given in the editions of Ayurvedic Pharmacopoeia of India for the time being in force.
2.	Asavas and Aristas	The upper limit of alcohol as self generated alcohol should not exceed 12% v/v except those notified by the Central Government from time to time.

Till date, only four volumes of Ayurvedic Pharmacopoeia having monographs of about 326 herbs have been published, which is quite inadequate with respect to the huge number of herbs used in the Ayurvedic system of medicines (IDMA, 2002). Mere mentioning of preparation method in a list of 57 texts, are sufficient for manufacturing such Ayurvedic drugs. All of these books are old texts except the Ayurvedic Formulary of India (Part I) and Ayurvedic Pharmacopoeia of India. There is ample scope of misuse of this provision, as 55 books out of 57 are not properly defined in the legislature.

The monographs cover only a few parameters, which are considered to be quite inadequate for standardization (Govt. of India, 1990; Govt. of India, 1999; Govt. of India, 2001; Govt. of India, 2004). Monographs of herbs in British Herbal Pharmacopoeia prescribe chemical characterization involving TLC, GC and PC electrophoresis, whereas no such modern methods are required in the Ayurvedic Pharmacopoeia. Minimum pharmacological characterization is required, which is quite inadequate, compared to characterization specified by other Pharmacopoeias.

No standards for combination products are prescribed in statute, except Asavas and Aristas. Only alcohol content of these two products is given in D and C Act.

Standards of Siddha Drugs

As per the Drugs Act, simply mentioning of manufacturing process in a list of 30 books allows production of Siddha Drugs. Amongst these 30 books, 29 are old texts and Siddha Formulary of India (Part I) is the only book published by the Govt. of India recently.

Standards of Unani Tibetian System of Drugs

As per the Drugs Act mere mentioning of manufacturing process in a list of 13 books allows production of Unani and Tibetian drugs. Amongst these 13 books, 12 are old texts and the only modern book is National Formulary of Unani Medicine (Part I) published by Govt. of India.

Schedule T for Good Manufacturing practice

To manufacture good quality Ayurvedic, Siddha and Unani medicines Good Manufacturing practices have been made mandatory by incorporation of revised Schedule T in the year of 2003 (Govt. of India, 2005). Important features of Schedule T are as follows:

i) Raw materials to be used in manufacture of medicines must be authentic, of prescribed quality and free from contamination.
ii) Manufacturing process is as prescribed to maintain the standard.
iii) Adequate quality control measures to be adopted.
iv) Drugs released for sale shall be of acceptable quality.
v) To achieve the objectives listed above, the firm is required to maintain the following conditions stringently—
   A) Well designed factory premises with sufficient space required to be provided.
   B) Proper machineries require to be provided.
   C) Quality control laboratory require to be provided with required instruments and well qualified personnel.
   D) Shall evolve methodology and procedures for following the prescribed process of manufacture.
   E) Which should be properly documented and kept for reference and inspection.

Standards of Homoeopathic Medicines

Standard of Homoeopathic medicines has been prescribed in Second schedule of the Drugs and Cosmetics Act, 1940, which is given in Table 3.1.III.

Table 3.1.III: Standards of Homoeopathic Medicines as per Drugs and Cosmetics Act.

Sl. No	Class of Drug	Standard to be complied with
1.	Drugs included in the Homoeopathic Pharmacopoeia of India	Standards of identity, purity and strength specified in the edition of the Homoeopathic Pharmacopoeia of India for the time being and such standards as may be prescribed.
2.	Drugs not included in the Homoeopathic Pharmacopoeia of India but which are included in the Homoeopathic Pharmacopoeia of the United States of America or the United Kingdom or the German Homoeopathic Pharmacopoeia.	Standards of identity, purity and strength prescribed for the drugs in the edition of such Pharmacopoeia for the time being in which they are given and such other standards as may be prescribed.
3.	Drugs not included in the Homoeopathic Pharmacopoeia of India or the Homoeopathic Pharmacopoeia of the United States of America or the United Kingdom or the German Homoeopathic Pharmacopoeia.	The formula or list of ingredients displayed in the prescribed manner on the label of the container and such other standards as may be prescribed by the Central Government.

In addition to this, three more parameters are required to be controlled for mother tincture, which are identification of crude drugs, total solids and alcohol content.

For the first category presently we have eight volumes of Pharmacopoeia prescribing the monographs including identity, purity and strength of several raw materials (Govt. of India, 1971). But no standard for finished product was included till publication of fifth volume in the year of 1987. Sixth and eighth volume included standards of few finished products of Mother Tinctures and Mother solutions (Govt. of India, 2000). Standards include a few preliminary criteria like pH, wt. per ml, alcohol percentage, λ max and identification, which are considered inadequate for proper quality control at this age when sophisticated techniques like HPTLC are easily available.

Schedule M1: In order to ensure proper quality of Homoeopathic medicines manufacture, Schedule M1 was introduced in 1987 specifying requirement of technical staff, manufacturing plants, testing equipments etc. (Govt. of India, 2005). Experts feel that this is quite inadequate in this age of science.

Recently Government of India has taken an initiative to implement Good Manufacturing Practices (GMP) and a guidelines has already been published, which is effective from 2nd October 2008. This guideline is more detailed and prescribed minimum requirement of manufacturing areas, equipments, minimum qualification required for the personnel engaged in manufacturing and quality control, documents to be maintained etc. for manufacturing quality medicines.

Patent Protection to be exploited fully

Despite possessing huge natural wealth, India has not shown promising performance in the field of the thriving $ 80-100 billion global herbal market. A few countries—China, Russia, Europe, Japan and even USA have marched ahead with numerous international patents on medicinal plants.

If India can fully exploit its natural resources, skilled manpower and potential traditional knowledge and couple them with its technical powers then India can march ahead to compete with global players by partly substituting costly modern medicines with modern herbal drugs. If India can concentrate her efforts to develop the heritage herbal products and processes it seriously, it will be hard to hold back the progress (Mandal and Mandal, 1999).

It is unfortunate that some of the Indian products have been patented by different companies which are being used in India since a long time like- Neem, Amla, Kurchi, Sarpagandha, Calendula, Sankhapushpi, Jamun, Anar, Bagbherenda, Karela. Fortunately, Government of India has taken initiative to challenge the patent granted on turmeric to an US University and as a result U.S. patent (No. 5,401,504) on the use of turmeric (Curcuma longa L., Zingiberaceae) for healing was invalidated because it was not a novel invention. This is an encouraging victory for Indian activists campaigning to protect indigenous wisdom. Under World Trade Organisation (WTO) rules, patents are provided for inventions that qualify for their novelty, non-obviousness, and utility. The turmeric patent failed to satisfy the criteria of novelty as turmeric paste has been used to treat wounds and stomach infections for centuries by Indians. The turmeric patent was just one of the hundreds that the developed countries have claimed by ignoring indigenous and existing knowledge.

In order to prevent grant of patents based on Indian traditional knowledge, Government of India has undertaken an ambitious project of creating a Traditional Knowledge Digital Library (TKDL). This is a joint venture of the Council of Scientific Research and Central Council for Research in Ayurveda and Siddha. This project is intended to cover about 35,000 formulations available in 14 classical texts of Ayurveda to convert the information into patent compatible format. The work has been initiated with a co-operative set up of 30 Ayurveda experts, 5 information Technology experts and 2 Patent examiners. The digital library will include all details in digital format about international patent classification, traditional research classification, Ayurveda terminology, concepts, definitions, classical formulations, doses, disease conditions and references to documents.

Steps to be taken to improve the existing efforts of standardization

Control on quality of raw materials: Quality of medicines of herbal origin mainly depends on quality of raw materials. Presently, a major part of the raw materials are procured from wild origin, which have almost no control on parameters of cultivation or collection etc. Controlled cultivation could be a parameter of the quality control. If Good Cultivation Practice and Good Harvesting Practices are developed and implemented raw materials of good quality can be ensured. European Guidelines for Good Agricultural Practice (G.A.P.) of Medicinal and Aromatic Plants, Good Agricultural and Collection Practice for Medicinal Plants (GACP), Japan, Good Agricultural Practice for Traditional Chinese Medicinal Materials, People's Republic of China etc. have been published for this purpose. Recently World Health Organization has also published Good Agricultural and Collection Practice (GACP) which may be practiced in case of cultivation and collection of Medicinal plants (20).

Research for developing quality control methods: It is a fact that quality control of herbal drugs is not developing sufficiently, especially for combination products. Research on developing standardization methods involving modern instrumentation is urgently required. Though a few attempts have already been made, more emphasis is required in this area. Monographs of more plants require to be incorporated in the existing Ayurvedic Pharmacopoeia. More stringent specifications including use of sophisticated instruments are to be incorporated. Research and development of marker compounds and Metabolomics are order of the day, and stress must be laid in this area.

Clinical trial: In the third world countries like India, there is always a lack of enthusiasm noted for conduction of clinical trials, and also there is a dearth of coordination and effort to translate and utilize the results of clinical trials within various working groups and professionals. While most modern clinicians and researchers believe in rigorous screening and clinical trials, most specialists in traditional medicine are convinced of 100% efficacy of their drugs and consider clinical trials as redundant. This attitude is much more prevalent in India than in China, where institutes of traditional medicine have established their drugs on scientific basis rather than on the rationale of drug (Roy Chaudhury, 1994). For proper conduction of clinical trials, there is a requirement of experienced clinical pharmacists, pharmacologists, as well as experts in traditional system of medicines.

CONCLUSION

Medicines of herbal origin are being used since time immemorial throughout the globe. This discipline has developed gradually in terms of its quality, safety and efficacy. Status of herbal medicines also varies from country to country e.g. in UK it is considered as drug where as Netherlands does not consider it as drug. Problem lies with framing a national legislation and its implementation, to maintain the quality, safety, efficacy and pharmaco-vigilence. Steps are being taken to resolve these issues currently. More well framed regulations require to be incorporated for maintaining good standards considering quality and safety. Serious initiatives require to be taken to harmonise the regulatory requirements throughout the globe to make available standard herbal medicines the world over. The latest scientific methods available for standardization of herbal medicines require to be adopted in the existing legislation.

ACKNOWLEDGEMENTS

Author is thankful to Dr. Moitreyee Mandal, Lecturer, J.C. Ghosh Polytechnic, Kolkata for her kind help in preparing the manuscript. Author is also thankful to Dr. S. K. Roy Chowdhury, Director, Directorate of Drugs Control, Govt. of West Bengal for his constant encouragement.

REFERENCES

Gohil KJ, Patel JA. Herb-drug interactions: a review and study based on assessment of clinical case reports in literature. Indian J Pharmacol, 39, 129-139, (2007).

Government of India, Ministry of Health and Family Welfare, Department of Indian System of Medicine and Homoeopathy. The Ayurvedic Pharmacopoeia of India, Part–I, Vol. I. The Controller of Publications, Delhi, (1990).

Government of India, Ministry of Health and Family Welfare, Department of Indian System of Medicine and Homoeopathy. The Ayurvedic Pharmacopoeia of India, Part–I, Vol. II. Delhi, The Controller of Publications, (1999).

Government of India, Ministry of Health and Family Welfare, Department of Indian System of Medicine and Homoeopathy. The Ayurvedic Pharmacopoeia of India, Part–I, Vol. III. The Controller of Publications, Delhi, (2001).

Government of India, Ministry of Health and Family Welfare, Department of Ayurveda, Yoga-Naturopathy, Unani, Siddha and Homoeopathy (AYUSH). The Ayurvedic Pharmacopoeia of India,

Part–I, Vol. IV, The Controller of Publications, New Delhi, (2004).

Government of India. The Drugs and Cosmetics Act 1940 and The Drugs and Cosmetics Rules, 1945. Ministry of Health and Family Welfare, (2005).

Government of India. The Drugs and Cosmetics Act 1940 and The Drugs and Cosmetics Rules, 1945. Ministry of Health and Family Welfare, 405- 413, (2005).

Government of India. The Drugs and Cosmetics Act 1940 and The Drugs and Cosmetics Rules, 1945. Ministry of Health and Family Welfare, 367- 369, (2005).

Government of India. The Food Safety And Standards Act. (2006).

Govt. of India, Ministry of Health and Family Welfare, Department of Indian System of Medicine & Homoeopathy. Homoeopathic Pharmacopoeia of India, Vol. 8. The Controller of Publications, Delhi, (2000).

Govt. of India, Ministry of Health. Homoeopathic Pharmacopoeia of India, Vol. I. Delhi, The Controller of Publications, (1971).

Indian Drug Manufacturers Association, Indian Herbal Pharmacopoeia. Mumbai, Indian Drug Manufacturers' Association, (2002).

Mandal M, Mandal SC. Shifting the Paradigm in Herbal research Approach for the New Millennium. Current R & D highlights, 22(4), 22-25, (1999).

Marwick C. Growing Use of Medicinal Botanicals Forces Assessment by Drug Regulators. JAMA, 273-609, (1995).

Mukherjee PK. Evaluation of Indian traditional medicines. Drug Information Journal. 35, 623-631, (2001).

Mukherjee PK, Wahile A. Integrated approaches towards drug development from Ayurveda and other systems of medicines. J Ethnopharmacol, 103, 25-35, (2006).

Roy Chaudhury R. Herbal Medicine for Human Health, WHO, 18-19, (1994).

World Health Organization. Legal status of traditional medicine and complementary / alternative medicine: a worldwide review (document WHO/EDM/TRM/2001.2). Geneva, (2001).

World Health Organization. National policy on traditional medicine and Regulation of Herbal Medicines. Geneva, (2005).

World Health Organization. Regulatory situation of herbal medicines: a world wide review (document WHO/TRM/98.1). Geneva, (1998).

World Health Organization. WHO guidelines on good agricultural and collection practices (GACP) for medicinal plants. World Health Organization, Geneva, (2003).

chapter 30

Approaching Bio/Pharmaceutical Equivalence from the Perspective of Herbal Drug Standardization

Mayank Thakur, C.S. Bhargava and Shilpi Bhargava

HERBAL MEDICINE: CORE CONCEPT

Usage of herbal medicinal agents dates back to the duration of human evaluation itself (Rose, 2006). As an excerpt from Wikipedia clearly illustrates by the definition 'Herbalism is a traditional medicinal or folk medicine practice based on the use of plants and plant extracts. Herbalism is also known as botanical medicine, medical herbalism, herbal medicine, herbology, and phytotherapy. The scope of herbal medicine is sometimes extended to include fungal and bee products, as well as minerals, shells and certain animal parts.' (http://en.wikipedia.org/wiki/Herbal_drug). The field or scope of herbal drug research are vast and pretty much span over all the living systems in general (Thakur and Dixit, 2007).

In the recent 20 years the therapeutic use of herbal medicines is gaining considerable momentum (Thakur et al., 2005). As an estimate drawn by the World Health Organization (WHO) nearly 75-80% of the world population is still dependent on the services of herbal medicine and local herbal healers for various ailments and diseases (WHO, 1996). Amongst various reasons cited for the acceptance of the herbal medicine a few major one's include a better cultural acceptability, better compatibility with the human body and lesser side-effects (Pakzad et al., 2007). Although the later two points have now become a matter of scientific debate and a lot needs to be evaluated before the last two points could be justified completely (Shakeel et al., 2008). The international market for herbal medicine is more than $ 90 billion a year and growing at the rate of 5.4% annually (Gupta, 2007). The recent downturn and global economic crisis has no affected the growth of herbal drug market. Interestingly, alternative therapies have now been recognized under the insurance cover for the major global economies, thus paving way towards an increasing growth and development in this field (Sawalha, 2007).

The growth when clustered across the segment of world population signifies a major growth of nearly 4% in European Union and Great Britain, followed by 3.6% in North America and US. Developing countries like India, China and Brazil continue to see an increasing interest in herbal drug research as well as consumption (Zaenker et al., 2009; Ndhala et al., 2009; Weina, 2008).

STANDARDIZATION OF HERBAL MEDICINAL PRODUCTS

Herbal drug standardization has been a topic of growing interest for modern scientists and concern for the traditional healers and practitioners of complementary medicine systems (Yadav et al., 2009). In general a summary of herbal drug standardization can be drawn from the following excerpt drawn from a European monograph for herbal drug standardization approach (EMEA 2001; EMEA 2002).

All herbal substances/herbal preparations are essentially defined by their production process and their specifications;

- Standardised herbal substances/herbal preparations are adjusted to a given content of constituents with known therapeutic activity within an acceptable tolerance; standardisation is achieved by adjustment of the herbal substances/herbal preparations with excipients or by blending batches of herbal substances and/or herbal preparations.
- Quantified herbal substances/herbal preparations are adjusted to a defined range of constituents (active markers); adjustment is exclusively achieved by blending batches of herbal substances and/or herbal preparations.
- Other herbal substances/herbal preparations are active substances for which neither constituents with known therapeutic activity nor active markers are known. These herbal substances/herbal preparations are not adjusted to a defined content of analytical marker.

Table 30.1 General Testing Parameters for Characterization and Standardization of Herbal Medicines

	Testing parameters	*Guidelines*
1.	General data • Geographical • Harvesting time • Harvesting process • Processing	Good Agricultural Practices (GAP)
2.	Description	
3.	Identity • Macroscopic • Microscopic • Chemical • TLC fingerprints	According to Pharmacopoeias
4.	Purity • Foreign matter • Ash/Sulfated ash • Content of extractable matter • Water content	According to Pharmacopoeias
5.	Assay • Constituents with known therapeutic activity (biomarker) • Constituents with unknown therapeutic activity (marker substances) • Titrimetric • Photometric • HPLC/GC/TLC	According to Pharmacopoeias
6.	Contaminants • Pesticides • Heavy metals • Aflatoxins • Microbiological purity • Radioactivity	• Ph. Eur. • Recommended limits for herbal drugs (oct. 91) • Regulation on aflatoxins (Nov. 90) • Ph. Eur. 1997 Suppl. 1999

Approaches for Herbal drug Standardization

There has been a tremendous upsurge in the overviews for the methodologies and approaches towards herbal drug standardization. Amongst various conventional and newer methods for standardization, which have been extensively published and reviewed, the major that needs a brief mention here are:

A. Chromatographic Techniques:

a. *High Performance Liquid Chromatography*: One of the most versatile and flexible technique with high throughput, a variation of column system enables a scientist to use one equipment for multifaceted and reasonably faster standardization (Bournot et al., 1992). The only general problem is in case of herbal drugs without and authenticated marker or complex herbal medicinal products. Preparative HPLC and use of sophisticated Ultra Pressure Liquid Chromatographic apparatuses UPLC's have started to revolutionize the concept of standardization using liquid chromatography. A vast array of detector modules also simplifies the extent as well as degree of detection and sensitivity (Annesley et al., 1992; Hussain et al., 2009; German et al., 2009).

b. *High Performance Thin Layer Chromatography*: HPTLC with the modern scanners for TLC plates have also improved the way this vastly used technique could be utilized in herbal medicinal research. It is now an acceptable form of standardization for most single as well as complex herbal mixtures (Yue et al., 2008; Pulpati et al., 2008; Rout et al., 2008).

c. Gas Chromatography with Flame Ionization or mass detection (GC-FID or GC-MS) is a well documented techniques for volatile herbal components as well as sugar complexes in standardization (Fischer and Buhl, 1992).

Apart from these vastly used techniques a lot of day to day modifications for individual herbal drugs are being experimented in various research laboratories globally, providing a growing evidence towards herbal drug standardization.

Biotechnological approaches to herbal drugs standardization

Biotechnology and use of biomarkers has facilitated the herbal drug standardization in more than one way, a brief look at the techniques available can shed better light on the future that these concepts may hold:

I. DNA FINGERPRINTING

Some of the newly emerging techniques for ensuring correct botanical identity and quality include Herboprint™, which in addition to chemoprofile also considers ayurvedic properties (Sangwan et al., 2002). Various types of DNA-based molecular techniques can be utilized to evaluate DNA polymorphism (Sharma et al., 2001; Vieira et al., 2001).

Hybridization-based methods

Hybridization-based methods include restriction fragment length polymorphism (RFLP) and variable number tandem repeats. Labelled probes such as random genomic clones, cDNA clones, probes for microsatellite and minisatellite sequences are hybridized to filters containing DNA, which has been digested with restriction enzymes. Polymorphisms are detected by presence or absence of bands upon hybridization (Lazarowych et al., 1998 ; Sharma et al., 2002).

a. *PCR-based methods*: PCR-based markers involve *in vitro* amplification of particular DNA sequences or loci, with the help of specific or arbitrary oligonucleotide primers and the thermostable DNA polymerase enzyme (Ha et al., 2001).

b. *Sequencing-based markers*: DNA sequencing can also be used as a definitive means for identifying species. Variations due to transversion, insertion or deletion can be assessed directly and information on a defined locus can be obtained (Welsh and McClelland, 1991).

Genetic variation/genotyping

This technique is useful for identifying gepgraphical variations in different plant drugs due to geographical variation.

Thus in a nutshell the usefulness of DNA based techniques can for herbal drug research can be identified as (Bhutani, 2000).

a. *Authentication of medicinal plants*
b. *Detection of adulteration/substitution*
c. *Marker assisted selection of desirable chemotypes*
d. *Genetic variation, cultivar variation, cross breeding studies and disease resistant gene identification in* foods and nutraceuticals.

Biopharmaceutical Equivalence: Perspectives and advantages

Achievement of a known therapeutic benefit is an important aim from a pharmacological point of view (Gryniewicz et al., 2009). Since herbal medicinal products may also fall under the category of phytogenerics, therefore, it is important to draw a detailed information about their pharmacological potential as well as pharmaceutical equivalence (Chauhan et al., 1994). An approach in this direction is not only important from standardization point of view, but also from the lookout towards rationalization of herbal medicine practice (Gao et al., 2009).

According to an excellent review on the perspective of bioequivalence of herbal medicinal products by Loew and Kaszkin, 2002, 'Herbal medicinal products (HMP) are medicinal products containing as active substances exclusively herbal drugs or herbal drug preparations (HDP), precisely defined by the botanical scientific name according to the binominal system (genus, species, variety and author). In contrast to chemically defined drugs, HMP contain complex mixtures of different compounds with active, synergistic, complementary, antagonistic or toxic substances (Messina, 2006). In many cases, the active constituents responsible for efficacy are at present unknown. This often makes a confirmation of pharmaceutical and biopharmaceutical quality difficult (Myhre, 2000). Due to the insufficient definition of the active ingredient, evidence of the therapeutic equivalence of different HDP in bioavailability studies is not possible. Therefore herbal drug preparations are considered as being active ingredients in their total form and do not relate to the active principle, thus underlining the problem of comparability of the results of clinical studies' (Zaenker and Entschladen, 2009). This clearly denominates the probable shortcomings as well as voids in the role of biopharmaceutical equivalence in herbal drug standardization.

Pharmaceutical and Biopharmaceutical Equivalents

According to the Note for Guidance on the investigation of bioavailability and bioequivalence (Loew et al., 2000) medicinal products are pharmaceutically equivalent if they contain the same amount of the same active substance(s) in the same dosage forms that meet the same or comparable standards. These principles of pharmaceutical similarity applied to chemically defined drugs should also be applied to HDP as far as possible. The quality and quantity of a HMP depends on different factors (Commission of the European Communities, 1988; EMEA, 2001; 2002): the starting material, effect of geographic origin on the composition of plant material, free as possible from pesticides and diseases in order to guarantee healthy plant growth, natural fluctuations, collection and/or cultivation, harvesting, primary processing, washing, cutting, fumigation, freezing, distillation, drying etc. GAP (good agricultural practice), in particular the solvents used for extraction, the manufacturing process, control of the finished products, stability and GMP (good manufacturing practice). In this context the quality of herbal medicinal products is characterized (Quality of Herbal Remedies, 1998) as follows.

Since a herbal drug product is comparable to an active pharmaceutical ingredient (API) (Handa, 1995; Dhawan et al., 2002), therefore in order to bring various API's under one umbrella a look out for the herbal drug ingredients has been categorized depending on the pharmaceutical, analytical, pharmacological-toxicological and clinical findings (Petrinin, 2002):

A. Extracts containing constituents (single or groups) that are solely responsible for the known and acknowledged/well documented therapeutic activity. Adjustment (standardisation) to a defined content is acceptable.

B1. Extracts containing chemically defined constituents (single or groups) possessing relevant pharmacological properties (active markers). These substances are likely to contribute to the clinical efficacy; however, evidence that they are solely responsible for the clinical efficacy is not yet available. The characterisation of these extracts should take into consideration as far as possible the particular state of knowledge concerning the documented efficacy, quality and safety of an extract. Standardisation by blending different lots of a herbal drug before extraction, or by mixing different lots of herbal drug preparations is appropriate. Adjustment using excipients is not acceptable.

B2. Extracts containing no constituents documented as being determinant or relevant for efficacy, or as having pharmacological or clinical relevance. In these cases, chemically defined constituents (markers) without known therapeutic activity may be used for control purposes. These markers may be used to monitor good manufacturing practice or as an indication for the assay/content of the drug product.

Therefore the category from 3(B2) to 1(A1) can be achieved if a standardization approach is appropriately adopted, depending on the recommended techniques adopted by the manufacturer of herbal API's. Although, there are only a very few plant drugs that can be placed in the category A and therefore unless most of the therapeutically used drugs are tested and brought under the level A, it would be a big question to answer for their complete bioequivalence determination (Quality control methods for medicinal plant, 1998).

Bringing these herbal drugs into the category of API also involve the following contentions:

a. Pharmaceutical equivalence, i.e. raw material quality, extraction, manufacturing process, standardization.

b. Biopharmaceutical equivalence, i.e. the same extract/extract fractions, the same presentation form, the same dose, *in vitro* qualitative and quantitative conformity.

c. Equivalence in bioassays with regard to the pharmacological profile, i.e. the same profile in cell cultures, isolated receptor systems, enzymes, isolated organs and in the whole animal.

d. Bioequivalence in pharmacokinetics with regard to the rate and extent of the active substance.

e. Bioequivalence in effect kinetics, i.e. in clinical and pharmacological models.

f. If none of these conditions are fulfilled then it is a requisite to conduct controlled clinical studies according to the accepted guidelines on clinical efficacy and safety, as per the Pharmacopoeia guidelines (Handa, 1995; Loew and Kadzskin, 2002; Waldesch, 2003;).

Limitations for a bioequivalence determination in HDPS

The search for an indirect evidence via bioequivalence studies with herbal drugs is a logical step specially in cases where such evidence is a prerequisite for registration of a product or an incluson in monogaph (DeSmet and Brouwers, 1991). Although, it is worth understanding that it is one of the prime requirements that the product under investigation is in itself well understood and defined (Zhang et al., 2008). In general, a bioequivalence study in herbal drugs encompasses the measurement of a surrogate end point, especially when the substance under investigation is a marker isolated from the herbal drug mixture or extract (Ozaki et al., 1993). As a burgeoning question in the modern scientific scenario is the lack of herbal drugs that have been studied systematically, a few well studied examples include *Silybium marianum, Piper longum, Aesculus hippocastanum* etc. However it is very clear in the studies conducted on these herbs as well as there are numerous other constituents having biological activity in comparison to their original markers (vanErp et al., 2005; Gurley et al., 2006; Kunz et al., 1998; Sirtori, 2001, Bassler et al., 2003).

As an example for the study conducted on horse chest nut, the extract was standardized to 16-20% if aescin content. In a single dose and four multiple dose immunological assay a variation based on steady state concentrations, clearly demarcated the tat that bioequivalence parameters especially from a immunological perspective holds serious limitations. (Schroedter et al., 1998).

A careful and well conceived use of bioavailability or bioequivalence data is very necessary, especially when regulatory considerations have to be kept in mind. In this context there has been a misleading concept about using the chemical markers towards standardizing the pharmacological activity and especially drawing out the bioequivalence (van Die et al., 2009). Markers are by definition chemically defined substances that are useful in calculating the quantity of herbal drug in a preparation or a finished herbal product. An example to this can be illustatered by discussing the case of *Hypericum perforatum* (Brattstorm et al., 2009). Hypericin, which is a chemical marker for standardization of *H. perforatum* extract was also considered as biological marker for the purpose of biorquivalence determination as it had potent anti-depressive properties. In later findings another component, hyperforin was found to be active as well, and therefore the whole question of corealting bioequivalence to hypericin content came under serious debate (Rahimi et al., 2009).

Since in herbal drugs the overall effectiveness may be a result of complex self regulatory components henceforth, in an attempt to rationalize the concept of bioequivalence in herbal drugs the following guidelines were laid out for oral immediate release form drugs not requring *in vivo* studies (Chaudhary, 1992):

a. The active substance does not have a narrow therapeutic range.

b. It has a first pass metabolism > 70% and linear pharmacokinetics within the therapeutic range.

c. It is highly water soluble.

d. It is highly permeable in the intestine.

e. The formulation is not expected to have effects on pharmacokinetic parameters.

It is prominent that an evidence based bioequivalence studies are very difficult if not impossible, and although use of ultramodern analytical apparatuses may have made the estimation easier, there is a lot that needs to be done for a universally acceptable approach to be developed. Therefore there are in general the following three issues of major concern while evaluating the bioequivalence paramters for herbal drugs (Indian Herbal Pharmaceopoeia, 1998).

Important parameters for bio/pharmaceutical equivalence of herbal product (Petrini, 2002; Hamburger, 2007)

a. Pharmaceutical equivalence, which is dependent on raw material quality, extraction methodology, chemical standardization of extraction procedure, manufacturing processes and machinery involved etc.

b. Biopharmaceutical equivalence: Effect of same dosages and heir biological effect relication.

c. Therapeutic equivalence.

Therapeutic Equivalene as a complimenting factor to bio-equivalence (Sirtori, 2001)

According to the European as well as WHO guidelines (1998) a medicinal product is therapeutically equivalent with another product if it contains the same active substance or therapeutic moiety and, clinically, shows the same effectiveness and safety as those products, whose effectiveness and safety have been established. To demonstrate the therapeutic equivalence. Therefore as a complementary evaluation for bioequivalence a therapeutic equivalence determination involves the following determinations (Loew and Kaszkin, 2002):

Direct evidence: Clinical studies with primary and secondary end points regarding effectiveness or clinical studies with pharmacodynamic and surrogates as end points.

Indirect evidence: Confirmation of bioequivalence in clinical pharmacokinetic studies via surrogates AUC (quantity of absorption), Cmax (maximum concentration) and *t*max (rate of absorption) located within the confidence interval. Pharmacological profiles in animal models. *In vitro* studies in cell systems regarding influence on receptors, enzymes, channels (Loew and Kaszkin, 2002).

In practice indirect evidence, using pharmacokinetic surrogates for bioequivalence, is generally the most appropriate procedure to substantiate the therapeutic equivalence between medicinal products. Two medicinal products are bioequivalent if they are pharmaceutically equivalent and their bioavailability (rate and extent) after administration in the same molar dose are similar to such a degree that their effects, with respect to both efficacy and safety, will be essentially the same. Bioequivalence is based on the measured concentrations of the parent compound or an active metabolite in plasma or urine. Parameters of importance for equivalence are Cmax (maximal concentration), the shape of and the area under the concentration versus time curves (AUC) or the cumulative renal excretion and excretion rate in multiplicative models. Bioequivalence is assumed, if the 90% confidence interval of the ratio (test/reference) for the parameters AUC and Cmax lies within the range of 0.80–1.25 (log transformed data). In the case of Cmax a broader interval may be acceptable and must be prospectively defined, e.g. 0.70–1.43 (Quality of Medicinal Herbal Drugs, 1998).

Examples for bioequivalence studies from natural products

Gingko biloba is one of the highly studied herbal medicinal plant and a very good example for the application of bioequivalence studies in herbal drug standardization. Gingko extracts are approved by the German Commission E monograph for usefuless in treatment of dementia, vertigo and tinnitus. In gerenal, the product specifications fort his plant include dry extract of the dried leaf, manufactured using acetone/water with subsequent purification Steps, without the addition of concentrates or isolated ingredients and with a drug/extract ratio of 35 to 67:1 an average of around 50:1 (Kressman et al., 2002).

A bioequivalence study carried out by Müller and Blume compared the bioavailabilities of two gingko extarcts, both characterized as containing 24% flavonol glycosides on their labels. While, product A released less than 33% of ist triterpene lactone contents in 60 minutes, product B released 99 per cent in 15 minutes. Both products were administered to 12 healthy individuals and using a crossover trial design. The concentration of ginkolides A, B and bilobalide were measured in blood. A statistically significant maximum plasma concentration, and area under the cuves were obtained for product B. Statistical analyis using 90% confidence interval clearly revealed that the two products were not bioequivalent.

Therefore, it is clear that a bioequivalence study could provide some important to the question like a similar claim composition leads to different biological profile and a biological activity as well (Saw et al., 2006).

CONCLUSION

The quality of herbal medicinal products is an indicator as well as governing authority for the pharmacodynamic activities of the herbal drug and thus the therapeutic effects (Kamboj, 2000). It is understandable that the effect arising from natural sources are unavoidable yet with modern analytical techniques equipped with state of the art manufacturing procedures, reproducible herbal medicinal products are not a dream any more (Powell et al., 1996). A complex-structure activity does exist but with the availability of molecular modelling strategies such problems can be circumvented (Owuse-Agyei et al., 2007). There is a much better chance to understand the herbal drugs at molecular levels with the advancements in microscopic, biotechnological and analytical techniques. As an addition, phytotherapy research has proceeded dramatically with respect to identification and isolation of plant constituents regarding effectiveness and toxicity (Ozaki et al., 1993). As a consequence the pharmaceutical quality of HMP has clearly improved, which has opened the possibility of investigating standardized HDP in experimental and clinical studies. With the proof of extract-specific effectiveness the question of transferability of effects obtained with well-studied extracts to phytogenerics arises. Bioequivalence/therapeutic equivalence determination is an excellent option to bypass this issue, however, this concept mostly failed for HDP because of the complexity of special extracts (Will-Shahab et al., 2009). A prerequisite for an effect is the presence of the substance in the circulation and at the place of action (British Herbal Pharmacopoiea, 1996). In contrast to chemically defined drugs bioequivalence studies for HDP are nearly impossible due to the complexity of herbal drugs (Yamamoto et al., 2003). In summary, more detailed studies on the qualitative and quantitative analysis of the active principle(s) in HMP (Blume and Schug, 2000; DeSmet and Brouwers, 1999) as well as biopharmaceutical, pharmacokinetic and effect-kinetic studies of extracts are necessary for the development of herbal drugs or their formulations to achieve repeatable excellent perfomances in clinical trials and clinical usage.

REFERENCES

Al-Akoum M, Maunsell E, Verreault R, Provencher L, Otis H, Dodin S. Effects of *Hypericum perfo-*

ratum (St. John's wort) on hot flashes and quality of life in perimenopausal women, a randomized pilot trial. *Menopause* 16, 307-314, (2009).

Amira OC, Okubadejo NU. Frequency of complementary and alternative medicine utilization in hypertensive patients attending an urban tertiary care centre in Nigeria. *BMC Complement Altern Med*, 7, 30, (2007).

Annesley TM, Matz K, Leichtman AB. High-performance liquid chromatographic analysis of cyclosporin G, (Nva2-cyclosporine) in human blood. *Ther Drug Monit* 14, 397-401, (1992).

Bassler D, Okpanyi S, Schrodter A, Loew D, Schurer M, Schulz HU. Bioavailability of beta-aescin from horse chestnut seed extract, comparative clinical studies of two Galenic formulations. *Adv Ther* 20, 295-304, (2003).

Bhutani KK. Fingerprinting of Ayurvedic Drugs, *The Eastern Pharmacist*, 21-26, (2000).

Blume HH, Schlag B. Biopharmaceutical characterisation of herbal medicinal products, are in vivo studies necessary? *Eur J Metabol Pharmacokinetics*, 25, 1-8, (2000).

Bournot P, Es-souni M, Ramirez LC. Chromatographic and mass spectrometric characteristics of 20-dihydroaldosterone. *Steroids* 57, 480-484, (1992).

Brattstrom A. Long-term effects of St. John's wort (*Hypericum perforatum*) treatment, a 1-year safety study in mild to moderate depression. *Phytomedicine* 16, 277-283, (2009).

British Herbal Pharmacopoeia, British Herbal Medicine Association, (1996).

Chaudhury RR. Herbal Medicine for Human Health, World Health Organization, New Delhi, 51-57, (1992).

Chauhan BL, Mitra SK, Mohan AR, Gopumadhavan S, Anturlikar SD. Development of high performance thin layer chromatography fingerprint technique and bioassay to establish the self life of a proprietary herbal formulation, (PHF), an Ayurvedi formulation containing multiple ingredients of herbal origin, *Indian Drugs*, 31, 333-338, (1994).

Dhawan K, Kumar S, Sharma A. Comparative anxiolytic activity profile of various preparations of Passiflora incarnata linneaus, a comment on medicinal plants' standardization. *J Altern Complement Med* 8, 283-291, (2002).

EMEA. Note for guidance on quality of herbal medicinal products, EMEA/CVMP/814/00, London. (2001).

EMEA. Points to consider on Good Agricultural and Collection Practises, (GACP) for starting material of herbal origin, EMEA/HMP-WP/3131/99Rev 3, London. (2002).

Fischer C, Buhl K. Gas chromatography/mass spectrometry validation of high-performance liquid chromatography analysis of flecainide enantiomers in serum. *Ther Drug Monit* 14, 433-435, (1992).

Fushimi R, Tachi J, Amino N, Miyai K. Chinese medicine interfering with digoxin immunoassays. *Lancet*, 339, (1989).

Gao XY, Jiang Y, Lu JQ, Tu PF. One single standard substance for the determination of multiple anthraquinone derivatives in rhubarb using high-performance liquid chromatography-diode array detection. *J Chromatogr A* 1216, 2118-2123, (2009).

German R, Bukowska B, Pajchel G, Grzybowska W, Tyski S. Extremely long time stability study of selected antibiotic standards. J Pharm Biomed Anal, (2009).

Good Agricultural and Collection Practices, Document No. WHO/TRM/91.4, World Health Organization, Geneva, (1991).

Gryniewicz CM, Reepmeyer JC, Kauffman JF, Buhse, L.F. Detection of undeclared erectile dysfunction drugs and analogues in dietary supplements by ion mobility spectrometry. *J Pharm Biomed Anal* 49, 601-606, (2009).

Gupta S. Buyer beware. Taking an herbal supplement can sometimes do more harm than it does good. *Time*, 169, 58, (2007).

Gurley BJ, Barone GW, Williams DK, Carrier J, Breen P, Yates CR, Song PF, Hubbard MA, Tong Y, Cheboyina S. Effect of milk thistle ,(Silybum marianum) and black cohosh ,(Cimicifuga racemosa) supplementation on digoxin pharmacokinetics in humans. *Drug Metab Dispos* 34, 69-74 (2006).

Ha WY, Yau FCF, But PPH, Wang J, Shaw PC. Direct Amplification of Length Polymorphism Analysis Differentiates *Panax ginseng* from *P. quinquefolius*, *Planta Med*, 67, 587-589, (2001).

Hamburger M. New approaches in analyzing the pharmacological properties of herbal extracts. *Proc West Pharmacol Soc* 50, 156-161, (2007).

Handa SS, Quality Control and Standardization of Herbal Raw Materials and Traditional Remedies, Pharmatimes, 13-21, (1995).

Hussain K, Ismail Z, Sadikun A, Ibrahim P. Standardization and In Vivo Antioxidant Activity of Ethanol Extracts of Fruit and Leaf of Piper sarmentosum. *Planta Med*, (2009).

Indian Herbal Pharmacopoeia, Vol. I, A Joint Publication of RRL, Jammu Tawi and IDMA, Mumbai, (1998) *J Laryngol Otol*, 122, 1360-1364, (2008).

Kamboj VP. Herbal Medicine, *Current Science*, 78,(1), 35-39, (2000).

Kamei A, Hisada T, Iwata S. The evaluation of therapeutic efficacy of hachimi-jio-gan ,(traditional Chinese medicine) to rat galactosemic cataract. *J Ocul Pharmacol* 3, 239-248, (1987).

Kidd P, Head K, A review of the bioavailability and clinical efficacy of milk thistle phytosome, a silybin-phosphatidylcholine complex ,(Siliphos). *Altern Med Rev* 10, 193-203, (2005).

Kressmann S, Biber A, Wonnemann M, Schug B, Blume HH, Muller WE. Influence of pharmaceutical quality on the bioavailability of active components from Ginkgo biloba preparations. *J Pharm Pharmacol* 54, 1507-1514, (2002).

Kunz K, Lorkowski G, Petersen G, Samcova E, Schaffler K, Wauschkuhn CH. Bioavailability of escin after administration of two oral formulations containing aesculus extract. *Arzneimittelforschung*, 48, 822-825, (1998).

Lazarowych NJ, Pekos P. Use of fingerprinting and marker compounds for identification and standardization of Botanical Drugs, Strategies for applying pharmaceautical HPLC analysis to Herbal Products, *Drug Information Journal*, 32, 497-512, (1998).

Linde K. St. John's wort for depression—development of a Cochrane review from 1993 to 1996, *Z Evid Fortbild Qual Gesundhwes* 102, 487-492, (1997).

Loew D, Kaszkin M. Approaching the problem of bioequivalence of herbal medicinal products. *Phytother Res* 16, 705-711, (2002).

Loew D, Schrödter A, Schwankll W. and März RW. Measurement of the bioavailability of aescin-containing extracts. *Methods and Findings in Experimental Clinical Pharmacology*, 22, 537-542, (2000).

Messina BA. Herbal supplements, Facts and myths—talking to your patients about herbal supplements. *J Perianesth Nurs* 21, 268-278; quiz 279-28, (2006).

Myhre MJ. Herbal remedies, nephropathies, and renal disease. *Nephrol Nurs* J 27, 473-478; quiz 479-480, (2000).

Owusu-Agyei S, Awini E, Anto F, Mensah-Afful T, Adjuik M, Hodgson A, Afari E, Binka F. Assessing malaria control in the Kassena-Nankana district of northern Ghana through repeated surveys using the RBM tools. *Malar J*, 6, 103, (2007).

Ozaki Y, Suzuki H, Satake M. Comparative studies on concentration of berberine in plasma after oral administration of coptidis rhizoma extract, its cultured cells extract, and combined use of these extracts and glycyrrhizae radix extract in rats. *Yakugaku Zasshi* 113, 63-69, (1993).

Pakzad K, Boucher BA, Kreiger N, Cotterchio M. The use of herbal and other non-vitamin, non-mineral supplements among pre- and post-menopausal women in Ontario. *Can J Public Health*, 98, 383-388, (2007).

Petrini O. Clinical development of phytopharmaceuticals. *Wien Med Wochenschr* 152, 204-208, (2002).

Powell W, Morgante M, Andre C, Hanafey M, Vogel J, Tingey S, Rafalski A. The comparison of RFLP, RAPD, AFLP and SSR (microsatellite) markers for germplasm analysis, *Mol. Breed*, 2, 225-238, (1996).

Pulpati H, Biradar YS, Rajani M. High-performance thin-layer chromatography densitometric method for the quantification of harmine, harmaline, vasicine, and vasicinone in *Peganum harmala. J AOAC Int* 91, 1179-1185, (2008).

Quality Control Methods for Medicinal Plants Materials, Document No.WHO/PHARMA/92.559/ rev.1, World Health Organization, Geneva, (1998).

Quality of herbal remedies. Directive 75/318/EEC. 1998, Part 2, London. (1998).

Rahimi R, Nikfar S, Abdollahi M. Efficacy and tolerability of Hypericum perforatum in major depressive disorder in comparison with selective serotonin reuptake inhibitors, a meta-analysis. *Prog Neuropsychopharmacol Biol Psychiatry* 33, 118-127, (2009).

Rose G Why do patients with rheumatoid arthritis use complementary therapies? *Musculoskeletal Care* 4, 101-115, (2006).

Rout KK, Pradhan S, Mishra SK. Estimation of berberine in ayurvedic formulations containing Berberis aristata. *J AOAC Int* 91, 1149-1153, (2008).

Sangwan RS, Sangwan NS, Jain DC, Kumar S, Ranade S.A. RAPD profile based genetic characterization of chemotypic variants of *Artemisia annua* L. ,(J.), *Biochem. Mol. Biol. Int.* 47, 935-944. (2002).

Savaiano J, The Top Issues & Opportunities in Dietary Supplements, Nutraceutical World, 9, 34-43, (2006).

Saw JT, Bahari MB, Ang HH, Lim YH. Herbal use amongst multiethnic medical patients in Penang Hospital, pattern and perceptions. *Med J Malaysia* 61, 422-432, (2006).

Sawalha AF. Complementary and alternative medicine, (CAM) in Palestine, use and safety implications. *J Altern Complement Med*, 13, 263-269, (2007).

Schrödter A, Loew D, Schwankl W. und Rietbrock, N. Zur Validität radioimmunologisch bestimmter Bioverfügbarkeitsdaten von â-aescin in Rosskastaniensamenextrakten. *Arzneim.-Forsch,* (1998).

Shakeel M, Newton JR, Bruce J, Ah-See KW. Use of complementary and alternative medicine by patients attending a head and neck oncology clinic.

Sharma HC, Crouch JH, Sharma KK, Seetharama N, Hash CT, Application of biotechnology for crop improvement prospects and constraints, *Plant Sci*, 163, 381-395, (2002).

Sirtori CE. Aescin, pharmacology, pharmacokinetics and therapeutic profile. *Pharmacological Research*, 44, 183-193 ,(2001).

Sirtori CR. Aescin, pharmacology, pharmacokinetics and therapeutic profile. *Pharmacol Res* 44, 183-193, (2001).

Van Die MD, Bone KM, Burger HG, Reece JE, Teede HJ. Effects of a combination of *Hypericum perforatum and Vitex agnus-castus* on PMS-like symptoms in late-perimenopausal women, findings from a subpopulation analysis. *J Altern Complement Med* 15, 1045-1048, (2009).

Van Erp NP, Baker SD, Zhao M, Rudek MA, Guchelaar HJ, Nortier JW, Sparreboom A, Gelderblom H. Effect of milk thistle, (Silybum marianum) on the pharmacokinetics of irinotecan. Clin Cancer Res 11, 7800-7806, (2005).

Vieira RF, Grayer RJ, Paton A, Simon JE. Genetic diversity of *Ocimum gratissimum* L. based on volatile oil constituents, flavonoids and RAPD markers, *Biochem. Syst. Ecol.*, 2001, 29, 287-304, (2001).

Waldesch FG, Konigswinter BS, Remagen HB, Herbal Medicinal Products Scientific and Regulatory Basis for Development Quality Assurance and Marketing Authorisation, Published by Medpharm Stuttagart and CRC Press, Washington D.C., 37-52, (2002).

Weina PJ. Artemisinins from folklore to modern medicine—transforming an herbal extract to life-saving drugs. *Parasitologia* 50, 25-29, (2008).

Welsh J, McClelland M. Genomic fingerprints produced by PCR with consensus tRNA gene primers, *Nucleic Acids Res*,19, 861-866, (1991).

WHO Expert Committee on specifications for pharmaceutical preparations. World Health Organ Tech Rep Ser 863, 1-194,(2006) WHO expert committee on specifications for pharmaceutical preparations. Fortieth report.

Will-Shahab L, Bauer S, Kunter U, Roots I, Brattstrom A. St John's wort extract (Ze 117) does not alter the pharmacokinetics of a low-dose oral contraceptive. *Eur J Clin Pharmacol* 65, 287-294, (2009).

Yamamoto Y, Majima T, Saiki I, Tani T. Pharmaceutical evaluation of Glycyrrhiza uralensis roots cultivated in eastern Nei-Meng-Gu of China. *Biol Pharm Bull* 26, 1144-1149, (2003).

Yue Y, Zhang R, Fan W, Tang F. High-performance thin-layer chromatographic analysis of selected organophosphorous pesticide residues in tea. *J AOAC Int* 91, 1210-1217, (2008).

Zaenker KS, Entschladen F. Paving roads for new drugs in oncology. *Recent Pat Anticancer Drug Discov* 4, 137-145, (2009).

Zhang SH, Zhou YD, He HX. Bioequivalence of enteric coated tablet of Zhengqing Fengtongning]. *Zhongguo Zhong Yao Za Zhi* 33, 683-685, (2008).

Zhao, G. Tests of non-null hypothesis on proportions for stratified data. *Stat Med* 27, 1429-1446, (2008).

chapter 31

Free Radicals and Human Diseases

Manjula Rai, Gunjan Biswas, Subhash C. Mandal and Krishnendu Acharya

INTRODUCTION

Over the past two decades there has been an almost overwhelming increase in the volume of scientific and medical literature relating nutritional factors to most of mankind's degenerative and killer diseases.

Paralleling this growth is the evidence that oxidation generated free radical reactions are involved in most, if not at all, of these disorders. Evidence is also mounting that co-existing with aging and degeneration, antioxidant defense mechanisms decline due to reduced intake, increased utilization and excessive loss. The hypothesis that excessive free radical oxidative reactions acting inappropriately in the cell and over consuming protective or buffering antioxidant nutrients is the molecular basis to degenerative disease, still remains to be fully tested. The contention that the use of antioxidants in the prevention and treatment of many diseases is not scientifically substantiated can not be upheld any longer in view of substantial body of epidemiologic, case control, cohort and double-blind studies published.

If there actually is a strong component of free radical activity in degenerative disease, and this can be shown to be caused by depletion of suitable antioxidant reserves and repletion of the reserves can be achieved by maintaining a suitable antioxidant balance with specific compounds, the future of medicine and healthcare may depend more on nutritional medicine.

Free radicals and there oxidation products have been detected in most diseased states. Free radicals are highly reactive unpaired electrons which cause oxidation of metabolites in the body resulting in cell death and tissue injury (Cheeseman and Slater, 1993). Electrons are more stable when paired together in orbitals: the two electrons in a pair have different directions of spin. Hence, radicals are generally less stable than nonradicals, although their reactivity varies. The free radicals are capable of reacting indiscriminately with any molecules with which they come in contact. Once radicals are formed they can either react with another radical or with another nonradical molecule by various interactions.

Formation of free radicals

Free radicals are basically formed as accidental and deliberate byproducts and phagocytosis from oxygen, H_2O_2, etc. Some of them are superoxide ($O_2^{-\cdot}$), hydroxyl ($OH^{\cdot}$), etc (Cheeseman and Slater, 1993). Independent on the identity of the cellular O_2-activator, the initial reduction product is always a super-oxide radical. SOD, which is present in all cells, destabilizes $O_2^{-\bullet}$ by a diffusion-limited dismutation of two $O_2^{-\bullet}$ to H_2O_2 and O_2 (Figure 31.1). Due to cellular compartmentation of SOD, $O_2^{-\bullet}$ radicals are not expected to be totally metabolized to H_2O_2 (Loschen *et al.*, 1973). This is also the case with H_2O_2 which is a substrate for both catalase and glutathione-peroxidase (GSH-POD). H_2O_2 which escapes detoxification by the latter enzymes may become subject to the transfer of a further electron thereby forming $OH^\bullet$ radicals; these are the most reactive metabolites known in biological systems.

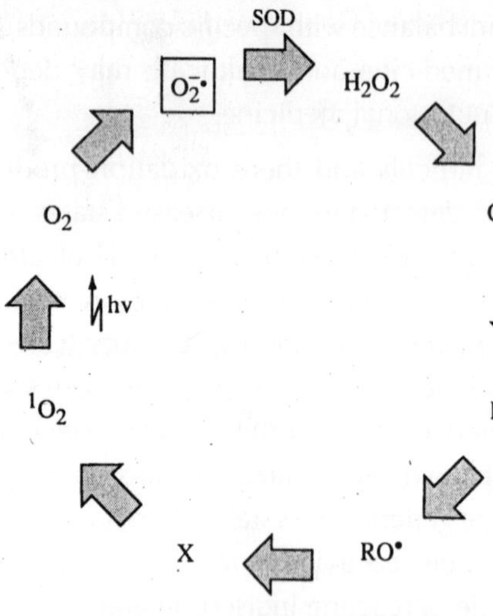

Fig. 31.1: Generation sequence of reactive oxygen species following univalent reduction of oxygen.

Due to its extremely high reaction potential, diffusion of $OH^\bullet$ from its site of generation can be excluded. Consequently respective reaction products are expected to be formed in close proximity to $OH^\bullet$ generation sites. The most frequent reaction product stems from an interaction of $OH^\bullet$ with membrane-phospholipids. The first step in this reaction sequence is a hydrogen-abstract from the divinyl-methane structure of polyunsaturated fatty acid and the subsequent addition of an O_2-molecule, resulting in the formation of peroxyl-radical. This peroxyl-radical can enter a chain reaction forming an alkoxyl-radical by a bimolecular reaction and O_2 in an excited state (singlet state). Vitamin E in cooperation with Vitamin C is able to terminate selfsustaining chain reaction either by a direct interaction with $OH^\bullet$ or by the chemical reduction of propagating organic radical intermediates. The excited state of singlet oxygen ($^1O_2$) is unstable and will lead to photo-emission by mono- or dimol reactions. Alternatively, the energy can be transmitted directly to other molecules such as carbonyl groups, which are in turn transferred into an excited state (singlet or triplet state) (Nohl, 1993).

Presence of transition metals is essential for free radical formation in most cases (Cheeseman and Slater, 1993). Antioxidants present in foods counter the action of oxygen free radicals which are produced under a number of circumstances. They are also formed as a part of body's normal metabolic process. Synthetic (xenobiotic) chemicals, radiation, x rays, pollution and even stress can produce these damaging entities. The chemicals known to produce free radicals include chlorinated hydrocarbons, aromatic hydrocarbons, industrial acids, solvents, most pesticides and herbicides, preservatives in foods, printing pigments and inks and other industrial chemicals, fragrances and perfume vehicles, cosmetic vehicles and cosmetics, pollutants in air and water, many if not all pharmacological agents used in medicine and anesthetics, which have a profound effect in producing radicals in the central nervous system. Even the transitional metal catalysts iron and copper, which are ubiquitous, have a most powerful generating effect on chain initiating radicals. Chemical mobilization of fat stores under various conditions such as lactation, exercise, fever, infection and even fasting, can result in increased radical activity and damage in particular to the immune and nervous systems.

Under conditions of continuing and excessive emotional stress, higher levels of the hormones adrenaline and nor adrenaline are secreted by the adrenal glands. As a natural part of their metabolic processing, these stress hormones are oxidized to simpler molecules and in doing so become free radicals. It is possible, through this increased production of hormone radicals that stress increased biological degenerative processes occur resulting in wide-spread molecular, cell and tissue damage (Sosa *et al.*, 2002).

In the living organism, free radical chain reactions are produced normally in the mitochondrial respiratory chain, liver mixed function oxidases, by bactericidal leucocytes, through xanthene oxidase activity, by atmospheric pollutants, and from transitional metal catalysts, drugs and xenobiotic chemicals.

Superoxide is formed by the reaction of oxygen with an electron.

$$O_2 + e^- \rightarrow O_2^{-\bullet}$$

Superoxide on reaction with hydrogen peroxide yields hydroxyl radical with the liberation of oxygen.

$$O_2^{-\bullet} + H_2O_2 \rightarrow OH^\bullet + OH^- + O_2$$

Oxygen on reaction with 2 electrons yields hydrogen peroxide.

$$O_2 + 2e^- + 2H^+ \rightarrow H_2O_2$$

Hydrogen peroxide is itself uncharged but is called reactive oxygen species (ROS) due to its highly reactive nature. Two superoxide ions may also react together to yield hydrogen peroxide and oxygen. This is known as dismutation reaction.

$$2O_2^{-\bullet} + 2H^+ \rightarrow H_2O_2 + O_2$$

Hydrogen peroxide in the presence of transition metals like Fe^{2+} forms hydroxyl radical which is known as Haber Weiss reaction (Halliwell and Gutteridge, 1990).

$$H_2O_2 + Fe^{2+} \rightarrow OH^\bullet + OH^- + Fe^{3+}$$

General effects of free radicals

Free radicals decompose enzymes, sequester proteins, scavenge different metabolic compounds. But they are hard to study due to their short life span. Their life-span may range from a few nanoseconds to one or two seconds only. However during the period of time they are present, they can do untold damage to biological systems including DNA, macromolecules such as proteins, lipids and intracellular organelles such as mitochondria, Golgi apparatus and lysosomes. They are also induced by several external agents. A classic example is carbon tetrachloride (CCl_4) (Poli *et al.*, 1987). It is believed that CCl_4 causes hepatic toxicity by free radical attack. Lipids are most susceptible to free radical attack. They cause extensive lipid peroxidation. Lipids are present in the cell membrane in the form of poly unsaturated fatty acids or PUFA. Lipid peroxidation triggers a chain of degenerating events. It directly leads to decomposition of membrane. Indirectly, they lead to formation of other highly reactive harmful aldehydes (Esterbauer *et al.*, 1990; Porter, 1990). Peroxidation is also believed to be responsible for atherosclerosis (Lang and Esterbauer, 1991). It has less effect directly on proteins. But formation of lens crystallin proteins in the eye by peroxidation is believed to be caused by peroxidation of lipid leading to cataract (Seccia *et al.*, 1991; Spector, 1985). It has a direct and more expansive effect on DNA which may be the cause of cancer (Fraga *et al.*, 1990; Kasai and Nishimura, 1991). Its effect on DNA may be considered to be causing indirect effect on the protein constituents of the cell.

Defences against free radical attack

Defences against the free radical attack may be basically categorized into two (Cotgreave *et al.*, 1988):

1. prevent the production of free radicals.
2. intercept or scavenge the produced free radicals.

One way of preventing the production of free radicals is to sequester transition metal ions required for their formation. Hydrogen peroxide, lipid peroxides formed during lipid peroxidation may be removed by catalase and glutathione peroxidase (GSH) enzymes found in peroxisomes and cytosol respectively leading to prevention of further damage.

Scavenging of preformed free radicals may be done by the enzyme super oxide dismutase (SOD). α-tocopherol (major unit of vitamin E), ubiquinol, ascorbic acid (vitamin C), uric acid, glutathione, etc. also perform this function (Burton *et al.*, 1983a; Burton *et al.*, 1983b; Burton and Ingold, 1986; Cotgreave *et al.*, 1988; Stocker *et al.*, 1991; Stocker and Frei, 1991). α-tocopherol is called chain breaking antioxidant.

ROLE OF FREE RADICALS IN HUMAN DISEASES

Free radicals and atherosclerosis

Free radicals have a profound link with atherosclerosis. The development of atherosclerosis is a multifactorial process in which both elevated plasma cholesterol levels and proliferation of smooth cells play a central role. Atherogenesis is an alteration of the artery wall that includes two major phases:

1. adhesion of monocytes to the endothelium, their migration to the sub endothelial space and differentiation into macrophages. These cells oxidized low density lipoproteins and through this process they are transformed into foam cells.
2. vascular smooth muscle cell migration from the media into the intima and their proliferation with the formation of atherosclerotic plaques.

Reactive oxygen species have been implicated as key processes of atherosclerosis, including oxidative modification of low density lipoprotein and endothelial dysfunction, thereby promoting a vascular inflammatory response. Angiotensin II is a major stimulator of vascular reactive oxygen species production. Angiotensin II stimulates the production of the ROS from both arterial smooth muscle cells and endothelial cells. Thus, there is substantial evidence implicating that vascular NADPH oxidase stimulated, at least in part, by angiotensin II is a major vascular source of ROS in atherosclerosis (Ishiro-Fukai *et al.*, 1996).

More recent data also show that ROS is critically involved in angiotensin II inducing pro-inflammatory effects in vascular cells. In endothelial cells, the expression of the leucocyte adhesion molecules VCAM–1 is potently induced by angiotensin II (Landmesser and Drexler, 2005). These data support the hypothesis that ROS formation is critical for vascular inflammation – basic pathogenetic mechanism of atherosclerosis.

Recently studies suggest that oxidative modification of low density lipoprotein is a critical factor for atherogenesis and designated as the "bad actor in the free radical hypothesis of atherosclerosis".

LDL may be oxidatively modified by all major cell types of the arterial wall, including endothelial cells, smooth muscle cells, and macrophages (Fruchart and Duriez, 1994; Parthasaratry and Rankin, 1992; Morel *et al.*, 1984) via their extracellular release of reactive oxygen species (ROS). Hydroxyl radical (thus formed) may initiate the peroxidation of long-chain polyunsaturated fatty acids within LDL molecule, giving rise to conjugated dienes and lipid hydroperoxy radicals ($LOO^{\bullet}$) This process is self-propagating, such that $LOO^{\bullet}$ can attack adjacent fatty acids until complete fatty acid chain fragmentation occurs. A number of highly reactive products then accumulate in the LDL particle, including malondialdehyde and lysophosphatides. These products interact with the amino side chain of the apoprotein B 100 and modify it to form new epitopes that are not recognized by the LDL receptor. OxLDL is avidly taken up by subendothelial macrophages via the "scavenger" receptor pathway which does not recognize native, unmodified LDL. Through the scavenger receptor, unlimited amounts of modified LDL are ingested by the monocyte/macrophage, which is now a "foam cell" in the arterial intima. The "foam cell" recruits more monocyte/macrophages to convert in foam cells (Figure 31.2). Accumulation of LDL-laden foam cells beneath arterial endothelium lays the foundation for the "fatty streak", the earliest histopathological evidence of the development of atherosclerotic plaque (Fruchart and Duriez, 1994). Oxidized LDL also stimulates the release of monocyte-derived TNFα and IL-1β, leading to smooth muscle cell proliferation. Elaboration of collagen and elastin by smooth muscle cells lays the foundation for plaque formation and ultimately fibrosis (Fruchart and Duriez, 1994; Morel *et al.*, 1984). Lipid peroxides also inhibit synthesis of prostacyclin, an antiplatelet-aggregation substance, which can result in platelet adherence and aggregation. Platelets release growth factors, subsequently leading to smooth muscle cell proliferation and migration to intima. Besides, aggregation of platelets lays the foundation for formation of thrombus (Fruchart and Duriez, 1994).

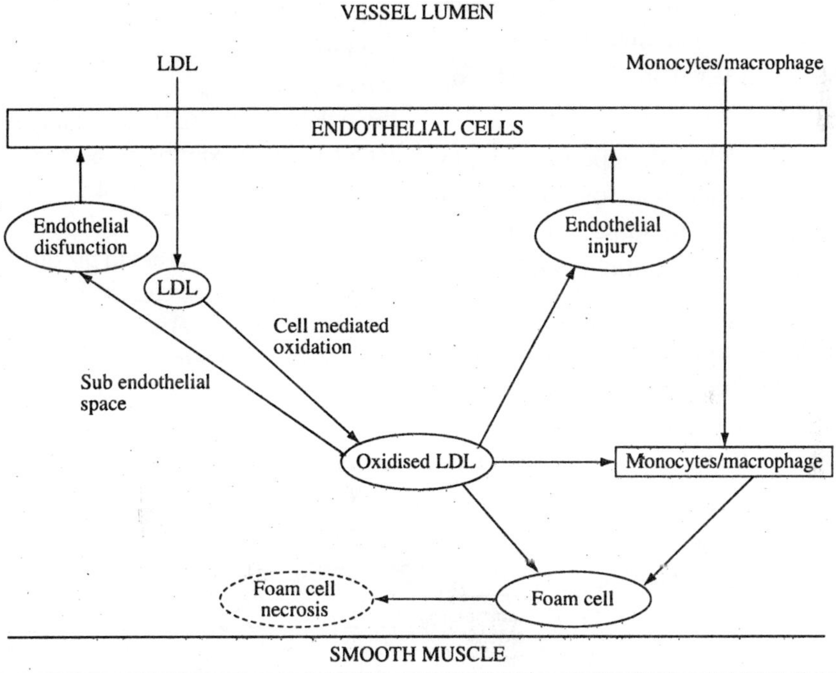

Fig. 31.2: Oxidative modification hypothesis of atherosclerosis

Free radicals in relation to ischemia and reperfusion injury

Myocardial ischemia occurs when myocardial oxygen demand exceeds oxygen supply. Unless reversed, this situation results in cell injury, and clinical event is myocardial infarction. Reperfusion of the ischemic myocardium can restore oxygen and substrates to the ischemic myocardial cells, but this process may create another form of myocardial damage, termed "reperfusion injury" (Bolli, 1992; Ferrari *et al.*, 1993; Bolli, 1991).

Evidence suggests that damage to the myocardial cell induced by the cycle of ischemia and reperfusion may be due, in part, to the generation of toxic, reactive oxygen species such as superoxide radical, hydrogen peroxide, and the hydroxyl radical (Bolli, 1991; Starkopf *et al.*, 1995; Fox, 1992; De Lorgeril *et al.*, 1993; Valen and Vaage, 1993). The active involvement of free radicals in the ischemia-reperfusion damage is demonstrated by direct and indirect experimental evidences. Direct evidences arise from the possibility of measuring radicals in myocardial tissue by electron spin resonance (ESR) and spin trapping methodology (Garlick *et al.*, 1987; Pietri *et al.*, 1989); indirect evidences by the measurement of the products of free radical attack on biological substrates (usually malondialdehyde as a measure of lipid peroxidation extent), and intracellular and extracellular antioxidant capacity (Ytrehus and Hegstad, 1991; Dousset *et al.*, 1983; Coghlan *et al.*, 1993; Tortolani *et al.*, 1993).

Reactive oxygen radicals in reperfusion injury can originate from intracellular sources, such as mitochondria and xanthine oxidase, or from extracellular sources, such as neutrophiles and macrophages.

The rapid decrease of oxygen in ischemic tissue causes a switch from oxidative to anaerobic metabolism. Within minutes of the onset of ischemia, energy demands exceed the heart's capacity to synthesize ATP anaerobically. Energy depletion has fundamental importance in the genesis of subsequent injurious events. Lactate and unbuffered hydrogen ions accumulate in tissue leading to the rapid change in tissue acid-base status. The failure of all energy dependent mechanisms leads to the deterioration of membrane ion gradients, opening of selective and unselective ion channels and equilibration of most intracellular and extracellular ions. As a consequence of this "anoxic depolarization", potassium ions leave the cell, sodium chloride and calcium ions enter. Cellular accumulation of ions causes formation of cytotoxic edema. Intracellular Ca^{2+} overload can also set off a cascade of events which may lead to the formation of ROS. The elevated Ca concentration activates proteases that can convert xanthine dehydrogenase to xanthine oxidase. During reoxygenation, xanthine oxidase can use O_2 as an electron acceptor, leading to formation of superoxide anion ($O_2^{\bullet-}$) and hydrogen peroxide (H_2O_2), which can react to produce hydroxyl radicals ($OH^{\bullet}$). These reactive species are responsible for the tissue damage. Xanthine oxidase production of oxygen free radicals plays a major part in generating tissue damage seen in ischemia/reperfusion injury (Figure 31.3) (Fox, 1992; Jeroudi *et al.*, 1994; Otani *et al.*, 1986).

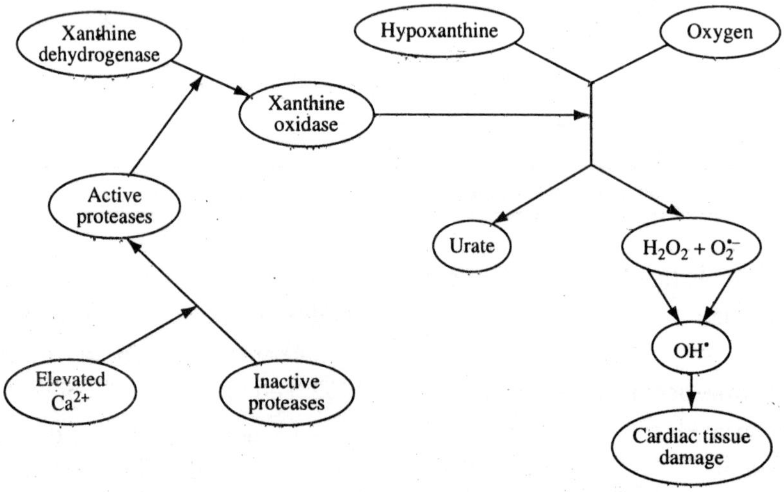

Fig. 31.3: ROS in ischemia/reperfusion

Free radicals and lung diseases

There is increasing evidence that ROS can be of importance of pathophysiology of several lung diseases like adult respiratory distress syndrome (ARDS), activated polymorphonuclear leucocytes, hyperactivity in asthmasis, oedema, lung fibrosis, emphysema etc. Lung injury induced by air pollutant, mineral dust, cigarette smoke, herbicides and anticancer agents since, at least partly, to be mediated by free radicals, these agents can affect epithecial, nasothecial and fibroblastic cells. These cells may rupture, releasing proteolytic enzymes and chemolytic mediators causing infiltration of other cells such as neutrophils, thus initiating an inflammatory process leading to an increase generation of ROS (Kehrer *et al.*, 1988).

One may divide ROS-induced oxidative damage into two categories: those which occur at rather high oxidative challenge and those occurring at relatively low oxidative challenge. Those events occurring at high oxidative challenge and which generally lead to acute cell and tissue injury are probably mediated through the hydroxyl radical. Such events include lipid peroxidation as well as protein sulfhydryl oxidation, which may lead to membrane destruction and altered enzyme activity respectively. An example related to the lung is the inactivation of α_1-antitrypsin through an oxidative modification of a methionine moiety in this enzyme. This inactivation may contribute to the development of emphysema, since α_1-antitrypsin inhibits the effects of several proteolytic enzymes, such as elastase and collagenase. ROS can also cause oxidative DNA damage of various types, cytoskeletal damage and disturbed calcium homeostasis (Sies, 1991).

With the limited oxidative stress, events such as modification of receptor activity and signalling as well as release of endogenous mediators (including AA metabolites), may occur. These events can lead to over expression of normal physiological processes and are probably more important than direct oxidative damage. In the lung, AA release and metabolism to eicosanoid agents can lead to vaso- and bronchoconstriction as well as to the development of oedema (Holtzman, 1991). Thus, the exposure of the lung to hydrogen peroxide and other hydroperoxide or systems generating $O_2^{\bullet}$ or H_2O_2 (xanthine/ xanthine oxidase; glucose/glucose oxidase) has been shown to result in vaso- and broncho-constriction as well as development of oedema (Tate *et al.*, 1988; Gurtner *et al.*, 1987; Olafsdottir *et al.*, 1991).

The free radical theory of aging

A free radical theory of aging was proposed by Harman in 1956 (Harman *et al.*, 1976). Multicellular organisms generally undergo qualitative changes with time (aging) that are associated with progressive degeneration of biological functions, increased susceptibility to diseases and increased probability of death within a given time period. The widely popular free radical theory of aging (Harman, 1956) states that the age-related degenerative process is to a large extent the consequence of free radical damage. Genetic evidence linking oxidative stress to life span has been obtained for different animal species (Honda and Honda, 1999; Ishii, 2000; Lin *et al.*, 1998; Melov *et al.*, 2000; Migliaccio *et al.*, 1999; Orr and Sohal, 1994; Parkes *et al.*, 1998; Taub *et al.*, 1999). Harman *et al* also proposed a slow progressive damage caused by unscavenged free radicals leading to failure of normal self recognition mechanisms. Autoantibodies may be produced leading to accumulation of phagocytes ultimately resulting in autoimmunity. Cutler, 1984 supported the theory by his findings of a direct correlation between SOD activity and lifespan. SOD extracted from liver of older rats was found to be less effective and thermolabile as compared to SOD extracted from younger rats. This theory may also explain the increased survivality of cold blooded animals at low temperatures as fewer radicals are produced at low temperature due to lower metabolic activity.

In 1978, Nohl and Hegner described an age-related increase in the release of $O_2^{\bullet -}$ and H_2O_2 from respiring mitochondria (Nohl and Hegner, 1978). In the same paper, it was also reported that the age-related stimulation of mitochondrial oxygen activation was responsible for an imbalance between prooxidants and antioxidants. The existence of this so-called 'oxidative stress' situation was surmised from the observed accumulation of oxidative damage to the structure and function of mitochondria isolated from old animals. Many papers have been published since that time which all supports the idea that in ageing the organism has to face an increasing imbalance between prooxidant formation and antioxidant defense systems.

ROS in hypertension

Up to date experimental evidence indicates that reactive oxygen species (ROS) play an important pathophysiological role in the development of hypertension. This is due, in large part, to $^{\bullet}O_2^-$ excess (oxidative stress) and decreased NO bioavailability in the vasculature and kidneys and to ROS-mediated cardiovascular remodeling (Touyz, 2003; Chabrashvili *et al.*, 2002; Kishi *et al.*, 2004). In human hypertension, biomarkers of systemic oxidative stress are elevated (Redon *et al.*, 2003). Treatment with superoxide dismutase (SOD) mimetics or antioxidants improves vascular and renal function, regresses vascular remodeling, and reduces blood pressure (BP) (Rodriguez-Iturbe *et al.*, 2003; Virdis *et al.*, 2004). Vascular ROS are produced in endothelial, adventitial, and vascular smooth muscle cells (VSMCs) and derived primarily from NAD(P)H oxidase: $2O_2$ + NAD(P)H $\rightarrow 2O_2^-$ + NAD(P) + H^+ (Lassegue *et al.*, 2003). Vascular NAD(P)H oxidase comprises at least 4 components: cell membrane–associated p22phox and gp91phox (or gp91phox [nox2] homologues, nox1 and nox4), and cytosolic subunits, p47phox and p67phox (Lassegue *et al.*, 2003; Touyz *et al.*, 2003). Vascular NAD(P)H oxidase is regulated by humoral (cytokines, growth factors, and vasoactive agents) and physical factors (stretch, pulsatile strain, and shear stress) (Lassegue *et al.*, 2003). Physiologically, ROS are produced in a controlled manner at low concentrations and function as signalling molecules (Touyz *et al.*, 2003) to maintain vascular integrity by regulating endothelial function and vascular contraction-relaxation. Under pathological conditions, increased ROS bioactivity leads to endothelial dysfunction, increased contractility, VSMC growth, monocyte invasion, lipid peroxidation, inflammation, and increased deposition of extracellular matrix proteins, important factors in hypertensive vascular damage (Diep *et al.*, 2002; Taniyama and Griendling, 2003).

Impaired endothelium-mediated vasodilation in hypertension has been linked to decreased NO bioavailability. This may be secondary to decreased NO synthesis or to increased NO degradation because of its interaction with $^{\bullet}O_2^-$ to form $ONOO^-$ (Landmesser *et al.*, 2003). Vasomotor tone is also modulated through direct ROS effects on calcium ion (Ermak and Davies, 2002; Tabet *et al.*, 2004). Whereas VSMC $^{\bullet}O_2^-$ is associated primarily with vasoconstriction, endothelial H_2O_2 has been described as an endothelium-derived relaxing factor (Morikawa *et al.*, 2003).

Molecular processes underlying ROS-induced vascular changes involve activation of redox-sensitive signalling pathways. Superoxide anion and H_2O_2 stimulate mitogen-activated protein kinases, tyrosine kinases, and transcription factors (NFκB, AP-1, and HIF-1) and inactivate protein tyrosine phosphatases (Touyz *et al.*, 2003; Chiarugi and Cirri, 2003). ROS also increase calcium ion and upregulate protooncogene and proinflammatory gene expression (Touyz *et al.*, 2003). These processes occur through oxidative modification of proteins by altering important amino acid residues, by inducing protein dimerization, and by interacting with metal complexes such as Fe-S moieties (Touyz *et al.*, 2003).

Free radicals and diabetes

Elevated ROS levels have also been implicated in diabetes mellitus (Baynes, 1991; Wolff, 1993). In this case oxidative stress is associated with a pro-oxidative shift of the glutathione redox state in the blood (De Mattia *et al.*, 1998). Hyperglycemia is a hallmark of both noninsulin-dependent (type 2) and insulin-dependent diabetes mellitus (type 1). Elevated glucose levels are associated with increased production of ROS by several different mechanisms (Baynes, 1991; Nishikawa *et al.*, 2000; Oberley, 1988; Sakurai and Tsuchiya, 1988; Van Dam *et al.*, 1995). In cultured bovine aortic endothelial cells, hyperglycemia was shown to cause increased ROS production at the mitochondrial complex II (Nishikawa *et al.*, 2000). Several independent strategies that ameliorate mitochondrial ROS production were shown to prevent some of the typical secondary complications of the disease, including the activation of protein kinase C or NF-κB and the formation of advanced glycation end products (Nishikawa *et al.*, 2000).

In addition, superoxide is generated by the process of glucose auto-oxidation that is associated with the formation of glycated proteins in the plasma of diabetic patients (Baynes, 1991; Oberley, 1988; Sakurai and Tsuchiya, 1988; Van Dam *et al.*, 1995; Wolf *et al.*, 1991; Wolff *et al.*, 1994). The interaction of advanced glycation end products with corresponding cell surface receptors stimulates ROS production and decreases intracellular glutathione levels (Yan *et al.*, 1994). The increase in ROS production contributes to the development of diabetic complications such as atherosclerosis and other vascular complications (Aragno *et al.*, 2000; Baynes, 1991). In addition, hyperglycemia enhances cell-mediated low-density lipoprotein (LDL) peroxidation in endothelial cells (Maziere *et al.*, 1995). Treatment with antioxidants ameliorates diabetic complications including the dysfunction of endothelial cells or increased platelet aggregation (Cameron *et al.*, 1993; Ceriello *et al.*, 1991; Ido *et al.*, 1997; Karpen *et al.*, 1982; Low and Nickander, 1991; Siman and Eriksson, 1997; Wohaieb and Godin, 1987).

In addition to O_2^-, hyperglycemia also stimulates the synthesis of NO via increased enzymatic activity of endothelial (Cosentino *et al.*, 1997) and inducible (Schonfelder *et al.*, 1996) isoforms of NOS. However, the NO generated in diabetic vasculature is rapidly scavenged by omnipresent O_2^- to form peroxynitrite [$OONO^-$] at a rate of $6.7 \times 109\ ms^{-1}$ (Huie and Padmaja, 1993). This rate is three times faster than the reaction between O_2^- and SOD (Beckman and Koppenol, 1996). Hence, the formation of $OONO^-$ is a double-edged sword; on one hand potentially deleterious O_2^- is neutralised, on the other hand the most potent vasodilator NO is consumed and $OONO^-$ is produced as a result (Lefer, 1995). It is therefore easy to comprehend why $OONO^-$ itself has been suggested as both a toxic compound eliciting tissue damage as well as a protective molecule improving cellular and organ vitality. $OONO^-$ has been shown to increase insulin secretion, DNA damage and cell death in human and rat islets of Langerhans (Hadjivassilou *et al.*, 1998). It has also been linked to attenuation of vascular responses in diabetic and preeclamptic human placentas (Kossenjans *et al.*, 2000). A recent report has also demonstrated that $OONO^-$ contributes to the destruction of pancreatic islet beta-cells of NOD mice developing autoimmune diabetes, suggesting that $OONO^-$ may play a pivotal role in the initiation of insulin-dependent diabetes mellitus (IDDM) (Suarez *et al.*, 1997). Proposed general theory of hyperglycemia resulting in the pathophysiology of diabetes via generation of ROS is presented diagrammatically in the Figure 31.4.

Free radicals and malignant diseases

ROS are potential carcinogens because they facilitate mutagenesis, tumor promotion and progression (Dreher and Junod, 1996; Ha *et al.*, 2000;

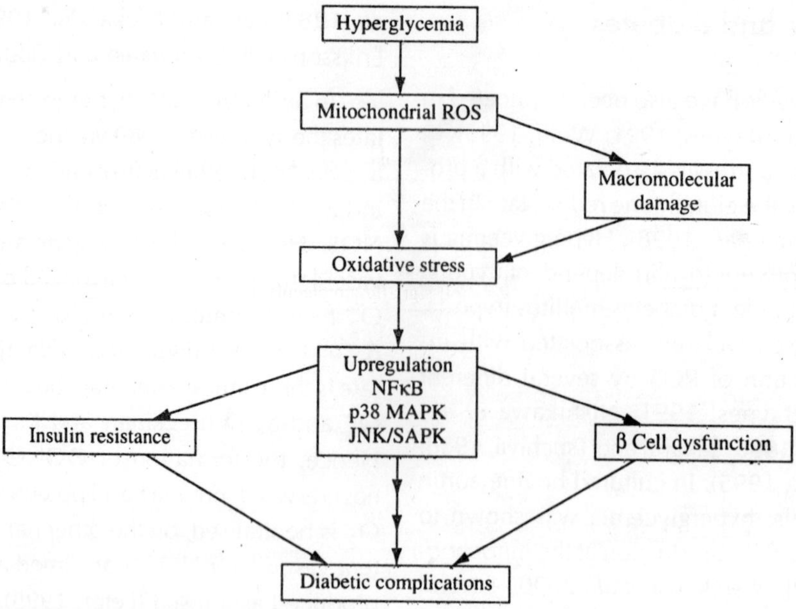

Fig. 31.4: Proposed general theory of how hyperglycemia result in the pathophysiology of diabetes via the generation of ROS. This diagram shows the proposed causative link between hyperglycemia, mitochondrial ROS generation, oxidative stress, activation of stress sensitive pathways (NFκB, p38 MAPK, JNK/SAPK, and others), insulin resistance, β-cell dysfunction, and diabetic complications.

Hussain *et al.*, 1994; Nakamura *et al.*, 1988; Salim, 1993). The growth-promoting effects of ROS are related to redox-responsive signalling cascades. A placebo-controlled clinical study of patients with previous adenomatous colonic polyps, i.e., a group with an increased risk for colon cancer and increased proliferative index of colonic crypts, revealed a significant decrease in the proliferative index after treatment with *N*-acetylcysteine (Estensen *et al.*, 1999). A pro-oxidative shift in the plasma thiol/disulfide redox state has been observed in patients with various types of advanced malignancies (Hack *et al.*, 1997). This shift is reminiscent of similar changes in diabetes mellitus, old age and intensive physical exercise. Because cancer patients commonly have decreased glucose clearance capacity (Marks and Bishop, 1957; Newman *et al.*, 1992; Pisters *et al.*, 1992; Rohdenburg *et al.*, 1919; Tayek, 1992) and, in addition, abnormally high glycolytic activity and lactate production (Shaw *et al.*, 1985; Shaw and Wolfe, 1987; Tayek, 1992; Warburg *et al.*, 1924), it is reasonable to assume that the observed pro-oxidative shift is mediated by an increased and basically uncontrolled availability of mitochondrial energy substrate.

Oxidative stress has many diverse cellular effects. As depicted in Figure 31.5, this ubiquitous stress can cause mutagenicity, cytotoxicity, and stimulate changes in gene expression (Harris, 1989). Furthermore, these effects are likely to interplay in the development of carcinogenesis by oxidants. Mutations induced by oxidants may initiate carcinogenesis; oxidative modification of the genetic material may also participate in the progression of benign to malignant neoplasms. Alteration of the pattern of gene expression by oxidants may function in the stimulation of the initiated cell during tumour promotion. Further, oxidant-induced toxicity in the normal population may facilitate the clonal expansion of the more resistant initiated cell during promotion.

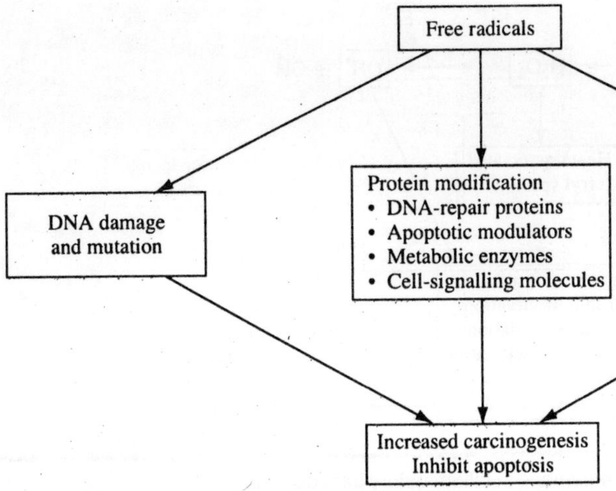

Fig. 31.5: Role or free radicals in the incidence of cancer

Free radicals in relation to inflammation and arthritis

In recent years it has become increasingly apparent that, in man, free radicals play a role in variety of normal regulatory systems, the deregulation of which may play an important role in inflammation. Inflammation represents the normal response to mechanical, chemical or infectious tissue injury. Whether acute or chronic, inflammation is dependent upon regulated humoral and cellular responses and if unchecked, leads to the generation of inflammatory diseases. The physiological function which may be perturbed in inflammation, include: the oxidative modification of low density lipoprotein, the oxidative inactivation of alpha-1-protease inhibitor, DNA damage/repair and heat shock protein synthesis. During phagocytosis neutrophils, eosinophils and mononuclear phagocytes consume increased amount of oxygen, i.e., the process termed as respiratory burst. Activation results in increased NADPH production and the generation of superoxide anion radical, hydrogen peroxide, hydroxyl radical and hypochlorous acid (HOCl); these ROS are capable of damaging cell membranes and wide variety of biomolecules. At the sites of inflammation, increased ROS activates neutrophil NADPH oxidase and/or the uncoupling of a variety of redox systems (Winrow *et al.*, 1993).

It has been proved that free radicals which were generated through the induction of DNA strand breaks activates transcription of genes c-fos, c-myc, c-jun and β-actin which are responsible for cell growth, differentiation and development (Amstad *et al.*, 1992). At low doses, ROS stimulate growth of fibroblast and epithelial cells in culture and thus play a role early in inflammation by promoting fibrosis and wound healing. The inflammation also takes place via an indirect route, through the lipid peroxidation products which promotes collagen synthesis (Murrell *et al.*, 1990; Chojkier *et al.*, 1989).

NFκB is an important transcription factor in inflammatory system because it controls the transcription of a number of cytokinin genes like IL-2, TNF α, etc. Recently, it has been shown that free radical generating systems also damage a variety of cellular and plasma proteins, e.g., immunoglobulin G (Figure 31.6) and α-1-proteinase inhibitor which are well documented examples relevant to inflammation.

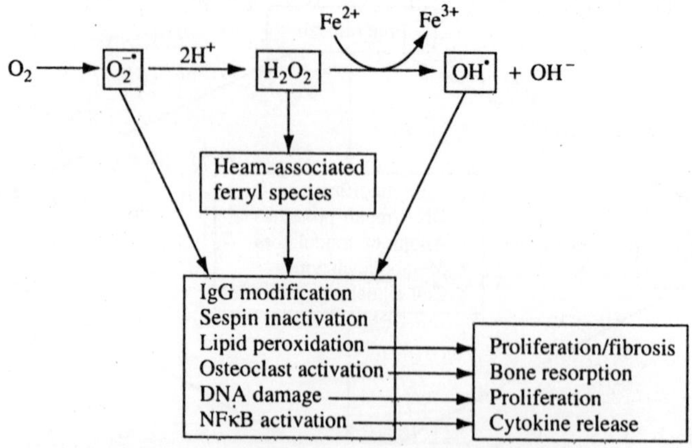

Fig. 31.6: Schematic representation of oxidative damage in inflammatory joint disease

CONCLUSION

The important role of ROS in the regulation of physiological responses is underscored by the apparent deregulation of physiological responses in various disease related oxidative stress conditions. Diabetes mellitus and cancer commonly show a prooxidative shift in the systemic thiol/disulfide redox state, similar to the shift seen in old age. These "mitochondrial oxidative stress" conditions are typically associated with skeletal muscle wasting. In diabetes mellitus ROS may also be generated by glucose auto-oxidation, which is associated with the formation of glycated proteins in the plasma. ROS are potential carcinogens because they facilitate mutagenesis, tumor promotion, and progression. The growth-promoting effects of ROS are related to redox-responsive signaling cascades. Another group of diseases designated as "inflammatory oxidative conditions" includes atherosclerosis and chronic inflammation and is typically associated with excessive stimulation of NAD(P)H oxidase activity. Some of the pathological complications are indicative of a redox mediated deregulation of signalling cascades and/or gene expression, e.g., the overproduction of cell adhesion molecules. ROS production by xanthine oxidase has been implicated in the pathology of ischemia and reperfusion injury. Similar mechanisms may also operate in obstructive sleep apnea. There are various indirect manifestations of oxidative stress in old age, including lipid peroxidation, DNA oxidation, protein oxidation, and a shift in the redox states of thiol/disulfide redox couples such as glutathione, cysteine, and albumin. The term *replicative senescence* describes the fact that somatic cells divide in cell culture only for a finite number of generations. Recent evidence suggests that the decrease in replicative capacity may be related to an increase in ROS levels and/or a pro-oxidative shift in the thiol/disulfide redox state. Mild oxidative stress was also shown to cause telomere shortening in fibroblasts.

Free radicals are also involved in Parkinson's disease, senile and drug induced deafness, schizophrenia, Alzheimer's disease, etc. The classic free radical syndrome, the iron storage disease-hemochromatosis, is typically associated with the constellation of free radical related symptoms including movement disorder, psychosis, skin pigmentary melanin abnormalities, deafness, etc. Because the free radicals are necessary for life, the body has number of mechanisms to minimize free radical induced damage. There are some encouraging recent reports about the use of SOD/catalase mimetics in certain experimental systems.

The development of procedures to ameliorate undesirable ROS production may be one of the central issues in research on aging and oxidative stress-related diseases in the near future. Flooding the system with antioxidants or the overexpression of antioxidative enzymes may be just as detrimental as excessive exposure to free radicals. To ensure ordered redox-mediated signalling, life requires a delicately balanced intermediate level of free radicals and radical-derived ROS.

REFERENCES

Amstad PA, Krupitza G, Cerutti PA. Mechanism of c-fos induction by active oxygen. *Cancer Res*, 52, 3952-3960, (1992).

Aragno M, Parola S, Tamagno E, Brignardello E, Manti R, Danni O, Boccuzzi G. Oxidative derangement in rat synaptosomes induced by hyperglycaemia: restorative effect of dehydroepiandrosterone treatment. *Biochem Pharmacol*, 60, 389-395, (2000).

Baynes JW. Role of oxidative stress in development of complications in diabetes. *Diabetes*, 40, 405-412, (1991).

Beckman JS, Koppenol WH. NO, superoxide and peroxynitrite: the good, the bad and the ugly. *Am J Physiol*, 271, C1424-C1437, (1996).

Bolli R. Oxygen-derived free radicals and myocardial reperfusion injury: An overview. *Cardiovasc Drugs Ther*, 5, 249-268, (1991).

Bolli R. Myocardial Protection: the Pathophysiology of Reperfusion and Reperfusion Injury. Raven Press, New York, pp 105-149, (1992).

Burton GW, Cheeseman KH, Doba T, Ingold KU, Slater TF. Biology of Vitamin E. Pitman Press, London, pp 4-18, (1983).

Burton GW, Ingold KU. Vitamin E: application of the principles of physical organic chemistry to the exploration of its structure and function. *Acc Chem Res*, 19, 194-201, (1986).

Burton GW, Joyce A, Ingold KU. Is vitamin E the only lipid-soluble chain-breaking antioxidant in human blood plasma and erythrocyte membranes? *Arch Biochem Biophys*, 221, 281-290, (1983).

Cameron NE, Cotter MA, Maxfield, E.K. Anti-oxidant treatment prevents the development of peripheral nerve dysfunction in streptozotocin-diabetic rats. *Diabetologia*, 36, 299-304, (1993).

Ceriello A, Guigliano A, Dello Russo P, Lefebvre PJ. Metabolic control may influence the increased superoxide generation in diabetic serum. *Diabetes Med*, 8, 540-542, (1991).

Chabrashvili T, Tojo A, Onozato ML, Kitiyakara C, Quinn MT, Fujita T, Welch WJ, Wilcox CS. Expression and cellular localization of classic NADPH oxidase subunits in the spontaneously hypertensive rat kidney. *Hypertension*, 39, 269-274, (2002).

Cheeseman KH, Holley AE. Measuring free radical reactions *in vivo*. *British Medical Bulletin*, 49(3), 494-505, (1993).

Cheeseman KH, Slater TF. An introduction to free radical biochemistry. *British Medical Bulletin*, 49(3), 481-493, (1993).

Chiarugi P, Cirri P. Redox regulation of protein tyrosine phosphatases during receptor tyrosine kinase signal transduction. *Trends Biochem Sci*, 28, 509-514, (2003).

Chojkier M, Houghim K, Solis-Herruzo J, Brenner DA. Stimulation of collagen gene expression by ascorbic acid in cultured human fibroblasts-A role for lipid peroxidation? *J Biol Chem*, 264, 16957-16962, (1989).

Coghlan JG, Flitter W, Holley AE. Detection of freeradicals and cholesterol hydroperoxides in blood taken from the coronary sinus of man during coronary of man during percutaneous transluminal coronary angioplasty. *Free Radic Biol Med*, 14, 339-342, (1993).

Cosentino F, Hishikawa K, Katusic ZS, Luscher TF. High glucose increases NOS expression and superoxide anion generation in human aortic endothelial cells. *Circulation*, 96, 25-28, (1997).

Cotgreave I, Moldeus P, Orrenius S. Host biochemical defense mechanisms against prooxidants. *Annu Rev Pharmacol Toxicol*, 28, 189-212, (1988).

Cutler RG. Free radicals in biology. Academic Press, New York, pp 371-428, (1984).

De Lorgeril M, Richard MJ, Arnaud J. Lipid peroxides and antioxidant defenses in the accelerated transplantation associated coronary arteriosclerosis. *Am Heart J*, 125, 974-980, (1993).

De Mattia G, Bravi MC, Laurenti O, Cassone-Faldetta M, Armeinto A, Ferri C, Balsano F. Influence of reduced glutathione infusion on glucose metabolism in patients with non-insulin-dependent diabetes mellitus. *Metabolism*, 47, 993-997, (1998).

Diep QN, Amiri F, Touyz RM, Cohn JS, Endemann D, Neves MF, Schiffrin EL. PPAR alpha activator effects on Ang II-induced vascular oxidative stress and inflammation. *Hypertension*, 40, 866-871, (2002).

Dousset JC, Trouilh M, Foglietti MJ. Plasma malondialdehyde levels during myocardial infarction. *Clin Chim Acta*, 129, 319-322, (1983).

Dreher D, Junod AF. Role of oxygen free radicals in cancer development. *Eur J Cancer*, 32A, 30-38, (1996).

Ermak G, Davies KJ. Calcium and oxidative stress: from cell signaling to cell death. *Mol Immunol*, 38, 713-721, (2002).

Estensen RD, Levy M, Klopp SJ, Galbraith AR, Mandel JS, Blomquist JA, Wattenberg LW. *N*-acetylcysteine suppression of the proliferative index in the colon of patients with previous adenomatous colonic polyps. *Cancer Lett*, 147, 109-114, (1999).

Esterbauer H, Zollner H, Schaur RJ. Membrane Lipid Oxidation. Boca Raton, CRC, pp 239-283, (1990).

Ferrari R, Ceconi C, Curello S. Myocardial damage during ischemia and reperfusion. *Eur Heart J*, 14, 25-30, (1993).

Fox KAA. Myocardial Protection: the Pathophysiology of Reperfusion and Reperfusion Injury. Raven Press, New York, pp 151-165, (1992).

Fraga CG, Shigenaga MK, Park JW, Degan P, Ames BN. Oxidative damage to DNA during aging: 8-hydroxy-2'-guanosine in rat organ DNA and urine. *Proc Natl Acad Sci*, 87, 4533-4537, (1990).

Fruchart JC, Duriez P. Free Radical Damage and its Control. Elsevier Science, pp 257-281, (1994).

Garlick PB, Davies MJ, Hearse DJ, Slater TF. Direct detection of free radicals in the reperfused rat heart using electron spin resonance spectroscopy. *Circul Res*, 61, 757-760, (1987).

Gurtner GH, Farrukh IS, Edkinson NF, Sciuto AM, Jacobson JM, Michael JR. The role of arachidonate mediators in peroxides-induced lung injury. *Am Rev Respir Dis*, 136, 480-483, (1987).

Ha HC, Thiagalingam A, Nelkin BD, Casero RA. Jr Reactive oxygen species are critical for the growth and differentiation of medullary thyroid carcinoma cells. *Clin Cancer Res*, 6, 3783-3787, (2000).

Hack V, Schmid D, Breitkreutz R, Stahl-Hennig C, Drings P, Kinscherf R, Taut F, Holm E, Dro GEW. Cystine levels cystine flux and protein catabolism in cancer cachexia, HIV/SIV infection and senescence. *FASEB J*, 11, 84-92, (1997).

Hadjivassilou V, Green MHL, James RFL, Swift SM, Clayton HA, Green IC. Insulin secretion DNA damage and apoptosis in human and rat islets of Langerhans following exposure to NO, peroxynitrite and cytokines. *Nitric Oxide: Biology and Chemistry*, 2, 429-441, (1998).

Halliwell B, Gutteridge JMC. Role of free radicals and catalytic metal ions in human disease: an overview. *Methods Enzymol*, 186, 1-85, (1990).

Halliwell B. Lipid peroxidation *in vivo* and *in vitro* in relation to atherosclerosis: some fundamental questions. *Agents Actions Suppl*, 26, 223-231, (1988).

Harman D, Eddy DE, Noffsinger J. Free radical theory of aging: inhibition of amyloidosis in mice by antioxidants; a possible mechanism. *J Am Geriat Soc*, 24, 203-210, (1976).

Harman D. Aging: a theory based on free radical and radiation chemistry. *J Gerontol*, 11, 298-300, (1956).

Harris, C. Individual variation among humans in carcinogen metabolism, DNA adduct formation and DNA repair. *Carcinogenesis*, 10, 1563-1566, (1989).

Holtzman MJ. Arachidonic acid metabolism, Implications of biological chemistry for lung function and disease. *Am Rev Respir Dis*, 143, 188-203, (1991).

Honda Y, Honda S. The daf-2 gene network for longevity regulates oxidative stress resistance and Mn-superoxide dismutase gene expression in *Caenorhabditis elegans. FASEB J*, 13, 1385-1393, (1999).

Huie RE, Padmaja S. The reaction of NO with superoxide. *Free Radic Res Commun*, 18, 195-199, (1993).

Hussain SP, Aguilar F, Amstad P, Cerutti P. Oxy-radical induced mutagenesis of hotspot codons 248 and 249 of the human p53 gene. *Oncogene*, 9, 2277-2281, (1994).

Ido Y, Kilo C, Williamson JR. Cytosolic NADH/NAD1 free radicals and vascular dysfunction in early diabetes mellitus. *Diabetologia*, 40, 115-117, (1997).

Ishii N. Oxidative stress and aging in *Caenorhabditis elegans. Free Radical Res*, 33, 857-864, (2000).

Ishiro-Fukai M, Zafari AM, Fukui T, Ishizaka N, Griendling KK. p22phox is a critical component of the superoxide-generating NADH/NADPH oxidase system and regulates angiotensin II-induced hypertrophy in vascular smooth muscle cells. *J Biol Chem*, 271, 23317-23321, (1996).

Jeroudi MO, Hartley CJ, Bolli R. Myocardial reperfusion injury: role of oxygen radicals and potential therapy with antioxidants. *Am J Cardiol*, 73, 2B-7B, (1994).

Karpen CW, Pritchard KA, Arnold JH. Jr Cornwell DG, Panganamala RV. Restoration of prostacyclin/thromboxane A2 balance in the diabetic rat. Influence of dietary vitamin E. *Diabetes*, 31, 947-951, (1982).

Kasai H, Nishimura S. Oxidative Stress: Oxidants and Antioxidants. Academic Press, London, pp 99-116, (1991).

Kehrer JP, Mossman BT, Sevanian A, Trus MA, Smith MT. Contemporary issues in toxicology. Free radicals mechanisms in chemical pathogenesis. *Toxicol Appl Pharmacol*, 95, 349-362, (1988).

Kishi T, Hirooka Y, Kimura Y, Ito K, Shimokawa, H, Takeshita A. Increased reactive oxygen species in rostral ventrolateral medulla contribute to neural mechanisms of hypertension in stroke-prone spontaneously hypertensive rats. *Circulation*, 109, 2357 2362, (2004).

Kossenjans W, Eis A, Sahay R, Brockman D, Myatt L. Role of peroxynitrite in altered fetal-placental vascular reactivity in diabetes and preeclampsia. *Am J Physiol*, 278, H1311-H1319, (2000).

Landmesser U, Dikalov S, Price SR, McCann L, Fukai T, Holland SM, Mitch WE, Harrison DG. Oxidation of tetrahydrobiopterin leads to uncoupling of endothelial cell nitric oxide synthase in hypertension. *J Clin Invest*, 111, 1201-1209, (2003).

Landmesser U, Drexler, H. Oxidative stress, the renin-angiotensin system, and atherosclerosis. *Europ Heart J Suppl*, 5, A3-A7, (2005):

Lang, J., Esterbauer, H. Membrane Lipid Oxidation. Boca Raton, CRC, pp 265-282, (1991).

Lassegue B, Clempus RE. Vascular NAD(P)H oxidases: specific features, expression, and regulation. *Am J Physiol Regul Integr Comp Physiol*, 285, R277-R297, (2003).

Lefer AM. Attenuation of myocardial ischaemia-reperfusion injury with NO replacement therapy [review]. *Ann Thorac Surg*, 60, 847-851, (1995).

Lin YJ, Seroude L, Benzer S. Extended life-span and stress resistance in the *Drosophila* mutant methuselah. *Science*, 282, 943-946, (1998).

Loschen G, Azzi A, Flohe L. Mitochondrial H_2O_2 formation: relationship with energy conservation. *FEBS Lett*, 33, 84-88, (1973).

Low PA, Nickander KK. Oxygen free radical effects in sciatic nerve in experimental diabetes. *Diabetes*, 40, 873-877, (1991).

Marks PA, Bishop JS. The glucose metabolism of patients with malignant disease and of normal subjects as studied by means of an intravenous glucose tolerance test. *J Clin Invest*, 36, 254-264, (1957).

Maziere C, Auclair M, Rose-Robert F, Leflon P, Maziere JC. Glucose-enriched medium enhances cell-mediated low density lipoprotein peroxidation. *FEBS Lett*, 363, 277-279, (1995).

Melov S, Ravenscroft J, Malik S, Gill MS, Walker, DW, Clayton PE, Wallace DC, Malfroy B, Doctrow SR, Lithgow GJ. Extension of life-span with superoxide dismutase/catalase mimetics. *Science*, 289, 1567-1569, (2000).

Migliaccio E, Giorgio M, Mele S, Pelicci G, Reboldi P, Pandolfi PP, Lanfrancone L, Pelicci PG. The p66shc adaptor protein controls oxidative stress response and life span in mammals. *Nature*, 402, 309-313, (1999).

Morel DW, DiCorleto PE, Chisolm GM. Endothelial and smooth muscle cells alter low density lipoprotein by free radical oxidation. *Arteriosclerosis*, 4, 357-364, (1984).

Morikawa K, Shimokawa H, Matoba T, Kubota H, Akaike T, Talukder MA, Hatanaka M, Fujiki T, Maeda H, Takahashi S, Takeshita A. Pivotal role of Cu, Zn-superoxide dismutase in endothelium-dependent hyperpolarization. *J Clin Invest*, 112, 1871-1879, (2003).

Murrell G, Francis N, Bromley L. Modulation of fibroblast proliferation by oxygen free radicals. *Biochem J*, 265, 659-665, (1990).

Nakamura Y, Gindhart T, Winterstein D, Tomita I, Seed J, Colburn N. Early superoxide dismutase-sensitive event promotes neoplastic transformation in mouse epidermal JB6 cells. *Carcinogenesis*, 9, 203-207, (1988).

Newman E, Heslin MJ, Wolf RF, Pisters PW, Brennan MF. The effect of insulin on glucose and protein metabolism in the forearm of cancer patients. *Surg Oncol*, 1, 257-267, (1992).

Nishikawa T, Edelstein D, Du XL, Yamagishi S, Matsumura T, Kaneda Y, Yorek MA, Beebe D, Oates PJ, Hammes HP, Giardino I, Brownlee M. Normalizing mitochondrial superoxide production blocks three pathways of hyperglycaemic damage. *Nature*, 404, 787-790, (2000).

Nohl H. Involvement of free radicals in ageing: a consequence or cause of senescence. *British Medical Bulletin*, 49(3), 653-667, (1993).

Nohl H, Hegner D. Do mitochondria produce oxygen radicals *in vivo*? *Eur J Biochem*, 38, 179-188, (1987).

Oberley LW. Free radicals and diabetes. *Free Radical Biol Med*, 5, 113-124, (1988).

Olafsdottir K, Ryrfeldt A, Atzori L, Berggren M, Moldeus P. Hydroperoxide-induced broncho-and vasoconstriction in the isolated rat lung. *Exp Lung Res*, 17, 615-627, (1991).

Orr WC, Sohal RS. Extension of lifespan by overexpression of superoxide dismutase and catalase in *Drosophila melanogaster*. *Science*, 263, 1128-1130, (1994).

Otani R, Engelman RM, Roussou JA. Cardiac performance during reperfusion improved by pretreatment with oxygen-free radicals scavengers. *J Thorac Cardiovasc Surg*, 91, 290-295, (1986).

Parkes TL, Elia AJ, Dickinson D, Hilliker AJ, Boulianne GL, John P. Extension of *Drosophila* lifespan by overexpression of human SOD1 in motorneurons. *Nature Genet*, 19, 171-174, (1998).

Parthasaratry S, Rankin SM. Role of oxidized low density lipoproteins in atherogenesis. *Progr Lipid Res*, 31, 127-143, (1992).

Pietri S, Culcasi M, Cozzone PJ. Real-time continuous-flow spin trapping of hydroxyl radical in the ischemic and post-ischemic myocardium. *Eur J Biochem*, 186, 163-173, (1989).

Pisters PWT, Cersosimo E, Rogatko A, Brennan MF. Insulin action on glucose and branched-chain amino acid metabolism in cancer cachexia: differential effects of insulin. *Surgery*, 111, 301-310, (1992).

Poli G, Albano E, Dianzani MU. The role of lipid peroxidation in lipid damage. *Chem Phys Lipids*, 45, 117-142, (1987).

Porter NA. Membrane Lipid Oxidation. Boca Raton, CRC, pp 33-62, (1990).

Redon J, Oliva MR, Tormos C, Giner V, Chaves J, Iradi A, Saez GT. Antioxidant activities and oxidative stress byproducts in human hypertension. *Hypertension*, 41, 1096-1101, (2003).

Rodriguez-Iturbe B, Zhan CD, Quiroz Y, Sindhu RK, Vaziri ND. Antioxidant-rich diet relieves hypertension and reduces renal immune infiltration in spontaneously hypertensive rats. *Hypertension*, 41, 341-346, (2003).

Rohdenburg GL, Bernhard A, Krehbiel O. Sugar tolerance in cancer. *JAMA*, 72, 1528-1534, (1919).

Sakurai T, Tsuchiya S. Superoxide production from nonenzymatically glycated protein. *FEBS Lett*, 236, 406-410, (1988).

Salim AS. The permissive role of oxygen-derived free radicals in the development of colonic cancer in the rat. A new theory for carcinogenesis. *Int J Cancer*, 53, 1031-1035, (1993).

Schonfelder G, John M, Hopp H, Fuhr N, van der Giet M, Paul M. Expression of inducible NOS in placenta of women with gestational diabetes. *FASEB J*, 10, 777-784, (1996).

Seccia M, Brossa O, Gravela E, Slater TF, Cheeseman KH. Exposure of α_L-crystallin to oxidizing free radicals enhances its susceptibility to transglutaminase activity. *Biochem J*, 274, 869-873, (1991).

Shaw JH, Klein F, Wolfe RR. Assessment of alanine, urea and glucose interrelationships in normal subjects and in patients with sepsis using stable isotopic tracers. *Surgery*, 97, 557-567, (1985).

Shaw JH, Wolfe RR. Glucose and urea kinetics in patients with early and advanced gastrointestinal cancer: the response to glucose infusion and TPN. *Surgery*, 101, 181-186, (1987).

Sies H. Oxidative Stress: Oxidants and Antioxidants. Academic Press, London, (1991).

Siman CM, Eriksson UJ. Vitamin E decreases the occurrence of malformations in the offspring of diabetic rats. *Diabetes*, 46, 1054-1061, (1997).

Sosa MC, Molina RV, Guinzberg R, Piña E. Adrenaline (via $_{\kappa 1B}$-adrenoceptors) and ethanol stimulate OH" radical production in isolated rat hepatocytes. *Life Sciences*, 71(21), 2469-2474, (2002).

Spector A. The Ocular Lens. Marcel Dekker, New York, pp 405-438, (1985).

Starkopf J, Zilmer K, Vihalemm T. Time-course of oxidative stress during open-heart surgery. *Scand J Thorac Cardiovasc Surg*, 29(4), 181-186, (1995).

Stocker R, Bowry VW, Frei B. Ubiquinol-10 protects human low density lipoprotein more efficiently against lipid peroxidation than does á-tocopherol. *Proc Natl Acad Sci*, 88, 1646-1650, (1991).

Stocker R, Frei B. Oxidative Stress: Oxidants and Antioxidants. Academic Press, London, pp 213-242, (1991).

Suarez Pinzon WL, Szabo C, Rabinovitch A. Development of autoimmune diabetes in NOD mice is associated with the formation of peroxynitrite in pancreatic islet beta-cells. *Diabetes*, 46, 907-911, (1997).

Tabet F, Savoia C, Schiffrin EL, Touyz RM. Differential calcium regulation by hydrogen peroxide and superoxide in vascular smooth muscle cells from SHR. *J Cardiovasc Pharmacol*, 44, 1-9, (2004).

Taniyama Y, Griendling KK. Reactive oxygen species in the vasculature: molecular and cellular mechanisms. *Hypertension*, 42, 1075-1081, (2003).

Tate PM, Morris HG, Schroeder WR, Repine JE. Oxygen metabolites stimulate thromboxane production in isolated saline- perfused lungs. *J Clin Invest*, 74, 608-613, (1988).

Taub J, Lau JF, Ma C, Hahn JH, Hoque R, Rothblatt J, Chalfie M. A cytosolic catalase is needed to extend adult lifespan in *C. elegans darf-C* and *clk-1* mutants. *Nature*, 399, 162-166, (1999).

Tayek JA. A review of cancer cachexia and abnormal glucose metabolism in humans with cancer. *J Am Coll Nutr*, 11, 445-456, (1992).

Tortolani A, Powell S, Misik V. Detection of alkoxyl and carbon-centered free radicals in coronary sinus blood from patients undergoing elective cardioplegia. *Free Radic Biol Med*, 14, 421-426, (1993).

Touyz RM, Tabet F, Schiffrin EL. Redox-dependent signalling by angiotensin II and vascular remodelling in hypertension. *Clin Exp Pharmacol Physiol*, 30, 860-866, (2003).

Touyz RM. Reactive oxygen species in vascular biology: role in arterial hypertension. *Expert Rev Cardiovasc Ther*, 1, 91-106, (2003).

Valen G, Vaage J. Toxic oxygen metabolites in reperfusion injury. *Scand J Thor Cardiovasc Surg*, 41, 19-29, (1993).

Van Dam PS, Van Asbeck BS, Erkelens DW, Marx JJM, Gispen WH, Bravenboer B. The role of oxidative stress in neuropathy and other diabetic complication. *Diabetes Metab Rev*, 11, 181-192, (1995).

Virdis A, Neves MF, Amiri F, Touyz RM, Schiffrin EL. Role of NAD(P)H oxidase on vascular alterations in angiotensin II-infused mice. *J Hypertens*, 22, 535-542, (2004).

Warburg O, Posener, K, Negelein E. über den Stoffwechsel der Carcinomzelle. *Biochem Z*, 152, 309-344, (1924).

Winrow VR, Winyard PG, Morris CJ, Blake DR. Free radicals in inflammation: second messengers and mediators of tissue destruction. *British Medical Bulletin*, 49(3), 506-522, (1993).

Wohaieb SA, Godin DV. Alterations in free radical tissue-defence mechanisms in streptozotocin-induced diabetes in rat. Effects of insulin treatment. *Diabetes*, 36, 1014-1018, (1987).

Wolf SF, Jiang ZY, Hunt JV. Protein glycation and oxidative stress in diabetes mellitus and ageing. *Free Radical Biol Med*, 10, 339-352, (1991).

Wolff SP, Crabbe MJC, Thornalley PJ. The autooxidation of simple monosaccharides. *Experientia*, 40, 244-246, (1984).

Wolff SP. Diabetes mellitus and free radicals. Free radicals, transition metals and oxidative stress in the aetiology of diabetes mellitus and complications. *Br Med Bull*, 49, 642-652, (1993).

Yan SD, Schmidt AM, Anderson GM, Zhang J, Brett J, Zou,YS, Pinsky D, Stern D. Enhanced cellular oxidative stress by the interaction of advanced glycation end products with their receptors/binding protein. *J Biol Chem*, 269, 9889-9897, (1994).

Ytrehus K, Heĝstad AC. Lipid peroxidation and membrane damage of heart. *Acta Physiol Scand*, S599, 81-91, (1991).

LIST OF CONTRIBUTORS

A K S Rawat
Pharmacognosy and Ethnopharmacology Division
National Botanical Research Institute
Lucknow 226 002, India

Amit Nayak
Lakshmi Narain College of Pharmacy
Kalchuri Nagar, Raisen Road,
Bhopal 462 021 (MP) India

Amit Srivastava
Pharmacognosy and Ethnopharmacology Division
National Botanical Research Institute
Lucknow 226 002, India

Ambarish Mukherjee
Department of Botany, Burdwan University
Golapbag, Burdwan 713 104, India

Anita Jain
Laboratory of Ethnobotany and Agrostology
Department of Botany, College of Science
M L Sukhadia University
Udaipur Rajasthan 313001

Ashok Kumar C K
Omar Al-Mukhtar University
Al-Bayda
P O Box-991, Derna, Libya

A Y Mensah
Faculty of Pharmacy and Pharmaceutical Sciences
Kwame Nkrumah University of Science and Technology (KNUST)
Kumasi, Ghana

B. Parimala Devi
School of Chemical and Biotechnology
SASTRA University, Thirumalaisamudram
Thanjavur 613 402, Tamilnadu, India

Brigitte Binneman
University of Pretoria, Medicinal Plant Science
Pretoria 0028, South Africa

C S Bhargava
Advance Group of Pharmacy Colleges
Naramau, G.T. Road, Kanpur 209217
Uttar Pradesh, India

Deepak P Belsare
College of Pharmacy
Gangapur Road
Nashik 422002, Maharashtra, India

Dinesh D Rishipathak
M E T, College of Pharmacy
Bhujbal Knowledge City
Adgaon, Nashik 422002, Maharashtra, India

Evan Prince Sabina
School of Bio-Sciences and Technology
V I T University, Vellore 632014, Tamil Nadu, India

E V S Subrahmanyam
N G S M Institute of Pharmaceutical Science
Paneer, Deralakatte
Mangalore 574 160, Karnataka, India

G Arunachalam
P G P College of Pharmaceutical Science and Research Institute
NH 7, Namakkal-Karur Main Road
Namakkal 637297, Tamilnadu, India

G David Lin
Faculty of Health
University of Canberra, Building 12D35
Canberra ACT 2601, Austrialia

Gunjan Biswas
Moledular and Applied Mycology and Plant Pathology Laboratory, Department of Botany
University of Calcutta
Kolkata 700 019, India

Hauzel Lalhlenmawia
Department of Pharmacy
Regional Institute of Paramedical & Nursing Sciences
Zemabawk, Aizawl 795 017, Mizoram, India

Joseph Adetunji Aladesanmi
Department of Pharmacognosy
Faculty of Pharmacy
Obafemi Awolowo University
Ile-Ife, Nigeria

Joydeep Acharya
Department of Botany, Burdwan University
Golapbag, Burdwan 713 104, India

Jyoti Kumar
Department of Botany, Ranchi University, Ranchi
Jharkhand 834 001, India

K Annan
Faculty of Pharmacy and Pharmaceutical Sciences,
Kwame Nkrumah University of Science and
Technology (KNUST)
Kumasi, Ghana

Kamini Kumar
Department of Botany, Ranchi University, Ranchi
Jharkhand 834 001, India

Krishnendu Acharya
Moledular and Applied Mycology and Plant
Pathology Laboratory, Department of Botany
University of Calcutta
Kolkata 700 019, India

Mahaboob Khan Rasool
School of Bio-Sciences and Technology
V I T University, Vellore 632014, Tamil Nadu, India

Manjula Rai
Moledular and Applied Mycology and Plant
Pathology Laboratory, Department of Botany
University of Calcutta
Kolkata 700 019, India

Manoranjan Adak
Department of Biochemistry
National Medical College and Teaching Hospital
Tribhuvan University
Birgunj, Nepal

Mayank Thakur
Charite University of Medicine
Campus Benjamin Franklin, Hindenburgdamm 30,
12200 Berlin, Germany

Mohammad Yaseen Khan
Lakshmi Narain College of Pharmacy
Kalchuri Nagar, Raisen Road
Bhopal 462 021 (MP) India

Mostafa Elachouri
Mohammed 1st University
Biology Department
Ethnopharmacological and physiological Laboratory
Bd. Mohammed VI, BP 717
Oujda 60000
Morocco

Moumita Gangopadhyay
Medicinal Plant Laboratory, Department of Botany
Bose Institute, 93/1 A P C Road
Kolkata 700 009, India

Nageswara Rao Thalapaneni
Department of Pharmaceutical Technology
Jadavpur University
Kolkata 700 032, India

Nimrita Lall
University of Pretoria, Medicinal Plant Science
Pretoria 0028, South Africa

Nilanjan Ghosh
Dr B C Roy College of Pharmacy and Allied Health
Science, Durgapur 713 206, India

Pharkphoom Panichayupakaranant
Department of Pharmacognosy and
Pharmaceutical Botany,
Faculty of Pharmaceutical Sciences
Prince of Songkla University
Hat-Yai, Songkhla, 90112, Thailand

Praveen Kumar Galav
Laboratory of Ethnobotany and Agrostology
Department of Botany, College of Science
M L Sukhadia University
Udaipur Rajasthan 313001

R Venkidesh
Caplin Point Laboratories Limited
3 Lakshmanan Street
T Nagar, Chennai 600 017

R A Dickson
Faculty of Pharmacy and Pharmaceutical Sciences
Kwame Nkrumah University of Science and
Technology (KNUST),
Kumasi, Ghana

Rabish Chandra
Department of Pharmaceutical Technology
Jadavpur University
Kolkata 700 032, India

Rajarajan Amirthalingam Thandavarayan
Niigata University of Pharmacy and Applied Life Sciences
Department of Functional and Analytical Food Sciences
265-1 Higashijima, Akiha-ku, Niigata City 956-8603,
Japan

Ranbir Sahu
Department of Pharmaceutical Technology
Jadavpur University
Kolkata 700 032, India

S A Nirmal
Pravara Rural College of Pharmacy
Loni, Rahata, Ahmednagar 413736
Maharashtra, India

S C Pal
College of Pharmacy
Gangapur Road
Nashik 422002, Maharashtra, India

S Mohanalakshmi
Department of Pharmacognosy
Sree Vidyanikethan College of Pharmacy
Tirupati 517 102,
Andhra Pradesh, India

S S Katewa
Laboratory of Ethnobotany and Agrostology
Department of Botany, College of Science
M L Sukhadia University
Udaipur (Rajasthan) 313001

Saikat Dewanjee
Department of Pharmaceutical Technology
Jadavpur University
Kolkata 700 032, India

Sabita Bhattacharya
Medicinal Plant Laboratory
Department of Botany
Bose Institute, 93/1 APC Road
Kolkata 700 009, India

Sanjay K Banerjee
Cardiovascular Institute
University of Pittsburgh, PA 15213, USA and
Indian Institute of Chemical Technology,
Hyderabad 500607
India

Sannah Patience Nkami Mativandlela
University of Pretoria, Medicinal Plant Science
Pretoria 0028, South Africa

Santanu Saha
N G S M Institute of Pharmaceutical Science
Paneer, Deralakatte
Mangalore 574 160, Karnataka, India

Shilpi Bhargava
Advance Group of Pharmacy Colleges
Naramau, G.T. Road, Kanpur 209217
Uttar Pradesh, India

Sharad Srivastava
Pharmacognosy and Ethnopharmacology Division
National Botanical Research Institute
Lucknow 226 002, India

Subhash C Mandal
Department of Pharmaceutical Technology
Jadavpur University
Kolkata 700 032, India

Subhash C Mandal (Sr.)
Directorate of Drugs Control
Government of West Bengal
Kolkata 700 073, India

V Kalaiselvan
Indian Pharmacopoeia Commission
Government of India (Ministry of Health and Family Welfare), Sector 23, Raj Nagar
Ghaziabad, Uttar Pradesh 201 002

Vimal Kumar
Lakshmi Narain College of Pharmacy
Kalchuri Nagar, Raisen Road
Bhopal 462 021 (MP) India

Vivekananda Mandal
Department of Pharmaceutical Technology
Jadavpur University, Kolkata 700 032, India

INDEX

Some exciting gifts are up for grabs with this book!!

HERBAL DRUGS

Dr Subhash C Mandal

FREE Gifts Rs. 1000/-

DEAR READERS

By now you must have gone through this book in the entirety. So we invite your assessment on this title with absolute impartiality and candid observations. After all, we publishers blindly depend on your benchmarking. Friends, please fill up the open spaces below with CAPITAL LETTERS. You may add some extra sheets of paper if the space provided is not sufficient for you.

i. What are the important topics of your syllabus which are not adequately covered in this book?

ii. In which chapters and on what topics the treatment of the subject-matter by the author is not satisfactory and why?

iii. Have you come across the typos, factual inaccuracies, inconsistencies, and other forms of mistakes in the book? If yes, then please specify the mistakes and page numbers.

iv. Name top three books on the same subject, which, in your consideration, are better than this book. Could you provide some reasons?

Your 1st Preference: ....

Your 2nd Preference: ....

Your 3rd Preference: ....

v. Any suggestion to improve the quality of illustrations, diagrams, etc.?

vi. How did you like the cover design? Any suggestion on colours?

vii. Suggestions for further improvement of production-standard:

viii. Who recommended you this book:

☐ Teacher ☐ Friend ☐ Parents ☐ Bookseller ☐ Librarian

ix. Name of the person who has recommended:

Designation: ....

Address: ....

Phone No.: ....

e-mail: ....

x. Name and address of the bookseller from whom you have purchased this book:

....

....

....

xi. Name and address of the library where you would like to find the book:

....

....

xii. Name and address of your institution (Please mention the University or Board):

....

....

xiii. Your name, e-mail, and complete postal address:

....

....

....

xiv. A few other titles published by us that you would like to read:

....

....

The best assessment will be rewarded half-yearly. The award will be in the form of our publications, as decided by the Editorial and Marketing Operations Division, amounting to Rs. 1000/- (Rupees one thousand) only.

....

Please mail the filled up coupon at your earliest to :

Editorial & Marketing Operations Division

NEW CENTRAL BOOK AGENCY (P) Ltd

8/1 Chintamoni Das Lane, Kolkata 700 009

West Bengal, INDIA

Phone + Fax: 033 + 2241 8411, 2241 8573, 2241 9094

e-mail: ncbapvtltd@eth.net, ncba@cal2.vsnl.net.in

Website: www.centralgroup.com